Essential Pediatrics for Nurses

Fourth Edition

Essential Pediatrics for Nurses

Fourth Edition

Meharban Singh

MD, FAMS, FIAP, FIMSA, FNNF, FAAP

Former Professor and Head
Department of Pediatrics and Neonatal Division
WHO Collaborating Center for Training and
Research in Newborn Care
All India Institute of Medical Sciences
New Delhi 110 029

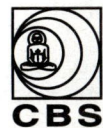

CBS

CBS Publishers & Distributors Pvt Ltd

New Delhi • Bengaluru • Chennai • Kochi • Kolkata • Mumbai
Hyderabad • Nagpur • Patna • Pune • Vijayawada

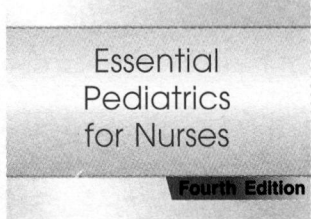

Essential
Pediatrics
for Nurses
Fourth Edition

ISBN: 978-93-86310-67-5

Fourth Edition: 2017
First Edition: 2004
Second Edition: 2008
Third Edition: 2014

Published by Satish Kumar Jain and Produced by Varun Jain for

CBS Publishers & Distributors Pvt Ltd
4819/XI Prahlad Street, 24 Ansari Road, Daryaganj, New Delhi 110 002, India.
Ph: 23289259, 23266861, 23266867   Fax: 011-23243014   Website: www.cbspd.com
e-mail: delhi@cbspd.com; cbspubs@airtelmail.in.
Corporate Office: 204 FIE, Industrial Area, Patparganj, Delhi 110 092
Ph: 4934 4934   Fax: 4934 4935   e-mail: publishing@cbspd.com; publicity@cbspd.com

Branches

- Bengaluru: Seema House 2975, 17th Cross, K.R. Road,
  Banasankari 2nd Stage, Bengaluru 560 070, Karnataka
  Ph: +91-80-26771678/79   Fax: +91-80-26771680   e-mail: bangalore@cbspd.com
- Chennai: 7, Subbaraya Street, Shenoy Nagar, Chennai 600 030, Tamil Nadu
  Ph: +91-44-26680620, 26681266   Fax: +91-44-42032115   e-mail: chennai@cbspd.com
- Kochi: Ashana House, No. 39/1904, AM Thomas Road, Valanjambalam,
  Ernakulam 682 016, Kochi, Kerala
  Ph: +91-484-4059061-65   Fax: +91-484-4059065   e-mail: kochi@cbspd.com
- Kolkata: 6/B, Ground Floor, Rameswar Shaw Road, Kolkata-700 014, West Bengal
  Ph: +91-33-22891126, 22891127, 22891128   e-mail: kolkata@cbspd.com
- Mumbai: 83-C, Dr E Moses Road, Worli, Mumbai-400018, Maharashtra
  Ph: +91-22-24902340/41   Fax: +91-22-24902342   e-mail: mumbai@cbspd.com

Representatives

- Hyderabad   0-9885175004
- Nagpur   0-9021734563
- Patna   0-9334159340
- Pune   0-9623451994
- Vijayawada   0-9000660880

Printed at Nutech Print Services - India

To

Florence Nightingale
an embodiment of compassion,
consideration, care and concern
and
a role model for all nurses

The Roles and Responsibilities of Nursing Professionals

"Nursing encompasses autonomous and collaborative care of individuals of all ages, families, groups and communities, sick or well and in all settings. Nursing includes the promotion of health, prevention of illness, and care of ill, disabled and dying people. Advocacy, promotion of safe environment, research, participation in shaping health policy and in patient and health system management and education are also key nursing roles."

International Council of Nurses

"The use of clinical judgement in the provision of care to enable people to improve, maintain or recover health, to cope with health problems, and to achieve the best possible quality of life, whatever their disease or disability, until death."

Royal College of Nursing, UK

"Nursing is the protection, promotion, and optimization of health and abilities, prevention of illness and injury, alleviation of suffering through the diagnosis and treatment of human responses, and advocacy in health care for individuals, families, communities and populations."

American Nurses Association

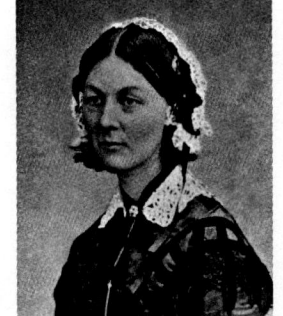

I solemnly pledge myself before God and in the presence of this assembly, to pass my life in purity and to practice my profession faithfully. I will abstain from whatever is deleterious and mischievous, and will not take or knowingly administer any harmful drug. I will do all in my power to maintain and elevate the standard of my profession, and will hold in confidence all personal matters committed to my keeping and all family affairs coming to my knowledge in the practice of my calling. With loyalty will I endeavor to aid the physician in his work, and devote myself to the welfare of those committed to my care.

(This is a modified Hippocratic Oath composed by a committee chaired by Lystra Gretter in 1893 as a token of esteem and reverence towards the founder of modern nursing)

International Nurses Day is celebrated globally on May 12, the birth anniversary of Florence Nightingale.

Preface to the Fourth Edition

The excellent acceptance accorded to the third edition of the book inspired the author to bring out an updated and revised version on the advise and recommendations of eminent nursing tutors of the country. The nursing process and communication as the key for successful nursing of sick children have been highlighted in a simple language. The basic health needs of children and care of both healthy and sick children by various nursing tasks and skills have been covered in depth. The triage of sick children and role of a nurse in the outpatient department have been covered. The compassionate role of a nurse in the care of chronically sick and terminally ill children has been covered in detail.

The book has been revised, updated and practically rewritten. Five new chapters have been incorporated and they include Organization of a Neonatal Intensive Care Unit, Immunity and Allergy, Mosquito-borne Diseases, Helminthic and Protozoal diseases, Musculoskeletal Disorders and Integrated Management of Neonatal and Childhood Illnesses. Bibliography has been provided at the end of each chapter to encourage the keen student to seek more information from the literature. In view of the importance of health preventive and promotive services for welfare of children, a new chapter on Preventive Pediatrics has been included. The supportive nursing care of sick children has been expanded to include several additional nursing procedures and therapeutic interventions. The important role of a nurse in delivery of school health program and combating various social issues like discrimination against the girl child, the beaten or battered child, child abuse and neglect, street children and procedure for adoption have been covered. The community and social health issues, national rural health mission, national urban health mission, and strategies for child survival have been covered in depth. The Glossary of Common Medical Conditions has been expanded. Apart from comprehensive coverage of contents, the greatest asset of the revised book is the clarity of language with a large number of practical tips and nursing alerts to highlight important child care messages.

I would like to take this opportunity to thank Mr YN Arjuna (Senior Vice-President Publishing, Editorial and Publicity), Mrs Ritu Chawla (AGM Production), Mr Ram Murti (Graphic artist) and Mr Vikrant Sharma (DTP operator) for inserting the manuscript in the word processor and to my friend Shri Satish Kumar Jain for his enthusiasm and commitment to publish the revised book in an improved style and format. The book has been written in a simple, easy-to-understand language without any medical jargon and is most suitable to serve the needs of nurses in developing countries. I am confident that **Essential Pediatrics for Nurses** would serve as a Bible of pediatric nursing to fulfill the felt needs of nursing students of general nursing and midwifery and graduate students of pediatric nursing.

Child Care Center
625, Sector 37, Arun Vihar, Noida
e-mail: drmbsk@gmail.com

Meharban Singh MD

Preface to the First Edition

The nurse has a stellar role to assist the nature and the treating doctor to augment the process of healing at all ages but her role is far more important and challenging to provide tender loving care to sick children who are totally dependent and at the mercy of their care takers. Nurse is perhaps the most important link between the child's family on one hand and the treating medical staff on the other. In our country, there is a considerable gap between the training facilities and opportunities provided to the doctors and the nurses to acquire an uptodate knowledge and skills to manage patients. There is an urgent need to narrow this gap so that nurses are well informed and have the confidence and expertise to discuss patients under their care with their doctor colleagues without any reservations or hesitation.

Most of the books for the nurses are written by the nurse educators in the west and there is a paucity of books by the Indian authors. In view of the marked differences in the environmental conditions, cultural background, family dynamics and quality of medical care between the developed countries and our own setting, the nursing books written by the foreign authors are often inappropriate to serve the needs of nurses in the developing world. There is thus a felt need to have state-of-the-art books for various medical disciplines for the nurses in Indian context. During my academic career at All India Institute of Medical Sciences, New Delhi, I had a long experience for over three decades in teaching diploma, graduate and postgraduate nursing students and providing in-service training to qualified nurses in pediatrics and neonatology.

The book has been written keeping in mind the recommendations of the Nursing Council of India for training of undergraduate and graduate students of general nursing and midwifery. The art of pediatric nursing has been discussed in the light of scientific basis of pediatrics. Children have special needs even when they are well and pediatric nurses must have good knowledge regarding growth and development of normal children as well as the specific needs of sick children. The special nursing requirements of children and desirable attributes of pediatric nurses have been discussed in detail. The differences between children and adults during health and disease have been highlighted because most of the available nursing books are adult-oriented.

In view of the emerging problems of newborn babies and the importance of enhancing their survival to reduce infant mortality rate in our country, the nursing care of healthy, high-risk and critically sick newborn babies have been discussed in detail. The basic components of child health like growth and development, evolution of behavior and developmental disorders, preventive pediatrics and immunizations, fluid and electrolyte balance, etc. have been discussed in detail. Feeding and nutrition from birth through adolescence of healthy and sick children and common nutritional disorders have been covered in depth. The common diseases of children have been covered briefly in a simple language to serve the needs of nurses. Accidents, poisonings, developmental defects and children with disability and handicaps have been accorded sufficient coverage and practical guidelines. Nursing routines, rituals and procedures conducted in the pediatric and neonatal intensive care units have been discussed extensively in the light of Indian constraints and conditions. The practical aspects of giving medications to children through various routes and complementary life-saving procedures and therapeutic modalities have been discussed in detail.

I am grateful to my charming and enterprising wife Kaushal for her support and encouragement and to my grand children Karan and Kabir for providing me the comic relief during the travails of my daunting task of writing this book. My special thanks are due to Ms Garima Grover for her help in typing the manuscript and to my friend Shri Narinder Sagar for his enthusiasm and cooperation in publication of this book in a record time.

We are all aware that the pediatric nurse has a challenging and daunting triple task of providing nursing care to sick children, educating the families to update their knowledge and skills of child care and to serve as a manager to improve the logistics of delivering compassionate care to sick children at all levels, i.e. community, ambulatory clinics, under-five clinics, emergency department, specialized in-patient and intensive care units. I hope the book would serve the comprehensive needs of both basic and graduate nursing students and serve as a standard reference book for the qualified pediatric nurses over the years to come.

Child Care and Dental Health Center
625, Sector 37, Arun Vihar, Noida

Meharban Singh MD

Contents

Other Popular Titles by Prof Meharban Singh

- **Care of the Newborn**
  (Revised 8th Edition, 2015)

- **A Manual of Essential Pediatrics**
  (2nd Edition, 2013)

- **Medical Emergencies in Children**
  (Revised 5th Edition, 2016)

- **Pediatric Clinical Methods**
  (5th Edition, 2015)

- **Medical Quotations by Eminent Physicians and Philosophers**
  (4th Edition, 2016)

- **Drug Dosages in Children**
  (9th Edition, 2015)

- **Celestial Principles: The Mystical Laws of Living**
  (1st Edition, 2016)

- **The Art and Science of Baby and Child Care**
  (4th Edition, 2014)

- **A to Z Child Care**
  (Ist Edition, 2015)

- *Bachon Ka Swasthya Aur Unki Dekhbhal* **(in Hindi)**
  (Ist Edition, 2015)

Introduction to Pediatrics

> "We are guilty of many errors and many faults. But our worst crime is abandoning the children, neglecting the foundation of life. Many of the things we need can wait, the child cannot. Right now is the time his bones and flesh are being formed, his blood is being made, and his senses are being developed. To him we cannot answer tomorrow, his name is TODAY".
> — **Gabriela Mistral**

Pediatrics is a branch of medical science that deals with health care and diseases of children from birth to 18 years of age. The word pediatrics (also spelled paediatrics) and its cognates means "healer of children", they derive from two Greek words *pais* (child) and *iatros* (doctor or healer). *The aim of pediatrics is to ensure that every child is able to achieve his full potential for physical growth and mental development.* It is the dream and wish of every parent that their child should be tall, mentally sharp or smart and endowed with a charming personality and good manners. Children are indeed foundation of a nation. There is an increasing evidence to suggest that seeds of most adult diseases namely obesity, metabolic syndrome X, type 2 diabetes mellitus, stroke and osteoporosis are sown in childhood. Healthy children grow to become healthy and strong adults who can actively participate in the developmental activities of the nation.

> "I wish you could realize that destiny of our beloved land lies not with us but in our children"
> — **Mahatma Gandhi**

Pediatrics deals with promotion of health and well-being of children and not merely diagnosis and treatment of diseases of children. Pediatricians and pediatric nurses should, therefore, provide health promotive, preventive, curative and rehabilitation services to children from birth through adolescence.

Differences between the Health Care of Children and Adults

1. Children are dependent and at the mercy of parents and health care professionals to look after their nutritional and health care needs. Educated, well-informed, economically independent and adjusted parents can provide better health care to their children.

2. Children cannot explain or express their discomfort and therefore identification and diagnosis of the diseases may be delayed if parents are not intelligent, observant and concerned. Pediatricians need greater clinical acumen and skills to diagnose diseases in children because they depend upon the second hand information or history provided by the parents or caretakers.

3. The children are not mini-adults. The differences in the nature and manifestations of illnesses in children and adults are based on the anatomic, physiologic and psychologic differences between the immature child and the mature adult.

4. Childhood period is characterized by rapid physical growth and mental development. Depending upon the developmental status, diseases behave differently at different age groups. Diseases produce non-specific symptoms and signs and take a more serious course in newborn babies and infants.

5. Diseases in children may adversely affect physical growth and mental development of children. Children with recurrent or chronic diseases are prone to develop nutritional problems and stunting.

6. Because of their wide range of body sizes (ranging in body weight from 1.0 kg at birth to over 50 kg at adolescence) and developmental status at different ages, they need medical equipment of different sizes and sophistication.

7. Nutritional and caloric needs of children per unit body weight are higher because they need extra

energy for rapid physical growth and higher level of their physical activity. Nutritional disorders are more common in children compared to adults. Their needs for fluids, electrolytes, calories and micronutrients are calculated on the basis of their age and body weight.

8. Children are more vulnerable to develop infections (especially diarrhea, respiratory infections, exanthematous illnesses) and parasitic infestations due to lack of immunity (because of their first contact with a pathogen), poor environmental sanitation and overcrowding. They are likely to develop frequent infections during first 6 months of their entry to a creche or play school because of contact with other children. In general, children are prone to fall sick frequently during first 5 years of life.

9. Congenital malformations, developmental disorders including genetic and chromosomal disorders are mostly seen in childhood. Cancer and malignant disorders do occur in children but they are more common among elderly people. Atherosclerosis, coronary artey disease and type 2 diabetes mellitus

> "Children are not merely small adults and to understand children it is not enough to extrapolate from adults."
> — John Apley

occur in adults but their seeds are often sown in early life due to poor fetal growth (intrauterine growth retardation) and over nutrition or unhealthy lifestyle during childhood.

10. Children are more likely to have accidents, poisonings, animal and insect bites due to their ignorance, innocence and curiosity.

11. Children are not mini-adults because they have anatomical and functional immaturity of various body organs at different stages of life. They rapidly develop life-threatening medical emergencies due

to their physiological instability. Children are like flowers, they can rapidly wither following an acute illness but are endowed with tremendous recuperative capabilities and when tended with love, care, compassion and due concern for their physiological handicaps, they bloom back to life with equal case.

12. The drug dosages in children are calculated on the basis of their age, body weight or surface area. In view of small doses in young infants, the safety margin of drugs is small and hence extra caution and care should be taken to administer drugs to children.

13. Vital signs vary in children depending upon their age. Body temperature is maintained within the narrow range of 98.2°F ±0.7°F (36.8°C ±0.4°C) at all ages. However, temperature is more labile and unstable in newborn babies and young infants. Vital signs at different age groups are shown in **Table 1.1**.

14. Above all, sick children should be treated as "children" because unlike adults children do not realise that they are "patients". You must adopt a non-structured approach and play attitude while providing nursing care to children to elicit their cooperation. Children are delicate and they should be handled with utmost care, compassion and tender love.

Age-Groups in Children

Pediatricians look after children from birth up to 18 years of age. Till recently, adolescents or children between 12 and 18 years were neither looked after by internists (adults physicians) nor by pediatricians. In most developed countries in the West, adolescents are being looked after by pediatricians and there are separate male and female wards for adolescent children. In India, many pediatricians provide ambulatory or OPD care to adolescent children but no adolescent wards have been created as yet.

Vital signs	Neonates (Term baby)	Infants (up to 1 year)	2 to 5 years	Above 5 years
Temperature (oral °F)	98.2 ± 0.7	98.2 ± 0.7	98.2 ± 0.7	98.2 ± 0.7
Heart rate (beats/min)	120–160	80–120	70–110	60–90
Respiratory rate (rate/min)	40–60	25–40	20–30	15–18
Blood pressure (mm Hg)	60/40	70/50	90/50	110/80

Table 1.1 Vital signs of children at different ages (Age groups)

Vital signs should be recorded when child is quiet and resting.
Heart rate and breathing rate in a neonate are double of an adult.
Blood pressure in a neonate is one-half of an adult.

Neonates Children between birth and up to 28 days of life are called newborn babies or neonates. They are delicate and have distinctive health problems with high morbidity and mortality demanding specialized healthcare facilities.

Infants Children between birth and up to their first birthday are called infants. They should be provided exclusive breastfeeding (not even water should be given) up to first 6 months of life and continued breast-feeding for at least one year but preferably longer.

Toddlers Children between 1 and 3 years are called toddlers because during this period they are crawling, cruising and walking with unsteady steps. They are most vulnerable to nutritional disorders and growth faltering because they are started on complementary or weaning foods and are exposed to a variety of infections with increased risk of diarrheal disorders. Adequacy of nutrition or optimal nutrition during 0–3 years of age is most crucial for optimal physical growth and brain development. It is believed that the linear growth or height achieved at the age of 3 years is a good predictor of ultimate adult height or stature.

Under-five children Children between the age of 0–5 years are called under-five or under-5 children. They are specially vulnerable to a variety of vaccine-preventable diseases, diarrheal disorders and respiratory infections.

Preschool children Children between 3 and 6 years are called preschool children when they go to a play school or crèche. They are vulnerable to nutritional disorders, respiratory and GI infections and vaccine-preventable diseases. Most of the brain growth is completed by 6 years.

School-going children Children between 6 and 12 years are called school-going children when they are in a regular school. After entry to the regular school, the risk of intercurrent infections among healthy children becomes minimal. During this period, their growth velocity is slow.

Adolescents Adolescence is a phase of childhood which is characterized by rapid physical growth, sexual maturation and emotional development. The physical changes and sexual maturation during adolescence are triggered by hormonal changes. Girls mature both sexually and emotionally earlier than boys by two years. In girls, pubertal changes take place between 10 and 16 years. A large majority of girls begin their sexual development at the age of 10 years and have their first menstrual period around 12 years of age. The average boy starts puberty around 12 years and achieves sexual maturity during 14–18 years. When full sexual matura-tion is achieved, the epiphyses of the long bones fuse with their diaphyses and there is no further linear growth or increase in height. After completion of puberty, the girl becomes a woman and a boy becomes a man.

BASIC NEEDS OF CHILDREN

Every human being has basic or fundamental needs for survival and fulfillment of his role in society. Depending upon their importance and relevance as the child grows, they can be depicted as a pyramid (**Figure 1.1**). The higher or celestial needs emerge as the lower needs are satisfied.

1. Love, Tender Care and Protection

We all need love from cradle to grave from different people throughout our lifespan. Love is the energizing elixir of life. Mother provides unconditional selfless love to her child without any expectation; which is the highest form of true love or compassion. Just as food is necessary for the body, love is necessary for the soul. The gentle touch, cuddling and caressing of the baby by her mother, transmits exhilarating electromagnetic messages to the baby. The nurse should visualize the mother as a role model to provide comfort and transmit healing thoughts and vibrations to the ailing child.

Unlike offspring's of other mammals, human baby is dependent and at the mercy of her caretakers during first 3 to 5 years of life. They need constant care and protection against environmental vagaries (heat or cold), physical comfort, relief of pain, toilet needs, bathing, personal hygiene, clothing, etc.

2. Physiologic Needs of Air, Water and Food

Human beings (rather all living beings) cannot survive without air, water and food. We cannot survive beyond

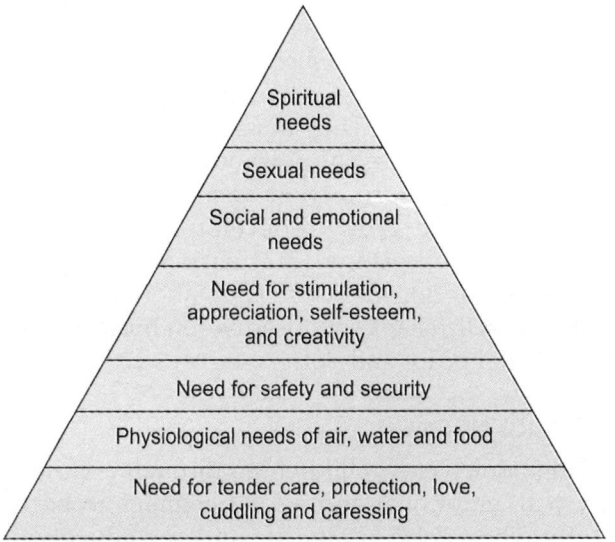

Figure 1.1 Pyramid of basic needs of children

1

few minutes without oxygen, few days without water and few weeks without food. And children are at the mercy of their parents or caretakers to look after these basic needs and they are at a greater risk to suffer from their ill effects earlier due to their lack or deficiency compared to adults. Children should be provided with unpolluted air, safe drinking water and balanced age-appropriate food with adequate amounts of macro- and micronutrients to ensure that they achieve their optimal physical growth and mental developmental potential.

3. Safety and Security

Because of their dependence, curiosity and lack of skills, children need close supervision and protection against hazards of physical injuries, accidents, choking, poisonings, animal bites, etc.

4. Stimulation, Appreciation and Creativity

Our brain is stimulated by virtue of our special senses, i.e. what we see, hear, feel through touch, smell and taste. Stimulation should begin from fetal life and continue throughout childhood both at home and school. Preschool years (birth–5 years) are most critical for maturation of brain and development of skills because almost adult size of the brain is achieved by the age of 5 to 6 years. Instead of bookish rote memory, children should be encouraged to develop self-confidence, power of observation, curiosity and creativity.

5. Social and Emotional Needs

Children learn various traits, habits and attributes by watching various role models in their vicinity like parents, relatives, friends, teachers, clerics and politicians. You can mold your child depending upon your own perceptions and values in life. You must have a vision and a dream as to what attributes and qualities your child should have as he or she grows up to become a responsible adult in the society which is full of virtues and vices. Parents must set a good example for their children to emulate. They must be reared with love, security and discipline without any rejection or favoritism, over-protection and over indulgence. Children should grow to develop a well-groomed personality, emotional maturity and necessary interactive or social skills. They should evolve as confident, self-reliant, self-assertive, enthusiastic adults with mental peace and poise.

6. Sexual Needs

During adolescence, children go through a variety of physical, emotional and sexual changes to become adults. They need family life and sex education to handle this crucial phase of life to become responsible adults having basic information regarding sexual anatomy, dangers of promiscuity, drug abuse, safe sex and importance of contraception and family planning. Sex is a fundamental need for procreation and promotion of human progeny.

7. Spiritual Needs

Health is not merely absence of disease, it is boundless energy, enthusiasm, happiness, peace of mind, success and loving relationships. It is achieved by a state of equilibrium between body, mind and soul. Spiritual awakening is the ultimate goal of human life, an awareness which distinguishes us from animals. Spirituality does not mean following any religion, rituals, symbols or code of conduct. Human values of spirituality are based on love, compassion, sharing and caring for fellow human beings and seeing God or super power in all living beings. Society is at commercial cross roads and what we need is that our children should become good human beings—caring and concerned for the needs of others. The nurse should be aware of all the aforementioned basic needs of children so that she is able to effectively look after children and guide their parents during different phases of life both in health and during the disease.

HEALTH CARE OF CHILDREN

Nurse should not be concerned merely to treat sick children but should have knowledge and skills to provide supportive health care for promotion and maintenance of health and prevention of illnesses in children.

Health Promotion and Maintenance

All children whether normal or high-risk, should be helped to achieve their optimal growth potential and wellness by providing health, family life and nutrition education to parents, school teachers, and community at large. During every contact with a health care worker, the family should be given advice for importance of balanced nutrition, need for nutritional supplements, safe drinking water, personal hygiene and environmental sanitation to promote health of children.

Prevention of Illness

Nurse should provide health and nutrition education and ensure administration of timely vaccinations to children and their families. She should have the knowledge and understanding about the common modes of occurrence of diseases (like air-borne, water-borne, blood-borne, close physical or sexual contact, through pathogens, pollutants, toxins, nutritional deficiency states, etc.) and underlying predisposing factors like poor personal hygiene, unsatisfactory environmental sanitation, breeding of mosquitoes, house flies and other vectors, lack of safe drinking water, poor housing facilities, and overcrowding.

Restoration of Health and Rehabilitation

Although promotion of health and prevention of illness are far more important to ensure welfare of a large number of children in the society but most of the time of a nurse in our country is spent in restoration of health of sick children by supporting their treatment and

> "Keep the patient under best conditions like fresh air, plentiful space, nutritious food, warmth, clean surroundings, solitude and allow nature to heal the patient."
> — **Florence Nightingale**

rehabilitation in the ambulatory clinic or hospital. She provides care and comfort to children with acute illnesses, life-threatening emergencies and chronic disease states demanding prolonged care, emotional support and rehabilitation. For effective delivery of curative services, the nurse works under direct guidance and supervision of a pediatrician or a pediatric superspecialist.

Child Health Problems

The leading health problems of children in developing countries include nutritional disorders such as low birth weight babies, infections and infestations, developmental and genetic disorders, behavior problems and conduct disorders. Children suffer from a large number of preventive disorders.

1. **Nutritional disorders** Malnutrition is the core health problem in children in developing countries. According to the State of World's Children, UNICEF 2012 data, 28% newborns are low birth weight (<2500 g), 43% of under-5 children are underweight and 48% are stunted in India. Children are vulnerable to develop nutritional disorders because they are dependent on their parents and caretakers to look after their nutritional requirements. Their caloric and protein requirements are much higher (3 times of an adult per unit body mass) to sustain their rapid growth velocity and meet the nutritional demands of physical activity and intercurrent infections. The various factors leading to high incidence of nutritional disorders include poor health status, education and dignity of mothers, increased risk of infections because of poor socioeconomic status, lack of healthy living conditions, overcrowding, pollution and

unsafe drinking water. Apart from nutritional deficiencies, other deficiency disorders include deficiencies of oxygen (hypoxia because of birth asphyxia, respiratory and cardiac disorders), water (dehydration due to vomiting and diarrhea), vitamins and trace minerals and hormones (deficiency of thyroxine and growth hormone). In affluent sections of society, overnutrition or obesity is emerging as a public health problem.

2. **Infections and infestations** In developing countries, children are vulnerable to develop frequent day-to-day infections because of greater opportunities (overcrowding, unhealthy living conditions, poor hygiene and sanitation) and greater vulnerability (poor immunity due to nutritional disorders) to develop infections. Undernourished children are more susceptible to develop infections and are likely to have slower recovery, increased severity and higher mortality. Occurrence of frequent infections, further compromises the nutritional status thus setting up a vicious cycle of malnutrition—infections—malnutrition. Infections may occur from a variety of pathogens including viruses, bacteria, spirochetes, fungi and parasites.

3. **Developmental disorders** Most of the developmental disorders manifest during infancy and childhood. They include genetic diseases or inborn errors of metabolism, chromosomal disorders, congenital malformations and learning disability.

4. **Accidents and poisonings** By virtue of their ignorance and innocence, children are vulnerable to develop home accidents (falls, burns, scalds, electric shock) and ingestion of poorly stored medicines and chemicals like kerosene, lye, insecticides, etc. There is increasing incidence of automobile accidents among adolescents because of drunken driving and macho behavior. Because of various social factors and unemployment, drug abuse is assuming public health relevance in certain societies.

5. **Allergic, hypersensitivity and autoimmune disorders** In developed countries, because of control of infections by virtue of better living conditions and environmental sanitation, allergic disorders are assuming greater importance. The common allergic disorders include skin allergy or atopy, food allergy, allergic rhinitis, bronchial asthma, post-infectious disorders, collagen vascular or connective tissue disorders.

6. **Degenerative disorders** Most degenerative disorders occur among aging population but their seeds are sown during childhood. Children with asymmetric intrauterine growth retardation and metabolic

syndrome X are more vulnerable to develop atherosclerosis, insulin resistance and coronary artery disease during adulthood. Rare degenerative disorders in children include progeria and degenerative disorders of central nervous system.

7. **Neoplasms** Benign cysts and neoplasms are common in children while malignant disorders are a leading cause of mortality in elderly subjects. Hematologic malignancies are common in children and can be managed effectively with modern chemotherapy and stem cell transfusion.

8. **Psychogenic and psychosomatic disorders** Children are prone to manifest a number of behavior abnormalities, habit and conduct disorders due to unsatisfactory parenting, marital discord and psychodynamic issues. Common behavior and developmental disorders include breath-holding spells, nocturnal enuresis, attention seeking behavior, food fussiness or "blackmailing" tactics, anxiety, depression, conversion reaction, attention deficit hyperactivity disorders (ADHD), autism spectrum disorders (ASDs), and substance abuse, etc.

Hospital Care of Sick Children

Children wards and hospitals for sick children should have their distinct identity with necessary facilities and features to make them child-friendly. There should be both small cots with railings as well as standard adult beds for older children. Each bed should be provided with a centralized source of oxygen and suction. Due to shortage of nurses and to avoid separation anxiety and fear of strangers and strange environment, mother or a lady attendant should be allowed to stay with the child round-the-clock. A comfortable padded bench and a locker should be provided next to the bed for the comfort of mother or attendant. Two bays adjacent to the nursing station should be provided to admit moderately sick children requiring intravenous fluid therapy and close monitoring by the nurses. These patients should be visible to the nurses from the nursing station through the glass walls. The ward should be decorated with colorful soft toys and innovative designs of indigenous cartoon characters on the walls. A procedure room should be available in each unit to undertake diagnostic and therapeutic procedures. Each pediatric unit should be provided with 3 to 4 independent rooms with an attached bathroom for isolation of children who are immunocompromised or suffering from contagious diseases. They should be provided with gowning and handwashing facilities. In each pediatric unit, provision must also be made for a

pantry and formula room to dispense special diets. A well-equipped Pediatric Intensive Care Unit (PICU) with all the essential monitoring and therapeutic electronic equipment should be provided to look after critically sick children with life-threatening medical disorders. On an average, 20% beds should be earmarked for pediatric emergencies, i.e. a 100-bedded children ward should have a 20-bedded PICU.

> "The art of medicine consists of amusing the patient while nature cures the disease."
> — Voltaire

Children should be provided with home-friendly ambience in the hospital. Efforts should be made to keep them busy and in good mood. A play room with necessary toys and indoor games should be available. Play room should be located in the corner of the ward so that the noise produced by the children while playing does not disturb the more sick children. There should not be any fixed times of play for the hospitalized children. A social worker or a play therapist (play lady) should organize and supervise the play activities. A dining room is an essential requirement because children do eat better in the company of other children. Children are fussy in their food habits and their fussiness becomes worse when they are sick. Dining room with a TV set and other ancillary facilities does encourage and motivate sick children to eat better. The washrooms and toilet facilities should cater to the needs of children as well as their mothers and attendants. Children should be provided with a colorful and clean dress from the hospital which should be changed daily. Bed linen and sheets must be changed daily because children are more likely to soil them. The colorful dress of the nurses and avoidance of white coat by the doctors are likely to enhance nurse–child and doctor–child relationship and cooperation.

THE CHILD IN THE HOSPITAL

Hospital stay is difficult and challenging for a child at any age. There is stress and discomfort of illness as well as stay in the unfamiliar surroundings of the hospital. They are exposed to unpleasant experience of bitter medicines, procedures and painful injections. They are likely to miss their friends and family members, they often get scared and bored. Children may not understand why they are in a hospital and may have false beliefs about what is happening to them. Both sickness as well as hospital stay are likely to adversely affect the growth and development of children. A hospital stay is likely to affect different children in different ways, depending upon the age, awareness, temperament or personality of the child, for example, whether child is easy-going and self-confident or shy and unsure in unfamiliar circumstances. There is a need for using a different approach in handling children of different ages to minimize the adverse effects of hospitalization and to ensure easier and faster adaptation to stressful mileau of the hospital.

Birth to 1 Year Old

- This is the age for fast development of skills like rolling, sitting, crawling and standing or walking with support.
- Infants need sensory-stimulation, e.g. music, body positions, touch, toys, interaction and sunlight.
- They are likely to have stranger anxiety, it is important that mother or a familiar member should stay with the child.

1 to 2 Years

- They are disturbed by change in their daily routines of bathing, feeding and sleeping.
- They continue to develop new gross and fine motor skills which are adversely affected both by the illness and hospital stay.
- Children of this age do not fully understand why they are in the hospital.
- They develop anxiety and stress due to contact with a number of strangers.
- Children are developing trust in their caregivers during this age period which is compromised because many new faces are involved in their care and they are exposed to several challenging experiences.

2 to 5 Years

- It is stressful to be away from home and familiar daily routines.
- Children may believe that they did something wrong and that is why they are in the hospital.
- They are afraid to go through unpleasant routines and procedures.
- They know more about their bodies but their understanding is limited.
- Language skills are developing fast but may misunderstand words they hear.

5–12 Years

- Being away from home, school and friend is stressful.
- There is anxiety, fear, and pain of injections and procedures.
- They are scared of surgical procedures.

12 Years and Older

- Being away from home, school and friend is often stressful.
- Adolescents need privacy which is adversely affected.
- Teenagers are more aware and concerned about the long-term effects of illness.

Role of Nurses and Parents in Handling Hospitalized Children

There are many ways that parents, nurses and health care professionals can help children cope with inconveniences and stresses of a stay in the hospital. When you provide assurance and comfort to reduce the anxiety and stress of hospital stay, it is associated with faster recovery and shorter stay in the hospital.

Getting Ready for the Hospital

In case of planned or elective admission to the hospital, parents can help their child to buffer or cushion the anticipated experience. Depending upon the age of the child, he or she can be explained about the need for hospitalization, the nature of health team and their roles, various routines and likely procedures to be conducted. The procedures can be explained on dolls, animals or simulators. Parents must exhibit stoic courage and confidence, to serve as role models to the child. Talk to the child about any anxiety, fears, various concerns and misunderstandings. They must be told about their likely experience in the hospital in a simple positive way without any deceptions and lies. Address their worries and queries in a simple matter of fact manner.

Visitors

In order to reduce the anxiety and stress, it is important that mother or a caretaker from the family is allowed to accompany the child in the hospital, which is a standard practice in India and many developing countries. Familiar faces are reassuring to build the confidence of the child. In view of shortage of nurses in developing countries, the attendant can be guided and trained to provide simple nursing chores. Phone calls, internet chats and visits by family members, siblings and friends help the child to stay connected to his or her world outside the hospital.

Familiar Objects from Home

The favorite objects, toys and stuffed animals should be packed and taken to the hospital along with other essential articles of daily care and need. These objects help to provide comfort and bonding to the child.

Play and Dining Room Facilities

The hospital environment should simulate the familiar home environment of the child. Hospitalized children should be provided with a variety of indoor games and fun activities in a dedicated play room under the supervision of a social worker. Play activities and interactive games can take the child's mind away from pain, anxiety and illness. It helps the child to stay stimulated and encouraged to have normal development. It is also a good idea to have a dinning room in children ward, where children are motivated to eat better and develop friendship with other inmates of the ward.

BIBLIOGRAPHY

Maguire P, Pitceathly C. Key communication skills and how to acquire them. *BMJ* 2002; 325(7366): 697–700.

Manojlovich M, DeCicco, B. Healthy work environment, nurse-physician communication and patients outcome. *Am J Child Care* 2007; 16(6): 536–543.

Singh M. The art, science and philosophy of child care. *Indian J Pediatr* 2009; 76(2): 171–176.

Singh M. Communication as a bridge to build a sound doctor-patient/parent relationship. *Indian J Pediatr* 2016; 83(1): 33–37.

Singh M. The Art and Science of Pediatric diagnosis. In: Pediatric Clinical Methods, 5th edition, *New Delhi, CBS Publishers and Distributors Pvt. Ltd.* 2016, p 1–13.

Singh M. Celestial Principles: The Mystical Laws of Living. *CBS Publishers and Distributors Pvt. Ltd, New Delhi*, 2016.

The Art of Pediatric Nursing

> *"The trained nurse has become one of the great blessings of humanity, taking a place beside the Physician and Priest."*
> — **Sir William Osler**

> *"Patients many forget your name, but they will never forget, how you made them feel."*
> — Maya Angelou

ATTRIBUTES OF A PEDIATRIC NURSE

Nursing is a noble profession and should be undertaken by those who are endowed with an inherent interest and inclination to provide care, comfort and solace to fellow human beings. Nursing is an art and act of devotion as it deals with care and healing of a living being, the temple of God's spirit. It is not an easy job but it is a worth doing job which gives immense satisfaction. *The nurse should not consider her job as a profession but as a mission in life to provide tender loving care (TLC) to the suffering humanity.* The pediatric nurse should have genuine love for children and a special knack to handle them in a playful manner to elicit their best cooperation. She should establish a good rapport with children under her care despite the fact that she has to perform certain unpleasant tasks like giving injections, setting up an intravenous line, inserting a catheter or a nasogastric tube. She should be caring, compassionate and considerate to look after children with love and delicate handling in a methodical and systematic way. She should interact and communicate both with children and their parents in a relaxed manner without showing any hurry, worry and anger. She should have the expertise to undertake all the pediatric nursing chores with due competence and confidence. Apart from having uptodate knowledge and skills to perform all the essential nursing tasks, she should be a good human being with a genuine concern for children and their parents. She must have an alert mind and a warm heart. The key attributes of a good pediatric nurse are listed in **Box 2.1**.

> *Remember the first dictum of patient care is "Do No Harm."*
> **Florence Nightingale**

Communication is the Key for Successful Nursing

The nurse should have the art of listening more and talking less to obtain information regarding the onset and evolution of the disease process and underlying environmental factors and family dynamics. She should have the ability to establish and maintain a sound rapport with the family. She should provide an opportunity to parents to ventilate their feelings and concerns in order to relieve their tension and anxiety, and assist them to understand and resolve their own problems. The key components of communication are listed in **Box 2.2**.

NURSING DUTIES AND SKILLS

> *"Observe, record, tabulate and communicate. Use your five senses".*
> — **Sir William Osler**

The objectives of pediatric nursing include promotion of health, prevention of illness, care of unwell, disabled and critically sick children. The key nursing roles include advocacy, promotion of safe environment, management of sick children, research, and participation in shaping health care policies for welfare of children.

1. **General nursing care** To provide a comfortable and a clean bed and to look after the needs of personal hygiene by daily sponging, brushing of teeth, changing the clothes, making the hair, etc. *Caring indeed is the essence of nursing.* She should supervise feeding and nutrition of sick children and provide them comfort, company and play activities. She should be an advocate for welfare of children, maintain privacy and confidentiality in all health matters.

2

> **Box 2.1** **The key attributes of a good pediatric nurse**

- Knowledge, skills and professionalism.
- Caring, empathetic and compassionate.
- Communication skills.
- Self-confidenec with emotional stability and serenity under all odds.
- Flexible and adaptable to acept responsibility with an attitute of "Never say never".
- Interpersonal skills, love for children and sense of humor.
- Physical endurance and stamina because nursing is a tough and demanding profession.
- Quick response with calm demeanor and problem solving skills.
- Respectful, disciplined and responsible.
- Attention to detail, competent and confident.
- Good record keeper.

> **Box 2.2** **Principles governing effective communication by the nurse**

- Interview should be conducted in a cordial and warm atmosphere with a genuine expression of concern and liking for the family. The tone of dialogue should be pleasant and poised without any tinge of abruptness and rudeness. She should be relaxed and endowed with patience.
- Speak in a simple language without any medical jargons and in keeping with the education and intellectual level of the parent or attendant.
- Communicate in a language with which the family is comfortable by asking simple short questions in a relaxed manner.
- Nurse should speak less and listen more (God has given us one mouth and two ears!).
- Establish empathy and genuine concern with parents and their children.
- Nurse should accept the parents and their child as they are without any judgement or evaluating their actions as 'bad' or 'wrong'.
- Nurse should assist parents to express their concerns, worries, anxiety and other negative emotions to enable them to get a sense of relief and release of pent up emotions and tension.
- School-going and adolescent children should be encouraged to talk and explain their health problems, concerns, worries and fears.

2. **Monitoring of vital signs** Temperature, pulse/ heart rate, breathing rate and blood pressure should be checked and monitored as per the frequency recommended by the attending doctor. She should be able to identify any deterioration in the condition of the child under her care and inform the pediatrician promptly and without any delay.

3. **Administration of fluids, electrolytes, blood and blood components and drugs** In newborn babies and young infants, there is an increased risk of over administration of fluids, electrolytes and drugs due to low margin of safety. They should be administered with the help of a mini-burette or infusion pump and mini-syringes (insulin, tuberculin syringe). The nurse should exercise due vigilance and caution to prevent avoidable therapeutic mishaps.

4. **Diagnostic and therapeutic procedures** She should be able to collect samples of blood and body fluids for screening and diagnostic purposes. She should make necessary arrangements and assist the doctor to undertake various diagnostic and therapeutic procedures like endoscopies, tissue biopsies, bone narrow aspiration, lumbar puncture, paracentesis, assisted ventilation, exchange blood transfusion, etc. Informed consent of the family should be taken before undertaking a procedure.

5. **Nursing procedures** She should have the specialized skills to perform various pediatric nursing procedures independently. A higher level of precision and skills are required in performing procedures in newborn babies and young infants. The common pediatric procedures include giving various injections, setting up an IV line, doing hydrotherapy, inserting a catheter, providing nasogastric feeds, undertaking bowel wash, pre- and postoperative care, dressing wounds, relieving pain, etc.

6. **Resuscitation skills** She should have the necessary training, expertise and confidence to resuscitate a child with apnea or cardiac arrest by providing bag and mask ventilation and chest compressions. She should be able to manage a child who develops anaphylaxis following administration of a drug or blood transfusion.

7. **Specialized nursing and monitoring skills** The critically sick children admitted in the pediatric and neonatal ICUs demand high levels of skills and competence by specially trained pediatric nurses. High quality of supportive and nursing care is mandatory to salvage children with life-threatening emergencies. She should be able to provide nursing care to children with coma, shock, status epilepticus, status asthmaticus and multi-organ failure.

> *"Constant attention by a dedicated nurse is as important as a major operation by a surgeon."*
> — Dag Hammarskjold

She should be able to provide nursing support and chest physiotherapy to children on assisted ventilation, peritoneal dialysis, phototherapy, etc. The critically sick children need comprehensive and frequent monitoring of vital signs, blood gases and acid-base parameters, input-output of fluids and electrolytes, medications, and body weight changes.

8. **Vaccinations** She should have an up-to-date knowledge and skills to administer various vaccines and store them under strict cold chain conditions. She should have the skills to take various anthropometric parameters and record them on the Road-to-Health cards.

9. **Prevention of nosocomial infections** Sick children admitted to the pediatric ward and especially those admitted to an intensive care unit are very vulnerable to develop life-threatening infections from health care professionals and other potentially infected patients. Strict handwashing, barrier nursing, asepsis and isolation strategies should be used to prevent nosocomial infections.

10. **Universal precautions** In view of the increasing incidence of acquired immunodeficiency syndrome (AIDS), it is recommended that every patient admitted to the hospital should be considered as potentially infected with HIV and "universal precautions" should be followed by the nurses and other health care professionals to safeguard against the risk of contracting HIV and Hepatitis B infection.

11. **Tutoring and record keeping** The registered nurse (RN) should provide "on the job" supervision and training to student nurses, organize their duties and workload responsibilities. She should maintain an accurate monitoring record of patients under her care and hand over a written report after completion of a duty shift.

12. **Advocacy for children** The nurse administrator should serve as an advocate for welfare of children at all levels—home, school, well child clinic, ambulatory clinic or doctor's office, hospital, intensive care unit and community at large. She should provide guidance and know how to patients and their families to maintain healthy living habits in order to promote optimal health and good quality of life.

13. **Evidence-based nursing competencies** The nurse should be conversant and aware of Cochrane databased evidence for care of healthy and sick children. She should be able to implement changes and strategies in her nursing practice on the basis of scientific evidence. The nurse must have knowledge and expertise to access latest information and critically analyze research data.

THE NURSING PROCESS

> "Nurses are the heart, soul and face of our healthcare system."
>
> — Meharban Singh

Nursing process is a coordinated plan or frame of work which is followed by a nurse in the care of all patients and is considered as a foundation of their practice by professional nurses. Nursing process is a continuous process or an algorithm which is followed in sequential steps for care of children. The rationale of each step is based on nursing theory. The five basic steps of nursing process include assessment, nursing diagnosis, planning of care, implementation or intervention and evaluation or monitoring (Figure 2.1). The nursing process provides an organized format to deliver holistic or comprehensive nursing care to sick children. Table 2.1 shows an example of nursing process in a child suspected to have poststreptococcal glomerulonephritis.

Assessment

Interview should be conducted with due courtesy and in a relaxed manner keeping in mind the education and understanding of the parent or attendant and age of the child. The child must be assessed along with his family, parents, friends and environment. History is taken to assess family dynamics, socioeconomic status, environmental conditions, concept of personal hygiene, educational status of parents, number of siblings, availability of safe drinking water, and living conditions, etc. The onset, duration and evolution of disease process are assessed. Physical examination is conducted to assess anthropometry (weight, length or height and head circumference), vital signs (temperature, pulse or heart rate, breathing rate, blood pressure), hydration and nutritional status. Developmental status of the child and presence of any neuromotor disability is recorded. Activity, behaviour, general well-being, level of consciousness, feeding behavior and excretory functions (stool consistency and frequency, urinary

> "Children should not be fragmented into systems, organs, tissues, cells and DNA. They must be viewed in totality (body, mind, heart and soul) and that too not in isolation but in context with the dynamics of environment, family, friends and society".
>
> — Meharban Singh

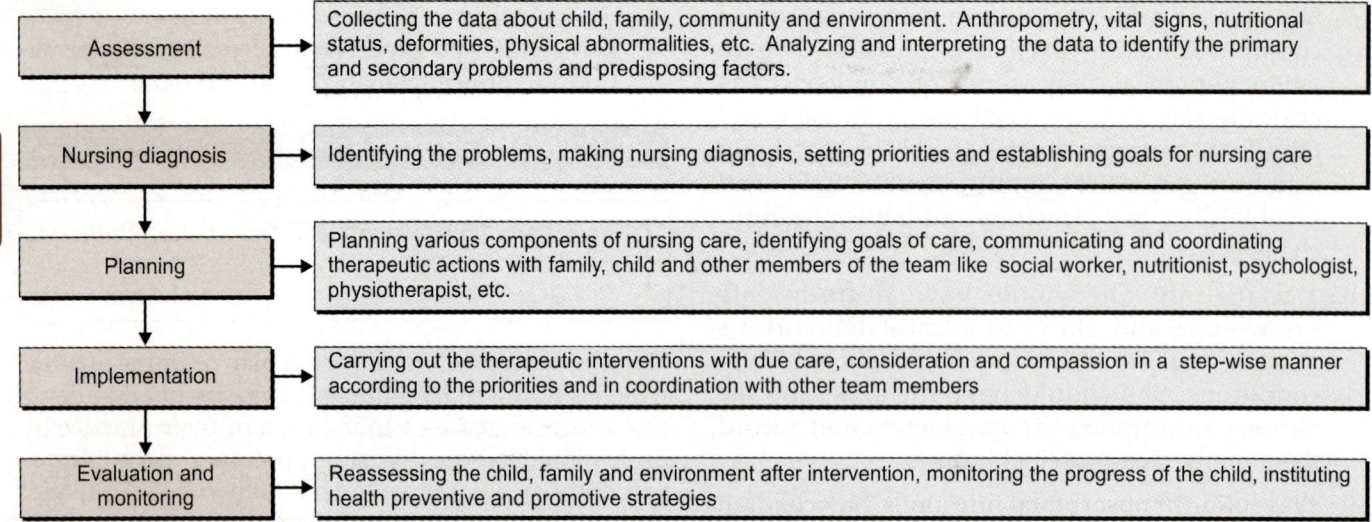

Figure 2.1 The nursing process

Day of illness	Assessment	Nursing diagnosis	Planning	Implementation	Evaluation and monitoring
	Table 2.1 Nursing process in a 5-year-old child with acute glomerulonephritis				
10th	• History of sore throat 2 weeks ago	• Accumulation of extracellular fluid	• To reduce fluid accumulation	• Bed rest and back rest	• Puffiness and pedal edema—less
	• Puffiness of face and edema feet	• Increased blood volume	• Treat hypertension	• Low salt and low protein diet	• BP—130/85 mm Hg
		• Hypertension			• Fluid intake— 800 mL/24 hr
	• Urine—coca-colored	• Hematuria	• Maintain adequate renal function	• Administration of furosemide and hydralazine	• Urine output— 300 mL/24 hr
	• BP—135/90 mm Hg	• Renal dysfunction		• Restriction of fluids	• Body weight— 21.0 kg
	• Fluid intake— 950 mL/24 hr, urine output— 250 mL/24 hr			• Intake-output chart	• Blood urea— 65 mg/dL
	• Body weight— 22.5 kg			• Urine testing and blood urea level	
	• Urine loaded with RBCs and hyaline casts			• Reassurance and emotional support to the family	
	• Blood urea— 85 mg/dL				
	• Decreased serum C_3 level				

Note: The nursing process is drafted everyday during the hospital stay of the patient.

volume and frequency) are assessed and recorded. The nurse must have knowledge regarding normal ranges of physical and physiological parameters of healthy children at different ages before she can interpret the abnormalities in a sick child. The salient abnormalities are listed and severity of disease process is graded into acute or insidious and chronic in nature and in case of acute disease process whether it is mild, moderate, severe or life-threatening in severity.

Nursing Diagnosis

The findings and data obtained on history, physical examination and laboratory evaluation are analyzed and synthesized into various diagnostic possibilities. The diagnostic possibilities for various diseases in children can be summarized into eight broad groups (**Table 2.2**).

According to North American Nursing Diagnosis Association (NANDA), 72 nursing diagnoses have been proposed by taking into consideration not only the disease states of children but by including all areas of health care like health promotion, health maintenance, health restoration and rehabilitation. The identified health problems and issues should be prioritized to plan therapeutic interventions. According to NANDA classification, the latest approved list of nursing diagnoses, in an alphabetical order, is shown in **Table 2.3**.

Planning of Care

Nursing strategies should be planned keeping in mind a time frame of achieving various goals. Priorities are established to tackle various health problems being faced by the child. In view of the fact that every child is unique and no two children are alike, the interventions are customized or individualized to serve the specific needs of every sick child. The nursing care plan is made available to all the members of the nursing team.

Implementation of Interventions

Depending upon the nursing diagnosis and desired goals, the nursing interventions are outlined and explained to all the team members, family and the child to seek their cooperation for effective implementation. It is important that family and child must participate and cooperate to facilitate the process of healing and recovery. The basic philosophy of interventions is to provide comfort to the child and reverse all the physiological and biological abnormalities of the child. Child must be treated like a child (not a patient) and handled with utmost care, consideration and love. The pediatric nurse must have genuine love for children and adopt a flexible, innovative and play centered approach for care of children. They must be nursed in a position of most comfort depending upon their underlying disease process. The prime goal of interventions is to provide comfort to the child and relieve tension and anxiety of the parents. And the guiding principle of all interventions, as extolled by Florence Nightingale is, "Do No Harm".

Evaluation and Monitoring

Evaluation and monitoring should be recorded on a predesigned proforma to assess the response of the child to various therapeutic interventions. During this phase, the data should reflect improvements in the health status of the child and achievement of goals. The management of health problems of children is a dynamic and continuous process. During intervention, as some existing problems resolve, new health problems or complications may appear. Therefore, the nursing process of assessment, nursing diagnosis, planning care, deciding interventions, and evaluation of outcome is a continuous process and is followed in a cyclic manner till child is completely recovered. After complete recovery, the strategies are formulated and discussed with the family to promote and maintain health and well being of the child by instituting health promotive, preventive and rehabilitative interventions. The supreme goal or philosophy of child care is to ensure that every child is assisted to achieve his/her full genetic

Table 2.2 The spectrum of diagnostic possibilities

Etiology	Spectrum of diseases
Infections	Viral, bacterial, fungal and parasitic, etc.
Exogenous toxins and injuries	Drugs, chemicals, foreign body, trauma, burns, scalds and electric shock
Deficiency disorders	Hypoxia, dehydration, protein-calorie malnutrition, deficiency of vitamins, minerals and hormones
Developmental disorders	Genetic diseases, chromosomal disorders and congenital malformations
Neoplasms	Benign or malignant
Allergic, hypersensitivity, or autoimmune disorders	Allergic diathesis, atopy, bronchial asthma, post-infectious disorders, collagen vascular disorders, etc.
Degenerative disorders	Atherosclerosis, progeria, CNS degenerative disorders
Psychogenic and psychosomatic disorders	Breath-holding spells, enuresis, recurrent abdominal pain, conversion reaction, drug addictions, conduct disorders, behavior disorder, autism spectrum disorders, attention deficit hyperactivity disorder, learning disability, etc.

Table 2.3 The list of common nursing diagnoses

- Activity intolerance
- Activity intolerance, risk of
- Adjustment, impaired
- Airway clearance ineffective
- Anxiety
- Aspiration, risk of
- Body temperature, altered risk of
- Bowel incontinence
- Breastfeeding, ineffective
- Breathing pattern, ineffective
- Cardiac output, decreased
- Communication, impaired, verbal
- Comfort, altered, pain
- Confusion
- Constipation
- Coping, ineffective, individual
- Coping, ineffective, family
- Diarrhea
- Diversional activity, deficit of
- Family process, altered
- Fatigue
- Fear
- Fluid volume, deficit, risk of
- Fluid volume, excess, risk of
- Fluid volume deficit
- Gas exchange, impaired
- Growth and development, altered
- Hopelessness
- Hyperthermia
- Hypothermia
- Infant feeding pattern, ineffective

- Infection, risk of
- Injury, risk of
- Knowledge deficit
- Memory, impaired
- Mobility impaired, physical
- Noncompliance
- Nurtrition, altered, less than body need
- Nutrition, altered, more than body need
- Oral mucous membrane, altered
- Pain, acute
- Pain, chronic
- Parenting, altered
- Parental role conflict
- Poisoning, risk of
- Post-trauma response
- Protection, altered
- Self-care deficit: feeding, bathing, dressing, toileting, hygiene
- Sensory alteration: visual, auditory, tactile, taste and smell
- Skin integrity, impaired
- Skin integrity, impaired, risk for
- Sleep pattern, disturbance of
- Social interaction, impaired
- Suffocation, risk of
- Swallowing, impaired
- Thermoregulation, ineffective
- Thought process, altered
- Tissue integrity, impaired
- Tissue perfusion, altered: cerebral, renal, cardiopulmonary, gastrointestinal, peripheral
- Urinary elimination, altered

Source: North American Nursing Diagnosis Association (NANDA), 12th annual meeting, 1996.

potential for physical growth and optimal mental, emotional, social and spiritual development to serve the needs of the society in a committed and humane manner.

NURSING MANPOWER

Nurses are the backbone of our healthcare system. They lead a demanding and challenging life while working with doctors, providing comfort and tender loving care to patients, guiding families and educating communities.

Most nurses in India are females because in the beginning the practice of nursing was mostly addressed to midwifery. In general, till recently the image of nurses has been rather low due to discrimination, nature of job, caste system, high workload and relatively low remuneration. According to 2012 data, India has 1,597 nursing schools, 833 BSc nursing

colleges and 97 MSc nursing colleges with a capacity to train 79, 850 diploma nurses, and 41,650 graduate nurses every year. According to WHO, there is a need to have 1:3 doctor–nurse ratio but the current ratio is only 1:1.5. Although concerted efforts have been made to increase the number of registered nurses in the country but to achieve the recommended allocation of one nurse for 500 population is a distant dream. Moreover, about 20% of graduating nurses head to foreign countries every year, in search of better salary, working conditions, better image, dignity and standard of living. According to recommendations of Indian Public Health Standards, one nurse is required for 2 hospital beds (225 nurses for a 500 bedded hospital) inclusive of 25% leave reserve to cover social exigencies, sickness, annual leave and maternity leave.

BIBLIOGRAPHY

Fenton K, Casey A. A tool to calculate safe nurse staffing levels. *Nursing Time* 2015, 111(3): 12–14.

Indian Public Health Standards (IPHS). Guidelines for District Hospitals (100 to 500 bedded). Director-General of Health Services. Ministry of Health and Family Welfare, Government of India, Revised 2012.

Navora A–M, Schlan R, Murray M, et al. Assessing nursing care need of children with complex medical conditions: The nursing-kids intensity of care surgery. (N–kids). *J Pediatr Nursing* 2016. DOI. http://dx.org/10.1016/jpedn.2015.11.012

Hodap RM. Effects of hospitalization on young children: implications of two theories. *Child Hlth Care* 1982, 10(3): 83–86.

Rush B, Cook J. What makes a good nurse? Views of patients and carers. *Brit J Nursing* 2006, 15(7): 382–385.

Sterling YM. Pediatric nurses as advocates. *J Pediatr Nursing* 2013, 28(3): 309–310.

2

Nomenclature and Health Statistics

The majority of health indices, definitions and terminologies described below are based on the standard sources such as tenth revision of International Classification of Diseases (ICD) by WHO, The State of the World's Children report of 2015 by UNICEF, and Government of India, Statistical Year Book 2015.

DEFINITIONS

Fetus

Fetus is product of conception, irrespective of the duration of pregnancy, which is not completely expelled or extracted from its mother. The fetus is designated as embryo during first 9 weeks of gestation.

Abortion

Early fetal death at a gestational age of less than 20 weeks or of a fetus weighing less than 500 g.

Stillbirth

Fetal death at a gestational age of more than 20 weeks or of a fetus weighing 500 g or more.

Birth Weight

Birth weight is the first weight of the baby which should preferably be taken within the first hour of life and certainly during the first day of life before any significant postnatal weight loss has occurred. The average birth weight of newborn babies in India is around 2.8 kg.

Birth Weight Groups

Low birth weight (LBW) babies Babies with a birth weight of less than 2500 g, irrespective of the period of gestation, are called LBW babies. About 28% of newborn babies in India weigh less than 2500 g at birth. About one-third of LBW babies are preterm or born early while two-thirds are born at term but have suffered from intrauterine growth retardation or fetal malnutrition.

Very low birth weight (VLBW) babies Babies with a birth weight of less than 1500 g are called VLBW babies.

Extremely low birth weight (ELBW) babies Babies with a birth weight of less than 1000 g are called ELBW babies.

Gestational Age Groups

Gestational age is calculated from the first day of the last normal period till the date of birth and is expressed in completed weeks, e.g. 34 weeks + 6 days is considered as gestation of 34 weeks only.

Preterm (born early or "premature") Preterm is defined as a baby with a gestation of less than 37 completed weeks (36 weeks or less). Around 10–15% babies in India are born preterm.

Near term or borderline preterm Babies with a gestational age between 35 and 36 completed weeks.

Term Babies with a gestational age between 37 and 41 weeks are called as term babies.

Post-term (postmature) Babies with a gestational age of 42 weeks or more are classified as post-term babies.

Classification by Birth Weight and Gestational Age Groups

Small-for-dates (SFD) babies (small-for-gestational age or SGA) Babies with a birth weight of less than 10th percentile for their gestational age are designated as SFD babies.

Appropriate-for-dates (AFD) babies (appropriate-for-gestational age or AGA) Babies with a birth weight between 10th and 90th percentile for the period of their gestational age are called AFD babies.

Large-for-dates (LFD) babies (large-for-gestational age or LGA) Babies with a birth weight of more than 90th percentile for the period of their gestation are called LFD babies.

By combining classification of babies on the basis of gestational age alone and gestational age with birth weight, the newborn population can be divided into the following 9 subgroups (**Figure 3.1**).

1. Preterm		I SFD
		II AFD
		III LFD
2. Term		I SFD
		II AFD
		III LFD
3. Post-term		I SFD
		II AFD
		III LFD

This classification is useful to assign a risk to newborn baby at birth. Term appropriate-for-dates babies have the best outcome while preterm small-for-dates babies have the worst chances of survival. Even when they survive they have an increased risk of neuromotor disability on follow-up.

Perinatal Period

Perinatal period extends from the 28th week of gestation (or more than 1000 g birth weight) to the 7th day of life (early neonatal period).

Perinatal Mortality Rate (PMR)

It is defined to include late fetal deaths plus early neonatal (first week) deaths of babies weighing more than 1000 g (or 28th weeks of gestation or more) at birth per 1000 total (stillbirths plus live births) births weighing more than 1000 g. The current PMR in India is around 50 per 1000 live births.

$$PMR = \frac{\text{Number of stillbirths + deaths during first week of life in a year}}{\text{Total number of births in a year}} \times 1000$$

Neonatal period Neonatal period extends from birth up to 28 days of life. Infant up to 28 days of life is called as a newborn baby or neonate. Early neonatal period refers to first 7 days of life while late neonatal period signifies period from 7 days to under 28 completed days of life.

Neonatal deaths First day death is defined as deaths occurring within 24 hours of age (exclude if baby had completed 24 hours of age).

Early neonatal deaths include deaths within 7 days (less than 168 hours) of age.

Neonatal deaths include all deaths within 28 days of age.

The leading causes of neonatal deaths include prematurity and low birth weight babies, bacterial infections, birth asphyxia and congenital malformations.

Neonatal Mortality Rate (NMR)

It is defined as deaths of newborn babies weighing over 1000 g during first 28 days of life per 1000 live births. The current NMR in India is around 29 per 1000 live births. Neonatal deaths account for 69% of all infant deaths (deaths within first year of life) and 56% of all deaths of children below 5 years of age.

$$NMR = \frac{\text{Number of deaths of neonates less than 28 days of age in a year}}{\text{Total number of live births in a year}} \times 1000$$

Infant Mortality Rate (IMR)

It is defined as deaths of infants between birth and first year of life expressed per 1000 live births. It is a useful index of socio-economic status and health status of the country. The current IMR of India is around 37 per 1000 live births but it widely varies in different states with highest in States of Bihar, Madhya Pradesh, Rajasthan, UP, Odisha and lowest of 10 in Goa and 12 in the State of Kerala. Female literacy of over 90%, empowerment of women and availability and accessibility of health

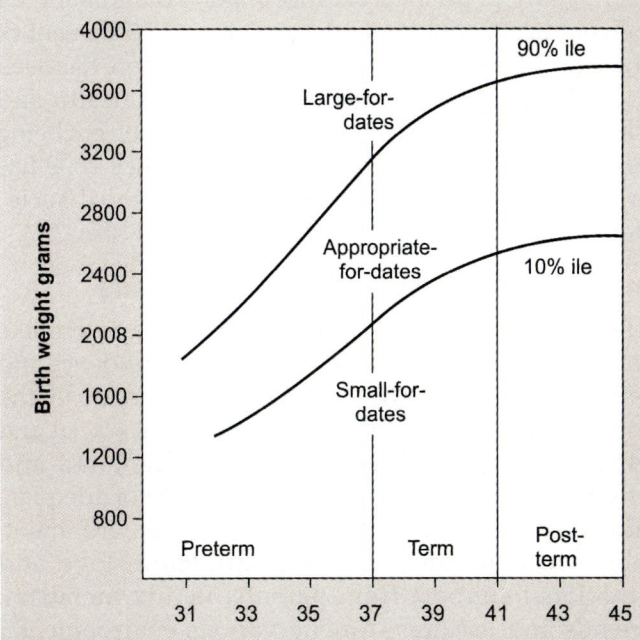

Figure 3.1 Classification on the basis of birth weight and gestational age

3

services within a short distance are important correlates of low IMR in Goa and Kerala.

$$IMR = \frac{\text{Number of deaths of infants less than 1 year of age in a year}}{\text{Total number of live births in year}} \times 1000$$

Neonatal deaths account for over 69% of all infant deaths. The main causes of post-neonatal deaths (28 days – 1 year) include GI infections, respiratory infections, vaccine-preventable diseases and accidents. Protein-energy malnutrition is the core health problem in preschool children which makes them vulnerable to suffer from a variety of infections. Malnutrition directly or indirectly account for a large number of deaths of under-5 children.

Under-five Mortality Rate (U5MR)

It is defined as number of deaths in children between birth and five years of age expressed per 1000 live births. The current under-five mortality rate in India is around 48 per 1000 live births.

According to UNICEF, U5MR is the single most important indicator of the state of the children of a country. India has 63rd rank among 194 countries of the world regarding U5MR. It depends upon a variety of health indicators like education and health status of women, income and food availability to the family, availability of clean water and safe environment, availability of maternal and child health services, coverage of immunizations, effective treatment of acute respiratory infections, and ORS use for treatment of acute diarrhea.

$$U5MR = \frac{\text{Number of deaths in children less than 5 years of age in a year}}{\text{Total number of live births in a year}} \times 1000$$

Total Fertility Rate

The number of children that would be born per woman if she were to live to the end of her child-bearing years and bear children at an age in accordance with prevailing age-specific fertility rates. The current fertility rate in India is 2.6, i.e. a couple is producing at least 2½ children which is leading to increase in population at a rapid pace. The fertility rate must come down to 2 or less for stabilization of population dynamics.

Maternal Mortality Ratio (MMR)

It is defined as annual number of deaths of women from pregnancy-related causes per 100,000 live birth. The current MMR in India is around 167.

Life Expectancy

Life expectancy is the number of years that the newborn children are likely to live if subjected to the mortality risks prevailing for the cross-section of population at the time of their birth. The current life expectancy in our country is around 64.1 years in men and 65.8 years in women.

Adult Literacy Rate

It is defined as percentage of people aged 15 years and older who can read and write. The current adult literacy rate of our country is around 88% in men and 74% in women.

SALIENT VITAL STATISTICS

Vital statistics refer to systematically collected data relating to vital national health events. In India, the main sources of vital statistics include the census, health registration records of vital events such as births and deaths and sample registration system (SRS). The SRS obtains annual information on birth and death rates, fertility rates, and age-specific mortality rates in the country through a combination of continuous registration and half yearly surveys. The current population of India is estimated to be around 1,252,140,000 (1.2 billion). The country is overcrowded and thickly populated because India, accounts for 2.4 percent of the globe's land area where 17.5 percent of the world's population lives (**Table 3.1**). There has been a gradual improvements in the status of health and health indices in our country but they are far from being satisfactory. The National Population Policy 2000 has laid down the health objectives and national socio-demographic goals to be achieved by 2010 (**Box 3.1**).

Interaction between Nature and Nurture

The growth and development (global parameters like intelligence, emotional, social, courage, confidence and enthusiasm quotients) of children depend on the interaction between their genetic potential (racial and ethnic background, constitution or genome) and environmental conditions like availability of adequate nutrition, safe drinking water, healthy environment, physical and fun activities, education, love and emotional support from parents, family members, friends and teachers. Among various environmental factors, adequate nutrition is most crucial for optimal growth and wellbeing of children.

Table 3.1 Salient demographic, maternal and child health indices*

Basic indicators		
Total population		1,252,140,000
Annual births		25,595,000
Neonatal mortality rate		29
Infant mortality rate		37
Under-5 mortality rate		48
Life expectancy at birth	Male	66 years
	Female	68 years
Adult literacy rate	Male	88%
	Female	74%
Nutritional status		
Low birth weight babies		28%
Under-5 children*	Underweight	44%
	Wasted	20%
	Stunted	48%
Maternal indicators		
Antenatal coverage	At least once	75%
	At least 4 times	51%
Skilled attendant at delivery		53%
Maternal mortality rate (per 100,000 live births)		167
Total fertility rate		2.5
Annual population growth rate		1.6

Source: The State of the World Children, UNICEF 2015

*Underweight: Below minus 2 standard deviation from median weight-for-age
Wasted: Below minus 2 standard deviation from median weight-for-height
Stunted: Below minus 2 standard deviation from median height-for-age

Box 3.1 National population policy goals to be achieved by India

1. Provide the essential unmet needs for basic reproductive and child health infrastructure, services and supplies.
2. Ensure free and compulsory school education up to 14 years of age.
3. Achieve 100% deliveries by the trained health personnel.
4. Achieve 100% of immunization coverage.
5. Achieve 100% registration of pregnancies, births and deaths.
6. Reduce infant mortality rate to below 30 per 1000 live births.
7. Reduce maternal mortality rate to below 100 per 100,000 live births.
8. Promote small family norm.
9. Achieve universal access to safe drinking water, health care, information and counseling.

Maternal Health and Child Survival

Health and wellbeing of children is intimately linked with health, nutrition, education and awareness of their mothers. Mothers are the creators and sustainers of human progeny. Health and wellbeing of a baby in the womb depends upon the health and nutrition of the mother (not the father!) because she provides both the seed as well as the soil where baby is nurtured for 9 months. Healthy mothers produce healthy babies and they are in a better position to look after the health and wellbeing of their children. Mother is the sole provider of nutrition when baby is in the womb and during first 6 months of life by virtue of exclusive breastfeeding. Therefore, it is important to provide life cycle approach for the care of girl children with a special focus for equal opportunities for their nutrition (from birth through infancy, childhood, adolescence, pregnancy and lactation), health care, education, dignity, empowerment, and status to have a say in the society.

STRATEGIES FOR CHILD SURVIVAL

The four pillars of good health are sound genetic constitution, safe environment, wholesome food and healthy lifestyle. National Population Policy and National Rural Health Mission have outlined several strategies to improve child survival and reduce avoidable human wastage by implementing the following strategies:

1. Health and wellbeing of children is intimately linked with health, education and nutrition of their mothers. Healthy and well-informed mothers produce healthy children and they are in a better position to look after the health and wellbeing of their children.

2. Girl child should be accorded essential health care, nutrition and formal education without any discrimination. Ensure 100% literacy rate and provide adequate nutrition throughout the life cycle of girls, i.e. infancy, childhood, adolescence, pregnancy and lactation. Women are the creators and sustainers of the progeny and they should be financially independent and empowered to have a say in the society.

3. Ensure availability of safe drinking water, satisfactory environmental sanitation and provide health and nutrition education to the community on a priority basis.

4. Provide adequate infrastructure and operative facilities for essential family welfare, reproductive and child health services.

5. Ensure availability of good quality antenatal care facilities and safe delivery (either at a health post or by a trained birth attendant) in 100% cases.

6. Ensure availability of essential newborn care facilities, promote exclusive breastfeeding, universal immunizations, early detection and management of common childhood illnesses by promoting ORS and rational use of antibiotics.

7. Health and social welfare activities should be further reinforced and integrated by active involvement of NGOs to improve the socioeconomic status and quality of life at the individual family level.

8. The World Health Organization and the United Nations Children's Fund have launched integrated management of neonatal and childhood illness modules by providing hands-on clinical skills to health workers to manage common health problems in children with the help of flowcharts. Apart from rational management of common diseases, health workers promote breastfeeding and provide immunization as well as health and nutrition education. The emphasis has shifted from purely curative services to a package of comprehensive health promotive and preventive services at each contact of the health worker with the families. Under the National Rural Health Mission, it has been proposed to create a cadre of community-based female health functionaries, named as accredited social health activists (ASHAs), to provide essential health care services at the doorstep of people.

MILLENNIUM DEVELOPMENT GOALS AND TARGETS

The various millennium development goals and targets based on the United Nations Development Program and Human Development Report 2003 are as follows:

1. **Goal 1** Eradicate extreme poverty and hunger.
   a. **Target 1** Halve, between 1990 and 2015, the proportion of people whose income is less than $1 a day.
   b. **Target 2** Halve, between 1990 and 2015, the proportion of people who suffer from hunger.

2. **Goal 2** Achieve universal primary education.
   Target 3 Ensure that by 2015 children everywhere, boys and girls alike, will be able to complete a full course of primary schooling.

3. **Goal 3** Promote gender equality and empower women.
   Target 4 Eliminate gender disparity in primary and secondary education, preferably by 2005, and in all levels of education no later than 2015.

4. **Goal 4** Reduce child mortality.
   Target 5 Reduce by two-thirds, between 1990 and 2015, the U5MR.

5. **Goal 5** Improve maternal health.
   Target 6 Reduce by three-quarters, between 1990 and 2015, the maternal mortality rate.

6. **Goal 6** Combat human immunodeficiency virus, acquired immunodeficiency syndrome, malaria, and other diseases.
   a. **Target 7** Have them halted by 2015 and begin to reverse the spread of human immunodeficiency virus/acquired immunodeficiency syndrome.
   b. **Target 8** Have halted by 2015 and begun to reverse the incidence of malaria and other major diseases.

7. **Goal 7** Ensure environmental sustainability.
   a. **Target 9** Integrate the principles of sustainable development into country policies and programs and reverse the loss of environmental resources.
   b. **Target 10** Halve the proportion of people without sustainable access to safe drinking water by 2015.
   c. **Target 11** Have achieved by 2020 a significant improvement in the lives of at least 100 million slum dwellers.

8. **Goal 8** Develop a global partnership for development.
   a. **Target 12** Develop further an open, rule-based, predictable, non-discriminatory trading and financial system (include a commitment to good governance, development, and poverty reduction—both nationally and internationally).

b. **Target 13** Address the special needs of the least developed countries (include tariff and quota-free access for exports, enhanced program of debt relief for and cancellation of official bilateral debt, and more generous official development assistance for countries committed to poverty reduction).

c. **Target 14** Address the special needs of land-locked countries and small island developing states (through the Program of Action for the Sustainable Development of Small Island Developing States and 22nd General Assembly provisions).

d. **Target 15** Deal comprehensively with the debt problems of developing countries through national and international measures to make debt sustainable in the long term.

e. **Target 16** In cooperation with developing countries, develop and implement strategies for decent and productive work for youth.

f. **Target 17** In cooperation with pharmaceutical companies, provide access to affordable essential drugs in developing countries.

g. **Target 18** In cooperation with the private sector, make available the benefits of new technologies, especially information and communication technologies.

The Millenium Development Goals and Targets are based on the Millenium Declaration signed by 189 countries including 147 Heads of State, in September 2000. The dead line for achievement of these goals was 2015 but many of the goals and targets have not been achieved. Source: www.un.org/documents/ga/res/55/a55r002.pdf_A/RES/55/2.

BIBLIOGRAPHY

Singh M. The art, science and philosophy of child care. *Indian J Pediatr* 2009, 76(2): 171–176.

Singh M. Nomenclature and definitions. In: Care of the Newborn. *CBS Publishers and Distributors Pvt Ltd*. Revised 8th Edition 2016, pp 7–10.

The National Family Health Survey (NFHS-4). Ministry of Health and Family Welfare, Government of India, New Delhi. 2015–16.

United Nations Children Fund. The State of the World's Children; New York: UNICEF 2015.

4

Preventive Pediatrics

In this best pediatric tradition, the approach in child health is oriented towards prevention of childhood diseases and disorders and promotion of child health. *The basic aim or goal of pediatrics is to ensure that every child is assisted to achieve his or her optimal genetic potential for physical growth and mental development.* Pediatrics deals with the promotion of health and well-being of children and not merely diagnosis and treatment of diseases of children. Pediatricians and nurses should provide global health care, i.e. preventive, promotive, curative and rehabilitative services. The health care professionals (HCPs) should be health *care* providers and not merely health *cure* providers. The four pillars of good health are sound genetic constitution (on which we have no control), safe environment, wholesome food and healthy lifestyle. The public health measures to promote community health are far more cost-effective than providing high-tech curative services once the person has become ill. This concept is beautifully summed up in a Chinese proverb, *"Treating someone who is already ill is like beginning to dig a well after you have become thirsty"*.

MATERNAL HEALTH AND CHILD SURVIVAL

Health and wellbeing of children is intimately linked with health, nutrition, education and awareness of their mothers. Mothers are the creators and sustainers of human progeny. Health and wellbeing of a baby in the womb depends on the health and nutrition of the mother (not the father !) because she is both the seed as well as the soil wherein the baby is nurtured for nine months. Mother is the sole provider of food, nutrition and protection of her fetus and young infant through transplacental parenteral nutrition and breastfeeding (transmaternal nutrition) and tender loving care. Healthy mothers produce healthy babies and they are in a better position to look after the health and wellbeing of their children.

The Girl Child

Girls are the future mothers and creators and sustainers of progeny. There is, therefore, a need to provide equal status and opportunities to girl children throughout their life cycle so that they grow to become healthy, literate, empowered and economically independent adults to look after their own health and wellbeing of their children. The concept of gender equity means that boys and girls should have equal access to food, health care, education and opportunities in life. The current dismal status and discriminatory practices against girl children should be eliminated by creating public awareness by active involvement of prominent public figures, religious groups and political leaders. The nurses have an important role to create awareness for ensuring gender equity during their one-to-one interactions with parents.

Premarital Health Check-up

The prospective couple (especially girl) should undergo complete medical check-up before getting married so that they are fully equipped to meet the health needs of their baby. Adequacy of nutritional stores (especially iron) should be ensured during adolescence rather than trying to correct the deficiency state during pregnancy. The adolescent girls should be given supplements of iron (to maintain hemoglobin above 12 g/dL and serum ferritin >35 mg/L), folic acid, calcium and vitamins. The ideal age of 25–35 years for bearing children needs to be emphasized to discourage too early and late marriages. It is a sad reality that almost 70% girls in our society are married off before the age of 18 years and without their consent.

In the urban areas, there is an increasing trend for late marriages or delayed pregnancy due to career concerns by the working couples. Advanced maternal age is associated with declining fertility, increased risk of abortions and stillbirths, chromosomal abnormalities, hypertensive complications and prematurity. Premarital genetic counseling and recognition of metabolic carrier states in the would-be couple helps to reduce the incidence of genetic disorders. A detailed systemic examination should be conducted to identify and treat any underlying systemic disorder like hypertension, heart disease, bronchial asthma, diabetes mellitus, hypothyroidism, urinary tract infection, pelvic inflammatory disease and any sexually transmitted disease. Prospective mothers should be informed about the harmful effects of smoking or chewing tobacco and indulgence of alcohol or drugs of abuse, on the growing fetus. All girls should preferably be immunized against tetanus, rubella and human papillomavirus (HPV) before they get married.

Care of the Mother during Pregnancy

Adequate antenatal care and maintenance of optimal nutrition by proper dietary advice and nutriton supplements are crucial for favorable outcome of pregnancy. She should avoid taking any drugs or exposure of radiation, as far as possible, during first trimester of pregnancy which is a period of organogenesis. After mid-pregnancy, the mother should eat for two, for herself and for her growing baby in the womb. She should take additional 350–500 kcalories and 20 g proteins by consuming fresh green leafy vegetables, pulses, legumes, milk and milk products and seasonal fruits. The pregnant woman is advised to take at least 2.6 g of omega-3 fatty acids and 300 mg of docosahexaenoic acid (DHA) to ensure optimal growth of fetal brain. Intake of folic acid during periconceptional period (before conception and during first 3 months of pregnancy) is recommended to reduce the risk of neural tube defects and cleft lip. There is some evidence that adequate intake of calcium, riboflavin, vitamin C, vitamin E and omega-3 fatty acids is associatd with reduced incidence of toxemia of pregnancy. Mothers should receive supplements of iron and folic acid to maintain their hemoglobin above 11 g/dL.

In order to conserve expenditure of energy, mothers should be advised adequate physical rest and relaxation during third trimester of pregnancy so that energy is spared for the growth of the fetus. Every pregnant woman should receive two doses of tetanus toxoid 4 weeks apart as a safeguard against development of tetanus neonatorum. Tetanus toxoid may be given any time durning the pregnancy, but the second dose must be received at least 4 weeks before the anticipated time of delivery. She should be emotionally and physically prepared and motivated for breast feeding by paying proper attention to her breasts and nipples during pregnancy. Mothers with high-risk factors should be identified early and provided with appropriate care and referred to a facility with higher level of maternal and neonatal care (**Box 4.1**).

HEALTH PREVENTIVE STRATEGIES

Prenatal Diagnosis

It is possible to make prenatal diagnosis of disabling or potentially fatal abnormalities in the fetus by ultrasound examination, cytogenetic, molecular (DNA probes) and biochemical studies on chorionic villus sample (CVS), amniocytes obtained by amniocentesis or fetal blood collected by cordocentesis. These studies are conducted in high-risk mothers with previous history of giving birth to a child with chromosomal abnormalities or inborn errors of metabolism. When fetus is affected, the family is counseled and offered the option of medical termination of pregnancy.

Reduction of Low Birth Weight (LBW) Babies

Most low birth weight (LBW) babies in the industrialized or developed countries are preterm. In India, about two-thirds of LBW babies are born at term but are small-for-dates due to intrauterine growth retardation. Over 80% of all neonatal deaths occur among LBW babies. Improvement in birth weight is thus the most important strategy to reduce the morbidity and improve the survival of newborn babies. The various strategies for reducing the incidence of LBW babies are listed in **Box 4.2**. There is a need to launch a national crusade to improve the health and wellbeing of neonates which account for more than 69% of all infant deaths and 56% of all deaths of children below the age of 5 years.

Reduction of Perinatal Hypoxia and Birth Trauma

Early recognition of pregnancy, adequate antenatal care, prompt recognition and management of pregnancy-induced disorders are crucial for reducing morbidity and mortality due to perinatal hypoxia. Most deliveries in developing countries are conducted by untrained traditional birth attendants. It is essential that they should be trained to conduct a delivery safely with reduced hazards to the mother and the baby. The knowledge and skills pertaining to basic care and resuscitation of newborn baby at birth should be taught with flip charts, simple colored illustrations and practical demonstrations. *As a long-term policy, it should be ensured that all deliveries are conducted in a health care facility.* A national crusade should be launched to spread the massage of "give a breath to save a life" to the grass root level health workers. Early recognition of signs of fetal hypoxia (clinically and by judicious use of

4

Box 4.1 High-risk pregnancies

Primary high-risk factors (early antenatal contact)

- Poor socioeconomic status and maternal illiteracy
- Maternal undernutrition: Short stature (<145 cm), under weight (<40 kg) and anemic (hemoglobin <10 g/dL) mother
- Primigravida or grand multipara (>4)
- Maternal age less than 20 years or more than 35 years
- Inter-pregnancy interval of less than 24 months
- Presence of chronic systemic disease and an endocrinal disorder
- Past obstetrical history of difficult or operative deliveries, abortions, stillbirths, neonatal deaths, low birth weight babies and developmental defects
- Rhesus negative or 0 group mother

Secondary high-risk factors (key time for their identification is 28th week of gestation)

- Pregnancy-induced hypertension
- Sever anemia (hemoglobin <8 g/dL)
- Rhesus isoimmunization
- Maternal infections
- Slow fetal growth
- Antepartum hemorrhage
- Multiple pregnancy
- Abnormal presentation like unstable lie, transverse or breech
- Poly- and oligohydramnios
- Cephalopelvic disproportion
- Fetal distress
- Premature and prolonged rupture of membranes (>12 hours)
- Early onset of labor (<34 weeks)

Box 4.2 Strategies to reduce incidence of LBW babies

- Women should be considered as the creators of progeny and accorded due health care, education, status and empowerment in society.
- Provide optimal nutrition and health care to girl children throughout their life cycle.
- Impart family life and mother-craft education to teenage boys and girls.
- Avoid early marriage and teenage pregnancy.
- Provide pre-pregnancy health check-up, general and nutritional guidance, and essential vaccines.
- Ensure inter-pregnancy interval of at least 3 years.
- Provide optimal and good quality antenatal care to all pregnant women.
- Enhance caloric intake, ensure balanced protein intake and provide supplements of iron, folic acid and micronutrients during pregnancy.
- Avoid smoking, tobacco chewing and substance abuse especially during pregnancy.
- Early recognition and management of incompetent os, pregnancy-induced hypertesion (PIH), placental dysfunction, malaria, tuberculosis, UTI, diarrhea, dysentery, genital colonization and bacterial vaginosis.
- Avoid physical labor, emotional stress and sex during third trimester of pregnancy.

monitoring equipment) and prompt measures to deliver the child with speed and safety are of fundamental importance. In borderline cases of cephalopelvic disproportion and malpresentation, the decision for instrumentation and cesarean section should not be unduly delayed. All deliveries in the hospital should be attended by a pediatrician and a nurse who are trained in the art of neonatal resuscitation.

Prevention of Neonatal Infections

Neonatal infections are one of the leading causes of neonatal mortality in developing countries. Measures for reducing neonatal infections deserve high priority and should be enforced at all levels where deliveries are conducted and newborn babies are being looked after. Most neonatal infections are preventable if asepsis is maintained in the nursery. A detailed housekeeping protocol for prevention of neonatal infections in the NICU is given in **Chapter 6**.

Prevention of Rhesus Isoimmunization

All unsensitized Rh-negative women (indirect Coomb's test negative) should be given prophylactic injection of anti-D immunoglobulins 300 μg IM within 72 hours of birth of Rh-positive baby or abortion of Rh-positive conception and following certain procedures (amniocentesis, chorionic villus biopsy, podalic version, manual removal of placenta) which are associated with increased risk of fetomateral hemorrhage. To further enhance its efficacy, it is recommended to administer 500 μg anti-D immunoglobulin around 28–32 weeks of gestation. If delivery occurs more than 4 weeks later and the infant is Rh-positive the mother should receive additional 500 μg anti-D immunoglobulin intramuscularly, within 72 hours of delivery.

Prevention of Congenital Malformations

Majority of congenital malformations are not associated with any predisposing etiologic factors and are not preventable with the current state of our knowledge. During first trimester of pregnancy, all medications and irradiation should be avoided as far as possible. Girls should be given rubella vaccine before they get married. The incidence of chromosomal disorders is high in infants of elderly mothers. These can be reduced by discouraging active reproduction beyond the age of 35 years. The incidence of genetic disorders or inborn errors of metabolism can be brought down by avoiding consanguineous marriages. There is evidence to suggest that administration of high doses of folic acid during periconception period may lower the incidence of neural tube defects and cleft lip. Prenatal diagnosis of genetic and chromosomal disorders and induction of therapeutic abortion of abnormal fetuses is being increasingly practised.

Reduction of Disability

Premarital health check-ups and counseling should be given to would-be couples. The prospective parents should be healthy, well nourished and free from any systemic disease. There is a greater risk to give birth to a child with a genetic or hereditary defects if parents are blood relatives (like first cousins). Elderly mothers (>35 years) have a greater chance to give birth to a child with a chromosomal disorder (especially Down syndrome). Mother should avoid cigarette smoking and drinking alcohol during pregnancy. During first 3 months of pregnancy, mother should avoid taking any medicines and exposure to X-rays unless advised by the obstetrician. Intake of nutritional supplements specially folic acid is associated with reduced risk of congenital malformations like neural tube defects and cleft lip. The delivery must take place in a health care facility having adequate facilities both for the mothers and there newborn babies. Pediatrician and a specially trained nurse must the present at the time of delivery to provide basic care and effective resuscitation to the neonate. *Many avoidable handicaps in childhood have their origin in the perinatal period.* Perinatal distress factors such as hypoxia, hypothermia, acidosis, hypoglycemia and hyperbilirubinemia should be prevented, identified early and managed promptly. All newborn babies (especially high-risk neonates) should be routinely screened for inborn errors of metabolism, deafness and visual defects. Early detection of the handicap, proper management and rehabilitation are essential to reduce the severity of disability.

Prevention of Infections and Infestations

Infectious diseases are a leading cause of morbidity and mortality in children. The infection may occur due to direct contact (skin infections, sexually transmitted disease) or contact with non-living objects (fomites) like infected clothes (handkerchief, towel, bed sheet), books, toys, medical and surgical instruments and appliances. Airborne and droplet infection occurs in a number of viral infections, exanthematous illnesses, whooping cough, diphtheria and tuberculosis. Food and water-borne diseases account for over 80% of infections namely food poisoning, diarrhea, dysentery, cholera, typhoid fever, viral hepatitis (hepatitis A and E virus) and worm infestations. Blood-borne infections may be transmitted through contaminated needles (abscess, hepatitis B and C virus, HIV), sexual contact (STDs) and transfusion of infected blood or blood products (malaria, HBV, HCV, HIV, CMV). Several infections are transmitted through living objects (like mosquitoes, sandflies, animals) which serve as intermediate hosts or vectors of infection.

Most infectious diseases can be prevented by improvement of environmental sanitation and standards of personal hygiene by using soap and water for frequent washing of hands. *According to Sir William Osler, "Soap and water and common sense are the best disinfectants".* The public health measures for control of water-borne diseases include availability of safe drinking water, environmental sanitation and effective disposal of waste through underground sewage, availability of latrines at every home, boiling and pasteurization of milk, avoidance of intake of food or juice from roadside vendors or *dhabas*, control of houseflies and mosquitoes. We preach through slogan that "cleanliness is next to godliness" but unfortunately we hardly practice it either at home or in public places. Children should be taught to cover their face or turn the face to one side while coughing and sneezing to prevent spread of droplet infections.

Immunization is the most cost-effective public health investment to prevent a large number of vaccine-preventable diseases. The dream of Jenner was realized in the year 1979 when smallpox was declared eradicated from the universe. Poliomyelitis has been eradicated and India was declared polio free on 13 January, 2014 by the success of Pulse Polio Immunization (PPI) program. The preformed antibodies or immuno-globulins, specific or non-specific, either from animal or human source, can be administered before or soon after the exposure (hepatitis A and B virus, chickenpox, rabies) to prevent or reduce the severity of disease. Chemoprophylaxis can be given to household members, staff members and children in a day care center or nursery school, where two or more children suffered from *H. influenzae type b* (Hib), meningococcal meningitis, pertussis and tuberculosis.

Mosquito-borne diseases are controlled by promotion of public health measures to improve environmental sanitation, reduce breeding of mosquitoes and by regular fogging with malathion during the transmission season. The personal protective measures for prevention of bites by mosquitoes namely use of nets, full sleeve shirts and *pyjamas* and use of mosquito repellents (like cream, spray, electrical vaporisers, patch, fumes) should be promoted. A protective vaccine against Japanese encephalitis is available while vaccines are in the pipeline for development for prevention of malaria and dengue fever.

Worm infestations are common in children due to poor standards of personal hygiene. Children should be taught the habit of handwashing with soap and water after defecation, on coming back home from school or play and before taking meals. Children need supervision to prevent eating of mud (Pica) and their toys should be kept washed and clean. Salads and raw vegetables should be thoroughly washed under running water and taken after peeling. The water used for drinking should be safe (boiled or filtered) and protected against contamination. The personal hygiene and cleanliness should be maintained by daily bath, change of undergarments, keeping nails trimmed and wearing shoes while playing or when stepping outdoors. Children should be worn tight underwears or *pyjamas* at night so that they have no direct access to the anus while itching. Intake of raw pork should be avoided and it should be consumed after proper cooking to prevent infection by tapeworms.

The transmission of diseases from animals to human beings (zoonosis) should be controlled by proper caring and handling of domestic animals like dogs and cats. The domestic animals should be effectively vaccinated under the guidance of a veterinary doctor.

Promotion of Optimal Nutrition

Undernutrition is the core health problem in children. Promotion of exclusive breastfeeding for first 6 months, weaning with home-based nutritious foods, prevention of day-to-day infections by ensuring adequate environmental sanitation and personal hygiene and timely administration of various vaccines are mandatory to improve nutrition of children and enhance their survival.

Children must receive a well-balanced diet and optimal nutrition to enable them to achieve their optimal potential for physical growth and neuromotor development. The following strategies should be promoted to improve nutritional status of children at the national level.

1. A special focus should be placed on providing health care, nutrition (life cycle approach for providing adequate nutrition during infancy, adolescence, pregnancy and lactation) and education to girl children.

2. Promotion of exclusive breastfeeding (even water should not be given!) during first 6 months of life and continuation of breastfeeding for at least one year and even longer. Nursing mother should be given adequate nutrition to maintain her own health and improve the quantity and quality of her breast milk.

3. Ensuring adequate intake of home-based complementary or weaning foods having adequate calories, proteins and micronutrients starting at the age of 6 months. Strict practices of personal hygiene should be maintained at this stage to prevent occurrence of food and water-borne infections.

4. Fortification of food products of universal consumption such as common salt and wheat flour with nutrients of public health importance such as vitamin A, iodine, iron and zinc.

5. Dissemination of practical knowledge and information about child nutrition through *anganwadis*, media, magazines and television. The young boys and girls should be taught basic principles of mother-craft skills and child nutrition in the school.

HEALTH PROMOTIVE SERVICES

Promotive health care services are aimed at monitoring parameters of physical growth and neuromotor development for early diagnosis of any abnormalities for early intervention and rehabilitation.

Follow-up Program for NICU Graduates

The aim and goal of newborn care is not only to reduce neonatal mortality but more importantly to ensure their intact survival. It is mandatory that every neonatal unit must have adequate facilities and a protocol to follow-up the nursery graduates to assess their health-related quality of life and contribution to the society. Infants with neuromotor disability should be provided with early stimulation and rehabilitation. The various components of assessment of NICU graduates is summarized in **Box 4.3**. Detailed neurological and neurodevelopmental assessment is undertaken at the corrected ages (post-conceptional ages) of 4 months, 8 months, 12 months and then every 6 months till 5 years of age.

EARLY INTERVENTION PROGRAM

Stimulation in the NICU

Neonates in the NICU should not be treated as "objects" but provided with developmentally supportive care. Babies should be protected against bright light, loud

4

- Anthropometry: Weight, length, head circumference
- Development screening: Milestones, early markers of cerebral palsy, formal scales of development, intelligence quotient (IQ)
- Specialized screening
  - □ Inborn errors of metabolism: Hypothyroidism, phenylketonuria, G6PD deficiency
  - □ Vision: Retinopathy of prematurity (ROP), squint, opticokinetic nystagmus, visual evoked responses (VER)
  - □ Hearing: Otoacoustic emissions (OAE), brainstem evoked response audiometry (BERA)
  - □ Sonography of brain
- Systemic assessment

sounds and painful procedures. They should not be unnecessarily disturbed and allowed to have peaceful and quiet periods as long as feasible without compromising their care. The bonding with mother should be promoted through kangaroo-mother care. Preterm babies can be provided non-nutritive sucking on the empty breasts of the mother. Gentle touch, massage and passive movements of joints are useful to improve muscle tone and prevent muscle spasm. Soothing music, taped voice or heart beats of mother can be played near the baby or through headphones. Rocking and oscillating water bed has been used to stimulate kinesthetic and vestibular senses.

Stimulation at Home

Early recongnition of neuromotor handicaps should be followed by a home-based stimulation program. There is evidence to suggest that early stimulation is associated with improved functioning of synapses and even regeneration of neurons because of plasticity of the brain. Gentle inputs of visual, auditory and tactile stimuli promote the maturation and development of specific areas of brain. Soothing music, soft voice, gentle touch and massage, rhythmic movements, eye-to-eye contact, caressing, cuddling and skin-to-skin contact provide useful sensory inputs to augment the process of neuromotor development. Most infants with CP are helped by passive stretching exercises and increasing the range of movements of limbs. *Massage is contraindicated as it may further increase the muscle tone.* Parents should be instructed about ideal or functional positioning of their baby to make most effective use of limited motor skills. At times, more intensive physiotherapy, occupational therapy, special shoes, braces or surgical intervention is required.

Mother is the best therapist for the child and she should be given the necessary guidance, skills and encouragement to stimulate the child at home. The stimulation is provided through various special senses, like touch (tactile, physical activities, kinesthetic), auditory and visual stimuli (Table 4.1). The stimulation should be done as matter of routine in the form of a play activity and not as a ritual. The interactive play activities that both the parents and the child enjoy, is the best way to stimulate the sensory system and brain of the baby.

In addition, the infant should be provided specialized stimulation services including physiotherapy and occupational therapy by specially trained personnel with the help of dedicated protocols, like Bobath neurodevelopmental stimulation program. The aim of therapy is to reduce the pathologic muscle tone and facilitate the development of integrated righting and equilibrium functions of the brain. Massage is generally contraindicated because in most cases of cerebral palsy muscle tone is increased. Early intervention is likely to prevent atrophy of muscles and reduce fixity or contractures of joints and promote functional capability of the child.

Well Child Clinics (under-5 clinics)

The first 5 years of life are most crucial and all children should be regularly followed up for timely administration of vaccines, guidance for ensuring optimal nutrition, monitoring their physical growth parameters (body weight, length or height and head circumference) and charting them on Road-to-Health cards during first 5 years of life. The measurements should be recorded every month (during visits for immunization) during first year, every 2 months during second year and every 3 months subsequently. The periodic and regular weight record provides valuable information regarding physical growth and wellbeing of the child as opposed to a single weight record. The trend or slope of the weight curve is more important than its location on the chart.

In preterm babies, the corrected age (post-conceptional age) is used for charting growth and development parameters during first year of life. For example, if a child is born on Jaunary 31, 2013, while the expected date of delivery was March 31, 2013, this means that his gestational age at birth was 32 weeks. The child would be 0-day old on March 31, 2013. Therefore, the corrected age of this child on May 31, 2013 will be only 2 months (not 4 months when calculated from the date of birth). His physical growth and mental development on May 31, 2013 will correspond to a normal 2 months old infant. The

4

Table 4.1 Guidelines for providing early stimulation to the infant by parents

0–2 months

Maintain eye-to-eye contact, talk and sing to the baby while doing daily chores, like bathing, dressing, feeding, nappy change, etc. Show bright light or object from the side, provide different sounds, like rattle, bell, and squeezing a toy. Place the baby on different surfaces and different positions and rock the baby gently while supporting the head.

2–4 months

Hold the baby at the shoulder, hang bright objects about 30 cm above the crib in an arc or semicircle, talk to the child and maintain an eye contact, show bright objets to encourage the child to reach out and grasp, cuddle and caress the child after placing him on different surfaces and positions.

4–6 months

Place the baby flat on the mattress and encourage him to roll over, make him sit in the lap, place hands under the child's feet to encourage him to press and make pedaling movements, show toy to reach out, sound a bell from the side to make him turn towards the sound.

6–8 months

Make the child to sit with support and place him in various positions, call him by name, encourage him to roll over by showing colorful toys from sides, give him pieces of paper to crumple and tear.

8–10 months

Encourage the child to stand with support, clap hands, look at a picture book and turn pages, drop objects into a box, put cubes one over the other.

10–12 months

Name the body parts while bathing, do simple tasks, like clapping, saying bye-bye, encourage him to pull to stand, make him stand with support, show him a mirror, let him play with other kids, show animals and birds in the park.

12–15 months

Give picture books and encourage him to turn the pages, ask him to put one cube over the other, hide a toy under a pillow and let him discover, encourage him to scribble on paper, encourage him to hold small objects (strictly under observation), put objects in a box and retrieve them, encourage him to walk with support by holding on to a three-wheeled cart.

Note: The type of activities to be encouraged may be modified on the basis of developmental age of the child.

concept of corrected age is used during first year of life for evaluation of growth and neuromotor development. The various responsibilities and components of care by the nurse are shown in **Figure 4.1**.

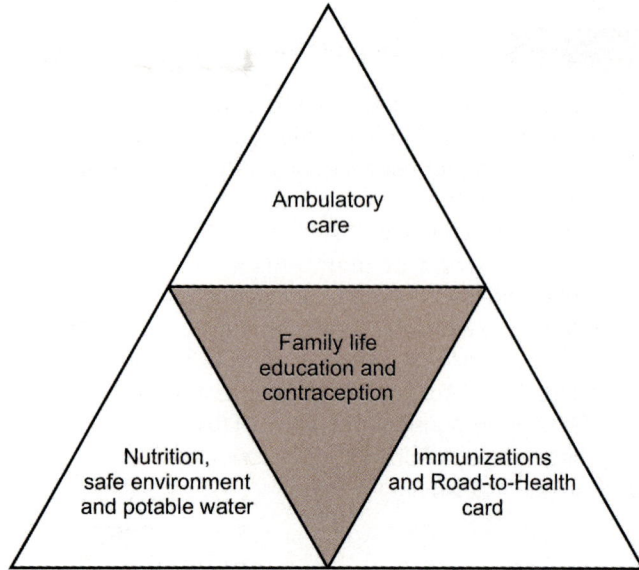

Figure 4.1 Role of nurse in under-5 clinic

SCHOOL HEALTH PROGRAM

The school nurse should maintain the health, anthropometry and immunization record of school children. She should provide the basic preventive, promotive and first aid curative health care to children. She should supervise the provision of healthy school environment such as environmental sanitation, safe drinking water, satisfactory toilets, adequate physical facilities (ventilation, proper lighting, comfortable furniture), size and weight of school bag, safety and quality of food provided by the canteen. Whenever any physical abnormality or deviation is detected, the child should be referred to the pediatrician or an appropriate specialist. The children with a learning disability should be assessed by a pediatric neurologist and developmental psychologist and managed under the direct supervision of a special educator.

Child Abuse and Neglect

Improvements in universal education, social skills and economic status of families is associated with improved interparental relationship. The promotion of life cycle approach towards girl children is the best investment for building a society. The government should provide adequate social services, universal education, employment skills and opportunities for employment, minimum wages, family life education and dissemination of knowledge and skills for mothercraft and fathercraft. The moral and spiritual values of the society needs to be promoted by teachers, religious leaders and politicians.

Sexually Transmitted Diseases (STDs)

There is a need to introduce a regular curriculum on family life and sex education in all the schools of the country. Adolescent boys and girls should be told about the safe sexual practices, avoidance of unwanted pregnancies and safeguard against the development of STDs. Blood and blood products should be effectively screened for various infective agents like human immunodeficiency virus (HIV), hepatitis B virus (HBV) and hepatitis C virus (HCV). Nurses should follow the *"universal precautions"* to prevent the risk of infections with HBV and HIV from contact with blood and body secretions of patients. The risk of HBV and human papillomavirus (HPV) infection can be reduced by timely administration of HBV and HPV vaccines.

Smoking and Substance Abuse

The addictive behavior like smoking, drinking alcohol and substance abuse usually has its onset during adolescence. It is prevalent in the extremes of social status, i.e. either extremely poor and illiterate or extremely rich families where children are not interested in studies. There is a need to inculcate social, spiritual and human values in society. Parents should be vigilant regarding the type of friends their teenagers have and the nature of outdoor or night activities they are indulging, but without being too nosy or interfering in their freedom. The teenagers must be nurtured to have full confidence in their capabilities and they should be encouraged to be assertive (not aggressive) to say "No" against unhealthy peer pressure (like smoking, drinking, gambling, drug abuse, etc.) and should be able to take independent decisions depending upon their personal perceptions and values in life. Their energy and enthusiasm should be channelized towards productive and image-building and confidence boosting activities like body building, creative hobbies, sports, yoga, music and dance.

Prevention of Adult-Onset Diseases

There is an increasing evidence to suggest that seeds of most adult diseases are sown in childhood. Children truly constitute the foundation of a nation because healthy children grow to become healthy and strong adults who can actively participate in the developmental activities of a nation. Major risk factors for cardiovascular diseases in adults include cigarette smoking, hypertension, dyslipidemia, type 2 diabetes mellitus, obesity, faulty dietary habits and sedentary lifestyle. Most of these risk factors have their origin in childhood and are amenable to modification, contributing to primary prevention of cardiovascular

diseases. Based on "thrifty gene" or developmental origins of adult diseases hypothesis by Barker, there is evidence to suggest that infants with intrauterine growth restriction are at an increased risk to develop certain adult-onset diseases like hypertension, coronary artery disease, metabolic syndrome X and type 2 diabetes mellitus.

Kawasaki disease in childhood may lead to coronary artery disease in adults. There is growing evidence of increased prevalence of vitamin D deficiency in our country which is a known predisposing factor for diabetes mellitus. Poor orodental hygiene and chronic gingivitis is a recognized risk factor for development of coronary artery disease. Above all, the seeds of integrity, character, confidence and discipline are sown in childhood. Parents and teachers have an important role in inculcating good *sanskars*, habits and etiquettes so that children grow to become well-adjusted adults with an wholesome personality. The successful adults have pleasant memories of happy childhood while maladjusted adults are constantly haunted by the emotional scars of early life.

CHILD WELFARE SERVICES

The government of India has launched a number of child welfare programs under the aegis of national policy for children to provide a network of health preventive, promotive and curative services (*see* **Chapter 46** for details). There are many urgent public health issues which need to be addressed. There is a need to improve environmental sanitation, availability of safe drinking water, construction of bore-hole latrines in all dwellings, proper disposal of waste and underground sewage drainage and effective control of vector-borne diseases. The availability and utilization of these public health interventions demand improvement of the socioeconomic status, narrowing the widening gap between the rich and poor and improving awareness and education of the community.

ROLE AND RESPONSIBILITIES OF NURSES

Nurses have a crucial role and responsibilities to work in close collaboration with parents and children in the family and community to provide them with safe environment and promote adequate facilities to prevent childhood illnesses and to assist them to attain their full genetic potential for optimal physical and mental development. The nurses have a unique opportunity to provide health and nutrition education, preventive and promotive health care services, teaching of mother-craft skills, providing tender loving nursing care and referral of sick children to an appropriate specialist when needed. The nurse should follow the well known steps of nursing process, viz. assessment, nursing diagnosis, planning, implementation or intervention and evaluation or monitoring while providing care to children to promote, maintain and restore their health. The salient nursing responsibilities for promotion of preventive pediatrics are summarized below:

1. Create awareness among the community regarding importance of health and nutrition of girl children who are the future mothers.
2. Providing family life and mothercraft education and nutritional supplements to adolescent boys and girls.
3. Ensuring that every pregnant woman receives optimal antenatal care through at least five contacts with a health care professional.
4. Providing essential care to the mother during delivery and newborn baby at birth. Early referral of high-risk mother or baby to a higher level of care, if needed.
5. Supporting and promoting exclusive breastfeeding during first 6 months of life.
6. Nutrition education, weaning with home-cooked nutritious semiliquid gruels, ensuring hygienic practices and preventing malnutrition.
7. Promotion of safe health care practices to reduce the risk of water-borne diseases, viz. personal hygiene, handwashing, environmental sanitation, safe drinking water and avoidance of foods from road-side vendors.
8. Promotion of immunization practices to prevent vaccine-preventable diseases.
9. Creating awareness for prevention of accidents and poisonings in children.
10. Health education to adolescent children for promotion of reproductive health and family planning.
11. Promoting public health measures to improve environmental sanitation in the community in rural and semiurban or slum areas by construction of latrines, proper disposal of waste and garbage and ensuring availability of safe drinking water.
12. Providing health care services in the well child or under-5 clinics and school health program for monitoring anthropometry, early identification and prompt management of common health disorders.
13. Promotion of beneficial traditional child rearing practices and avoidance of harmful cultural practices.
14. Involvement and motivation of families to participate in various child health services devoted towards prevention of childhood diseases.
15. Providing support for implementation of various national child health programs.
16. To serve as a key functionary to coordinate and cooperate with a large number of specialists to provide holistic health care to children, viz. preventive, promotive, curative and rehabilitative services.

BIBLIOGRAPHY

American Academy of Pediatrics. Committee on Genetics. Prenatal genetic diagnosis for pediatricians. *Pediatrics* 1994, 94: 1010–1015.

Berry AM, Davidson PM, Masters J, Rolls K. Systematic literature review of oral hygiene practices for intensive care of oral hygiene practices for intensive care patients receiving mechanical ventilation. *AM J Crit Care* 2007, 16(6): 552–559.

Campbell S, Pearce JM. Ultrasound vizualization of congenital malformations. *Brit Med Bull* 1983, 39: 322–331.

Gilbert F, Marinduque B. DNA prenatal diagnosis. *Curr Opinion Obst Gynecol* 1990, 2: 226–235.

Singh M. Preventive neonatology. In: Care of the Newborn. *CBS Publishers and Distributors Pvt. Ltd.* Revised 8th Edition 2016, pp 46–74.

Vohr B, Wright LL, Hack M, et al. Follow-up care of high-risk infants. *Pediatrics* 2004, 114 (Suppl): 1377–1397.

Nursing Care of Sick Children

Children are dependent and at the mercy of their caretakers to look after their needs of love, protection, stimulation, nutrition, personal hygiene, safe environment and prevention of diseases by timely immunizations. When they become sick they further regress demanding more tender loving care (TLC) and attention to relieve their anxiety, discomfort, pain and disability. They become irritable, cranky and fussy demanding more cuddling and caressing for their comfort. Their feeding behavior becomes worse because of loss of appetite due to illness demanding lot of ingenuity to look after their basic needs of fluids and food. When an adult becomes sick he looks towards a doctor with respect and admiration as a saviour and a nurse as a compassionate care giver. But unlike adults, sick children do not perceive themselves as "patients" and they behave like children. And infact they demand more care and concessions from their caretakers as a matter of their right and without any special consideration, obligation or appreciation.

THE LEVELS OF NEWBORN CARE

Based upon birth weight and gestational age, a three-tier system is proposed to provide optimal neonatal care.

Level I Care

Over 80 percent of newborn babies require minimal care which can be provided by their mothers under the supervision of basic health care professionals. Neonates weighing above 1800 g or having gestational maturity of 34 weeks or more belong to this category. The care can be provided at home, subcenter and primary health center level. Basic care at birth, provision of warmth, maintenance of asepsis and promotion of breastfeeding form the mainstay of level I care. Traditional birth attendants and community health workers must be trained in the art of essential perinatal care.

Level II Care

Infants weighing between 1200 and 1800 g or having gestational maturity of 30 to 34 weeks need specialized neonatal care supervised by trained nurses and pediatricians. First referral units, district hospitals, teaching institutions and nursing homes should be equipped to provide intermediate or special neonatal care. Equipment for resuscitation, maintenance of thermoneutral environment, intravenous infusion and gavage feeding, phototherapy and exchange blood transfusion should be available. There should be no compromise on the basic needs of adequate space, trained nursing staff and maintenance of asepsis including provision for disposable gamma-irradiated suction catheters, feeding tubes, endotracheal tubes, small-vein infusion sets, etc. Intermediate neonatal care is needed for about 10 to 15 percent of newborn population and should be available at all hospitals catering to 1000 to 1500 deliveries per year.

Level III Care

Intensive neonatal care is required for babies weighing less than 1200 g or those born before 30 weeks of gestation. Apex institutions or regional perinatal centers equipped with centralized oxygen and suction facilities, servo-controlled incubators, vital sign and trans-cutaneous monitors, ventilators and infusion pumps, etc. are required to provide intensive neonatal care (**Figure 5.1**). Skilled nurses and neonatologists especially trained in the art of neonatal intensive care are required to organize this service. About 3 to 5 percent of newborn population qualify for intensive care. Establishment of intensive care neonatal unit demands a sound infrastructure and should be envisaged only when optimal intermediate neonatal care facilities have already been in existence for some time. The capital and recurring expenditure for level III care is exorbitant and it is not cost-effective unless service is regionalized.

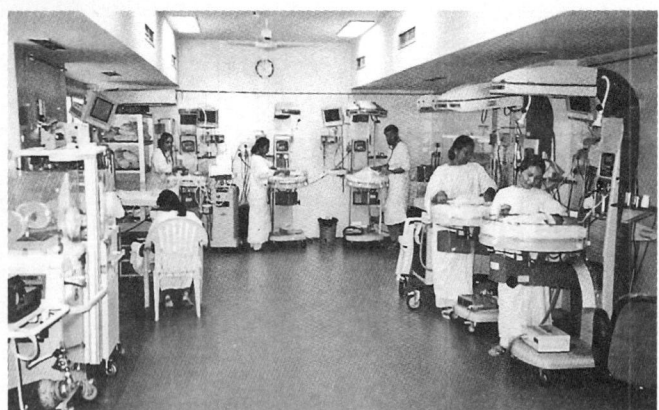

Figure 5.1 Neonatal intensive care unit (NICU) of All India Institute of Medical Sciences, New Delhi

5 TRIAGE OF A SICK CHILD

Triage is defined as a process of rapid screening of sick children when they first report to the hospital. In a busy out-patient department, an experienced nurse should be able to categorize sick children into following 3 groups so that acutely sick or critically sick children are allowed to by pass the queue in order to provide them with urgent medical attention. *Effective screening demands a keen sense of observation and a tender and sensitive touch without any tools.*

1. Critically Sick Child

i. *Hyperpyrexia or hemorrhagic skin rash.*
ii. *Ineffective breathing or ventilation.* Extremely labored and rapid or noisy breathing with cyanosis.
iii. *Severe dehydration.* Sunken eyes, markedly inelastic skin (skin pinch over the chest or abdomen goes back slowly), Kussmaul breathing (rapid deep breathing due to metabolic acidosis), non-passage of urine for >6 hours and shock (*vide-infra*).
iv. *Shock.* Cold and clammy (wet) hands and feet, rapid and thready (weak) radial or brachial pulse, non-passage of urine for more than 6 hours in an infant and >12 hours in an older child and capillary refill time (CRT) of more than 2 seconds. Pulp of the finger or front of the chest is blanched by pressure and time noted till it gets flushed or pink on withdrawal of pressure.
v. *CNS manifestations.* Children with seizures and loss of consciousness (unresponsive to a strong pinch) demand urgent attention. These children should be given immediate first aid and escorted to the emergency department or pediatric intensive unit for institution of immediate life-support measures.

2. Moderately or Acutely Sick Child

These children should be accorded priority and sent to the doctor without wasting time in the queue.

i. High-grade fever as assessed by touching the trunk and forehead.
ii. Sick infants below 2 months.
iii. Rapid breathing with chest retractions and working of alae nasi.
iv. Unconsolable crying or drowsy child with refusal to take feeds.
v. Persistent vomiting and watery diarrhea with some dehydration.
vi. Severe wasting, marked pallor, and edema feet.

3. Ambulatory Patients

Most children that report to the out patient department either need an immunization shot or have a mild acute illness or a chronic disorder and they can be handled in a routine manner. The common ambulatory disorders include cough and cold, persistent cough due to nasobronchial allergy, chest infection, acute gastroenteritis, constipation, skin infections or allergy, worm infestations, failure to thrive or being a fussy, picky or a finicky eater.

ROLE OF A NURSE IN THE OPD

Nurse has an important role to play in the pediatric out-patient department (OPD) to provide comprehensive health care to children.

1. **Screening of patients** Nurse should have the expertise to quickly screen the patients to identify critically sick children needing emergency care and acutely sick children for immediate attention without unnecessary delay as explained *vide-supra* under triage of sick children.

2. **Anthropometry** Depending upon the protocol being followed in the OPD, periodic record of weight, head circumference and length/height should be recorded and charted on the Road-to-Health card. Weight should be recorded on every visit to the hospital. There is no need to completely undress the child and weight can be taken with minimal clothes and without shoes. Temperature should be recorded if fever is the main complaint for reporting to the hospital.

3. **Health education and counseling** Nurse can impart health education and counseling to parents and attendants while children are waiting for their turn to see the doctor. Health and nutrition education DVDs can be screened for the benefit of parents and attendants. The nurse should talk to the parents to

relieve their anxiety by providing emotional support. The availability of a play area is useful to keep the children busy and in good mood before they enter the consultation chamber of the doctor.

4. **Assistance to the consultant** The nurse should assist the doctor for undressing or restraining the child during clinical examination. The presence of a female nurse is mandatory when an adolescent girl is being examined by the pediatrician. She should explain the details regarding medications prescribed, dosages and frequency of their administration to prevent any errors and improve the compliance. The details about investigations and supportive care like importance of personal hygiene and balanced nutrition should be explained to the mother. The date of next visit and if there are any warning signs to be watched should be explained to the caretaker.

5. **Immunizations and maintenance of records** The nurse provides immunizations, administers any intradermal diagnostic tests (Mantoux test, Casoni's test), gives parenteral and nebulized medications as and when needed. She should explain to the mother the importance of maintaining a file to keep the hospital records, immunization card and Road-to-Health or growth chart of the child. In specialized follow-up clinics, the patient's records are maintained and filed by the nurse for easy retrieval at each subsequent visit of the patient.

REACTIONS OF CHILDREN TO HOSPITALIZATION

Every child is unique and no two children are alike. Depending upon their genetic background and upbringing they respond differently to various situations of stress in life. Children's reaction to visit to the hospital or hospitalization depends upon their previous experience or contact with a health care professional and whether it was pleasant or unpleasant.

The child may manifest separation anxiety (if mother or attendant is not allowed with the child), regression, negativism, depression, unrealistic fear or phobia and at times suppression or denial of symptoms to facilitate early discharge from the hospital.

Hospitalization leads to separation from siblings and grandparents but fortunately in our setting an attendant, usually mother or a female attendant, is allowed to stay with the hospitalized child. The presence of a mother is desirable for care of hospitalized children as it greatly reduces the anxiety and stress in a sick child and attendant learns the basic nursing chores for looking after the child after discharge from the hospital. Moreover, because of shortage of nurses in our country, the availability of an attendant can be

harnessed effectively to undertake certain nursing chores like sponging the child, dressing, combing, toilet care, administration of oral drugs, and feeding the sick child. Infact the policy of allowing an attendant with a hospitalized child is being encouraged and emulated by the children's hospitals in western countries.

Hospitalized children may feel scared of white aprons, gowns, masks, gloves, electronic machines, shouting and howling kids, grieving and growling attendants and parents. The general atmosphere and ambience of most children wards in our country is unsatisfactory and often dismal. The confidence of the child is further compromised when she is administered parenteral medications, intravenous fluids and attached to the monitoring or therapeutic devices. The diagnostic procedures are likely to cause pain and further anxiety unless due caution is taken to make the procedures pain-free and tolerable by proper handling and pre-medications or local anesthetics. In general, children do experience lot of stress, anxiety, discomfort, and pain during hospitalization. Unless handled properly, they are likely to cry, show agitation, anger and violent behavior, and may lose their self-esteem and trust in adults.

Nosocomial Infections

Children admitted to the hospital, especially neonatal (NICU) and pediatric intensive care units (PICU), are at an increased risk to develop nosocomial or hospital-acquired infections (HAIs). Sick children, especially those with an acute life-threatening illness or a chronic disabling systemic disease, are more vulnerable to develop nosocomial infections. Children receiving chemotherapy, corticosteroids and broad-spectrum antibiotics are immunocompromised and at an increased risk to develop life-threatening superinfections with multidrug-resistant bacteria and fungi. The infection may occur through direct contact (and droplet or air-borne) with the infected patient or through indirect routes like contaminated hands of doctors and nurses, syringes and needles, suction, urinary and vascular catheters, infusates (especially TPN), life-saving equipment and contaminated linen. The infection may occur due to a variety of Gram-positive and Gram-negative pathogens including Candida species which are likely to be multi-drug-resistant causing serious morbidity and high mortality.

A strict protocol for asepsis as outlined in **Chapter 6** should be followed to reduce the risk of nosocomial infections. *Handwashing is the single most important and effective strategy to reduce the risk of hospital-acquired infections.* Adequate cot-spacing and avoidance of overcrowding are crucial to reduce the risk of infections. There should be no compromise in the liberal use of gamma-irradiated disposables. Immunocompromised children should be isolated, advised to wear a mask and provided with individualized care and barrier nursing. Universal precautions should be taken to prevent the risk of blood-borne infections (HIV, HBV and HCV) to health care professionals and patients. The diagnostic and therapeutic procedures should be performed under strict aseptic conditions by wearing a gown, mask and surgical gloves. The intensive care units should be provided with the highest standards of cleanliness and asepsis akin to the protocols being followed in the operation theaters. The hospital should have an Infection Control Committee to formulate, implement and monitor infection control measures.

Effects of Hospitalization on the Family

Hospitalization is not only a source of stress for the sick child but may adversely affect the family dynamics. The parents and siblings may show anxiety, anger, uncertainty, disappointment, self-blame and feeling of guilt due to lack of confidence and ability to look after their child. There are many factors that increase their anxiety and stress such as separation from the child, suffering or pain of the child, and uncertainty about the outcome. There is a constant fear of complications of the disease and risk of nosocomial infections. Parents may face difficulties in their place of work and loss of wages. Due to exorbitant cost of medical care in the private sector, the family is faced with the financial difficulties by seeking a loan or mortgaging the land or property. The parents may perceive that the illness is due to their faulty actions or *karma* and consider child's illness as punishment or curse of God. This may lead to feeling of guilt, depression, hopelessness, hostility and aggressive behavior towards health care professionals.

Role of a Nurse

1. Children's hospitals or children wards of a general hospital should have a unique child-friendly ambience and an identity. They should have brightly colored walls, child-friendly furniture, cartoon characters, plenty of soft cuddly toys in the play room, dining room and library. Child should be allowed to bring some home toys or any other article (like a blanket) with which he or she is emotionally attached.
2. The nurse should provide "customized care" to the child depending upon her age, developmental level, socioeconomic background, family dynamics, interests, hobbies and nature of illness. The anxiety

and stress of the family should be handled with compassion and due concern. Nurse should patiently listen to the concerns of the family and try to give pragmatic answers to relieve their anxiety and instill positive vibes of hope and healing. She should show utmost patience and restraint to answer the queries of parents even if they are repetitive or irritating.
3. The nurse must explain the procedure or intervention to the family or directly to an older child before it is conducted to allay their anxiety and fear and improve their cooperation. The procedure can be explained on a doll, cuddly animal or a simulator.
4. In case of a chronic illness, the nurse should explain the nature of disease process, duration of treatment, likely outcome and possibility of any long lasting disability. The nurse should try and encourage the parent and child to develop a positive mental attitude towards the illness. They should be told that faith, trust and will power are great healers and should be exploited to achieve best dividends. The family can be encouraged to join parent support groups for emotional support and sharing information.
5. In case of prolonged hospitalization, the child should be involved in therapeutic play activities and encouraged to participate in role-plays and story telling to accept the reality of his illness and develop a positive mental attitude to accept it as a challenge. The child must be encouraged to continue with his academic studies at home with the help of parents or a professional coach. The child should be encouraged to maintain his contacts with his school mates and friends by organizing get-togethers at home. Healthy siblings should not be neglected and they may feel jealous of the parental attention given to the sick child. They should be informed and involved in the care of sick child as an integral part of family system.

Informed Consent

Children are minors and are incompetent to make a decision. Informed consent is taken from the parents as a matter of routine because of the present era of Consumer Protection Act and the community becoming more aware of their rights. Informed consent is also mandatory before carrying out any diagnostic or therapeutic procedure and before surgery.

Informed consent is a written consent which is preferably taken in the presence of a witness in which parents are explained in detail about the disease of the child, and risks of the diagnostic and therapeutic or surgical interventions which may be required to treat it. The nurse must explain and give answers to various queries and doubts raised by the parents. The parent or legal guardian is required to sign the consent form. In case they are not available, the attendant or a relative who brought the child to the hospital is asked to sign the consent form.

Principles Governing Nursing Care of Hospitalized Children

1. Welcome the family and child with a greeting and a smile.
2. The sick child should be *"handled as a child and not as a patient"*.
3. Call the child by name and approach him/her with sensitivity, concern and compassion. Nurses must develop the art of providing "gentle healing touch".
4. The cultural, social and religious beliefs of the family should be accepted and respected without any judgement or condemnation.
5. Take parents and patients into confidence while discussing the nursing process like assessment, diagnostic procedures and interventions. School-going children can participate in decision making process and feel comfortable when they are taken into confidence.
6. During communication, avoid any use of medical jargon, come down to the level and language of understanding of the parents and maintain an eye contact.
7. Provide physical comfort by appropriate positioning, provision of warmth and protection against any accident and physical injury. Guide and help the mother to look after the toilet needs of the child.
8. During various nursing procedures, divert the attention of the child by offering a toy, telling a story or simply talking to the child to distract him.
9. Praise the child for giving cooperation and never give any threats to seek cooperation. Avoid the use of lies or negative statements to seek cooperation.
10. Restraints should be used only when they are necessary and unavoidable.
11. In adolescent children, honor their privacy, confidentiality and dignity.
12. Patience, tenderness, sensitivity and gentleness are essential attributes for nurses working in children's ward and hospitals. Establish a rapport with the family and sick child which is crucial to gain their cooperation and confidence to help them relax. *The nurse should work not only with her brain but also with her heart!*

Role of a Nurse in the Care of Terminally Sick Children

It is a most challenging task to provide emotional support to the parents of children with terminal illnesses (AIDS, malignancy, genetic disorder, single or multiorgan failure). Though death is an ultimate truth but it is difficult to accept this reality especially when

> *"He whom the gods favour, dies in youth"*
> — **Plantus**
>
> *"Whom the gods love, dies young"*
> — **Menander**

death is anticipated and victim is a child who has not played his part or fulfilled the purpose of life. The news of a terminal or life-threatening illness should preferably be communicated to both the parents simultaneously with stoic calmness and conviction. When diagnosis of a potentially incurable disease is told to the parents there is a sudden shock, anger and denial on the part of parents. They can't accept the situation as to why their child is afflicted with this tragic disease. What wrongs they have done in this life or their past lives for this punishment? They have lots of questions and they should be encouraged to talk and ventilate their pent up emotions of helplessness, anxiety, fear and guilt. The nurse should patiently listen while parents raise their doubts and ask questions. The answers should not be blunt but should be pragmatic and based on known facts regarding the nature and outcome of the disease process. The nature of treatment, possible complications, modes of treatment and its cost, adverse effects of drugs and duration of follow-up, etc. should be explained. Never give a time frame that "Your child is likely to live for so many months". There are many variables and no body can estimate the duration of life or predict the time when the last breath will be taken.

The news of "gloomy prognosis" must be tempered with due optimism and godly benevolence to keep the hope alive in order to augment the process of healing. *Hope is the greatest healer and glimmer of hope should never be extinguished.* Parents should be told that miracles do happen and advances in the availability of newer drugs and therapeutic options are happening so fast that a breakthrough may save or prolong the life of their child.

The nurse should provide *tender loving care* (TLC) to all sick children but much more so to those with terminal illnesses. She should provide emotional support and courage to the family and siblings to accept the reality. The child should be provided with comfort and freedom from discomfort and pain. Efforts should

5

be made to make rest of the child's life more meaningful and assist the family to tide over the crisis with equanimity and mental peace. The child should be helped and encouraged to live each day to the fullest.

The Dying Child

The death may be anticipated when child is suffering from a terminal illness or it may occur suddenly as a bolt from the blue in case of an acute life-threatening disease or an accident. In case of a sudden unexpected death, there is a state of shock and bewilderment because family is denied any time for preparation and acceptance of the tragedy and the process of subsequent

> *Death is not an end. Everything in the world is moving from one form to the other in a cycle. Despite all the technological advances, medicine can never achieve immortality. It is as natural to die, as to be born.*
> — **Meharban Singh**

grief is likely to be prolonged. When a diagnosis of a fatal or terminal illness is communicated to a family, there are five well recognized emotional phases or feelings that the family is likely to experience.

1. **Shock and denial** In the first stage, the parents are shocked or numbed and are not willing to accept that their child is afflicted with a fatal illness. When the diagnosis is confirmed and fool proof, the nurse can help the family to face and accept the reality. Parents should be encouraged to ask questions and their doubts and dilemmas should be clarified.

2. **Anger** After the reality of doom and helplessness has sunk-in, there is a stage of anger against health care professionals, other family members and society at large. There is a constant nagging question "Why this tragedy has been targeted against our child?". The nurse at this stage should try to help the parents to ventilate their feelings and anger in a reasonable manner without blaming anybody. Silent listening and support at this stage is valued more than unnecessary talking.

3. **Bargaining** In this stage, the parents would start praying and "bargaining" with God demanding a cure for their child at any cost. They are willing to sacrifice their own life and stake all their belongings in exchange for the life of their child. It is true that the life cannot be bartered in exchange for anything but parents should be encouraged to have faith in their prayers and power of supreme miracles.

4. **Depression and grief** As the disease process continues, parents become depressed and aloof and do not want any visitors. They want to spend most of their time either with their child or crying alone. The nurse should try to gain the confidence of the parents, sit by their side and comfort them gently by her actions or touch rather than by loud talking or chattering.

5. **Acceptance** Finally, the parents enter the stage of acceptance and develop courage to face the reality as the will of God or divine destiny. The parents should be offered all possible support and help by the nurse in the event of death.

Diagnosis of Death

The determination of death has become complex because most dying patients are supported on a life support system. Death is diagnosed when child has either (i) irreversible cessation of circulatory and respiratory functions or (ii) there is irreversible cessation of all functions of the brain including the brainstem.

1. *Cessation of circulation and breathing.* Absence of heart beats (or flat ECG) and lack of spontaneous breathing efforts during an observation period of at least 30 minutes despite vigorous cardiopulmonary resuscitation.

2. *Child on assisted ventilation.* The following criteria should be present before declaring death.

   a. Flat EEG for 30 minutes

   b. Lack of spontaneous respiratory movements when ventilator is switched off for 3 minutes.

   c. *Brain death*
   - Dilated and fixed pupils on both sides without any response to bright light.
   - Absence of corneal reflex.
   - No conjugate movements of eyeballs or dysconjugate movements of eyeballs when tested for Doll's head-eye movements response.
   - Absence of vestibulo-ocular reflex (No nystagmoid movements or conjugate movements of eyes) when ice-cold water is injected into the auditory canal to stimulate the tympanic membrane.
   - Absence of facial grimace when firm pressure is applied over the supraorbital ridge.
   - Absence of gag reflex while doing oropharyngeal or tracheal suction.

Handling of Death

The desire of parents that death should occur in the familiar atmosphere of home rather than hospital should be honored. The family's wishes for religious support (amulets, mantras, holy water, etc.) and

> *Death should not be viewed as a tragedy but a peaceful acceptance, a loving entry into the unknown, a blissful acceptance of ultimate truth and a joyful good-bye to all friends and foes.*
>
> **— Sir William Osler**

presence of a priest at bedside should be allowed. The family should be emotionally and spiritually prepared before declaration of death. The news of death should be conveyed with utmost compassion but in no unmistakable terms that the child has died despite our best intentions and efforts. When a child is conscious and dying, the parents should be at his bedside holding his hand and talking with him to allay his fears and assist him to express his concerns, desires and emotions.

During the emotionally charged atmosphere of the process of dying, some resident doctors and nurses may feel extremely frustrated, upset and demoralized due to their inadequacy and inability to save life despite sincere and maximal efforts. They also need emotional support, guidance and advice to avoid unnecessary identification and attachment with the family. They should be encouraged and assisted to learn the art of detachment, imperturbability and poise at all odds. After taking relevant postmortem biopsies, family

> *"Death is certain for the born, and rebirth is inevitable for the dead. You should not, therefore, grieve over the inevitable".*
>
> **— The Bhagvad Gita**

should be approached with caution and tact to seek permission for an autopsy.

After completing urgent formalities, the death certificate should be prepared. The family should be provided with necessary courtesy, compassion and conveyance for a dignified journey of the dead child to the mortuary or home. The coping of death of a child in the hospital is a painful and challenging experience for everybody, the family and team of doctors, nurses and health care professionals. Death deflates our ego and teaches us humility and provides strength to face and accept the greatest reality and truth of life which we should handle with equanimity, peace and poise.

BIBLIOGRAPHY

Glasper EA, McEwing G, Richardson J. Oxford Handbook of Children's and Young People's Nursing. *London, Oxford University Press* 2nd Edition, 2010.

Hockenberry M, Wilson D. Wong's Essentials of Pediatric Nursing. *St. Louis, Mosby* 9th Edition 2013.

Nakagawa TA, Ashwal S, Mathur M, Mysore MR, et al. Guidelines for the determination of brain death in infants and children. An update of the 1987 Task Force Recommendations: *Crit Care Med* 2011, 39: 2139–2155.

Singh M. The diagnosis of death. In: Pediatric Clinical Methods. *CBS Publishers and Distributors Pvt Ltd* 5th Edition 2016, p 320–324.

The Nursing Council of Hong Kong. Core-competencies for Registered Nurses (Sick children); March 2015.

(http://www.nchk.org.hk/filemanager/en/pdf/core_comp_english.pdf)

Organization of a Neonatal Intensive Care Unit

The organization of a neonatal intensive care unit (NICU) is essential for reducing the neonatal mortality and improving the quality of life among the survivors. During the past three decades, improvements in the diagnostic and therapeutic approaches in the care of high-risk infants have influenced their prognosis favorably. Unfortunately, many neonatal centers in the developing countries are unplanned and merely improvised. The pediatrician and nurse incharge of neonatal services should be taken into confidence during the planning stage so that the special care neonatal unit is based on their opinions for meeting the special needs of these infants. It is a welcome move that Government of India has launched an initiative to establish special care newborn units (SCNUs) at district hospitals. The SCNU at the district hospital is envisaged to provide; (i) care at birth including resuscitation of asphyxiated newborns, (ii) management of sick newborns, (iii) referral and transport services for babies needing mechanical ventilation and major surgical intervention, (iv) postnatal care and immunization services and (v) follow-up of high-risk newborns.

Adequate space, availability of running water round-the-clock, centralized oxygen and suction facilities, maintenance of thermoneutral environment and ready availability of plenty of linen and disposables is mandatory to provide optimal level II newborn care. Facilities for prevention and management of common neonatal problems, viz. perinatal hypoxia, hypothermia, LBW babies, respiratory distress syndrome, septicemia, hyperbilirubinemia and life-threatening congenital malformations, should be established. The emphasis should be laid on developing a sound infrastructure to ensure safe delivery, promote asepsis, provide warmth and adequate nutrition with human milk. The lop-sided enthusiasm to acquire sophisticated electronic gadgetry including ventilators, in the absence of basic infrastructural facilities, must be discouraged. Effective and optimal management of newborn babies at birth, prevention of hypothermia and bacterial infections and

feeding of all babies with human milk should be ensured before establishing neonatal intensive care facilities. Intensive care of the newborn is highly cost-intensive and demands considerable inputs of staff, equipment and time. The philosophy of specialized conservative management of high-risk newborn babies should be fully exploited to bring down the neonatal mortality rate to less than 20 per 1000 live births before intensive care facilities are launched **(Figure 6.1)**.

PHYSICAL FACILITIES

Space

The size of the unit is related to the expected population intended to be served. In India, about 15 to 20% of newborn babies need special care, depending upon the criteria for antenatal booking for confinement. In addition, if the center is to serve as a referral unit for the infants born outside the hospital (extramural babies), allowance should be made for additional physical facilities and space. In a maternity unit having 2,000 deliveries per year, facilities for special care of

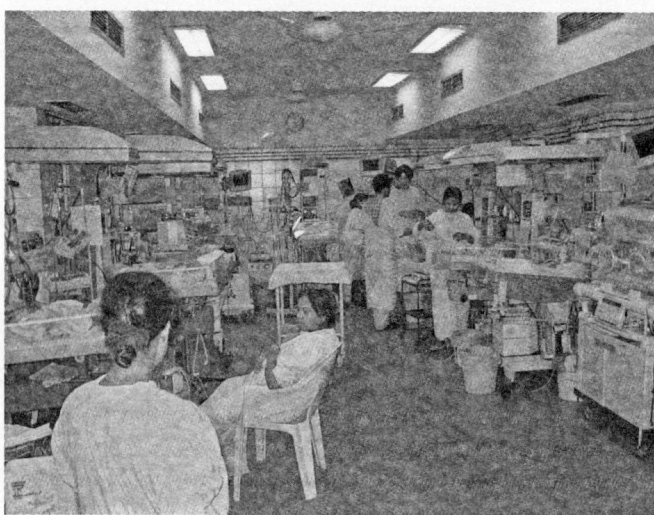

Figure 6.1 NICU of All India Institute of Medical Sciences, New Delhi

6–8 high-risk infants should be available. Each infant should be provided with a minimum area of 100 sq. ft. or 10 m². However, additional space would be needed to provide for special facilities as outlined below in the floor plan. There should be no compromise on space and its adequacy is crucial for reduction of nosocomial infections. Space should be allocated within the nursery complex for promotion of breastfeeding, expression of breast-milk and its storage.

Location

The neonatal unit should be located as close as possible to the labor rooms and obstetric operation theatre, to facilitate prompt transfer of sick and high-risk infants. The presence of an elevator in close proximity is desirable for transport of outborn infants. In tropical countries, the nursery should not be located on the top floor of the hospital but there should be feasibility for the sunlight to peep into the nursery to enhance brightness and provide ultraviolet rays to augment asepsis.

Nursery Design

The unit design may be in a square space or a single corridor-based rectangular unit. A split unit, i.e. on either side of the hospital corridor, should be avoided for ease of mobility and for prevention of infections. A unit design occupying one side of the corridor with a nurses control room in the centre, from where all the babies can be viewed, is preferred **(Figure 6.2)**. Apart from constant surveillance of all babies, the design should ensure minimal walking distance for the staff.

Baby Care Area

The unit should be provided with areas and rooms for inborn or intramural babies, stepdown nursery, outborn or extramural babies, examination area, mother's area for breastfeeding and expression of breast-milk, nurses station and charting area. The floor and walls should be made of washable glazed or vitrified tiles and windows should have two layers of glass panes to ensure some measure of heat and sound insulation. The obviously infected infants with open sepsis (especially those with diarrhea and abscesses) should be isolated in a septic nursery, which should be located away from the NICU and manned by different nursing and resident staff.

A large number of ancillary services are needed and should be designed and earmarked during the planning stage.

Handwashing and gowning room Handwashing and gowning facility should be located at the enterance. It

should be provided with abundant space with self-closing doors. A positive air pressure should be maintained in the NICU so that corridor air does not enter the NICU. Street shoes are changed with nursery slippers, followed by handwashing and gowning. The use of mask is controversial and is best avoided. Hand-free elbow-operated handwashing sink with liquid soap dispenser is recommended. Sink should be made of porcelain or stainless steel. Pictorial handwashing instructions should be provided on the wall next to the sink. Hands should be dried with single use or disposable napkins. The use of hot air dryer is not recommended due to risk of dissemination of pathogens. Walls adjacent to the sink should be made of non-porous or non-absorbent material to prevent growth of molds. Sinks should not be provided with slabs or countertops which are a potent source of infection. The unit should be provided with 24-hour uninterrupted water supply by having dedicated over head tank with a capacity of 1000–2000 liters.

Examination area A small comfortable room with examination table, comfortable seating, sufficient light, and warmth is needed for assessment of baby before admission to the nursery. The baby is cleaned and provided with nursery garments in this room.

Mother area The room should be provided with comfortable seating and privacy to the mother to breastfeed and express the breast-milk with the help of a lactation nurse.

Handwashing stations Handwashing sinks should be provided within 20 feet (6 meters) of every newborn bed. The sink should be large and deep (24" wide × 16" front-back and 10" deep) and made of porcelain or stainless steel and without any counter or shelf. Single use cotton or disposable paper napkins should be available for drying the hands. Alternatively, antiseptic sanitizing solution (sterillium) can be used for disinfection of hands in-between the babies.

Preparation of intravenous fluids A separate area should be earmarked and provided with a laminar flow system for preparation of intravenous fluids, parenteral nutritional formulations, enteral feeds and medications. Boiling and autoclaving facilities should be available next to this area.

Nurses station Nursing station and charting area for nurses and residents should be located in a central area from where all the babies can be observed. Newborn charts, hospital forms, computer terminals, telephone lines should be located in this area. It is preferable to use electronic medical recording of clinical notes and retrieval of laboratory reports.

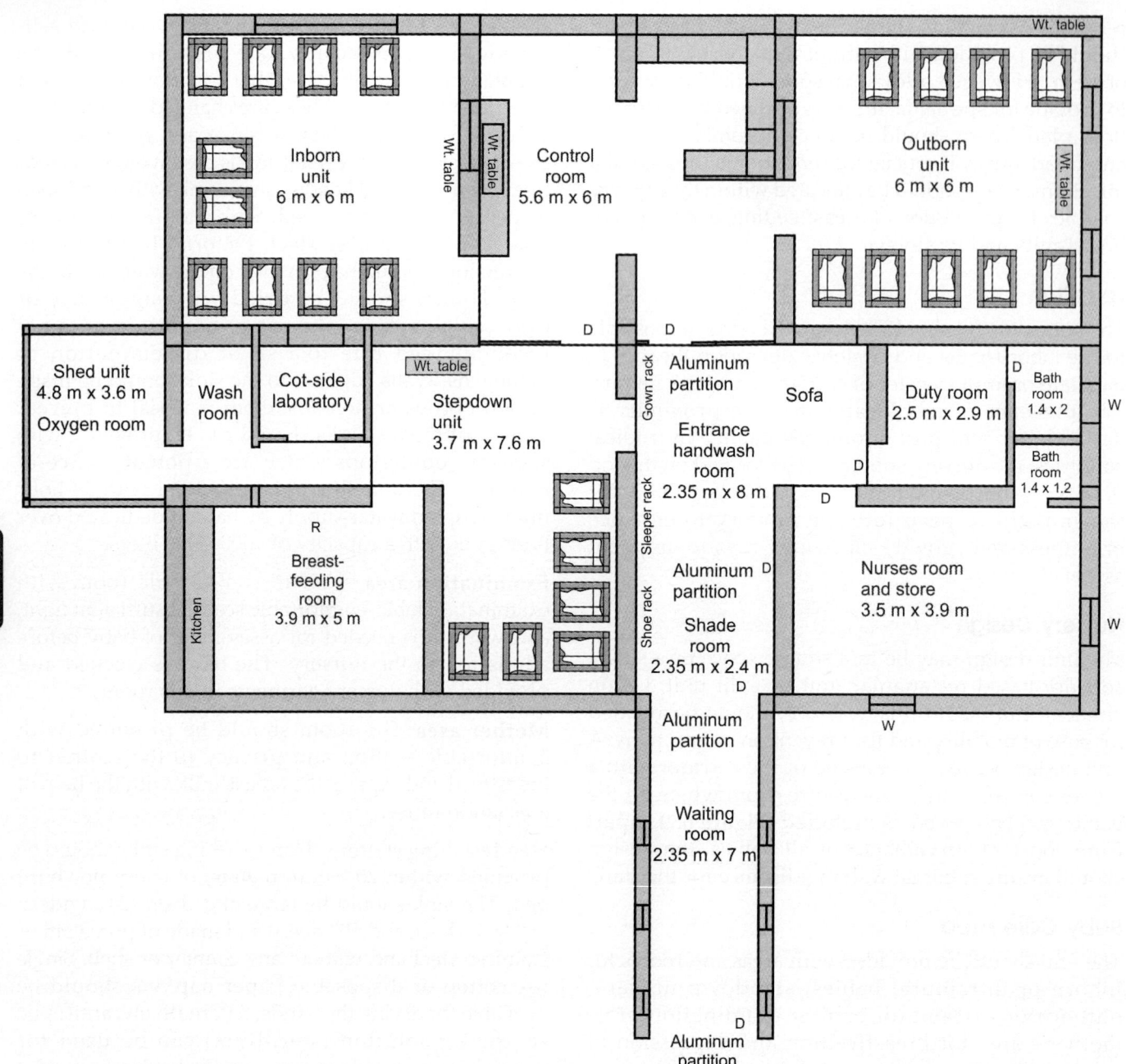

Figure 6.2 The conceptual layout for a special care neonatal unit for 25 babies. Adapted from tool kit for setting up special care neonatal unit, UNICEF

Clean utility and soiled utility holding rooms There should be enough space for stocking clean utility items and sterile disposables, and for disposal of dirty linen and contaminated disposables. Built-in wall wooden cabinets with foldable covers are useful for stacking purposes. The ventilation system in the soiled utility or holding room should be engineered to have negative air pressure with all air being exhausted to the outside. The soiled utility room should be so located that it enables removal of soiled material without passing through the baby care area.

Staff rooms Space should be provided within the unit to meet the professional, personal and administrative needs of resident staff on duty. A comfortable room with intercom, telephone and computer terminal and WC facilities is mandatory. Nurse's change room is required for changing from formal street clothes to a smart shirt and trouser dress as stipulated by the NICU.

Growing nursery A separate bay in the lying-in ward should be earmarked for transitional care of high-risk babies by their mothers before they are discharged from the hospital. The entry of visitors to this area should be restricted and it should be kept adequately warm. Facilities for monitoring asepsis and weighing the babies should be available in the transitional care room (TCR) or growing nursery (GN). The growing nursery is used with advantage for educating the mothers in child craft activities and promoting the practice of exclusive breastfeeding.

Ventilation

Effective air ventilation of nursery is essential to reduce nosocomial infections. The most satisfactory ventilation is achieved with laminar air flow system which is rather expensive. When centralized air-conditioning is used, minimum of 12 changes of room air per hour are recommended. There should be no draughts of air on and near the newborn beds. The air-conditioning ducts must be provided with millipore filters (0.5 µ) to restrict the passage of microbes. A simple method to achieve satisfactory ventilation consists of provision of exhaust fan in a reverse direction near the ceiling for input of fresh uncontaminated air and fixation of another exhaust fan in the conventional manner near the floor for air exit. A constant positive air pressure should be maintained in the nursery so that contaminated air from the corridors does not gain access into the nursery. The use of chemical air disinfection and ultraviolet lamps is no more recommended.

Lighting

The nursery must be well illuminated and painted white or slightly off white to permit prompt and early detection of jaundice and cyanosis. It is best achieved by cool white fluorescent tubes or LED (light-emitting diodes) to provide at least 100 foot-candle, shadow-free illumination at the infant's level. The number and exact location of fixtures can be worked out taking into account size of the nursery, height of the ceiling, and availability or otherwise of sunlight. Spot illumination for various procedures can be provided by a portable angle-poise lamp having two 15 watt fluorescent bulbs which when held at a distance of about one foot from the infant, produce about 100 foot-candle intensity of light. Most open care systems are equipped with in-built source of overhead spot lights. In places where electrical failure is frequent and prolonged, the electrical system of the nursery complex must be attached to a generator. Exposure of preterm babies to strong light has been incriminated as a risk factor for the development of retinopathy of prematurity. The nursery light should be dimmed at night to simulate day-night pattern to promote hormonal surge and growth of babies. Bedside lights with dimmer switches should be provided to create specialized microenvironment for each baby.

Environmental Temperature and Humidity

The temperature of the nursery complex must be maintained between 26°C and 28°C (78.8 and 82.4°F) in order to minimize effects of thermal stress on the babies. This is best achieved by centralized air conditioning having temperature control knobs in the nursery. The air movement should be so designed that draught is minimized. In places where air conditioning is not feasible, room temperature can be reasonably well maintained in winter by use of radiant heaters and hot air blowers. Portable radiant heater, infrared lamp or bakery bulb can be used to provide additional source of heat to an individual infant. The external windows of nursery should be glazed to minimize heat gain and heat loss and baby beds should be located at least 2 feet (0.6 meter) away from the wall or window. In most parts of India, relative humidity averages above 50%, which is quite satisfactory for routine needs of newborn babies. Humidity level can be raised for preterm babies nursed in an incubator. High and effective humidity level is useful to reduce insensible water loss but is associated with increased risk of nosocomial infection.

Acoustic Characteristics

The ventilation system, incubators, air compressors, suction pumps and many other devices used in the nursery produce noise. Sound intensity in the nursery should not exceed 75 dB to protect hearing of nursery personnel and infants. Excessive noise may lead to hearing loss, physiological and behavioral disturbances, such as sleep disturbances, startles and crying episodes, hypoxia, tachycardia and increased intracranial pressure. The fabrication and redesigning of nursery equipment should take into account the desirability of minimizing noise by dampening the sounds by acoustic or other means. It is desirable to have effective sound-proofing of ceilings, walls, doors and floor when a new nursery is designed. Telephone rings and equipment alarms should be replaced by blinking lights. Instead of air compressors, centralized sources of compressed air, oxygen and suction should be provided. Decibel meters should be installed to monitor sound levels in the nursery. The beneficial and soothing effects of meaningful sounds, such as gentle music or recordings of parent voice, should be harnessed to provide physiologic stability to the babies.

Handling and Social Contacts

Excessive and rough handling of delicate newborn babies is associated with several adverse physiological consequences, such as excessive crying, sleep disturbances, tachycardia or bradycardia, hypoxia and rise in blood pressure and intracranial pressure.

6

Handling should be gentle and kept to the barest minimum without compromising care. Soothing words, gentle stroking and rocking should be practised after a painful procedure. Gentle caressing, cuddling and touching by the mother are desirable to provide comfort and confidence to the baby and aid the process of healing. Infants should be exposed to gentle and soothing tactile, kinesthetic, vestibular, motor, auditory and visual experiences to provide opportunities for early learning and improvement in behavior. Parents should be allowed unrestricted entry to the nursery to provide these useful sensorimotor stimuli. It enhances the process of bonding between the baby and the family.

Communication System

The nursery complex should be provided with an intercom system so that additional person can be called for help in case of emergency without leaving the sick infant. A direct line external telephone is mandatory so that parents have an easy access to inquire about welfare of their infants and in turn they can be readily contacted whenever needed. Mobile phones should not be used near the vicinity of the nursery because the electromagnetic waves are likely to interfere with the functioning of the electronic equipment. The family should be kept constantly informed about the condition of their baby including therapeutic interventions being given. They should be given emotional support and pragmatic view of the likely outcome.

Electrical Outlets

There should be adequate number (8–12 electrical points at the height of 4–5 feet) of 5 amperes and 15 amperes electrical points attached to a common ground. Each infant must be provided with at least eight electrical outlets, 4 should be 5 amperes and another 4 of 15 amperes. The use of adapters and extension boards should be discouraged. The electrical equipment used in the nursery must be checked at least once a month for leakage of current and adequacy of grounding. If possible, special fittings with safety devices should be installed. The unit should have round-the-clock uninterrupted servo-stabilized power supply. There should be round-the-clock power back-up including provision of UPS system for the sensitive equipments.

PERSONNEL

It is important, that while allocating nursing, medical and paramedical staff to the hospital, the needs of the neonatal unit are not ignored. It is unfortunate that newborn babies are not counted as patients requiring nursing and medical care while expressing the bed strength of a hospital. The census of the hospital bed is administratively based on dieted beds. In fact, the situation is paradoxical because the neonates need rather specialized and sophisticated nursing and medical care. Therefore, the highest priority in the organization of the NICU is the availability of sufficient number of adequately trained personnel especially the nurses. *The survival of newborn babies depends upon the availability of specially trained nurses.* The Nursing Council of India has not outlined any special guidelines for this purpose. It has been recommended by the American Academy of Pediatrics that one nurse is needed to offer special or intermediate nursing care to 3 babies or intensive care to one infant. In countries where monitoring devices are not routinely available, relatively larger number of nurses are necessary for undertaking manual monitoring. It is generally not appreciated by the hospital administrators that a considerable time of the nurse is spent in rigorous housekeeping rituals to maintain asepsis in the nursery. The frequent toilet care, expression of breast-milk, formula preparation and feeding are time consuming and unassisted by any attendant. Whenever adequate number of nurses are not available, these rituals are compromised resulting in outbreak of epidemic of infection in the nursery. The nursery complex must, therefore, be considered as an independent nursing unit under the charge of a fully qualified nursing sister.

The National Neonatology Forum of India has recommended that at least one trained nurse should be allocated to provide coverage to four babies in the special care neonatal unit. The allowance should be kept for additional 25% staff to provide for the exigencies of day off and leave. Therefore, for an 8-bedded NICU, eight nurses should be sanctioned to ensure availability of two nurses in each shift along with one additional sister incharge in the morning shift. In a case of a baby on ventilator, one nurse should be allocated for one baby, while two critically sick babies without assisted ventilation can be looked after by one nurse. The continuity of service can be maintained, if at least 50% of the nurses are rather permanent and not transferred frequently as is the usual practice in general hospitals. There must be equal distribution of nurses in the three duty shifts during 24 hours. The nurses must be imparted continuing in-service training in the art of neonatal nursing and preventive maintenance of a variety of electronic equipment used in the NICU. They should participate in the monthly perinatal morbidity and mortality meetings. It is desirable to have services of public health nurses and social workers for follow-up and home care of low birth weight babies after their discharge from the hospital.

A pediatrician specially interested in the care of newborn babies should devote his full time to improve the existing standards of neonatal special care services in the country. The unit must also have an independent senior resident and one junior resident round-the-clock for every 8 babies requiring special care. The resident doctors must work in these units for at least 3 months to maintain continuity of medical care. All deliveries in the hospital should preferably be attended by a physician trained in the care of newborn. A laboratory technician should be available to operate bilirubinometer, glucometer, microcentrifuge, CRP kits and blood gas analyzer. A biomedical technician or a link person is essential to maintain a liaison with suppliers of equipment to ensure their smooth functioning, prevent breakdowns and reduce the downtime. The resident staff and nurses working in the NICU must be trained to properly handle and use the equipment. When ventilatory facilities are established, respiratory therapist is a useful member of the neonatal team to monitor ventilatory settings, provide tracheal suctioning and chest physiotherapy. A pediatric pathologist, who is specially trained for conducting and interpreting neonatal autopsies, is desirable to complement the functioning of the neonatal team.

EQUIPMENT

During the last 2–3 decades, a large number of monitoring devices for diagnostic and therapeutic use for the high-risk newborn infants have been developed. These have considerably improved their intact survival. Several basic prerequisites must be fulfilled before any center invests in purchase of expensive equipment involving foreign exchange. The fundamental needs of the unit are availability of adequate space, freedom from congestion and presence of a sufficient number of adequately trained nurses. A reasonable level of asepsis must be achieved and facilities for maintaining thermoneutral environment should be established. The feeding of babies should be associated with minimal risk of aspiration.

Acquisition of new equipment does not necessarily ensure better services and outcome. *Machines cannot replace men. The best monitors with us are dedicated nurses and resident doctors involved in the care of newborn babies with their observational skills sharpened by experience.* Therefore, they need continued in-service training, teaching and encouragement for obtaining the best results. In view of the exorbitant cost of imported equipment and problems faced in their maintenance, there is a constant need to promote indigenous fabrication of equipment required for neonatal care.

The maintenance of the existing equipment in proper working condition is more important than acquiring new and sophisticated gadgets. Before placing an order, check with existent consumer/s regarding reliability of the equipment and quality of after sales service provided by the local dealer. The supplier must install the equipment and provide training to the staff for proper use and maintenance of the equipment. Date of installation and expiry of warranty period should be recorded. After expiry of mandatory warranty period, you should enter into a yearly maintenance contract with the local dealer for preventive maintenance and emergency repairs in the event of breakdowns. In case of sophisticated and expensive equipment, a counterguarantee of service should also be taken from the foreign principals. Inventory of spares should be maintained and essential spares should be purchased and kept in stock while ordering new equipment. Photocopies of working and service manuals should be available in the NICU while original documents should be kept in a safe custody. Maintain a log book containing postal and e-mail addresses, telephone and fax numbers of local dealers and suppliers of equipment. When telephonic complaints are not heeded by the local supplier, you should send a written complaint and endorse a copy to the foreign principals.

Preventive Maintenance and Emergency Repairs

After-sales technical services including annual maintenance contract (AMC) should be a mandatory requirement at the time of purchase of the equipment. At the time of installation, the supplier should provide technical training, hands-on training for clinical use of the equipment and its proper maintenance to the nurses and resident doctors. A qualified in-house biomedical technician should be available to maintain an inventory of equipment and spares, ensure optimal preventive maintenance and take prompt action to call the service engineer to ensure maximum uptime of the life saving medical equipment. The in-house technician should have up-to-date information regarding the proper use of the equipment, should be able to undertake firstline corrective intervention that does not require any spare parts and when required he should be able to report correctly the nature of technical malfunctioning of the equipment to the on-call service engineer of the company.

The objectives of preventive maintenance include that the equipment should be functional most of the time and should operate with accuracy, efficiency and safety. The maintenance engineer should undertake at least two technical visits per year to check the wear and tear, and performance of the device as per manufacturers technical check list. The equipment should be cleaned and defective components replaced by spare parts. He should interact with in-house technician and end-users to provide necessary guidance for correct use of the equipment to ensure effective preventive maintenance and upkeep.

Despite careful use of the equipment, the average lifetime of most electronic equipment is about 7 years. In the event of breakdown, when contacted the service engineer should report to the NICU without delay to ensure that the downtime of the equipment is minimum. In case the device cannot be repaired on-site and the machine is taken to the workshop, a replacement model should be provided by the company for the period of the repair.

COT-SIDE LABORATORY FACILITIES

Satisfactory facilities for routine radiological examination should be available in the nursery round-the-clock. A good portable 3-phase generator X-ray machine of at least 200 milliamperes with extremely short exposure time (1/120 seconds) should preferably be housed in a small room adjacent to the NICU. In-house ultrasound, EKG and aEEG facilities should be available.

A side laboratory for routine analysis of blood, urine, amniotic fluid, gastric aspirate for shake test and cytology, Kleihauer-Betke count, glucose, bilirubin, hematocrit and blood gases and acid-base parameters should be available. Centralized facilities for microbiochemical techniques especially for estimation of total and direct serum bilirubin, blood glucose, arterial PO_2, PCO_2, pH and base deficit are desirable. Facilities for analysis of serum sodium, potassium, calcium and total serum proteins, and albumin should be at hand. The collection of venous blood is often difficult and hazardous in sick preterm babies. These babies often require frequent biochemical estimations. *It is generally not appreciated that removal of 10 mL of blood from a 1,500 g infant amounts to about 8% of his total blood volume. This is equivalent to removal of about 400 mL of blood in an adult.* Thus a micro-chemical laboratory which can carry out investigations on very small samples of blood obtained in heparinized capillary tubes or microcentrifuge tubes from heel puncture, should be considered as an essential facility for NICU. Preterm, high-risk and sick newborn babies are admitted to the neonatal intensive care unit (NICU). High quality nursing and supportive care is essential to improve the survival of high-risk neonates. Indications for admission of babies to the NICU are

Indications for admission to the NICU

1. Infants with a birth weight of less than 1800 g or gestation of less than 35 weeks
2. Severe birth asphyxia or birth trauma
3. Rhesus-isoimmunization
4. Respiratory distress or apneic attacks
5. Maternal diabetes mellitus
6. Major congenital malformations
7. Sick baby
8. Sick mother
9. Abandoned baby

listed in **Box 6.1**. The NICU manual should be available giving details of various policy guidelines for nursing routines and rituals.

ASEPSIS ROUTINES AND RITUALS

Neonatal bacterial infections are one of the leading causes of neonatal mortality in developing countries. Most neonatal infections are preventable if strict asepsis is maintained in the NICU. The vigilance and strict aseptic routines enforced in the operating theatres must be followed in the NICU. The NICU environment should be clean and dry with 24 hours water supply and electricity supply with a backup generator. There should be adequate ventilation and lighting. The temperature of the NICU should be maintained between 28°C ±2°C. Overcrowding must be avoided.

The basic requirements and principles for ensuring asepsis in the NICU are listed in **Box 6.2**.

Entry Guidelines for Personnel and Parents

1. Remove shoes, socks, full sleeve woolens, watch, bangles and rings
2. Put on half-sleeved sterile gown and slippers. There is no need to wear a mask.

Essential requirements to ensure asepsis

- Running water supply round-the-clock .
- Strict and compulsive handwashing policy.
- Promotion of feeding with human milk.
- Availability plenty of disposables without any compromise.
- Rational policy for entry and admission to the NICU.
- Avoidance of overcrowding.
- Avoidance of prophylactic antibiotics and promotion of rational antibiotic policy.
- Obsession with good housekeeping and asepsis routines

3. The nurse should preferably be provided with a sterile smart NICU dress such as a T-shirt and pants.
4. Parents and personnel with active infection or those who had recent exposure to chickenpox should not enter the NICU.
5. Apart from parents of the babies, no other visitors should be allowed entry. They should be instructed about the guidelines for entry and proper handwashing technique.

Handwashing

1. It is the single MOST IMPORTANT strategy for prevention of infections.
2. Two minutes of handwashing with soap and water is advised before entering the NICU. Subsequently, handwashing for 15 seconds is recommended before and after touching the baby and after touching any unsterile surfaces and fomites (inanimate objects and articles). Handwashing is done using liquid soap and running water.
3. The following steps for effective handwashing should be followed:
   i. Roll the sleeves above the elbow.
   ii. Remove wrist watch, bangles and rings, etc.
   iii. The nails should be kept trimmed. Wash various parts of the hands with soap and water in the following sequence: Palms, fingers and web spaces, back of hands, fingers and knuckles, thumbs, finger tips, wrist and forearm up to the elbow (**Figure 6.3**).
   iv. Close the tap using elbow handle or foot pedal.
   v. Dry hands by using a single-use sterile cotton or paper napkin. The use of a common towel, which is used by everyone for drying the hands is strongly condemned.

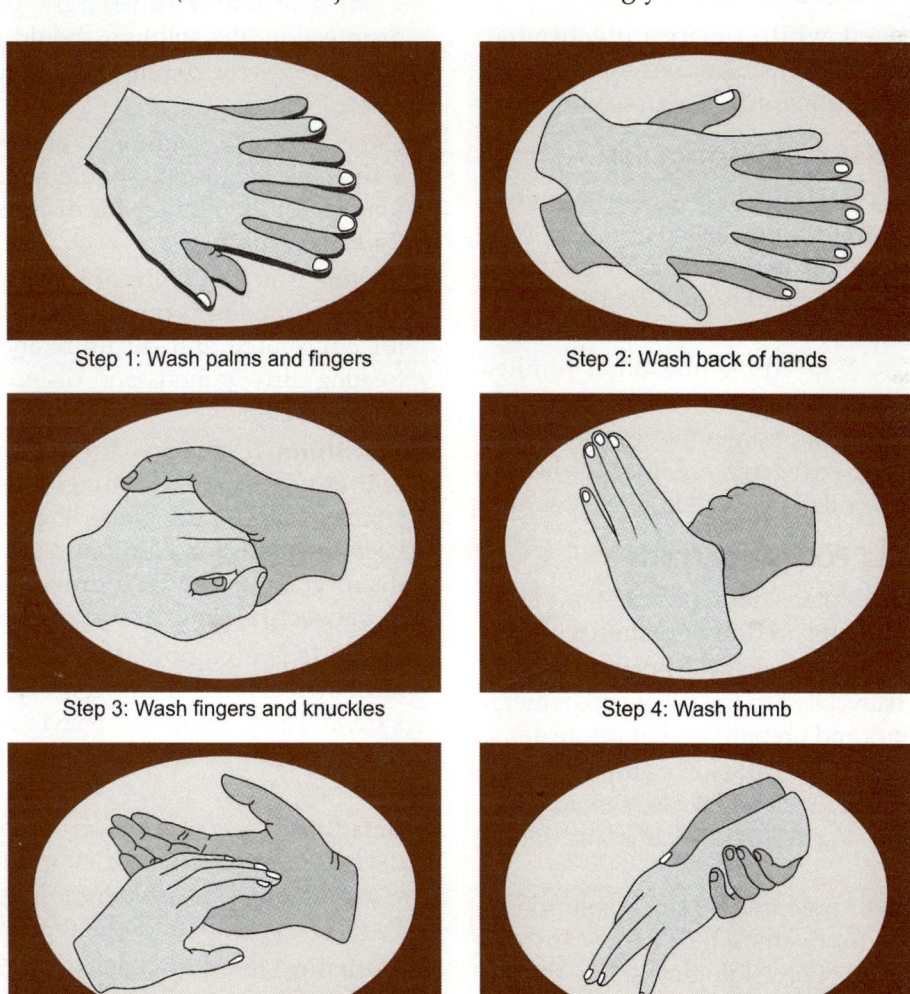

Step 1: Wash palms and fingers

Step 2: Wash back of hands

Step 3: Wash fingers and knuckles

Step 4: Wash thumb

Step 5: Wash finger tips

Step 6: Wash wrists

Figure 6.3 Steps and guidelines for effective handwashing. Handwashing should be done diligently and with a sense of purpose

Scrupulous handwashing before feeding, after napkin changing and before providing any nursing care to the baby must be followed strictly in the NICU.

Sterile Gloves

1. Always use sterile gloves for all invasive procedures like blood sampling, establishing IV line, lumbar puncture, exchange blood transfusion, endotracheal suction and administration of parenteral fluids and medications.
2. Wash the gloved hands to remove blood stains and secretions from the gloves and then discard them in a container of polar bleach. Wash hands again.
3. If gloves are being recycled, they should be cleaned, dried and packed for re-autoclaving at least in two shifts by the NICU orderly and adequate number of gloves should be prepared everyday.

Mask and Sterile Drapes

They should be used while performing lumbar puncture, exchange blood transfusion, arterial vascular catheter placement and other invasive procedures.

Barrier Nursing and Use of Disposables

1. Keep separate tape, stethoscope, thermometer, alcohol, betadine swabs for each baby.
2. The disposables should be available in plenty to avoid their prolonged use and reuse. Change suction catheter, feeding tubes, ET tube and IV line daily.
3. Do not keep files, X-ray films and other fomites alongside the baby.
4. Change the antiseptic solution in the suction bottles and sterile water in the oxygen humidification bottles and chambers of incubators everyday.

Stock Solutions and Parenteral Fluids

1. Parenteral fluids and total parenteral nutrition (TPN) solutions should be prepared under laminar flow.
2. Keep a separate parenteral fluid bottle properly labelled for each baby. Discard the left over parenteral fluids after 24 hours and prepare fresh infusate daily.
3. Change the syringe of the infusion pump or micro-burette set atleast once in 24 hours. Use separate sets for administration of parenteral drugs and blood products.
4. There is no need to prepare the stock solution of heparinized saline for flushing the IV lines. Instead single-use ampoules of physiological saline should be used for flushing.

Housekeeping Routines

Strict housekeeping routines for washing, disinfection, cleaning of cots, and incubators should be ensured and these policy guidelines should be available in the form of a manual in the NICU (**Table 6.1**).

Disinfectants and Germicides

Disinfection is defined as the process of destruction of all pathogenic microorganisms and their toxins. Sterilization is the process of killing all microorganisms including their vegetative forms like spores.

1. **Bacillocid** It contains formaldehyde, glutaraldehyde, alkylurea derivative and benzalkonium chloride. Use 2% solution by dissolving 200 mL of the concentrate in 10 liters of water. It is used for disinfecting surfaces and for spraying rooms. The fans and air conditioners should be put off for 30 minutes and surfaces should be kept wet with bacillocid for 30 minutes for effective disinfection.
2. **Korsolex** It contains formaldehyde and glutaraldehyde. One part of the concentrate is mixed with 9 parts of water to prepare 10% solution. For disinfection, the solution should remain in contact with fomites for 20 minutes and for sterilization for at least 4 hours.
3. **Cidex** It is a 2% solution of glutaraldehyde with an activator. The solution should remain in contact with fomites for 20 minutes for disinfection and 4 hours for sterilization.
4. **Savlon** It is a mixture of cetrimide, chlorhexidine gluconate and isopropyle alcohol. Use 1:100 solution for equipment and furniture and 1:30 solution for treating dirty wounds and disinfecting catheters or thermometers.
5. **Sterillium** It contains 2-propanolol, 1-propanolol and ethyl-hexadecyle-dimethyl-ammonium ethyl sulfate. Rub 2–3 mL of sterillium on the palms and backs of hands for 30 seconds and allow it to dry for disinfection of hands. It can be used as a sanitizer in-between nursing care or after handling the babies.
6. **Lysol** It is a combination of ethanol, isopropyl alcohol, p-chloro-o-benzylphenol, potassium hydroxide, and alkyl dimethyl benzyl ammonium chloride. It is useful for disinfection of floors, walls and wash basin.
7. **Betadine** It is 7.5% solution of povidone iodine and used for preparation of skin and disinfection of wounds. For skin preparation, leave it to dry for 60 seconds before undertaking the procedure.
8. **Formalin** (40% formaldehyde aqueous solution) is used for fumigation. For routine fumigation, 30 mL of 40% formalin is dissolved in 90 mL of water and for intensive fumigation, 90 mL of 40% formalin is dissolved in 90 mL of water. The fans and air conditioners are put off. Formalin is poured in a

Table 6.1 Housekeeping and disinfection routines

Area/item	Disinfection method and frequency	Other measures and remarks
▪ Floors	Use chlorophore cleanser (3% phenol or 5% lysol) during every shift. Pesticide spray and anti-cockroach measures should be used once a week.	Do not sweep or do dry dusting. Avoid use of cidex. The holes and crevices in the floors, walls and ceilings should be sealed.
▪ Walls	Wipe with 2% bacillocid once in two weeks.	Fumigation is done when infection rate goes up.
▪ Fans	Wet mop with soap and water once a month.	
▪ Air conditioner	Vacuum cleaning is done once in two weeks. Window AC should be sprayed with 2% bacillocid once a week.	Thorough cleaning and change of filters by AC maintenance staff twice a year.
▪ Sinks	Clean once a day with detergent powder and chlorophore cleanser.	Tiles under the sink should be cleaned daily.
▪ Entrance wash area	Daily mopping with chlorophore cleanser and 2% bacillocid spray twice a week.	Switch off fans and AC and close the area for one hour after spray.
▪ Refrigerator	Defrost and clean with soap solution once every 2 weeks.	
▪ Buckets and dustbins	Wash daily with soap and water.	The buckets and bins should be lined with polythene bags which should be changed after each disposal.
▪ Baby linen, cotton, gauze, etc.	Wash and autoclave.	
▪ Baby blankets and blanket covers	Wash or dry clean and autoclave between the babies.	
▪ Feeding bottles	Boil for 15 min or sterilize before each use.	
▪ Swab containers, injection and medicine trays	Clean daily with soap or cleanser.	Use a separate tray for each baby.
▪ Steel drums	Autoclave after every 48 hours.	They should be kept closed properly and replaced if broken.
▪ Cheatle forceps	Autoclave daily and keep in a sterile bottle containing 5% savlon or dry sterile cotton.	
▪ Stethoscope, measuring tape, thermometer, cuff of sphgygmomano-meter, electronic probes, etc.	Clean daily with 70% isopropyle alcohol or sterillium.	Keep a separate stethoscope for each baby. Keep thermometer in a bottle containing sterile cotton.
▪ Laryngoscope blade	Clean with 70% isopropyle alcohol or sterillium after each use.	Never use cidex because it may be harmful to the baby.
▪ Oxygen bood	Wash daily with soap and water. Dry with an autoclaved linen.	
▪ Face mask	After each use, clean with a detergent and immerse in cidex for 20 min. Rinse in sterile water and dry it with autoclaved linen.	
▪ Ambu bag and its reservoir, ventilator tubings, oxygen tubings, water traps, humidifier bottles, bottle and tubings of suction machine	Dismantle and clean with a detergent. Keep immersed in korsolex or cidex for 4 hours, rinse in sterile water, dry it and reassemble. Ambu bag and its reservoir should be cleaned once a week while other items should be cleaned daily.	Change ventilator circuit and oxygen tubing daily. Use distilled water in the humidifier and change it daily. Discard suction catheter after single use. Put 100 mL savlon in suction bottle upto the blue line. Keep the the suction connector covered with a sterile gauze piece.

(Contd.)

Table 6.1 Housekeeping and disinfection routines (*Contd.*)

Area/item	Disinfection method and frequency	Other measures and remarks
■ Weighing machine and radiant warmer	Mop daily with 2% bacillocid.	Place an autoclaved sheet on the scale before weighing the baby.
■ Incubator	Clean daily with a detergent and water followed by 2% bacillocid. Do not use alcohol to clean the canopy because it will make the perspex foggy. After discharge or death of a baby, fumigation is done by adding 50 mL of formalin in 50 mL of water in the humidity tank of the incubator and plugging it on for 4 hours.	Do not keep the baby in the same incubator for more than one week.
■ Nursery equipment and machines	Wet mop with sterile water once a day.	Keep them covered with a clean polythene sheet when not in use.

Note: Always discard disposables after a single use and do not compromise. The liberal use of disposables is the most effective strategy to reduce the risk of hospital acquired infections. Terminal disinfection should be done after discharge or death of a baby.

vaporiser which is plugged on for 6 hours after snuggly closing all the doors, windows and crevices.

After 6 hours, 4–6 ounces of ammonium hydroxide can be poured in the vaporiser after discarding left over formalin and machine is put on to get rid off the formalin fumes for earlier reuse of the nursery. If a vaporiser is not available, add 10 g of potassium permanganate to 35 mL of 40% formalin for fumigation. The formalin should not be poured over potassium permanganate as this may lead to explosion. This method takes about 10 hours for effective fumigation.

Surveillance

The incidence of infection, prevalence of various pathogens in the NICU and their antibiotic sensitivity pattern should be reviewed every 3 months. Room air, surfaces of various equipment that come in contact with babies and various solutions (water in the humidifier, cold sterilization solutions) should be cultured once a week or in the event of an increased incidence of infection or epidemic. Hands, nose and throat swabs of personnel are cultured as and when needed.

Universal Precautions

In view of increasing incidence of acquired immunodeficiency syndrome (AIDS) globally, every patient and every sample of body fluid and blood should be considered as potentially infected with human immunodeficiency virus (HIV). The risk of acquiring the infection through a needle-stick injury is about 1 : 300. Therefore, certain principles have been laid down to help reduce the risk of infection and they have been referred to as "Universal Precautions" which are listed in **Box 6.3**. These guidelines are useful for

Box 6.3   Universal precautions

- Treat every specimen of blood or body fluid as potentially infectious.
- Wear gloves for handling all bodily fluids and while performing phlebotomy.
- For all procedures where splashing of body fluids or droplets may occur, wear waterproof gown, mask and goggles.
- Avoid re-capping, bending or breaking of needles, but when recapping is unavoidable it should be done with a single hand to avoid accidental needle stick injury to the finger (**Figure 6.4**).
- Wear gloves for patient care if exudative or weeping dermatitis is present.
- Handwashing is a must in-between examination of patients, after any procedure and on removal of gloves.
- Promptly clean any blood spills or bodily fluids by pouring 1% bleach solution or 0.5% sodium hypochlorite over the spill and leave it on for atleast 10 minutes.
- Disinfect or sterilize re-usable devices as recommended.
- Ensure safe disposal of needles and other sharps into puncture resistant containers. Dispose puncture resistant disposable container for decontamination or incineration when three-quarters full.
- Wear heavy-duty rubber gloves for cleaning instruments, handling soiled linen or dealing with spills of blood and body fluids.

prevention of transmission of Hepatitis B virus (HBV) as well. Infact potential risk of transmission of HBV is much higher than HIV.

Post-Exposure Prophylaxis

If there has been a breach in the universal precautions or despite all precautions a needle-stick injury has

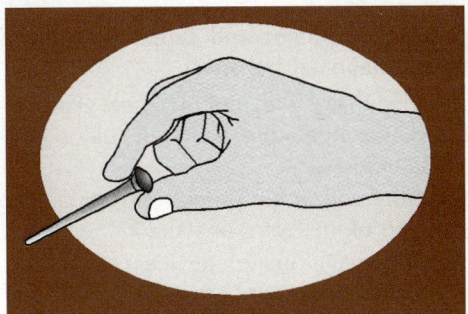

(a) Place needle cap on a flat surface

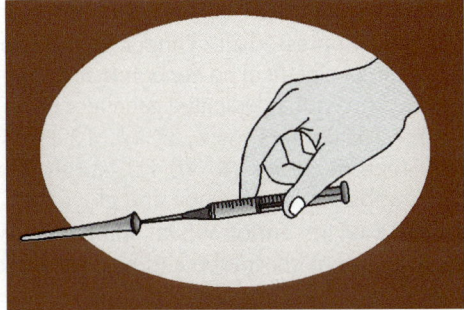

(b) With one hand, hold syringe and use needle to scoop up the cap

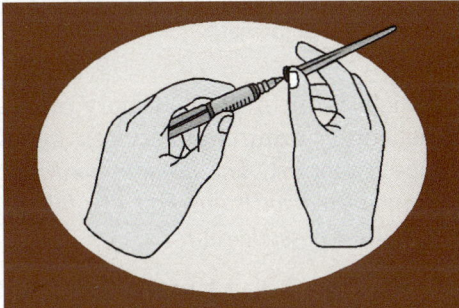

(c) When the cap covers the tip of the needle, use the other hand to place cap firmly on the needle hub

Figure 6.4 The steps for recapping the needle with one hand to avoid needle stick injury to the finger

occurred accidentally, post-exposure prophylaxis is advised. The aim of the post-exposure prophylaxis is to reduce or eliminate the risk of viral replication.

1. Encourage bleeding by squeezing, wash the wound thoroughly with soap and water and cover it with a waterproof sticking tape.
2. Determine the HIV status of the patient.
3. Counsel and check HIV status of the healthcare worker at baseline, 6 weeks, 3 months and 6 months after the incident.
4. *Low risk of infection.* Administer two nucleoside reverse transcriptase inhibitors namely zidovudine 300 mg twice a day or 200 mg three times a day plus lamivudine 150 mg twice a day for 4 weeks.

5. *High risk of infection.* Administer two nucleoside reverse transcriptase inhibitors plus protease inhibitors namely zidovudine 300 mg twice a day plus lamivudine 150 mg twice a day plus indinavir 800 mg three times a day or nelfinavir 750 mg three times a day for 4 weeks.

It is important to initiate the medications early, preferably within a few hours of exposure. However, it may be effective even if prophylaxis therapy is delayed for 1–2 weeks though its efficacy decreases. It is also important to monitor for drug toxicity by doing a complete blood count, renal and liver function tests at the baseline and 2 weeks after the start of therapy.

Isolation

Babies with thrush, diarrhea and draining abscesses should be isolated. Infants with certain congenital infections like cytomegalovirus (CMV) infection, congenital rubella syndrome, chickenpox and syphilis are highly contagious and should be isolated. Infants with congenital rubella syndrome may excrete the virus upto two years posing a special hazard to pregnant health care professionals. If a mother had developed chickenpox five days before or within two days after delivery, the baby should be isolated for three weeks.

6

TRANSPORT OF SICK NEONATES

Satisfactory transportation facilities are needed, whether a baby is being transported from one hospital to a regional or referral intensive care unit or simply within the hospital from NICU to the operation theater, imaging department or diagnostic laboratory. The short distance transport within the hospital can be accomplished in a transport incubator. The use of a plastic basket with perforated sides coupled with careful placing of hot water bottles or warm gel matresses is recommended for use in the rural setting. The baby can be wrapped in tin foil or covered with several layers of cotton and carried next to skin. Thermocole (polystyrene) box is an effective insulator and can be used in the community for transport of babies. Skin-to-skin contact with mother or a caretaker is a useful modality for transport in rural setting and resource poor situations. It is a sad reality that most transports in India are accomplished either by parents

Practical Tip

It is best to identify a high-risk mother during pregnancy and transfer her to a center having good perinatal services and NICU facilities because uterus is an ideal transport incubator.

in their own vehicle or by utilizing private ambulances without any dedicated equipment or trained staff. It is no wonder that most babies are cold, blue or hypoglycemic when they reach the referral NICU. Regionalization of perinatal services cannot be achieved unless a network of efficient neonatal transport services are established.

Indications for Neonatal Transport

When a high-risk mother is identified, it is best to transfer her to a center having NICU facilities because uterus is an ideal transport incubator. It is desirable that delivery should take place in a tertiary care center so that a sick or high-risk baby is not exposed to the risks of neonatal transport. The neonate is transferred to the nearby NICU, if the parent hospital is not equipped to look after the health care needs of the infant. Depending upon the facilities available at the birthing hospital, the following neonates are transferred to NICU providing tertiary care facilities.

- Preterm infants with a birth weight <1500 g or gestation <32 weeks.
- Respiratory distress requiring CPAP or assisted ventilation.
- Severe hypoxic–ischemic encephalopathy.
- Life-threatening sepsis.
- Intractable seizures.
- Severe jaundice with a need for exchange blood transfusion.
- Bleeding neonate.
- Major congenital anomalies or surgical neonate.
- Infants suspected to hence inborn errors of metabolism.
- Severe hyperbilirubinemia.
- Procedures or diagnostic facilities unavailable at the parent hospital.

Transport Team and Equipment

The neonates needing special or intensive care should preferably be transported by a skilled transport team. The receiving tertiary care NICU should have a dedicated team and a protocol for providing transport services. At least one senior resident and a specially trained neonatal nurse should report to the referring hospital to pick up the baby. The transport vehicle should be checked for availability of all equipment which should be in working order and essential supplies, disposables and life-saving drugs (Box 6.4). Customized transport ambulance should be equipped like a "mini-NICU" and should have a multi-channel vital sign monitor, portable incubator and a ventilator. The ambulance should be air conditioned, smooth in motion without any shaking and draughts of air. In India, most neonatal transports are achieved

Box 6.4 Equipment and supplies required during neonatal transport

- Transport incubator with multi-channel vital sign monitor for recording temperature, heart rate, blood pressure and oxygen saturation.
- CPAP facility with nasal prongs and portable ventilator (integral part of incubator or stand alone system).
- Airway equipment: Suction device, oral airway, T-piece device, nasal prongs, self or flow inflating bag and mask, laryngoscopes (size 00,0 and 1 blades) and endotracheal tubes (2.5, 3.0, 3.5, 4.0 mm).
- Infusion facilities: Infusates, infusion pumps, glucometer.
- Oxygen and compressed air cylinder, oxygen hood, heat and light source, electrical power points and adaptors and a power backup with a dedicated generator or an inverter.
- Disposables: Catheters (5, 6, 8, 10, 12 Fr), syringes, needles, feeding tubes (8, 10 Fr), surgical alcohol, betadine swabs, micropore tape and gloves, etc.
- Instrument tray for endotracheal intubation, vascular access, insertion of chest tube and nasogastric tube.
- Life-saving drugs.

1. All the equipment should have a battery backup and should be kept fully charged all the time.
2. Enough oxygen supply should be carried which should last during the duration of journey.

in a road vehicle; while in some tertiary care centers in the West, helicopter or aircraft services are used for a long distance transport. *The neonate needing transport should be transported with quickest available transport through the shortest possible route.*

Stabilization of the Baby before Transport

The condition of the baby should be assessed before transfer. The goal of every transport is to bring a sick neonate to a specialized neonatal center in a stable condition. To avoid complications during transport, the infant should be as stable as possible before leaving the referring hospital. Hypothermia, hypovolemia, hypoglycemia, acidosis and seizures should be treated before baby is transferred. Oral feeding should be stopped and an IV line established at a peripheral site or through umbilical vein for administration of 10% dextrose. Add 1 unit of heparin per mL of fluid, if infusion is given through an umbilical catheter. The infant with history of frequent apneic spells or severe respiratory distress syndrome should be decompressed by nasogastric aspiration and intubated before the start of journey. The baby should be placed in a prewarmed transport incubator and administered oxygen. The portable incubator provides an ideal micro-environment during transport. It is battery operated and has built-in system for oxygen supply (Figure 6.5).

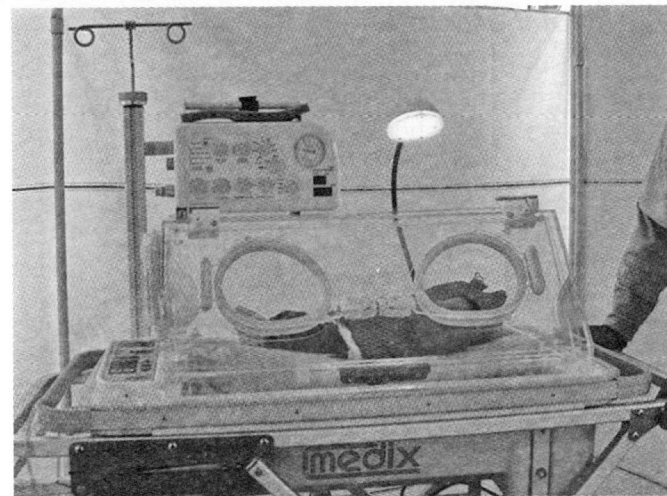

Figure 6.5 Battery-operated transport incubator with built-in oxygen supply and portable ventilator

The transport incubator should be light in weight but sturdy and should allow sufficient access to manage a critically ill baby. The transport team should estimate the amount of oxygen and air required during transport by assessing the distance, time required for journey and needs of the infant. The ambulance should be warm and well illuminated for observation of the baby. Temperature and color of the baby should receive due attention. Early transfer of a mildly ill baby is preferable to the transfer of a baby, whose condition has deteriorated to a state, when there is little hope for survival.

The principles of safe transport of sick babies are expressed by a number of mnemonics like **STABLE** where each alphabet stands for **S**ugar, **T**emperature, **A**irway, **B**lood pressure, **L**ab work and **E**motional support, **SAFER: S**ugar, **A**rterial circulatory support, **F**amily support, **E**nvironment, **R**espiratory support and **TOPS: T**emperature, **O**xygenation (airway and breathing), **P**erfusion and **S**ugar.

Protocol to be followed by the Referring Hospital

The neonate should be stabilized under the guidance of transport team of the referral NICU. The following management steps should be implemented and recorded.

- Maintain airway, oxygenation, thermal stability and tissue perfusion. In infants with RDS requiring long-distance transport, it is desirable to start CPAP through nasal prongs or nasopharyngeal catheter. It is recommended to intubate the baby before transport, if (i) infant with RDS needs ambient oxygen concentration of more than 40% (FiO_2 >0.4), (ii) recurrent apneic attacks, (iii) persistent seizures,

(iv) shock, (v) infant receiving prostaglandin E1 infusion for congenital heart lesion and (vi) congenital diaphragmatic hernia.
- Ensure umbilical or peripheral venous access and insert a nasogastric tube and decompress the stomach.
- Circulatory volume deficits of fluids and electrolytes should be replenished.
- Maintain adequate blood glucose level.
- Obtain culture samples and administer first dose of an appropriate antibiotic.
- Obtain a recent chest skiagram as a baseline and to check the position of catheters and tubes.
- Take the family member or parents along with the baby whenever feasible.
- When required, the transport team should undertake life-saving procedures (like endotracheal intubation, drainage of pneumothorax) and administer life-saving drugs, like surfactant and prostaglandin E1.
- The referring hospital should prepare a detailed transport note including copies of obstetric and neonatal charts for the transport team **(Box 6.5)**.

Care of the Baby during Transport

It is desirable to have a dedicated transport vehicle which should be adequately equipped to function like a mini or a portable NICU. The transport incubator and portable ventilator or stand alone CPAP facility

Box 6.5 | **Salient data to be recorded in the referral note prepared by the referring hospital**

- Name, address and contact details of the referring hospital.
- Detailed perinatal history, labor, delivery and neonatal resuscitation.
- Name of the baby (mother's name), date and time of birth, mode of delivery, gestational age, birth weight and weight at transfer.
- Neonatal problems, complete diagnosis, and treatment given before transfer.
- Condition of the baby at the time of transfer: Vital signs, arterial blood gases (ABG), complete blood counts (CBC), blood sugar, bilirubin, blood urea nitrogen (BUN), imaging studies, supportive care and medications given before transfer.
- The possible needs for emergency procedures during the transport.
- Reason/s for transport.
- Duly signed consent form by parents.
- The name/s and contact number/s of key personnel at the referral NICU.

should be securely fixed to the vehicle rails to avoid unnecessary jolts and jumps. The oxygen cylinder/s, air tank and monitoring equipment should be securely fastened. Depending upon the condition of the baby and duration of the journey, there should be sufficient supply of oxygen and air. There should be uninterrupted power source (dedicated generator, inverter, batteries) to operate the incubator, ventilator and monitoring equipment. Necessary adapters should be available to access the ambulance power source. The ambient conditions in the vehicle should ensure temperature stability, avoidance of excessive noise and vibrations and prevention of infection. The transport journey should be rapid and smooth without compromising the safety.

The ambulance temperature should be maintained above 26°C. In order to ensure optimal thermal control, availability of a transport incubator is ideal. When transport incubator is not available, thermal stability can be ensured through various improvisations like skin-to-skin contact, polythene covering, thermocole box or basket and use of phase-change warm gel mattress. Enteral feeds should be avoided in critically sick infants and they should preferably be given intravenous fluids. Infant should be positioned with slight extension of neck to maintain patency of the airway. Depending upon the respiratory studies and arterial oxygen saturation, infant may be provided with nasal CPAP through a T-piece resuscitator or attached to a ventilator. If tissue perfusion is poor (cold extremities, capillary refill time >2 sec or low blood pressure), infant should receive intravenous fluids with inotropes. The transport team should carefully observe the infant and various monitoring parameters so that corrective intervention/s are undertaken without any delay. The transport team should remain in constant touch with the nodal staff of the referral NICU to inform them about the latest condition of the baby and seek their expert guidance and advice during the course of transport.

Arrival at the Receiving NICU

The transport team should remain in constant touch with the referral NICU during the course of journey. The referral center should have a dedicated communication facility with mobile helplines operating 24 hours a day for ease of constant communication. The team should brief the NICU caregivers regarding the status of the baby and immediate clinical concerns. The clinical documents including referral note, copies of charts, consent form, radiographs, investigation reports, etc. should be handed over to the receiving unit. The referring hospital and parents of the baby (if not accompanying during transport) should be informed about the safe arrival and latest condition of the baby. The inventory of transport equipment should be checked, medications and essential supplies should be restocked for the next transport service. When infant has recovered from the underlying emergency and is stable for several days and he does not require intensive care, he is discharged or transported back (reverse transport) to the referring hospital.

BIBLIOGRAPHY

Deorari AK, Paul VK, Sachdeva A. Neonatal Equipment: Everything that you would like to know! *New Delhi, CBS Publishers and Distributors Pvt Ltd.*, 5th edition, 2017.

Gluck L (Ed.). Organization of perinatal care. *Clin Perinatology* 1976, 3: 267.

Gluck L. Design of perinatal center. *Pediatr Clin N Amer* 1979, 17: 777.

Malhotra AK, Deorari AK, Paul VK, Bagga A, Singh M. A new transport incubator for primary care of low birth weight babies. *Indian Pediatr* 1992, 29: 587–593.

Segal S, Pirie GE. Equipment and personnel for neonatal special care. *Pediatr Clin N Amer* 1970, 17: 793.

Singh M. Neonatal care perspectives in India (Editorial). *Indian J Pediatr* 1998, 65: 243–247.

Tyne MD. Concepts for improved nursery design. *Hospitals* 1974, 48: 66.

Woodward A, Insoft R, Kleinman N (Eds). Guidelines for Air and Ground Transport of Neonatal and Pediatric patients. 3rd edition, *American Academy of Pediatrics* 2007.

Care of Normal Birth Weight Newborns

The average birth weight of a newborn baby in India is around 2.8 kg. About 90 percent of babies are born after full term (37–41 weeks) while 10 to 15 percent of babies are delivered prematurely (less than 37 weeks of gestation). A large number of newborn babies (around 85%) require minimal care which can be effectively provided by the mother under the supervision and guidance of a nurse or health worker. The basic care of a healthy newborn baby can be provided at home, subcenter, primary health center or rooming-in ward of a hospital or nursing home. *It is desirable that normal babies should not be kept in a separate nursery but roomed-in along with their mothers.* Rooming-in policy is conducive to promote better emotional rapport between the mother and the baby. The mother can participate in the day-to-day chores and nursing care of her baby. This policy infuses self-confidence in the mother and reduces the demands on the nursing personnel. The risk of cross-infection is reduced and breastfeeding can be established more readily.

Practical Tip

Healthy babies above 2 kg and babies born by elective cesarean section should not be kept in the nursery but roomed-in with their mothers to promote bonding and breastfeeding.

ESSENTIAL NEWBORN CARE

There should be equitable distribution of resources for care of mothers and babies in the community and establishment of high-tech newborn care facilities by creation of a network of special care and intensive care neonatal units in a phased manner. The components of essential newborn care services include good quality antenatal care (at least 5 ANC contacts), safe delivery and optimal care at birth, prevention and early treatment of hypothermia and bacterial infections, and promotion of exclusive breastfeeding. The delivery should be conducted by a skilled health worker in a nearby health care facility or hospital. The moderately low birth weight babies (birth weight >1800 g and/or gestation >34 weeks) account for 90% of LBW babies and they should be provided essential newborn care at home or primary health care facility. The detailed components of essential newborn care are listed in **Box 7.1**. *There is a need for greater focus on the preventive rather than curative strategies because a large number of neonatal deaths occur due to potentially preventable disorders like birth asphyxia, hypothermia, hypoglycemia and septicemia.* The provision of essential newborn care in the community is the most urgent priority in our country and saving newborn babies is a national priority in order achieve further reduction in infant and under-5 mortality rate.

Care at Birth

After having ensured that the baby has established effective breathing, it is essential that all efforts are made to prevent the occurrence of hypothermia. The baby should be promptly dried and effectively covered with pre-warmed clothes. The neonate should be placed under a radiant warmer during the procedure of resuscitation. A sterile disposable delivery kit should be used for each baby to prevent cross-infection. The eyes should be cleaned with sterile normal saline using one swab for each eye. When prophylaxis against gonococcal ophthalmia is required, it can be ensured either by instillation of 1.0 percent silver nitrate drops or 0.5 percent tetracycline or erythromycin ophthalmic ointment. The umbilical cord should be tied using two ligatures or rubber band or a disposable clip. The clip or ligature should be applied at least 2 or 3 cm beyond the base of the cord to avoid inadvertent incision of gut contained in minor exomphalos. The base and tip

Nursing Alert

Efforts should be made to keep the babies effectively dried, covered and warm at birth. Baby bath should not be given in the labor room.

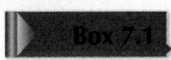

Box 7.1   **Essential components of perinatal and neonatal care**

Antenatal Care

- Provide at least four good quality antenatal check-ups.
- Improve the caloric and protein intake and provide anemia prophylaxis to the mother.
- Screen and treat infections especially syphilis, AIDS and malaria.
- Administer two doses of tetanus toxoid, the second dose should be given at least 4 weeks before delivery.
- Provide information and counseling for birth preparedness, awareness of danger signs, preparation and promotion of early and exclusive breastfeeding.

Care at Birth

- Ensure facility-based delivery or delivery by skilled birth attendant.
- Ensure five cleans: Clean hands, clean delivery surface, clean blade, clean cord tie, clean undressed cord without application of any home remedies.
- Early referral to a higher level of care if required.

Essential Newborn Care

- Keep the newborn warm: Dry and wrap the baby including head, dress the baby, provide skin-to-skin contact, avoid exposure.
- Give prophylactic eye care
- Avoid bath till cord has fallen
- Initiate immediate and exclusive breastfeeding within one hour of birth without any prelacteal or supplementary feeds. Promote exclusive breastfeeding (even water should not be given during hot summer months) during first 6 months of life.
- Maintain hygiene to prevent infections: Provide guidance to mother on personal hygiene, handwashing with soap and water, avoidance of unnecessary handling.
- Provide guidance to mother to identify and manage common developmental disorders.
- Early postnatal contact by health worker to identify and manage common illnesses.
- Provide immunizations such as BCG, OPV and hepatitis B vaccines soon after birth.
- Promote birth spacing.

Care of Future Mothers

- Equal opportunities for education and health care to girls.
- Improve the nutrition of girls throughout their life cycle: Infancy, childhood, adolescence, pregnancy and lactation.
- Discourage early marriages and teenage pregnancies.
- Improve the status and financial independence of women in the society.
- Improve women's health and family planning services.
- Promote safe sexual practices.

Adapted from State of the World's Newborns, 2014.

of the umbilical stump should be painted with triple dye or surgical alcohol. The cord should be inspected 2–3 hours after birth for bleeding because the ligature may become loose as the cord shrinks. Vitamin K 0.5 to 1.0 mg is administered intramuscularly to all babies to prevent occurrence of hemorrhagic disease of the newborn. The baby must have an identification tag before it is transferred out of the labor room.

Identification of Congenital Malformations

Quick but thorough clinical screening is essential to identify any life-threatening congenital anomalies and birth injuries. The cut end of the umbilical cord should be inspected for the number of blood vessels. Normally there are two umbilical arteries and one umbilical vein. The presence of a single umbilical artery is associated with internal congenital malformations in 15 to 20 percent of cases. The commonly associated malformations include esophageal atresia, imperforate anus and genitourinary anomalies. Single palmar crease (Simian crease) has increased association with additional anomalies including Down syndrome. The face and head should be closely observed for any asymmetry and dysmorphic features. *The infant should be examined for location and patency of all the orifices because anomalies are frequently encountered around the orifices.* The oral cavity must be examined to exclude the cleft palate. The patency of the esophagus should be checked by passing a stiff rubber catheter into the stomach in the following situations:

1. Small-for-dates baby
2. Single umbilical artery
3. Polyhydramnios
4. Excessive drooling of saliva
5. Choking during feeding

If there is no esophageal atresia and the catheter has reached the stomach, gastric contents should be aspirated. When gastric aspirate exceeds 20 mL in volume, it is strongly suggestive of high intestinal obstruction due to pyloric or duodenal atresia. The anomalies are also concentrated over the midline areas in front and back, e.g. spina bifida, meningomyelocele, pilonidal sinus, ambiguous genitalia, hypospadias, exomphalos, cleft lip, cleft palate, etc. The abdomen should be palpated for any masses and heart examined

Practical Tip

Examine the location and patency of all the body orifices and screen the midline areas of the baby both infront and back because congenital malformations are located at these sites.

for its position and any murmurs. The presence of abdominal distension with three masses, enlarged kidneys and distended urinary bladder, are suggestive of bladder neck obstruction. Displacement of the heart towards the right side in association with respiratory difficulty and resuscitation problems, is suggestive of either diaphragmatic hernia or pneumothorax on the left side.

Breastfeeding

Breastfeeding is natural and instinctive. The preparation and motivation for breastfeeding should begin during the antenatal period. The cracked and retracted nipples should be managed before the baby is born. The baby should be placed on the abdomen of the mother immediately after delivery to provide warmth and contact with the mother which helps to promote bonding and breastfeeding. The mother is advised to put the baby to the breast as soon as she has recovered from the exhaustion of labor. Most babies can be put to the breast within one hour of birth. There is no need for any prelacteal feeds like glucose water, honey or tea. For details regarding breastfeeding and nutrition of babies, refer to **Chapter 15**.

Maintenance of Body Temperature

Newborn babies are homeothermic but their thermoregulatory mechanisms are physiologically unsatisfactory. They are very prone to develop hypothermia unless adequate precautions are taken to protect them. The environmental temperature that may feel relatively uncomfortable to an adult may impose serious thermal stress to a newborn baby. The baby must be kept dried and effectively clothed using a cap and socks. The ritual of bathing babies at birth must be condemned. The baby bath should be delayed till the next day when his temperature has stabilized. During winter, the linen and clothes of the baby should be prewarmed before dressing. The room should be kept warm in winter with the help of a heater. The baby should be nursed in close proximity to the mother so that the baby is kept warm by maternal warmth. When a baby is effectively covered, his hands and feet are likely to be warm and pink. The cultural practice of keeping the mother and baby isolated for 40 days is useful and needs to be promoted. It prevents exposure of the baby to cold and safeguards against the

Nursing Alert

When hands and feet of a baby are cold, it means that baby has cold stress or is unwell. The baby must be provided with warmth and examined for any evidences of infection.

occurrence of infections. In summer months, depending upon the environmental temperature, the baby should be dressed in loose cotton clothes and kept indoors as far as possible. Exposure of the baby to direct sunlight during the hot summer months can lead to serious hyperthermia and skin damage.

Body Massage

In India, body massage is popular and is credited to provide various health benefits. Massage improves circulation, increases muscle tone and relieves fatigue. Some oil may get absorbed through the thin skin of the baby to serve as a source of nutrition. It improves the texture of the skin and reduces dryness. Touch is believed to send stimulatory messages to the brain to enhance neuromotor development of the baby. The baby should be at least 3 kg in weight before massage is given. Any mild non-irritating non-scented vegetable oil like olive oil or coconut oil can be used. Mustard oil should preferably be avoided in infants because it is pungent to the eyes and irritating to the skin. The use of almond oil or mineral oil is not recommended as they may clog the skin pores. Massage should be given before bathing the baby. The room should be warm and without any draughts. The oil should be rubbed between the palms to bring it to the body temperature. Massage should be done by using gentle pressure and smooth rhythmical movements (**Figure 7.1**).

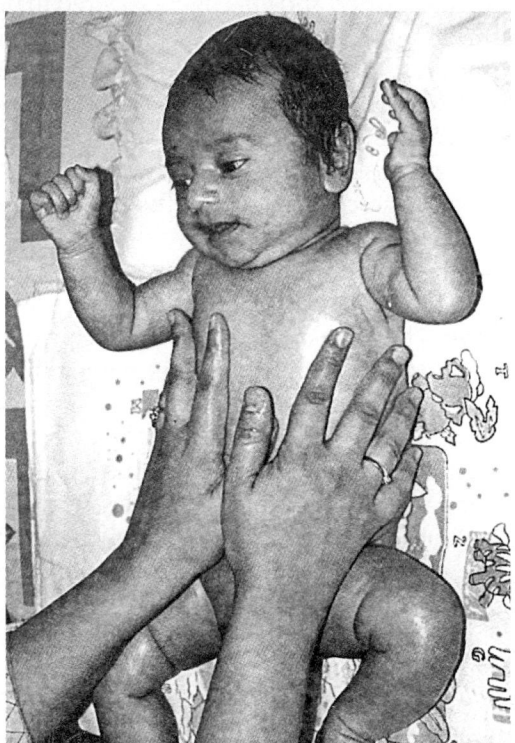

Figure 7.1 The baby is being given an oil massage before the bath

Massage the baby first while he is lying on his back and then when he is made to lie on his tummy. Begin from trunk and move towards the limbs. The direction of massaging movements should be in both the directions from center towards periphery of the body and limbs, and *vice versa*. You should make passive exercising movements of all the limbs during the massage. Mother must talk with her baby or let him listen to melodious music during the massage session. Most children love to be massaged and they often giggle and make various sounds during the procedure. When weather is pleasant and not windy, baby can be massaged in the sun to provide additional benefit of vitamin D, which is produced in the skin under the influence of ultraviolet rays of the sun.

Bathing of Babies

There is no hurry to give a bath to a baby at birth because she has been swimming for 9 months in a warm pool of water (amniotic fluid). At birth the baby should be immediately dried and effectively covered to prevent exposure. However, babies born to HIV-positive or HBsAg-positive mother should be bathed as soon as possible after birth to remove the maternal blood and secretions covering the skin of the baby. Gloves should be worn to bathe such a baby. Babies are usually coated with a protective cheezy light-yellow material called vernix caseosa particularly in the folds of neck, armpits and groins. No vigorous attempts should be made to clean it off to prevent any damage to the delicate skin of the baby. The skin should be gently cleaned off any blood, mucus or meconium (some babies may pass meconium in the womb) by a soft towel. Scalp should be effectively dried. The baby should not be unnecessarily disturbed after birth. He should be effectively clothed and provided with the closeness and warmth of his mother. The bath can be given on the second or third day. In many hospitals, no baby bath is given during the hospital stay of the baby.

Sponge Bath

As long as the umbilical stump is attached to the navel, dip baths should be avoided. The baby can be sponged. The diaper areas should be gently but thoroughly cleaned during every diaper change. Take warm water in a basin and two soft sponge towels. Place the baby on a large fluffy towel in a warm and comfortable room. Keep the baby wrapped in a towel and expose only those parts of his body, which are being sponged. The face should be sponged first by using a dampened cloth without any soap. Then sponge rest of the body by using damp sponge soaked with a mild liquid soap by paying special attention to creases like neck, behind the ears, armpits and groins. Wash the skin with a wet towel to remove all traces of soap. Diaper area showed by washed in the end, first with a soapy sponge towel followed by a towel soaked in plain water.

Dip Bath

When umbilical cord has fallen and navel has healed, mother or nurse can give dip baths. Depending upon the weather, liking and health status of the baby, there is no need to give a bath everyday. The bath should be given in a room which is warm and free of draught. The fan and airconditioner should be switched off. You should collect all the items needed during and after the bath and keep them by your side (**Box 7.2**). The plastic basin or baby tub should be filled up to half to two-thirds with comfortably warm water. The baby's skin is very delicate and only a mild acidic soap solution (pH 5.5) should be used. The soap bar should not contain any alkaline detergent that can destroy the skin barriers and cause flaking, scaling and dryness of skin. The newborn baby can be straddled on the legs and his head should be supported. After a couple of months, the baby can be placed in the water tub and his back and head are supported on your left hand and arm. The baby's bottom should be cleaned if it is soiled with stools before placing the baby in the tub.

Box 7.2　Items for baby bath

- Bath tub or a wide plastic basin of a bright color.
- Bucket of warm water or put the geyser on.
- One large fluffy towel and two baby napkins and soft towels.
- Baby oil, shampoo, soap, talcum powder, moisturizing lotion.
- Cotton balls and cotton buds.
- Surgical alcohol or triple dye or betadine lotion.
- Baby dress, napkin and safety pins.

First the baby's head should be washed by using a no-tear baby shampoo (**Figure 7.2**). When there is cradle cap, apply coconut oil or milk cream (*malai*) over the scalp followed by shampoo after half an hour. The lather should be rinsed by pouring water with a mug after placing your hand over his forehead so that soapy water drains out from the sides and does not enter the eyes. Do it several times to remove all traces of shampoo. Dry the scalp with a baby towel before proceeding further. If some soap manages to enter the eyes and baby cries, clean them with a damp towel soaked in warm plain water till all traces of soap are removed. Baby's face should be washed next, taking care to thoroughly clean the creases behind the ears and neck. This is followed by washing the trunk and extremities by paying special attention to armpits, groins and hands. Baby's bottom and diaper area should be thoroughly washed with soap and water in the end. Most babies enjoy taking their bath and hate being taken out of the tub. A couple of plastic toys floating around in the tub water add to the fun and joy of the bath.

After the bath, baby should be covered in a large fluffy towel (**Figure 7.3**). The skin should be dabbed dry with a baby towel instead of firmly wiping it. There is no virtue in using talcum powder but it does impart a pleasing odor to the baby. *Never sprinkle powder over the baby because she can get choked by inhaling it or it can enter the eyes.* Take a small amount of powder on your finger tips and dab it over the neck, chest, armpits and groins.

Bottom Care

Bottom is constantly soiled by urine and stools and must be kept clean at all times. As soon as the baby has passed urine or stool, the bottom should be cleaned with wet cotton and dried immediately. If the diaper area remains soiled by stools for a long time, the baby may develop nappy rash. In girls, there is a potential risk of development of ascending urinary tract infection. In order to prevent contamination of vulva with feces, water should be poured from front and washing hand stroked from front to backwards. In boys, soakage of penis with urine and stools may lead to development of scarring of the prepuce (foreskin) which may lead to difficulty in passing urine.

Care of Skin and Nails

Skin of a newborn is delicate and should be washed with a mild acidic detergent (pH 5.5) containing two gentle surfactants, alkyl carboxylate (soap) and acyl isethionate (syndet) which help in maintaining 'acid mantle' of the skin and reduce transepidermal water loss. The soap bar should not contain any alkaline

7

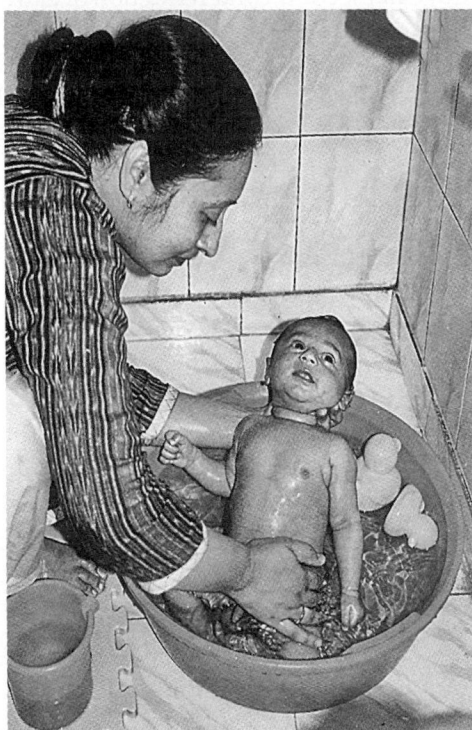

Figure 7.2 The baby enjoys being placed in a plastic basin filled with luke warm water. Floating rubber toys adds to the fun

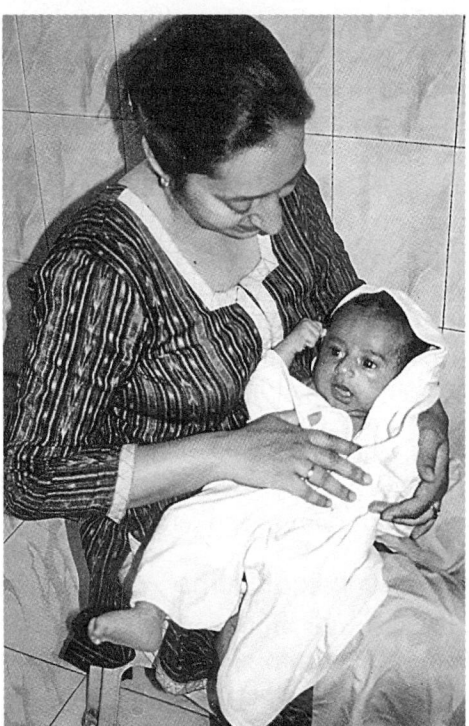

Figure 7.3 The baby should be dried and completely covered with a fluffy cotton towel to avoid exposure after the bath

detergents (pH 9–11) that can destroy the skin barriers and cause flaking, scaling and dryness of the skin. A baby skin lotion or moisturizer cream can be applied to keep the skin supple. During winter, woolens stored with moth balls (naphthalene balls) must be exposed to the sun for several hours before use. The baby with G6PD deficiency may react to naphthalene leading to development of hemolysis and severe jaundice.

The nails should be kep trimmed so that baby can't scratch himself. Nails can be trimmed with a blunt-nosed baby scissors or infant nail clippers when baby is asleep. During early life, the finger nails grow so quickly that they need to be trimmed twice a week. By contrast the toe nails grow rather slowly and need to be trimmed once or twice a month.

Care of Eyes, Mouth, Nose and Ears

Nature takes care to keep these organs and orifices clean. Tears keep the eyes wet and shining. In newborn babies, instillation of few drops of colostrum has been shown to reduce the risk of development of sticky eyes. Lids should be cleaned with a damp soft cloth during bathing. There is no need to put *surma* or *kajal* in the eyes as it can cause irritation, cross infection and even lead intoxication. There is no scientific basis to the commonly held belief that putting *kajal* or *surma* in the eyes improves eye sight or make the eyes bigger and beautiful. Home-made *kajal* or eyeliner can be used by girls later on as an inherent part of Indian tradition.

Clean the outside and back of the ears with a clean damp cloth. No effort should be made to remove any wax from the ear with a cotton bud or hair pin. Wax provides protection to the ear canal. The nostrils should be cleaned with a damp cloth or cotton bud. The dry crusts in the nose can be removed with a moistened cotton bud or a wisp of damp cloth. *The custom of pouring oil in the baby's nostrils and ears is dangerous and not recommended.* It may lead to development of aspiration pneumonia and fungal infection. The tongue usually does not need any cleaning. The whitish patch on the tongue due to sticking of milk is quite normal. If mother is concerned, you can ask her to clean it with a wet piece of gauze or damp handkerchief.

Care of the Umbilical Stump

The umbilical cord is an important portal of entry for *Clostridium tetani* in domiciliary midwifery. Health personnel must be told the importance of using a sterile disposable *dai-kit* to prevent the occurrence of tetanus neonatorum. Even when a new shaving blade is used for cutting the cord, it must be sterilized by boiling before it is used. Umbilical stump must be inspected

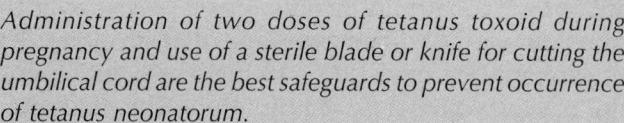

Nursing Alert

Administration of two doses of tetanus toxoid during pregnancy and use of a sterile blade or knife for cutting the umbilical cord are the best safeguards to prevent occurrence of tetanus neonatorum.

after 2 to 4 hours of clamping. Bleeding may occur at this time due to shrinkage of cord and loosening of the ligature. The use of a rubber band or disposable clip safeguards against this hazard. Triple dye, betadine or ethyl alcohol should be applied at the tip and around the base of the umbilical stump every day to prevent colonization. The cord must be left open without any dressing. The cord usually falls after 5 to 10 days but may take longer if it has been kept moistened or when it gets infected or the baby is having an immunodeficiency disorder.

Weight Record

Most healthy term babies loose weight during the first 2 to 3 days of life. The weight loss is usually up to 5 to 7 percent of birth weight. The weight remains stationary during next one to two days and birth weight is regained by the end of first week. The factors contributing to physiological weight loss include removal of vernix caseosa, mucus and blood from the skin, passage of meconim and reduction of extracellular fluid volume. Delayed feeding and unsatisfactory feeding schedule is associated with excessive weight loss. Babies who are given exclusive breastfeeding are likely to have greater weight loss due to poor lactation during first few days after delivery.

They is no need to monitor early weight changes in a healthy newborn baby because it can cause unnecessary anxiety to the mother and may lead to lactation failure. Babies who are adequately fed, they are contented, playful, have good sleep and are satisfied for at least two to three hours after a feed. The adequately fed baby passes urine at least 5 to 6 times during the day while many babies may pass urine (even stools) after each feed during the first 3 months of life. The average daily weight gain is around 30 g, 20 g and 10 g during the first, second, third 4 months periods

Practical Tip

Early administration of hepatitis B vaccine (within 72 hours of birth) can reduce the risk of vertical transmission of hepatitis B virus from mother to her infant. When mother is HBsAg-positive (especially hepatitis e antigen positive), she must also receive hepatitis B-specific immunoglobulins along with hepatitis B vaccine.

respectively during the first year of life. Most infants double their birth weight by 4 to 5 months of age and triple it by their first birth day.

Immunizations

It is recommended to give BCG and a first dose of hepatitis B and oral polio vaccine as early as possible preferably within the first week of life. The mother should be explained that the child must receive all the vaccinations at the proper time as recommended by the physician. For details of immunization schedule, refer to **Chapter 21**.

Early Identification of Disease

Most mothers do observe their babies carefully and are often worried by minor physical peculiarities and developmental problems which are of no serious consequence. She must be adequately informed and appropriately advised regarding minor health problems to prevent undue anxiety, concern and worry. The baby-mother dyad should be approached twice a day to enquire about any feeding problems, vomiting, bowel disorders, physiological jaundice, adequacy of body temperature and relieve the anxiety of the mother regarding various developmental peculiarities and minor physical problems which may be bothering her. The onset and intensity of jaundice should be watched in good natural day light. The infant should be closely watched for danger signs which should be brought to the attention of the physician for prompt management (**Box 7.3**).

Box 7.3 | Danger signs

1. Bleeding from any site
2. Appearance of jaundice within 24 hours of age or deep yellow staining of trunk, palms and soles
3. Failure to pass meconium within 24 hours or urine within 48 hours of birth
4. Persistent vomiting or diarrhea*
5. Poor feeding
6. Undue lethargy or excessive crying
7. Drooling of saliva or choking during feeding
8. Respiratory difficulty, apneic attacks or cyanosis
9. Sudden rise or fall in body temperature (cold extremities)
10. Seizures
11. Evidences of superficial infections such as conjunctivitis, pustules, umbilical sepsis, oral thrush, etc.

---

*Passage of stool after each feed may occur in some babies due to increased gastrocolic reflex and should not be labeled as diarrhea.

HOME CARE

The following guidelines should be given and explained to every mother when a newborn is discharged from the hospital.

1. **Promotion of exclusive breastfeeding** The mother should be advised to give exclusive breastfeeding (no water should be given even during hot summer months) to the baby on demand both during the day and night. She should be in a relaxed state of mind and take a nutritious balanced diet with nutritional supplements to promote lactation and improve the nutritional quality of the breast-milk. When the baby is jaundiced at discharge, the mothers should be asked to breastfeed the baby frequently. The practice of exposing the jaundiced baby to sunlight is neither useful nor safe and is not recommended.

2. **Temperature regulation** Room temperature should be maintained between 28°C and 30°C and baby should be clothed in accordance with weather conditions. In winter, the baby must be worn a cap, socks and mittens and kept effectively covered with woolens and should lie next to mother or provided with skin-to-skin contact. The mother should be explained how to assess the temperature of a baby by touch. When trunk and extremities of the baby are warm to touch, it indicates that the baby is healthy and without any cold stress. When trunk is warm but extremities are cold and pale, the baby has cold stress and will not have satisfactory weight gain because calories will be consumed for metabolic thermogenesis.

3. **Prevention of infections** Mother-baby dyad should be kept isolated in one room for a month. Visitors should be discouraged to touch or kiss the baby. The baby should be picked after washing hands with soap and water. Baby massage should be started after one month and when baby weight is more than 3 kg.

4. **Provide guidance for vaccinations** Bacillus Calmette-Guerin (BCG), hepatitis B and oral polio vaccines are given to the baby before discharge. Early administration of hepatitis B vaccine (within 72 hours

---

Nursing Alert

The practice of exposing a jaundiced neonate to direct sunlight is not recommended because it is neither effective nor safe for the baby.

of birth) can reduce the risk of vertical transmission of hepatitis B virus from the mother to her infant. When mother is hepatitis E antigen positive, the baby must also receive hepatitis B-specific immune globulins along with hepatitis B vaccine at two different sites. The mother should be given the vaccination schedule and explained about the timely administration of vaccines and monitoring of growth parameters on the "Road-to-Health" card.

BIBLIOGRAPHY

Lix, Zhong Q, Tang L. A meta-analysis of the efficacy and safety of using oil massage to promote infant growth. *J Pediatr Nursing* 2016. DOI: http://dx.doi.org/10.1016/jpedn2016.04.003.

Singh M. Care of a newborn baby. In: The Art and Science of Baby and Child Care. *New Delhi, CBS Publishers and Distributors Pvt Ltd* 4th Edition 2015, p 37–53.

Singh M. Care of normal newborn babies: Some practical points. *Indian J Pract Pediatr* 1993, 1:6–13.

7

Resuscitation of an Asphyxiated Newborn

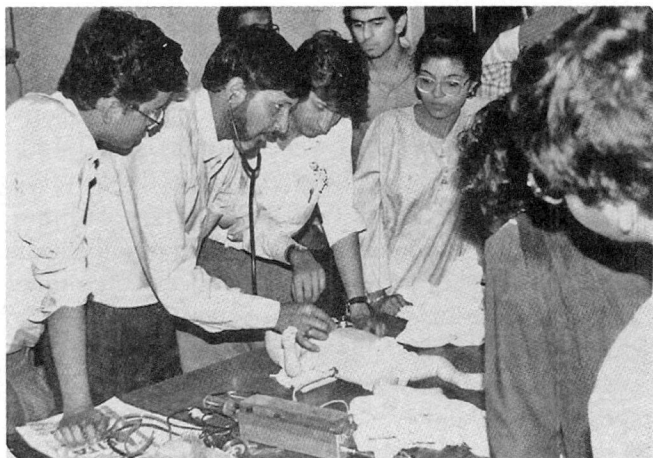

> *"Every birth must be considered as a medical emergency and we must be prepared to handle 26 million emergencies every year in our country."*
> — **Meharban Singh**

Every birth must be considered as a medical emergency and labor room must be provided with adequate infrastructure and facilities for resuscitation of babies who fail to establish spontaneous breathing. Perinatal hypoxia is one of the leading causes of perinatal mortality in developing countries. Most babies have a smooth transition from fetal to neonatal life and they are able to establish spontaneous breathing without any assistance. But 5.0–7.5% of neonates are likely to face difficulties in initiating spontaneous breathing at birth and they need active resuscitation. Every nurse must have the training and expertise to resuscitate an apneic or asphyxiated newborn baby (**Figure 8.1**).

Figure 8.1 Neonatal resuscitation workshop being conducted for training of medical students

FETAL HYPOXIA

The existence of certain high-risk factors during pregnancy and labor should be looked for because they provide a warning to the labor room staff that they should be fully prepared to resuscitate an asphyxiated baby (**Box 8.1**). All high-risk pregnancies should be monitored for fetal growth, presence of congenital malformations, adequacy of placental functions and evidences of fetal hypoxia. Mother should be advised to maintain fetal activity record by counting the number of fetal "quickenings" or movements during third trimester of pregnancy. The mother is asked to watch for fetal movements during morning, noon and evening for a period of one hour each. The total fetal count is multiplied by 4 to get a fetal movement count for 12 hours. The fetus is considered as healthy and well if it produces at least one movement per hour.

Fetal biophysical profile (Manning score) is a useful non-invasive parameter of fetal well being and is assessed by ultrasound examination during third

High-risk conditions associated with fetal hypoxia and birth asphyxia

1. Fetal distress
2. Placental insufficiency (Pregnancy-induced hypertension, toxemia, poor fetal growth, post maturity)
3. Premature labor
4. Ante-partum hemorrhage
5. Malpresentation, difficult and abnormal or operative delivery
6. Cord prolapse
7. Rhesus-isoimmunization
8. Multifetal gestation
9. Bad obstetrical history
10. Use of anesthetics, analgesics and narcotics during labor.

trimester of pregnancy. A combination of five fetal biophysical variables like fetal posture, fetal breathing movements, gross body movements, reactive fetal heart rate (acceleration of fetal heart rate with fetal body movements) and volume of amniotic fluid are used to assign fetal risk.

During labor, nonstress test is used to simultaneously and continuously monitor fetal heart rate in response to fetal movements and uterine contractions with the help of a cardiotocometer. Fetus is considered as "reactive" and without any distress if he can demonstrate acceleration of his heart beats by 15 or more beats for 15 seconds in association with fetal movements at least twice in a 20-minute recording period. A persistently slow fetal heart rate without any variability in response to fetal movements or uterine contractions is indicative of fetal hypoxia.

In addition to technology-based monitoring of the fetus, the following time-honored clinical parameters of fetal distress offer useful guidelines to an experienced nurse.

Exaggerated fetal movements The asphyxiated fetus behaves like a strangulated individual and makes desperate physical efforts or movements. After some time, this is followed by slow or reduced fetal movements which finally stop when fetus dies in utero.

Fetal heart rate Due to release of catecholamines, initially there is tachycardia followed by bradycardia and slow or irregular heart beats. The heart rate should be checked during later phase of uterine contraction with a fetoscope.

Passage of meconium in utero The passage of meconium in the uterus in a vertex presenting baby is an important and ominous sign of fetal distress. It is fraught with the risk of aspiration of meconium by the gasping fetus.

Assessment of the Infant at Birth

Despite its limitation, Apgar scoring system is conventionally used for assessing the condition of a newborn baby at one minute after birth (**Table 8.1**). The respiratory efforts and heart beats are the most critical components of Apgar scoring system because muscle tone, response to reflex stimulus and color are dependent upon the gestational maturity and cardiorespiratory status of the baby.

When one-minute Apgar score is 3 or less, it should be checked after every 5 minutes till score is atleast 7 or above. *Apgar score does not provide any useful guidelines for providing resuscitation to the baby but it is useful to predict future outcome of the baby*. When 10 minutes Apgar score is 3 or less, or there are no spontaneous breathing movements by 10 minutes, the baby is likely to develop neuromotor disability during follow-up.

Basic Care of a Normal Baby at Birth

There is no consensus regarding the ideal time for clamping the umbilical cord. In most deliveries, a relaxed approach should be followed for clamping the cord, neither immediate nor deliberate delay, should be practiced. Delayed clamping of the cord is associated with smoother transition from dependent fetal to independent neonatal cardiorespiratory physiology, lower risk of respiratory distress and iron deficiency anemia in the baby. Early clamping of the cord is advocated in babies with severe birth asphyxia, cord around the neck and rhesus isoimmunization. Holding the baby in an inverted position by the feet and slapping over the buttocks or squeezing the stomach or chest should be avoided. Nearly 90% of newborns are vigorous term babies with no risk factors and clear amniotic fluid. They can be directly placed on the mother's abdomen or chest, dried effectively and covered with dry linen. Warmth is maintained by direct skin-to-skin contact with the mother which also facilitates bonding and promotion of breastfeeding. The baby's mouth and nose should be wiped with a gauze piece or suction bulb to clear the upper airways. In regions with high risk of gonococcal ophthalmia, silver nitrate 1% or

---

Plea of a baby at birth

"I have come from an extremely warm, clean, quiet and comfortable abode, protect me at birth from microbes and cold. I am born wet and naked, dry me, cover me and place me under a heater.

I do not know how to smile, let me announce my arrival with a cry. Do not hurt me but gently clean my wind pipe to let me cry.

Do not give me injection but give me a breath to save my life. I have been swimming for 9 months in the womb, do not be in a hurry to bathe me in the labor room."

— **Meharban Singh**

Table 8.1 Apgar scoring system			
	Score		
Criteria	0	1	2
1. Breathing	Nil	Slow or gasping	Crying
2. Heart rate/min	Nil	Up to 100	More than 100
3. Tone	Flaccid	In-between	Flexed
4. Reflex response	Nil	Grimace	Cry
5. Color	Blue or pale	Peripheral cyanosis	Pink

tetracycline/erythromycin ophthalmic ointment are instilled in the eyes. Injection vitamin K 0.5–1.0 mg is given by intramuscular injection. Identification tag is affixed and an effectively dressed baby is shifted to the rooming-in ward along with the mother. No bathing facilities should be available in the labor room and bath should be delayed to the next day except when a baby is born to a mother who is either HBsAg-positive or HIV-positive.

Resuscitation Kit

The resuscitation table or trolley must be available in the same room where the mother is being delivered. Each delivery room should have a well lighted and warm micro-environment to receive the newborn baby. The resuscitation tray must contain a pencil handle laryngoscope with infant blade, Ambu bag and mask, De Lee suction trap, gamma-irradiated disposable endotracheal tubes with internal diameters of 2.0, 2.5, 3.0, 4.5 mm mounted with adapters, suction catheters, syringes and needles, 7.5 percent sodium bicarbonate solution, epinephrine 1 in 10,000 solution, nalorphine or naloxone, physiological saline solution and 5 percent dextrose (**Figure 8.2**).

Electrical points and the suction machine should be in working order. The oxygen cylinder should be checked for its contents. Sterile neonatal packs containing a bowl, scissors, cotton swabs and umbilical ties or clamp should be available for each delivery. The bassinet on which the baby is received should be kept warm and provided with an overhead radiant heat source and a stop clock to accurately time the sequence of events after birth (**Figure 8.3**). It is mandatory that the resuscitation kit should be checked by the staff nurse on every duty shift and rechecked by the physician before each delivery. It is essential that the equipment for resuscitation should be maintained in a sterile condition and baby should be received in a sterile and warm sheet with due aseptic precautions. Above all, the physician and nurse attending the delivery must be skilled and experienced in the art of cardiopulmonary resuscitation.

Care of a Meconium-Stained Baby

The amniotic fluid is meconium stained in 10–15 percent of deliveries. As soon as the head is delivered, when rest of the baby is still in utero, the oral cavity, oropharynx and hypopharynx should be sucked with a wide bored 12 Fr or a larger sized catheter. The

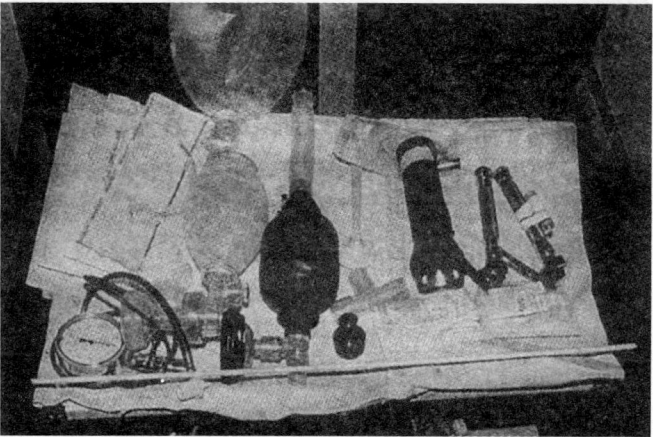

Figure 8.2 Resuscitation kit. Note corrugated tube attached at the inlet of Ambu bag to enhance concentration of oxygen delivered to the infant

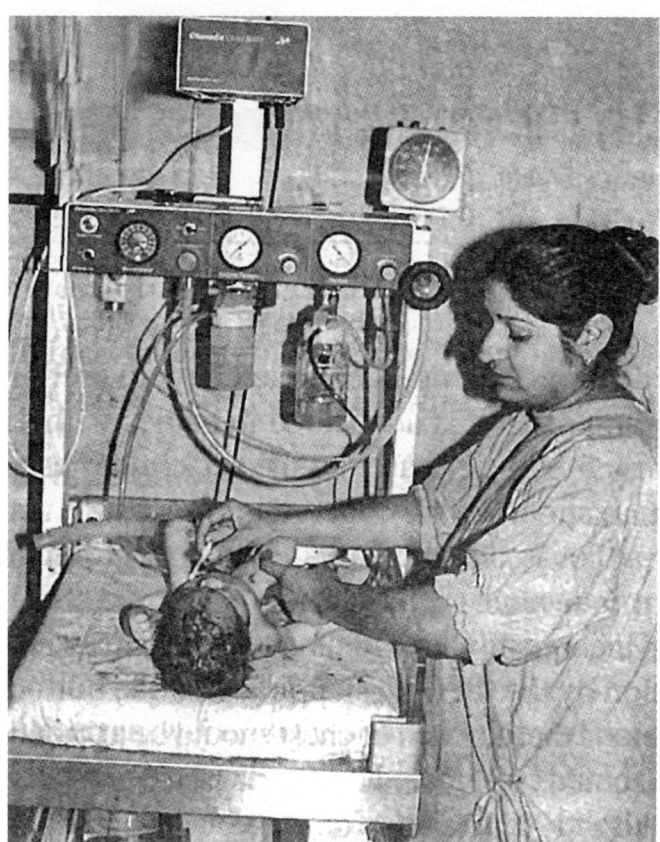

Figure 8.3 Resuscitation with overhead warmer and in-built facilities for suction, oxygen supply and intermittent positive pressure ventilation

practice is no longer followed because there is evidence to suggest that most meconium-stained babies aspirate meconium in-utero before they are born. After separation of the baby from mother, thorough suction of the oropharyngeal area should be done under direct vision with the help of a laryngoscope. If the baby is active, crying vigorously, having good muscle tone and

---

Nursing Tip

No facilities should be available in the labor room to bathe the newborn babies.

a heart rate of >100 beats/min, no further resuscitation is needed. When a baby is sluggish, depressed, not crying or having heart rate of <100 beats/min, endotracheal intubation should be done. Endotracheal tube (ET) is directly attached to a gentle intermittent suction source for providing negative pressure of 80–100 cm of water. Use a suction device to which ET tube connector will fit directly. The connector should have two openings wherein one opening can be intermittently blocked. During suctioning, the ET tube is gradually withdrawn while suction is being applied. When meconium is aspirated directly through the ET tube, check the heart rate. If the heart rate is >100 beats/min, the baby should be reintubated and suction done to remove all traces of meconium. When heart rate is slow (<100 beats/min) after first intubation and suction, it is recommended to provide bag and mask ventilation without repeating the procedure of endotracheal intubation.

RESUSCITATION PROTOCOL

Initial Steps of Resuscitation

The resuscitation kit should be checked before the baby is born. The radiant warmer should be put on to warm the bassinet. Due to increasing prevalence and risk of AIDS, the pediatrician or nurse resuscitating the baby must wear gloves. The baby should be received in a warm sheet and head kept slightly low **(Figure 8.4)**.

The baby should be placed under the radiant warmer and positioned properly by keeping the head end

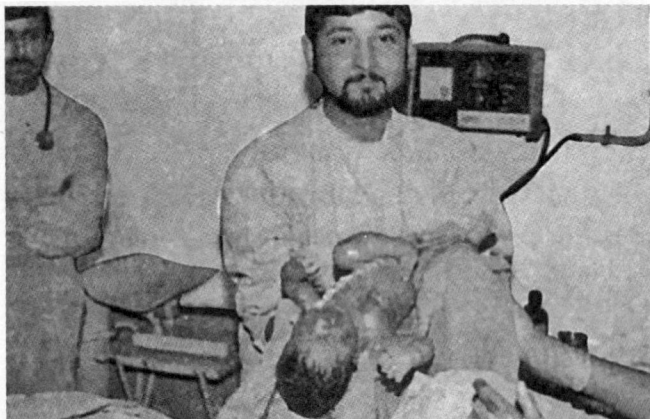

Figure 8.4 The correct method of holding the baby at birth

Nursing Alert

Due to potential risk of HIV and HBsAg infections always wear gloves while attending a delivery. Never suck the endotracheal tube with your mouth.

slightly low. The infant's mouth, oropharynx, hypopharynx and nose are sucked, in that order, using a thick-bored 12 Fr suction catheter with gentle intermittent suction with the help of a suction machine or a De Lee suction trap. If the baby is active, breathing or crying lustily, is pink and having a heart rate of >100 beats/min, no further active resuscitation is required. When a baby is blue despite having good respiratory efforts and heart rate is >100 beats/min, he should be given free flow oxygen till baby is pink. The baby should be promptly dried from top to toes and covered with a dry sheet. Head accounts for a large surface area of the newborn baby and must be dried thoroughly.

If after initial suction, the baby is not breathing or the breathing efforts are slow or gasping in nature, he should be stimulated by flicking at the soles or rubbing the back. The stimulation should not be continued beyond 3 to 4 flicks and when it is ineffective, the baby should be promptly ventilated with a bag and mask.

Most babies have a smooth transition from fetal to neonatal life and are able to establish spontaneous breathing without any active intervention. About 5.0 to 7.5% babies are likely to have difficulty in establishing spontaneous breathing at birth and need active resuscitation. At every deilvery, there should be at least one person, who is adequately trained in the art of neonatal resuscitation. When the delivery is high risk, at least two trained personnel should be available to perform complete resuscitation including bag and mask ventilation, endotracheal intubation, chest compressions and administration of medications. When mother is having multiple gestations, separate teams of trained personnel and equipment should be available to handle and resuscitate each baby. The procedure of resuscitation must be carried out by skilled and experienced persons with a sense of urgency but without any panic. The revised neonatal resuscitation program (NRP) guidelines of the Technical Committee of National Neonatology Forum of India recommends that the newly born baby should be assessed at birth by asking a single question, **Is baby breathing or crying?**

When answer to above question is **YES**, the baby needs routine care. But when baby is neither breathing nor crying, the baby is provided initial steps of resuscitation. The baby is correctly positioned, airway is cleared and neonate is effectively dried, covered and kept warm. When a baby is breathing but is cyanosed, she is administered free-flow oxygen at a rate of 5 liters/min till she becomes pink. Free-flow oxygen is administered through an oxygen mask or flow-inflating bag or a hand cupped around the oxygen tubing. If a baby is not breathing or having gasping breaths, she is provided tactile stimulation by flicking the soles or rubbing the back to promote breathing. Avoid prolonged tactile stimulation in an apneic baby, because it is likely to waste valuable time. The baby is simultaneously assessed for respiration, heart rate and color to take further decisions for resuscitation **(Figure 8.5)**.

Bag and Mask Ventilation

When despite stimulation, the baby is not breathing or having ineffective ventilation as evidenced by heart rate of less than 100 beats/min, he should be given bag and mask ventilation. Position the infant properly with slight extension of neck by placing a towel roll under the shoulders. Use an appropriate sized rounded mask

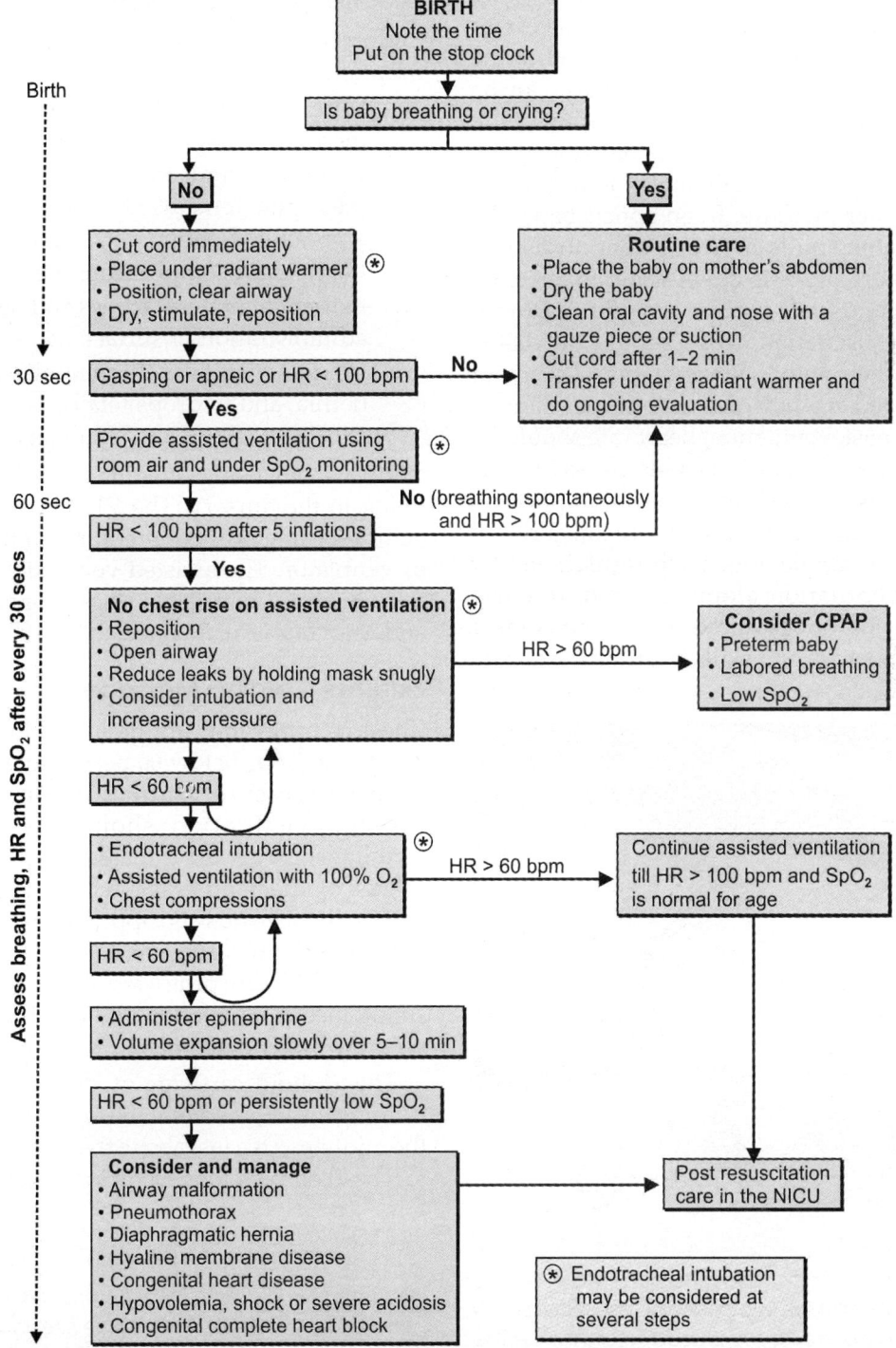

Figure 8.5 Algorithm for resuscitation of an asphyxiated newborn baby. Adapted from NRP-India guidelines

Nursing Alert

In community setting, when oxygen is not available, infant can be successfully resuscitated with room air with the help of bag and mask or tube and mask.

having cushioned edges. The mask should snugly fit on the face enclosing both the nose and mouth of the baby (**Figure 8.6**). Connect inlet of the mask to an oxygen source and attach an oxygen reservoir to increase the concentration of oxygen delivered to the baby. When oxygen in not available, baby can be effectively resuscitated with room air as shown by a number of multicentric studies. To avoid rupture of alveoli, the operator should train herself to deliver air at 15–20 cm of water pressure. In an apneic baby, the initial 2–3 ventilatory puffs may be strong to deliver oxygen at a pressure of 30–40 cm of water to open the collapsed alveoli and force out the lung fluid. During bag and mask resuscitation, there should be visible expansion of the chest with each ventilation. The infant should be ventilated at a rate of 40 breaths per minute. During bag and mask ventilation, heart rate should be closely monitored every 20–30 seconds. To save time, heart rate is counted for 6 seconds and multiplied by 10 to get the heart rate per minute. A large majority of asphyxiated babies can be effectively resuscitated by bag and mask ventilation alone and endotracheal intubation is usually not required. Every nurse must have necessary expertise and skills to provide effective

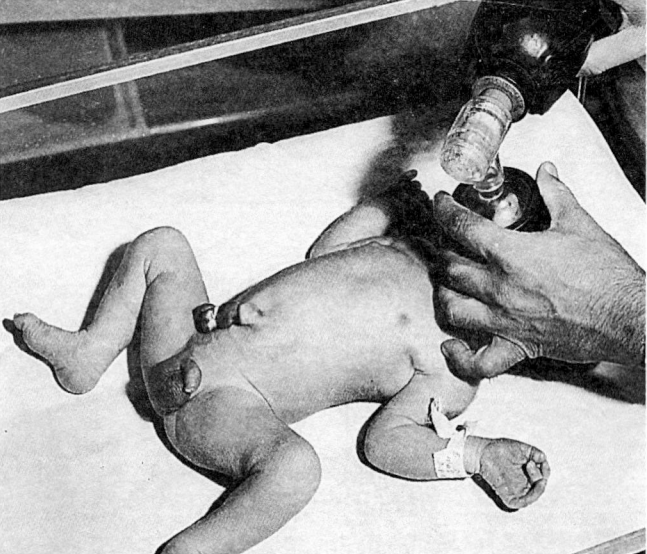

Figure 8.6 Bag and mask resuscitation. Most of the asphyxiated infants can be successfully resuscitated by this technique. Oxygen reservoir is used to enhance the concentration of oxygen in the inspired air

bag and mask ventilation. If despite effective bag and mask ventilation, heart rate is not improving or it further slows and drops below 60 beats/min, the infant should be intubated. At this stage, nalorphine 0.2 mL per kg or naloxone 0.1 mL per kg should be administered intravenously through the umbilical vein if mother had received pethidine or morphine within 4 hours of delivery.

Endotracheal Intubation

Endotracheal intubation is indicated in following situations:

i. When tracheal suctioning is required in a meconium-stained baby who is depressed.
ii. When bag and mask ventilation is ineffective (heart rate remains <80 bpm) or it is required for a prolonged period.
iii. When chest compressions are required.
iv. Extremely preterm babies and neonates requiring administration of surfactant.
v. Infants with airway anomalies, diaphragmatic hernia, and hydrops fetalis.

The art of intubation cannot be taught and must be learnt by practising on stillborn babies and neonates dying in the nursery. The ET tube must be suctioned before starting positive pressure ventilation with a bag or ventilator. The assisted ventilation can be stopped as soon as the baby establishes spontaneous breathing and heart rate is maintained above 100 beats per minute.

External Cardiac Massage

Chest compressions are indicated in babies in whom heart rate drops below 60 per minute despite effective positive-pressure ventilation for 30 seconds. The assisted ventilation should be continued and simultaneously heart is massaged either by using two fingers of one hand or encircling the chest of the baby with both the hands and applying sternal compressions with two thumbs (**Figure 8.7**). At least two specially trained health care professionals are required to provide simultaneous ventilation and chest compressions in a severely asphyxiated baby.

The xiphoid cartilage of sternum is identified by running the fingers along the lower edge of ribs towards the midline. Area just above the xiphoid catilage is used for chest compressions. Depress the sternum by one-third

Nursing Alert

A large majority of asphyxiated babies can be effectively revived and resuscitated by using bag and mask ventilation alone and intubation is usually not required.

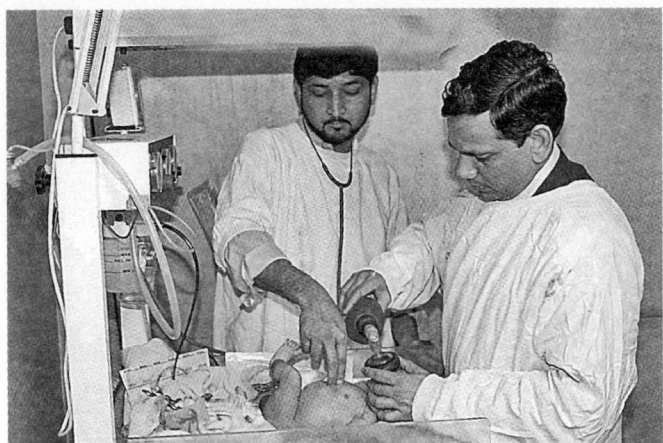

Figure 8.7 External cardiac massage with two fingers. Index and middle fingers are placed vertically over the lower third of sternum to provide cardiac compressions at a rate of 120/min. Bag and mask or bag and endotracheal tube ventilation should continue during chest compressions

of the anteroposterior diameter of the chest at a rate of 120 per minute. The thumbs or tips of fingers (depending upon the method used) should remain in contact with the sternum all the time and they should not be lifted off the chest after each compression. Check the heart rate after every 20–30 seconds and chest compressions are stopped when heart rate goes above 60 per minute.

Medications

Epinephrine is indicated when the heart rate remains below 60 beats per minute despite 30 seconds of assisted ventilation and another 30 seconds of coordinated chest compressions and ventilation. Administer 0.1–0.3 mL of 1:10,000 solution of epinephrine through the umbilical vein or endotracheal tube. The dose of epinephrine may be repeated every 3–5 minutes up to three doses. Intracardiac administration of epinephrine is not recommended due to increased risk of complications. When the baby is in shock, consider administration of plasma or normal saline in a dose of 10 mL per kg intravenously as a bolus. Sodium bicarbonate 5–10 mL of 7.5% solution (adequately diluted with an equal volume of distilled water or double volume of 5% dextrose) is administered through the umbilical vein slowly at a rate of 1.0 mL per minute

---

Nursing Alert

Sodium bicarbonate should not be administered till effective ventilation has been established. Never administer sodium bicarbonate as a bolus due to risk of causing intraventricular hemorrhage.

---

if effective spontaneous ventilations are not established by 10 minutes or later. There is no role of corticosteroids, atropine, calcium and respiratory stimulants during resuscitation of a newborn. **Box 8.2** highlights some of the don't during the procedure of resuscitation to prevent iatrogenic or procedure-related hazards to the baby.

Whole Body or Selective Brain Cooling

There is an experimental and clinical evidence to suggest that mild to moderate whole body or selective brain cooling with a cold cap is neuroprotective against the adverse effects of birth asphyxia. Cerebral hypothermia reduces ATP production and lowers metabolic rate of the brain with increase in the levels of inhibitory neuromodulators like glycine, taurine, GABA and adenosine which are neuroprotective. There is reduced alterations in ion flux and preservation of blood–brain barrier. Cooling is begun within 1–6 hour after hypoxic insult by maintaining brain or core body temperature between 33 and 34°C for 48–72 hours.

Whole body cooling is recommended in term infants (>36 weeks), if three of the following five inclusion criteria are fulfilled.

  i. Apgar score ≤5 at 10 minutes.
 ii. pH of cord blood or infant's blood ≤7.0 within one hour of age.
iii. Base deficit of cord blood or infant's blood within one hour age of ≥16 mEq/L.
 iv. Need for continued assisted ventilations at birth for at least 10 minutes.
  v. History of seizures or CNS abnormalities suggestive of grade 3 or more hypoxic–ischemic encephalopathy (HIE).

Box 8.2 | **Dont's in resuscitation**

- Do not give heavy sedation to the mother.
- Do not keep head of the baby too low for two long.
- Do not do vigorous and continuous suction.
- Do not allow the baby to become hypothermic.
- Do not continue with the tactile stimulation, if baby does not respond to 2–3 flicks.
- Do not delay bag and mask ventilation in a gasping or apneic baby.
- Do not blow your lungs into baby's mouth.
- Do not use full palmar grasp for giving bag to mask ventilation.
- Do not give sodium bicarbonate till ventilation is established.
- Do not give respiratory stimulants.

These infants should be given adequate sedation and excellent supportive care. There is evidence to suggest that neuroprotective effect of moderate hypothermia can be enhanced by coadministration of topiramate. However, inadvertent excessive cooling with fall in core body temperature is associated with adverse metabolic and physiologic effects with higher risk of morbidity and mortality. It would appear that hypothermia and selective cooling of brain after perinatal asphyxia is still an experimental intervention and cannot be recommended for routine clinical use till more data is available regarding its safety and efficacy in developing countries.

Post-Resuscitation Management

Infants with a 5-minute Apgar score of less than 4 or those who fail to establish spontaneous breathing at 5 minutes, should be admitted to the NICU. They should be placed in the open care system and attached to a multi-channel vital sign monitor. The infant should be nursed in a thermoneutral environment and started on 10% intravenous glucose and no electrolytes should be administered during first 48 hours of life. Urine output should be monitored and maintained above 2 mL/kg/hr. Shock, arterial oxygen saturation (SaO$_2$), acidosis, hypoglycemia, hypocalcemia and hyperkalemia should be looked for and treated appropriately. The onset of seizures within 24 hours of life are suggestive of severe birth asphyxia leading to hypoxic–ischemic encephalopahy. They are managed by intravenous administration of diazepam and phenobarbitone.

Systemic Manifestations of Severe Birth Asphyxia

Seeds of neonatal morbidity and neuromotor disability are sown in the labor room. A variety of clinical problems are encountered during early neonatal period among babies who are severely asphyxiated at birth (Table 8.2). Hypoxia can cause damage to almost every tissue and organ of the baby. During hypoxia, series of protective mechanisms collectively called as 'diving sea reflex' attempt to redistribute available blood flow from lesser to more vital organs. The blood flow to brain, heart and adrenal glands of the newborn is preserved at the expense of reduction of perfusion to kidneys, lungs, gastrointestinal tract, liver, spleen and skeletal muscles.

Prognosis

Severe birth asphyxia is the commonest cause of death on the first day of life. Depending upon the gestational maturity and quality of newborn care facilities, 15 to 50% of neonates exhibiting manifestations of HIE die

Table 8.2 Systemic manifestations of severe birth asphyxia

Organ/system	Features
Brain	Hypoxic–ischemic encephalopathy, intracranial hemorrhage, apneic attacks, seizures and neuromotor disability
Heart	Persistent fetal circulation, dysrhythmias, myocardial damage, tricuspid regurgitation, and congestive cardiac failure
Lungs	Meconium or liquor aspiration, hyaline membrane disease, transient tachypnea, persistent pulmonary hypertension, pulmonary hemorrhage, pneumonia, pneumothorax, and shock lung
Kidneys	Hematuria, renal failure, acute tubular necrosis, and renal vein thrombosis
Hematologic	Coagulopathy (DIC), thrombocytopenia, hyperbilirubinemia, and sepsis
Gastrointestinal	Necrotizing enterocolitis, GI bleeding, paralytic ileus and and hepatic dysfunction
Endocrinal	Syndrome of inappropriate secretion of antidiuretic hormone, adrenal hemorrhage, and transient hypoparathyroidism
Immunologic	Septicemia
Metabolic	Acidosis, hypoglycemia, hypocalcemia, hyponatremia and hyperkalemia

during neonatal period. Effective management of the baby at birth with early establishment of breathing, prevention of hypothermia and hypotension are associated with improved survival and outcome. The brain of a newborn baby, especially that of a preterm, is relatively resistant to the damaging effects of hypoxia and can withstand oxygen lack upto 5 to 7 minutes without any apparent sequelae. In an individual baby it is difficult to prognosticate for future mental development. It is amazing that several severely asphyxiated babies achieve fairly normal development without any neurological handicaps. Therefore, as a general policy, a guarded rather than hopeless prognosis should be communicated to the parents to cushion the anxiety and to avoid deliberate neglect of the child.

Following severe birth asphyxia 25% infants are likely to develop evidences of HIE. Relatively adverse outcome is anticipated if the infant was in terminal apnea especially when heart beats were absent at birth or 10-minute Apgar score was less than 3. Arterial blood pH of less than 7.0, plasma lactate level of more than 60 mg/dL, hypoglycemia, occurrence of neonatal convulsions, brainstem signs (poor sucking, pooling of oral secretions, pupillary changes, etc.) or abnormal neurological behavior for more than 5 days and multiple diffuse chaotic spike pattern or isopotential amplitude integrated electroencephalogram (a-EEG) are associated with unfavorable outcome. Multi-organ failure especially development of acute renal failure is associated with poor outcome.

The American Academy of Pediatrics has proposed that the terminology of perinatal or birth asphyxia should be reserved to describe an infant who manifests all of the following features: (i) Cord umbilical artery pH >7.0 with a base deficit of >10mEq/L; (ii) neonatal neurologic manifestations suggestive of hypoxic–ischemic encephalopathy (HIE); (iii) Evidences of multisystem organ dysfunction involving cardio-vascular, renal, gastrointestinal, hematologic or pulmonary system.

The incidence of cerebral palsy following birth asphyxia varies between 6.5 and 18.5 percent. Infants with evidences of intraventricular or parenchymal hemorrhage and extensive areas of infarction (hypo-density) on CT scan during early neonatal period are often associated with neurological handicaps on follow-up. Brainstem auditory, visual and somatosensory evoked responses by and large are of limited prognostic utility. Inferior colliculi which are credited to produce wave V are specially damaged by hypoxia. In normal infants, wave V obtained during brainstem auditory evoked response is bigger in amplitude as compared to wave 1. The ratio of wave V (actually waves IV and V which are often merged) to wave 1 gets reversed when there is hypoxic damage to the inferior colliculi which is associated with increased mortality and poor late neuromotor outcome among the survivors.

BIBLIOGRAPHY

Deorari AK. New guidelines for neonatal resuscitation: How my practice needs to change? *Indian Pediatr* 2001, 38: 496–499.

Gluckman PD, Wyatt JS, Azzopardi D, et al. Selective head cooling with mild systemic hypothemia after neonatal encephalopathy: Multicentre randomized trial. *Lancet* 2005, 365: 663–670.

Kattwinkel J, Perlman JM, Aziz K, *et al*. American Heart Association. Neonatal Resuscitation: 2010 American Heart Association Guidelines for Cardiopulmonary Resuscitation and Emergency Cardiovascular Care. *Pediatrics* 2010, 126(5): e1400–13. Epub 2010, Oct 18.

Marlow N. Do we need Apgar score? *Arch Dis Child* 1992, 67: 765–767.

Neonatal Resuscitation: *National Neonatology Forum of India*, second edition 2014.

8

Common Neonatal Problems

Most mothers observe their babies carefully and are often worried because of minor physical or physiological peculiarities which are of no consequence. It is important that her complaints are listened to carefully by the nurse and they are not ignored lightly without doing proper evaluation of the baby. She must be given reassurance and advice regarding the minor problems and difficulties that may be bothering her. Adequate explanation and reassurance is necessary to allay her anxiety which may otherwise lead to lactation failure.

REGURGITATION OF FEEDS AND VOMITING

Vomiting is common on the first day of life due to swallowed amniotic fluid. It usually resolves spontaneously but when it is persistent, it is relieved following stomach wash with normal saline. Regurgitation of feeds often occurs due to faulty technique of feeding and swallowing of air while feeding (aerophagy). All mothers must be given proper advise on the technique of feeding and burping after each feed. The baby must be held upright against the shoulder or made to sit up in the lap for at least 3 to 5 minutes to eructate the air swallowed during the feeding before she is put back to the cot **(Figure 9.1)**. Most babies enjoy being placed in the prone position which is associated with less risk of regurgitation as it relieves abdominal distension. *When vomiting is persistent, projectile or bile-stained or there is failure to pass meconium during the first 24 hours and or abdominal distension, the baby should be investigated for intestinal obstruction.*

In gastroesophageal reflux and hiatus hernia, vomiting occurs when the baby is returned to the cot after the feed. It does not occur if the baby is held upright or kept at an angle of 60 degrees. In hypertrophic pyloric stenosis, vomiting characteristically occurs after 2 weeks of age. This condition is more common in first born male infant and is characterized by nonbilious projectile vomiting, poor weight gain and

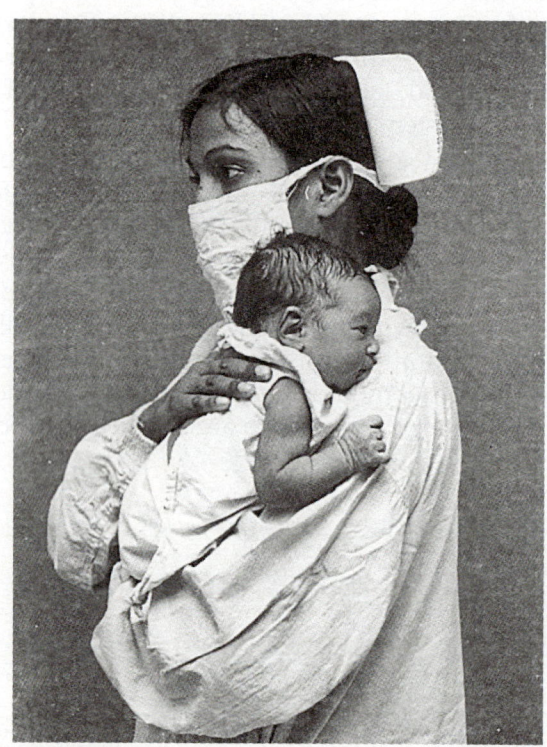

Figure 9.1 The infant should be put on the shoulder after feeds to facilitate burping

constipation. Visible peristaltic waves may be seen moving from left-to-right in the upper abdomen. Vomiting may occur due to raised intracranial tension because of intracranial hemorrhage, birth asphyxia, meningitis, urinary tract infection, sepsis, cardiac failure and metabolic disorders such as galactosemia and salt losing variety of congenital adrenal hemorrhage. Blood-tinged vomiting may occur due to swallowed blood and hemorrhagic disease of the newborn.

BOWEL DISORDERS

The baby may pass meconium in utero or soon after birth but all healthy newborn babies must evacuate within 24 hours of age. During the first two to three days, the baby passes black, tarry meconium stools which are followed by greenish (transitional) stools for the next one or two days. The breastfed baby usually passes 4 to 8 semisolid sticky golden-yellow stools every day. Some babies may pass stool after each feed due to exaggerated gastrocolic reflex. It does not need any treatment and baby will continue to gain weight satisfactorily. The breastfed babies may develop increased frequency of stools if the mother is taking certain antibiotics (cephalexin, ampicillin, and tetracyclines) and laxatives. Milk of magnesia, bulk laxatives and a glycerin suppository are safe for a nursing mother for treatment of constipation. *When a baby is exclusively breastfed, he is unlikely to develop infective diarrhea.* A sudden change in the baby's established bowel pattern leading to greater frequency and change in the character of stools should be taken seriously. Infective diarrhea occurs in bottle-fed babies. The stools are often watery with mucus and plenty of pus cells. Neonatal diarrhea may also occur in association with septicemia, necrotising enterocolitis, Hirchsprung's disease and phototherapy.

Babies fed on cow's milk are often constipated due to hard casein curds. Constipation may also occur because of inadequate feeding or gastrointestinal obstruction. Infants with congenital hypothyroidism, Hirschsprung's disease and anal stenosis are often constipated. Constipation in the absence of any underlying disease process is best managed by giving glucose water, and orange or sweet lemon juice. Intake of honey should be avoided due to potential risk of botulism. The insertion of a lubricated rectal thermometer or a rubber catheter often initiates reflex peristaltic activity resulting in evacuation. *The use of laxatives should be avoided in newborn babies.*

Delayed Passage of Urine

Fetus passes urine regularly in the womb after 12 weeks of gestation and amniotic fluid is contributed mostly by fetal urine. After birth most newborn babies pass urine during the first day of life but all must void within the first 48 hours of birth. If a baby has not passed urine by 48 hours, he should be examined to rule out renal agenesis and obstructive uropathy. However, the commonest cause of the alleged non-passage of the urine is that the baby has actually passed urine but it has been over looked by the mother. The normal frequency of micturition in a newborn baby varies between 7 to 10 times per day. *Some babies may cry before passing urine due to discomfort of a full bladder, they become quiet and dazed while passing urine and start crying again after having passed urine because of wet napkins.* This should not be considered as an evidence of obstructive

uropathy. The narrow stream of urine, straining and crying during the act of micturition, dribbling in the end and presence of palpable urinary bladder and enlarged kidneys are suggestive of obstructive uropathy.

Physiological Jaundice

About 60 to 70 percent of healthy term newborn babies develop jaundice on the second or third day of life. The serum bilirubin level does not cross 15 mg/dL. Jaundice disappears within 7 to 10 days. Physiological jaundice does not need any treatment and the mother should be reassured that it will disappear spontaneously. It is not indicative of any infection and does not require administration of extra fluids and feeds. *The occurrence of jaundice within the first 24 hours of life or when it is deep and intensely staining the trunk or causing yellow discoloration of the palms and soles or if it persists for more than 2 weeks, it is pathological and needs investigations and management.*

Jitteriness

Most normal babies are jittery or tremulous on touch and handling. They are easily startled by loud noise or rough handling. When jitteriness is excessive and persists even during feeding, it is important to exclude hypoglycemia and hypocalcemia.

Superficial Infections

Sticky eyes or purulent conjunctivitis is common during the newborn period. Gonococcal ophthalmia should be suspected if there is history of gonorrhea in the mother and conjunctivitis is marked with abundant purulent discharge and swelling of eyelids. It should be confirmed by microscopic examination of a Gram-stained preparation of conjunctival discharge. It is best treated by parenteral administration of ceftriaxone or cefotaxime and topical instillation of crystalline penicillin eye drops and frequent cleaning of eyes. Non-gonococcal purulent conjunctivitis is usually caused by staphylococci but other pathogens may be responsible depending upon the spectrum of microbes in the lying-in ward and NICU. It is best treated with local instillation of chloramphenicol or gentamicin eye drops every one hourly. After 24 hours, intervals between local medications can be gradually increased. The chlamydial conjunctivitis characteristically manifests as purulent conjunctivitis during second week of life. It is managed by topical instillation of 10 percent sulfacetamide eye drops or 0.5 percent erythromycin ophthalmic ointment and oral administration of erythromycin for two weeks. The eyes should be cleaned with sterile wet cotton swabs prior to the instillation of eye drops by using one swab for each eye.

Pyoderma It manifests as multiple pustules especially over the scalp, neck, axillae and groins. The infection is usually transmitted by the hands of personnel and is caused by staphylococci. The large pustules can be punctured with a sterile needle to drain the pus. The skin should be washed with hexachlorophene lotion and medicated soap. The skin lesions should be painted with triple dye or an antibiotic cream two to three times a day. When despite this therapy, the skin lesions are increasing in size or number, oral administration of erythromycin or cloxacillin is recommended.

Umbilical sepsis It manifests as redness and edema at the base of the cord and foul smelling purulent discharge. The presence of mucoid discharge on the stump and even isolation of bacteria are not indicative of umbilical sepsis unless there are clinical evidences of periumbilical inflammation or presence of pus cells in the exudate. The umbilical stump should be cleaned with spirit and treated with local application of triple dye or betadine lotion. If periumbilical inflammation is spreading or the infant is showing features of systemic spread of infection as evidenced by fever, lethargy, and poor feeding, she should be managed with parenteral antibiotics like a case of neonatal septicemia.

Oral thrush It manifests as white patches with erythematous margins which are distributed over the tongue and buccal mucosa. Unlike milk curds, the patches of thrush are adherent and they often bleed when attempts are made to remove them. Local application of 0.5 percent aqueous solution of gentian violet or nystatin or ketoconazole after each feed is followed by prompt recovery. The mother should be examined for vaginal and breast nipple candidiasis and given appropriate treatment.

Dehydration Fever

During the summer months, when the environmental temperature approaches 40°C, some healthy newborn babies may develop transitory fever during the second and third day of life. The fever is usually moderate in intensity (up to 38.5°C) and the child is active and keen to feed. The condition is transient and is best managed by lowering the environmental temperature and by providing hydrotherapy. *There is no role of giving an antipyretic agent.* Once the lactation is established and adequate feeding is ensured the infant becomes afebrile.

Excessive Crying

During the first few weeks, most newborn babies sleep during the day and they are awake, playful and troublesome during the night. This behavior is due to continuation of their in utero pattern of activity. During pregnancy when the mother is up and about during daytime, the baby is rocked in the pool of amniotic fluid and sleeps. During the night when mother is resting the fetus is active and playful. This pattern of activity or behavior spontaneously disappears after 4 to 6 weeks of postnatal age. Most babies usually cry when they are either hungry or are having discomfort. The cry may be a signal of an unpleasant sensation due to a full bladder before passing urine, painful evacuation of hard stools or discomfort of wet napkins. The experienced mother and nurse are able to differentiate between the cry used as a signal for feed and the cry of discomfort. An infant with abdominal colic would have audible gurgling sounds in the abdomen and usually feels comfortable when placed in a prone position which facilitates the expulsion of gas. The presence of excessive inconsolable crying or a high-pitched cry is always indicative of a serious disorder like intestinal colic, meningitis or a painful inflammatory condition, like acute otitis media and osteomyelitis. Crying may occur due to insect bites, exposure to cold, loneliness and boredom. Most babies are cranky or fussy while dozing off to sleep. Night crying with arching of back is a symptom of gastroesophageal reflux disease. The crying baby should be handled with patience, common sense and good humor.

Evening Colic

It is a distinct entity which is characterized by sudden bouts of unexplained spells of crying in the evening or night after a few days of birth. There are sudden episodes of screaming with flexion of thighs and flushing or frowning of face usually at a precise time in the evening in a clockwise regularity. The crying episodes may last for several minutes or for a couple of hours causing extreme anxiety and stress to the mother and other family members. The exact cause of evening colic is unknown but apparently it occurs due to intestinal colic as evidenced by excessing gurgling or peristaltic sounds on palpation of abdomen. Excessive crying due to colic leads to further swallowing of air thus initiating a vicious cycle of colic–crying–colic. The condition is more common in first born wiry and restless babies of anxious parents or grandparents. The condition is common both in exclusively breastfed or formula fed babies.

A variety of therapeutic measures have been suggested to handle the condition but nothing seems to work. Holding the baby close to chest, rocking, swaddling, cuddling, patting, kissing taking him for a drive or placing in a prone position with elevated hips may provide relief. A number of home remedies like application of asafoetida (*hing*) around the navel and administration of decoction of *ajwain* and *saunf* may provide relief. Administration of antispasmodic drops 30 minutes before the anticipated time of colic may break the cycle of misery. Probiotics have been shown to provide relief in some babies. Avoid making unnecessary changes in the feeding regime of the baby. The condition resolves spontaneously after one to two months.

Breath Holding Spells

Episodes of temper tantrums with breath holding spells are classically seen after the age of six months. Rarely, episodes of crying with holding of breath in expiration and cynosis may be seen during newborn period. The baby is fussy or over active and lacks patience while parents and grandparents are over indulgent and over anxious. The condition must be differentiated from anoxic spells due to tetralogy of Fallot and excessive crying in brain-damaged infants.

Excessive Sleepiness

During the first few days of life, many infants keep their eyes closed most of the time and they readily go to sleep after taking only a few sucks at the breast. The excessive sleepiness may be aggravated by heavy maternal sedation during labor. Barbiturates and opium derivatives when taken by the nursing mother may cause drowsiness in her suckling infant. Infants with Down syndrome and hypothyroidism are often lazy and lack activity due to generalized hypotonia.

Cephalhematoma

It is a subperiosteal collection of blood secondary to injury during vaginal delivery. It may occur both following an obstructed or a precipitate delivery. The swelling is not present at birth and it manifests after a couple of hours when sufficient amount of blood has extravasated (**Figure 9.2**). It is characterized by a fluctuant swelling which is limited by suture lines. It

Nursing Alert

The sudden appearance of lethargy or lack of interest in feeding, in a baby who had been feeding adequately in the past, is an important and may be the only manifestation of a serious illness like septicemia or a metabolic disorder.

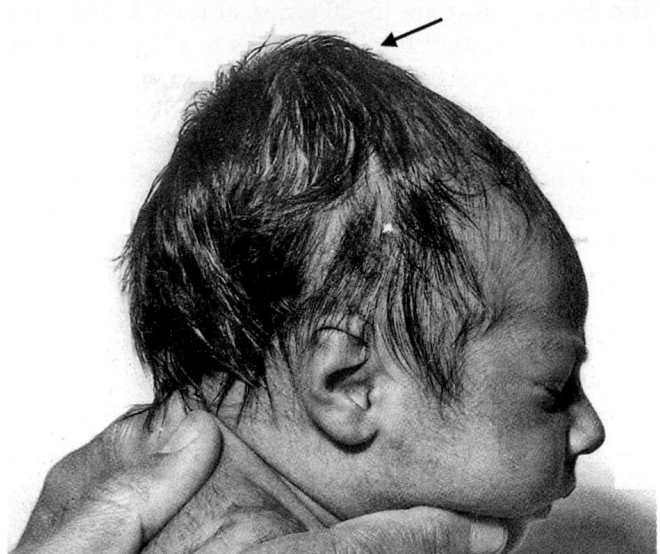

Figure 9.2 Arrow points to cephalhematoma over parietal region in an infant born following spontaneous vaginal delivery

gradually resolves over a period of several days or weeks depending upon the size of swelling. It may be associated with linear fracture of skull and severe jaundice. Incision or aspiration are contraindicated unless it gets infected or is associated with critical hyperbilirubinemia.

Cephalhematoma should be differentiated from *caput succedaneum* which manifests as a diffuse boggy pitting edema of the scalp on the presenting part. It is a non-fluctuant swelling and is not limited by the suture lines. The caput succedaneum is present right at birth and rapidly disappears during the next 24 to 28 hours.

Cradle Cap

It is characterized by presence of seborrheic flakes with crusting over the scalp due to excessive secretion of sebum. It is treated by application of coconut oil or milk cream (*malai*) over the scalp followed one hour later by shampoo with cetavalon or cetrimide.

Obstructed Nasolacrimal Duct

There is persistent wetness or watery discharge (epiphora) from one or both the eyes starting soon after birth. There is blockage of nasolacrimal duct which drains tears from the eyes into the nostrils. It is treated by massage of tear glands (lacrimal sacs) and nasolacrimal duct. Mother is asked to firmly press the lacrimal sacs (located at the inner corners of eyes) with her index finger and thumb and massage the nasolacrimal duct by exerting inward pressure from above downward along the lateral walls of the nose.

9

The massage is done 15–20 times, at least 3 times in a day and continued for 1–2 months or till watering of eyes disappear. After the massage of nasolacrimal duct, antibacterial eye drops should be instilled for one week to treat any associated conjunctivitis. The epithelial debris is often squeezed out and patency of the duct is restored. If the nasolacrimal duct does not open up by 5–6 months, probing and syringing through the punctum is indicated.

Umbilical Granuloma

It manifests as a flesh-colored or pale nodule at the base of the umbilical stump with persistent discharge. This can be managed by cautery with silver nitrate or application of common salt for 3 to 4 days.

Napkin Rash (Diaper Rash)

The perineal skin may become red, indurated and excoriated due to ammoniacal dermatitis if infant is not promptly cleaned and dried after the passage of urine or stools. Occurrence of diarrhea and the use of nylon or water-tight soakable diapers aggravate the condition. The bottom should be kept dried and exposed to air or sunlight. Application of coconut oil or a bland zinc-based ointment is promptly followed by recovery. The causative factors should be identified and eliminated. In resistant cases, infection of the skin by *Candida albicans* should be ruled out. It is characterized by marked erythema, maceration and erythematous papules or vesicles at the periphery. It is treated by local application of skin cream containing nystatin or ketaconazole 3 to 4 times in a day for 15 days.

Sneezing

Sneezing is common in healthy newborn babies due to irritation of the nose by amniotic fluid, meconium, blood, or debris. It should not be considered as a sign of a common cold. The nostrils should be cleaned with sterile wet cotton buds if sneezing is excessive.

Hiccups

Most newborn babies develop hiccups especially after the feeds. The distension of stomach may cause irritation of the diaphragm which leads to hiccups. They do not indicate any disease process in a newborn baby and the mother should be reassured regarding the benign nature of the hiccups.

> **Practical Point**
> *Yawning, sneezing and hiccups are physiological responses of the baby and their presence is reassuring that the neonate is healthy.*

Yawning

Many babies yawn before going to sleep or on waking up. It is important to remember that hiccups, yawning and sneezing are physiological responses of the baby and their presence should be considered as an indicator that the baby is healthy.

DISORDERS DUE TO TRANSPLACENTAL PASSAGE OF HORMONES

Engorgement of Breasts

Term babies of both sexes may develop engorgement of the breasts on the 3rd or 4th day due to the effect of transplacentally transferred progesterone and estrogens (**Figure 9.3**). The hypertrophy of the breasts may last for a few days to several weeks, but it disappears, spontaneously. Administration of metoclopramide to the baby or nursing mother can aggravate hypertrophy of the breasts. No effort should be made to massage the breast or express the milk, as it may lead to infection or mastitis.

Vaginal Bleeding

About 20 to 25 percent female babies may develop menstruation-like withdrawal vaginal bleeding after 4 to 5 days of birth. The bleeding is usually mild and lasts for 2 to 4 days. It does not need any specific therapy apart from local aseptic cleaning of genitals.

Mucoid Vaginal Secretions

Most female babies have copious grayish-white slimy vaginal secretions due to presence of maternal female sex hormones. This should not be confused with purulent vaginal discharge. The genitals should be cleaned gently during bathing.

Acne Neonatorum

Typical acne-like lesions with comedones may be seen over the forehead, nose and cheeks at birth in term babies. They occur due to transplacental passage of

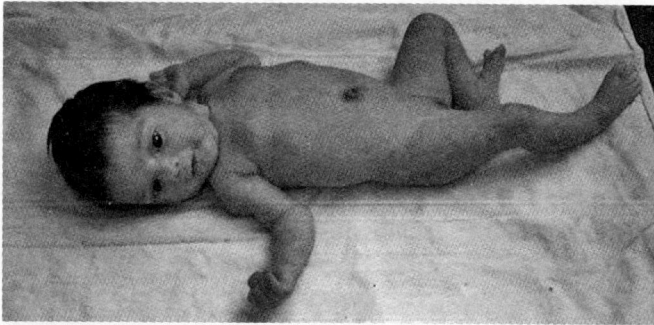

Figure 9.3 Enlargement of both the breasts in a term baby at the age of 5 days

maternal androgens to the fetus. The skin lesions gradually resolve spontaneously within next few days without any treatment.

MINOR DEVELOPMENTAL PECULIARITIES

Toxic Erythema (Urticaria Neonatorum)

About one-third healthy term newborn babies may develop an erythematous rash with a central papule on the second or third day of life. The rash usually starts on the face and spreads to the trunk and extremities in about 24 hours. The rash disappears spontaneously after two or three days without any specific treatment. The exact cause is not known but it is considered as an early marker of atopy or allergic diathesis. The rash should be differentiated from pyoderma and skin lesions of congenital syphilis.

Odd-Shaped Skull

Neonate may be born with an asymmetric or odd looking head because of space constraints in the uterus. Occiput or one of the parietal areas may become flat and bald. If head size is normal, there is no cause for concern. Proper positioning and support to head with soft pillows is followed by gradual rounding of the head shape.

Craniotabes

When skull bones are soft and they can be pressed like a table tennis ball, it is called craniotabes (soft skull). The condition should be looked for away from the sutures and fontanels. Localized craniotabes may be present due to in-utero pressure of the skull against mother's pubic bone. Craniotabes is suggestive of prematurity, hydrocephalus, congenital rickets, congenital syphilis, and osteogenesis imperfecta.

The Setting-Sun Sign

The eyes are rolled down and the sclerae become visible as they are uncovered by the upper eyelids. Most neonates may show transient episodic setting-sun sign which is of no significance. Persistent and constant setting-sun sign is seen in infants with hydrocephalus and kernicterus.

Tongue Tie

A thin frenulum under the tongue is normal and does not need any treatment. A thick and tight fibrous frenulum producing notch at the tip of the tongue is abnormal and may have to be snipped at around the age of 6 months to one year. Tongue tie seldom interferes with sucking or delay the development of speech in a child. Most parents wrongly blame tongue tie for delayed development of speech.

Non-Retractable Prepuce

The prepuce is normally non-retractable in all male neonates and it should not be diagnosed as phimosis. The mother should be advised against forcible retraction of the foreskin. The foreskin becomes retractable after the age of two years.

Mongolian Blue Spots

Almost all newborn babies of African and Asian origin have irregular blue patches of skin pigmentation especially over the sacral area and buttocks. At times they may be widespread and may involve other parts of the body including limbs. These patches have no relationship to Down syndrome and they usually fade or disappear after the age of 6 months.

Congenital Teeth

Some newborn babies may be born with one or two lower incisor teeth. They do not interfere with feeding but cause considerable anxiety among the parents and relatives due to the mistaken cultural belief that they are a bad omen. The loose teeth should be extracted as a safeguard against the risk of aspiration.

Stork Bites (Salmon Patches)

These are discrete pinkish-gray capillary hemangiomata commonly located at the nape of the neck, upper eyelids, forehead and root of the nose. They invariably disappear after a few months.

Milia

Yellow white pinhead-sized papules on the nose are seen in practically all neonates. They occur due to the retention of sebum and disappear spontaneously.

Excessive Scales and Peeling of Skin

Dried scaly skin with peeling and increased transverse skin creases are seen in post-term and some term small-for-dates babies. Dryness of skin occurs due to the paucity of amniotic fluid. Application of an emollient cream or oil provides relief.

Subconjunctival Hemorrhage

In some babies, semilunar spots of subconjunctival hemorrhage may be seen over the outer canthus of the eye. They are seen in babies born by vaginal delivery following vertex presentation. The hemorrhage gets resorbed within a few days.

Prominent Xiphisternum

The spear-shaped xiphisternal cartilage may stand out prominently in some babies and it is not indicative of any disease process.

9

Bowed Legs

In normal babies, when legs are extended, they form a concavity inwards due to genu varum giving an appearance of bowed legs. It is not indicative of rickets or bony deformity. After first birthday, bowing of legs is replaced by physiological knock knees.

Umbilical Hernia

When the cord has fallen off, the gut may protrude through the navel after the age of two weeks or later (**Figure 9.4**). Umbilical hernia is more common in infants with hypotonia because of cretinism, rickets and Down syndrome. Most of these usually disappear spontaneously by 6 months to one year of age. Application of coin and bandage over the hernia is not recommended, as it may further weaken the anterior abdominal wall and may cause necrosis of gut. If there are any associated conditions which are recognized to increase the intra-abdominal pressure like excessive crying, constipation and persistent cough, they should be identified and managed appropriately. Rarely when hernia is large or it persists beyond 3 years, surgical closure is advised.

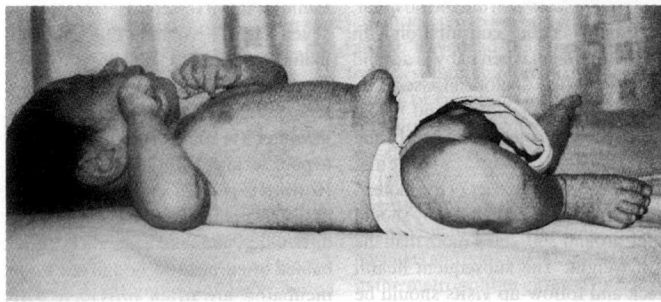

Figure 9.4 Umbilical hernia. No bandage should be applied as hernia spontaneously disappears after a few months

BIBLIOGRAPHY

Illingworth RS (Ed.). The Normal Child. *London, Churchill Livingstone*, 10th Edition 1991.

Singh M., Krishnamoorthy KS, Sinclair S, Ghai OP. Some developmental characterisitcs in the newborn. *Indian Pediatr* 1970, 7: 378.

Singh M. Care of the normal newborns. In: Care of the Newborn. *New Delhi, CBS Publishers and Distributors Pvt Ltd*. Revised 8th Edition, 2016 pp 152–165.

9

Birth Injuries

Due to advances in obstetrical practices and by conducting timely or early operative delivery whenever labor is prolonged or difficult, the incidence of birth injuries has become low in hospital practice. Most neonatal injuries during the process of delivery are now limited to domiciliary obstetric practice because most deliveries at home are conducted by untrained birth attendants or relatives. They have scant knowledge and skills to diagnose and handle cases of cephalopelvic disproportion and referral to a hospital is often delayed after a trial of difficult or complicated labor. Most of the times birth asphyxia and birth injuries co-exist. The incidence of birth injuries varies between 6 and 8 per 1000 live births. The high-risk factors for occurrence of birth injuries include primigravida mothers, prematurity, large babies (macrosomia) breech extraction with shoulder dystocia, cephalopelvic disproportion, malpresentation, and prolonged labor. It is important that high-risk pregnancy should be identified before onset of labor and woman is referred well in time to a health center or hospital for confinement.

SUPERFICIAL INJURIES

Superficial abrasions and swellings may occur over the sites of forceps or vacuum application. When delivery is prolonged, the presenting part may show petechiae, bruises and traumatic cyanosis. Spontaneous recovery occurs within 2 to 3 days. These babies are more prone to develop severe jaundice. Subconjunctival hemorrhages are commonly seen in healthy babies and they disappear spontaneously. Accidental incision of the baby may occur during cesarean section. The gaping incised wound may need stitching and local application of betadine.

Caput Succedaneum

There is baggy, diffuse, edematous swelling on the presenting part of the scalp. The swelling is present at birth and its size and severity are related to the duration of labor. The swelling is pitting, non-fluctuant and not limited by sutures unlike cephalhematoma. The swelling and ecchymosis may be present on the face in babies born by brow or face presentation. The swelling disappears spontaneously during next few days.

Cephalhematoma

There is subperiosteal collection of blood on the scalp which is limited by sutures and occurs following a difficult or precipitate delivery. Refer to **Chapter 9** for details

Sternomastoid 'Tumor'

During second week of life, a firm mass 1–2 cm diameter may be noted in the mid-portion of the sternocleido-mastoid muscle on one side of the neck. It is believed to be due to a small hematoma because of injury to the muscle at birth or due to fibromatous malformation of the muscle. The baby may develop torticollis on the affected side. Head is tilted toward the affected side while chin is rotated to the opposite side. The mother should be advised to overextend the affected muscle by rotating the infant's head in the opposite direction and flexing the neck towards unaffected side. These manipulations or passive exercises should be done about 3 to 4 times in a day by doing 20 repetitions of each exercise at a time. Crib toys should be so positioned that the infant would stretch the neck while reaching for them. The majority of these 'tumors' resolve spontaneously by six months to one year of age. If torticollis persists beyond one year, surgical correction is advised.

FRACTURES OF BONES

Skull Linear skull fractures may be associated in infants with cephalhematoma and they do not need any treatment. The depressed fractures may occur due to compression because of forceps or pressure against maternal symphysis pubis and sacral promontory. These also disappear spontaneously but at times surgical elevation may be required if they are associated with neurological manifestations.

> **Practical Tip**
>
> *In neonates with multiple fractures in different stages of healing and with deformities of limbs, osteogenesis imperfecta should be strongly suspected.*

Clavicle Fracture of the clavicle is most common and often follows breech extraction or shoulder impaction. The baby cries due to pain when handled and movements of the limb on the affected side are limited (pseudoparalysis). Moro reflex is likely to be asymmetrical. The arm on the affected side should be immobilized by pinning the infant's sleeve to the shirt or by strapping the limb. Paracetamol (15 mg/kg/dose) is the analgesic of choice for relief of pain in newborn babies. The prognosis is excellent and callus is formed within one week.

Humerus During shoulder impaction when the baby's arm is forcibly pulled, fracture of humerus may occur. The commonest site of fracture is the junction between upper one-third and the lower two-thirds of humerus. The diagnosis is suspected by pain and limitations of movement of the affected limb, asymmetric Moro response and crepitus at the site of fracture. It may be associated with fracture of clavicle and brachial plexus palsy. The arm should be strapped by the side of chest for immobilization.

Femur Fracture of femur is rare and caused by forcible manipulation of legs during breech extraction. The affected limb may show deformity, crepitus and pain on handling the limb. Paracetamol is useful for relief of pain. Healing occurs spontaneously without any splintage. In infants with multiple fractures, osteogenesis imperfecta should be ruled out.

Dislocation of joints The common sites of dislocation are hips, shoulders and cervical vertebrae. Dislocation of hips is more often due to dysplasia rather than traction or birth injury. The infant should be evaluated by an orthopedic surgeon and managed by immobilization.

PERIPHERAL NERVE INJURIES

Brachial Plexus Palsy

Avulsion of brachial nerve roots may occur during difficult breech extraction or shoulder impaction. Erb's palsy occurs when upper cervical roots (C_5 and C_6) are affected. The arm on the affected side hangs limply, adducted and internally rotated with elbow extended **(Figure 10.1)**. Pronation of the forearm with flexion of wrist gives an appearance of "policeman's bribe". Arm recoil is lost. The Moro reflex is asymmetric with lack of spontaneous movements of the limb. Associated phrenic nerve injury may lead to paralysis of diaphragm with respiratory distress and elevation of the leaf of diaphragm on the affected side.

When lower cervical roots (C_7, C_8 and T_1) are affected, it is called Klumpkes palsy. It is characterized by wrist drop and flaccid paralysis of hand with absent grasp reflex. The presence of meiosis (constriction of pupil), ptosis (paralysis of eyelid) and anhydrosis (absence of sweating) may occur on the affected side when there is associated damage to the cervical sympathetic chain and the condition is called Horner syndrome.

In infants with Erb's palsy, the arm should be kept in the position of abduction, external rotation at the shoulder and flexion of elbow. When there is respiratory distress due to phrenic nerve paralysis, neonate is placed on the affected side and given oxygen if indicated. The infant is fed intravenously or by gavage followed by oral feeding as the condition improves. In Klumpke's palsy, cotton ball should be placed in the

> **Practical Tip**
>
> *Paracetamol (15 mg/kg/dose) is the drug of choice for relief of pain and discomfort due to birth injuries and fractures. NSAIDs are not recommended in newborn babies.*

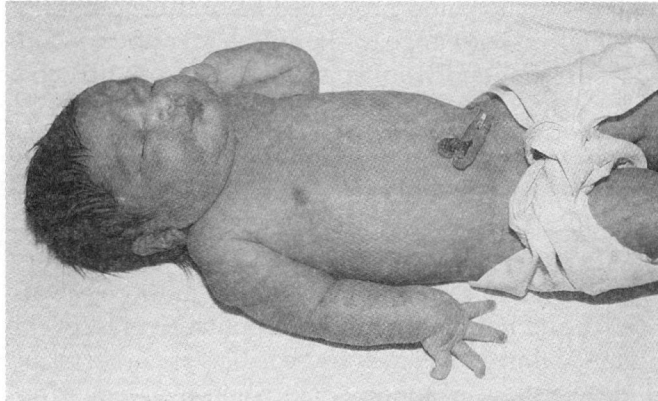

Figure 10.1 Erb's palsy on the right side in a large-for-dates baby of a mother with diabetes mellitus

10

baby's hand to avoid contractures. Massage and passive movements of the muscles would aid recovery. In severe cases when there is laceration of nerves, as evidenced by lack of recovery by 3 months, neuroplasty is indicated to facilitate recovery.

Facial Palsy

It is more common following delivery assisted by application of forceps but may occur in babies born by spontaneous delivery. There is facial asymmetry, inability to close the eye and absent rooting reflex on the affected side **(Figure 10.2)**. If infant is unable to suck effectively, gavage feeding may be required. When eye is kept open on the affected side, it can be covered with an eyeshield to prevent dryness of conjunctiva and cornea. The recovery is usually complete without any intervention. Neuroplasty may be required if facial nerve is torn and paralysis persists.

Partial facial palsy or congenital abscence or hypoplasia of depressor anguli oris muscle is a relatively frequent developmental condition which is not related to birth injury. During crying, the angle of mouth is pulled downwards on the normal side **(Figure 10.3)**. Eye closure is unaffected but nasolabial fold becomes flat on the normal side. The condition may be associated with cardiovascular, genitourinary and skeletal anomalies.

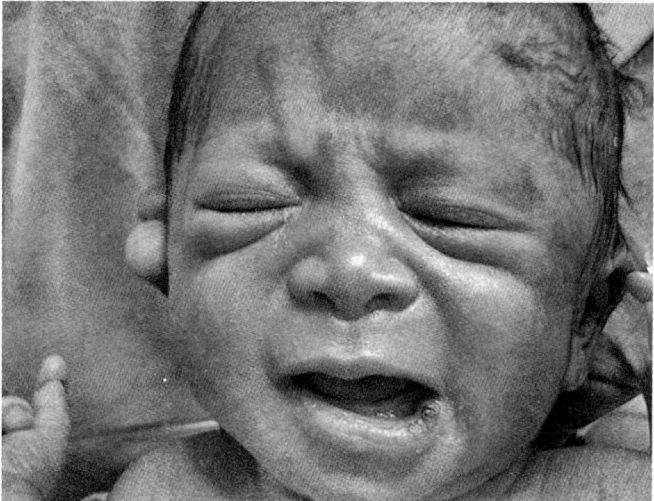

Figure 10.3 Congenital absence of depressor anguli oris muscle on the left side

Phrenic Nerve Palsy

It is rare but often associated with Erb's palsy. Diaphragmatic paralysis results in irregular labored thoracic breathing without any visible movements of abdomen. The diaphragm is elevated on the affected side and breath sound are diminished. The characterisitc see-saw movements of two sides of diaphragm during breathing is evident on fluoroscopic examination. The paradoxical movements of diaphragm (upward movement with each inspiration) on fluoroscopy or ultrasonography is diagnostic.

There is no specific therapy but baby should be nursed in lateral decubitus by turning towards the affected side. When there is respiratory insufficiency, oxygen therapy, CPAP and gavage feeding are often required. The recovery is usually complete but course may be complicated by respiratory infections. At times when recovery is incomplete, the weak and flabby leaf of diaphragm may manifest as eventration during infancy. In symptomate cases of eventration, surgical plication of diaphragm is recommended.

10

BIRTH TRAUMA TO CENTRAL NERVOUS SYSTEM

Intracranial Injury

Precipitate delivery or difficult forceps and vacuum extraction in a large baby, extraction of breech and other abnormal presentations may be associated with traumatic intracranial bleeding. The hemorrhage may be extradural, subdural, subarachnoid or intracerebral. Extradural hemorrhage is normally associated with fracture of skull bones. Subdural hemorrhage usually occurs following rupture of inferior sagittal sinus or small veins of cortex. Massive hemorrhage may result

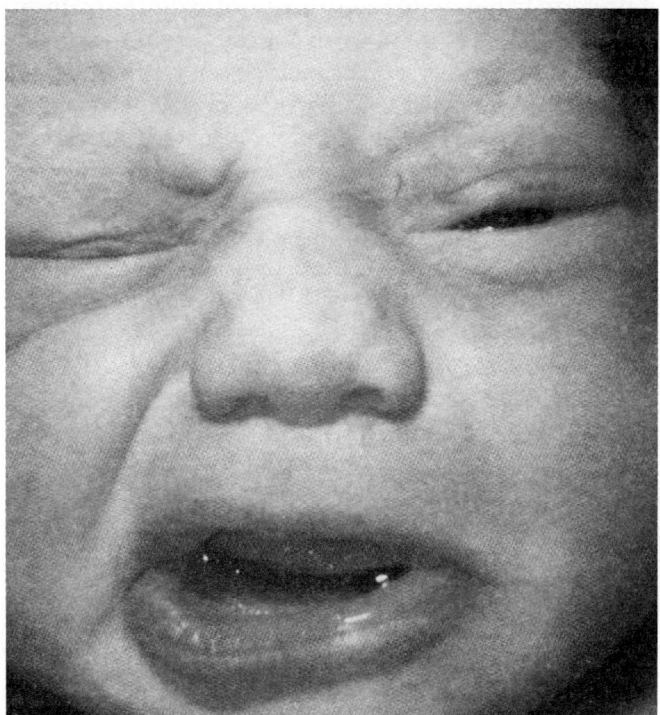

Figure 10.2 Facial palsy on the left side. Infant is unable to close the eye and there is no nasolabial fold on the affected side

from tear of the tentorium cerebelli and injury to the superior sagittal sinus. Intraventricular hemorrhage is limited to preterm babies and is non-traumatic. The baby manifests with abnormal neurological behavior within first 48 hours by cerebral depression, irritability, seizures, bulging anterior fontanel and unilateral neurological signs. There may be evidences of acute blood loss (pallor, shock) and aggravation of jaundice. It is difficult to differentiate between perinatal hypoxia and CNS trauma and both may co-exist. Ultrasound examination and CT scan of the brain may help to confirm the diagnosis of intracranial hemorrhage.

Treatment is mostly supportive and symptomatic. Infant should be nursed in a thermoneutral environment and head kept elevated to decrease intracranial pressure. Vitamin K 0.5–1.0 mg is administered IV or IM and fresh blood transfusion is given if there is hypotension. Phenobarbitone is given for prevention and control of seizures. Spinal puncture is indicated to relieve intracranial pressure in infants with subarachnoid hemorrhage. A subdural tap is done through anterior fontanel or coronal suture to drain subdural hematoma. Head circumference should be monitored to make an early diagnosis of hydrocephalus and neuromotor disability. Severely affected infants may die and survivors may develop hydrocephalus, recurrent seizures, cerebral palsy and mental retardation.

Spinal Transection

Avulsion of cervical cord with fracture of cervical spine may rarely occur following difficult breech extraction. At times a click or crack may be heard during delivery. It is characterized by flaccid paraplegia with retention of urine and overflow incontinence. Respiratory failure may occur due to paralysis of diaphragm by involvement of phrenic nerve. Prognosis is grave.

Visceral Injuries

Capsular laceration of liver, spleen and adrenals may follow difficult breech extraction. The damage to viscera may also occur because of over-zealous attempts at external cardiac massage. The hemorrhage may remain concealed as subcapsular hematoma or capsule may rupture with leakage of blood into the peritoneal cavity. The baby may manifest severe pallor, tachycardia and evidences of shock. The presence of shifting dullness may suggest the existence of blood in the peritoneal cavity which can be aspirated for diagnostic purposes. The diagnosis can be confirmed on ultrasonography of abdomen. Hyperbilirubinemia may occur due to breakdown of red blood cells of extravasated blood. Early recognition and administration of vitamin K and blood transfusion may salvage some of these babies.

Adrenal hemorrhage is rarely diagnosed in life but when detected on autopsy, it is difficult of say whether it was the result of direct trauma, anoxia or endotoxin shock due to sepsis.

PREVENTION

Modern practice of obstetrics and early resort to operative deliveris have reduced the incidence of birth injuries as well as birth asphyxia. Skilled antenatal care, early identification of high-risk pregnancies and evaluation of pelvic abnormalities and size of outlet are crucial to reduce the risk of birth trauma. During intranatal care, fetus should be monitored so that early decision is taken to deliver the baby by cesarian section if there is fetal hypoxia or discrepancy between the size of the fetus and pelvic outlet. Infants with breech presentation, especially in primigravida mothers, should be handled with utmost care and skill by an experienced obstetrician. When indicated, episiotomy should be carefully done to prevent incision of scalp. Instrumental deliveries with difficult forceps or vacuum extraction should be avoided or done with utmost care. During vaginal delivery of breech presenting baby, care should be taken to prevent shoulder dystocia and excessive stretching of neck to prevent the risk of brachial palsy and injury or hematoma in the sternomastoid muscle. Special care should be taken during vaginal deliveries of preterm babies to reduce the risk of trauma and birth asphyxia. Most cases of birth injuries are preventable by skilled midwifery practice which can reduce the risk of neonatal morbidity and permanent disability.

BIBLIOGRAPHY

Abedzadeh-Kalahrondi M, Talebian A, Mohammadzadeh M. Incidence of neonatal birth injuries and related factors in Kashan, Iran. *Arch Trauma Res* 2015, 4(1):C22831.

Borna H, Rad SM, Borna S, Mohseni SM. Incidence of and risk factors for birth trauma in Iran. *Taiwan J Obstet Gynecol* 2010, 49(2):170–173.

Nasab SAM, Varziri S, Arti HR, Najafi R. Incidence and associated risk factors of birth fractures in newborns. *Pak J Med Sci* 2011, 27(1):142–144.

Parker LA. Part 1: Early recognition and treatment of birth trauma: Injuries to the head and face. *Adv Neonatal Care* 2005, 5(6):288–297.

Pressler JL. Classification of major newborn birth injuries. *J Perinat Neonatal Nurs* 2008, 22(1):60–67.

Vhing MR. Management of birth injuries. *Clin Perinatol* 2005, 32:19–38.

Warker C, Malik S, Chokhandre, Saboo A. Birth injuries—A review of incidence, perinatal risk factors and outcome. *Bombay Hosp J* 2012, 54(2):202–207.

10

Temperature Regulation in Neonates

Neonates are physiologically homeothermic and are equipped with a thermostat in the hypothalamus but their thermoregulatory efforts are often insufficient with an increased risk of development of hypothermia in preterm and LBW babies. Heat is produced by muscular activity and shivering which are minimal in LBW babies. Non-shivering or metabolic thermogenesis occurs in the brown fat of newborn babies. Brown fat is located in nape of the neck, upper back, axillae, groins and around kidneys and adrenals. Preterm and small-for-dates babies have poor quota of brown fat and hence poor ability to keep themselves warm. Infant consumes lot of oxygen and glucose during metabolic thermo-genesis leading to hypoxia and hypoglycemia. When a baby is not nursed in a warm environment, his weight gain would be slow because glucose would be consumed for metabolic thermogenesis and denied for physical growth. Newborn babies, especially those who are preterm, LBW or sick, must be provided with a warm micro-environment to minimize or prevent metabolic thermogenesis. *The environmental temperature at which a baby consumes minimal oxygen and energy for metabolic thermogenesis is called as thermoneutral temperature.* When babies are nursed in a thermoneutral temperature, they are likely to have satisfactory growth velocity and enhanced survival.

MECHANISMS OF HEAT LOSS

In uterus, fetus bathes in a warm amniotic fluid which is maintained at 37°C. Infant is born naked, wet and partially asphyxiated in a labor room which is maintained at a temperature which is geared to provide comfort to the mother and is not satisfactory to serve the biological needs of the baby. Infant loses heat due to evaporation (latent heat of evaporation is 540 kcal per gram of water that evaporates) and through other avenues of heat loss (radiation, convection and conduction) as shown in **Figure 11.1**. After birth, skin and core temperature of the baby is likely to fall by

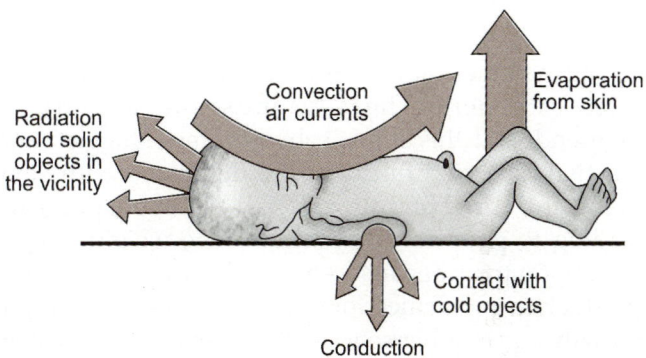

Figure 11.1 Four ways a newborn baby may lose heat to the environment

0.3°C and 0.1°C per minute respectively if attempts are not made to keep the baby warm. It is estimated that 15 percent of newborn babies develop hypothermia at birth in developing countries.

HYPOTHERMIA

Hypothermia in a newborn baby is defined as a skin temperature of <35.5°C or core temperature of <36.0°C.

Causes

Hypothermia may occur because of excessive heat loss, poor ability to conserve heat or poor ability to produce metabolic heat. The conditions leading to excessive heat loss include cold environment, wet or naked baby, cold linen, during transport and various procedures such as bath, blood sampling, imaging studies, intravenous infusion, diagnostic and surgical procedures, etc. Neonates are unable to conserve heat because of large surface area, poor insulation, paucity of fat and inability to reduce effective surface area by assuming flexed posture. The metabolic heat production is poor, especially in preterm and low birth weight babies because of deficiency of brown fat, greater risk of hypoxia and hypoglycemia, and poor integrity neurogenic pathways.

Clinical Manifestations

Hypothermia is far more common in newborn babies (especially preterm and LBW babies) than fever or hyperthermia.

The severity of hypothermia is graded on the basis of core or rectal temperature as follows:

1. *Cold stress* The core temperature varies between 36.0 and 36.4°C. The difference between the core and peripheral skin temperature is more than 1.5°C and extremities are cold and pale.
2. *Moderate hypothermia* Temperature between 32.0 and 35.9°C
3. *Severe hypothermia* Temperature of less than 32.0°C

The hypothermic baby is uncomfortable, restless and cries to generate heat by muscular activity. If unattended at this stage, baby becomes sluggish and inactive. The vital functions are depressed with slow breathing, bradycardia and fall in blood pressure leading to poor tissue perfusion. The weight gain is unsatisfactory because energy is wasted for heat production and denied for physical growth. Even brain growth may be adversely affected as evidenced by slow increase in head size. The immunologic system is also depressed with increased susceptibility to develop septicemia, sclerema and disseminated intravascular coagulation (DIC). Preterm babies nursed in a cold environment have a significantly increased risk of morbidity and mortality as compared to those nursed in a thermoneutral environment.

Recording Temperature

Rectal temperature should be recorded with a low-reading thermometer (range 30°C – 40°C) because otherwise the severity of hypothermia may be overlooked. *To safeguard against rectal perforation, thermometer should be directed slightly posteriorly and should not be inserted beyond 2 cm.* The thermometer should be left in place for at least 2 minutes before reading the temperature. Each baby should have a separate thermometer. Axillary temperature is reliable and should be taken after drying the axilla. The temperature should be recorded manually after every 2–3 hours to check that it coincides with the temperature displayed by the thermister probe. The temperature is best monitored with the help of an electronic thermister probe which is affixed over the skin of abdomen above the umbilicus. *The thermister probe must remain in close contact with the skin, otherwise baby would get inadvertently overheated.*

ROLE OF A NURSE IN KEEPING THE BABIES WARM

Labor room The baby should be received in a pre-warmed bassinet having a radiant heat source. He should be immediately dried and effectively covered with a prewarmed sheet or blanket. The head constitutes a large surface area of the baby and must be dried effectively. *Bath should be delayed to the next day and no baby should be bathed in the labor room except babies born to HBV or HIV positive mothers.* The low birth weight baby must be immediately transferred by the nurse to the warm environment of the nursery and housed in an incubator or open care system when indicated.

Lying-in ward During winter months, the baby should lie next to the mother rather than a separate cot. The warm body of the mother serves as a useful biologically controlled source of heat. In extreme winter, the room can be kept warm with a heater or hot air blower. A basin of water should be placed infront of hot air blower to increase the humidity. The oil-filled radiant warmer is preferred as it gives controlled heat and does not reduce humidity. The baby should be adequately clothed with woolens and head, feet and hands should be covered with a cap, socks and mittens **(Figure 11.2)**. There is no need to bathe the baby in winter, instead sponging can be done on alternate days.

Neonatal intensive care unit (NICU) *The high-risk and LBW baby must be transferred from the labor room to the NICU by the nurse (not an ayah!) and kept in the incubator or open care system if birth weight is less than 1800 g or gestation is below 35 weeks.* The baby is hooked to a servo-controlled open care system to maintain his mid-epigastric skin temperature around 36.5°C. This system is so geared that it would automatically maintain the temperature of the baby by increasing or decreasing the heat output depending upon the needs of the baby. When the temperature and clinical condition of the baby has stabilized he should be enclosed in a perspex heat shield or clothed and provided with a cap to reduce radiant heat loss. Application of oil or liquid paraffin to the skin reduces both heat and evaporative losses.

Nursing Alert

When a baby is under cold stress, he is likely to have poor weight gain because glucose is being used for metabolic thermogenesis and denied for physical growth.

Practical Tip

It must be remembered that hypothermia is an important symptom of septicemia in preterm babies and hypothermia per se is an important risk factor for development of bacterial infection.

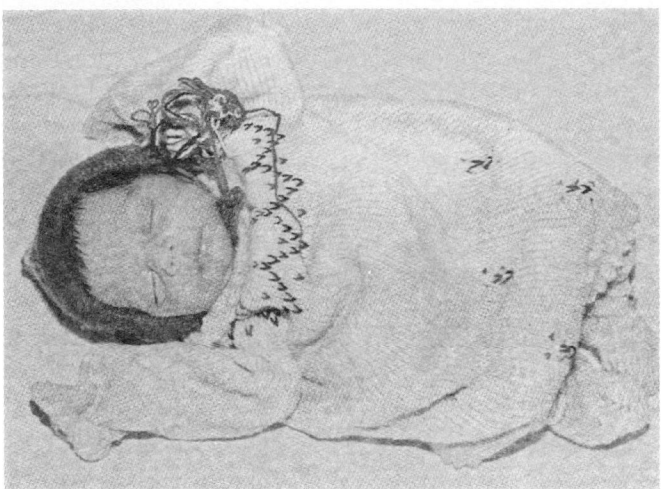

Figure 11.2 Effectively clothed baby to prevent hypothemia

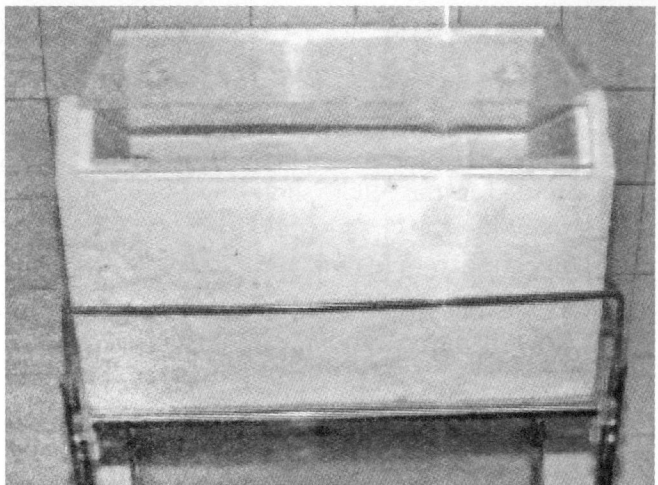

Figure 11.3 Thermocole box for transport of babies in developing countries

The temperature of the NICU should be maintained around 28°C ±2°C. The nursery babies should not be given a bath and they can be sponged. *During various diagnostic, therapeutic and surgical procedures, radiant heat source should be used to keep the baby warm.* When NICU facilities are not available, preterm babies can be kept warm with hot water bottles or electric blankets but these heat sources should never come in direct contact with the skin of the baby.

Operation theater Infants are at grave risk to develop severe hypothermia during surgery because of low temperature of operation theater, prolonged exposure, evaporative losses following skin preparation and administration of cold anesthetic gases. Infant should be placed on a circulating water mattress and over head radiant warmer should be affixed at a height of 45 cm above the infant. Fiberoptic "hot pipe" system can be used to effectively provide the baby with warm microenvironment from all sides. Rectal temperature of the infant should be continuously monitored with the help of a telethermometer.

Transport Availability of a transport incubator is ideal but it is available in selected hospitals and nursing homes due to high cost. The baby should be effectively covered with woolens (cap, socks, mittens) or wrapped with cotton or tin foil. Skin-to-skin contact during transport is useful to keep the baby warm. A padded cane basket with handle and hot water bottles in side hampers can be improvised. *The hot water bottle should never come in direct contact with the baby due to risk of burns.* A thermocole box with a transparent plastic lid can be used as a cheap, safe and effective transport incubator in developing countries. The thermocole box can be warmed with hot water bottle before the start of journey **(Figure 11.3)**.

Home care The mother must be explained about the risk of changes in the environmental temperature to the health and wellbeing of her infant. She should be trained to assess the temperature of the baby with her hands. *In a healthy baby nursed in thermoneutral environement, the trunk should feel warm to touch and hands and feet should be reaonably warm and pink.* The baby should be kept dried, effectively clothed and covered with woolens and provided with a cap, socks and mittens. The clothes should be pre-warmed by holding them infront of a heater or placing them on a hot water bottle or a hot *tawa*. Swaddling is useful to keep the baby warm in winter. The cot of the mother and baby should be kept away from the wall and baby should lie next to the mother to receive maternal warmth. The room should be kept warm with a heater or 'angeethi', taking due care to safeguard against accumulation of carbon monoxide. The culturally accepted practice of giving oil massage to the baby is useful because it reduces both heat as well as insensible water loss. Mother should be explained to avoid exposure during the procedure of bathing the baby. In winter months, daily sponging with warm water is better than dip bathing.

Prevention of Hypothermia

The goal of good thermal care is to achieve a core temperature between 36.8°C and 37.3°C. The following guidelines and strategies should be implemented to prevent hypothermia which is likely to reduce morbidity and improve survival of newborn babies.

1. High-risk mother should be identified during antenatal period and referred to a center equipped to provide good quality obstetrical and neonatal care services.

2. In the labor room, a warm microenvironment should be created to provide a warm welcome to the baby at birth. The baby should be dried promptly and covered effectively at birth.

3. Do not give bath to the baby at birth and babies admitted in the NICU should not be bathed but sponged.

4. The nursery or room temperature should be maintained around 28°C ±2°C. A standby incubator should be kept warm and ready all the time to receive a small, sick or cold baby.

5. The babies should be effectively covered and clothed with a cap, socks and mittens.

6. The fomites (inanimate objects) that come in direct contact with the baby should be prewarmed viz., cot, linen, clothes, infusates, X-ray film, etc.

7. Nurse should take special care to prevent hypothermia during the procedures and transport.

8. Application of oil or liquid paraffin to the skin reduces the risk of evaporation and heat loss.

9. Skin-to-skin contact or kangaroo-mother care (KMC) provides an excellent source of biologically controlled heat source. Apart from providing warmth, it promotes bonding and breastfeeding. The details of kangaroo-mother care are discussed in **Chapter 13**.

Key Message

The ambient temperature that feels uncomfortable or 'hot' to an adult, is most suitable to serve the biological needs of a newborn baby.

---

10. Mothers, health care workers and nurses should be provided with knowledge and skills to assess the baby's temperature by touch and prevent hypothermia. *When trunk is warm to touch and extremities are reasonably warm and pink, it indicates that baby is well and has a satisfactory body temperature. However, when trunk feels warm to touch but extremities are cold or pale, it suggests that baby has cold stress. But when both the trunk as well as the extremities are cold to touch, the baby has hypothermia.*

COLD INJURY

Preterm infants and neonates with birth asphyxia and damage to central nervous system are more vulnerable to develop features of cold injury. After initial restlessness and irritability, the baby becomes sluggish, inactive and refuses to take feeds. The skin becomes cold to touch. Facial erythema because of failure of dissociation of oxyhemoglobin at lower temperatures,

gives a false impression of wellbeing. Vital signs are depressed as evidenced by bradycardia, slow breathing with apneic attacks and hypotension. In advanced cases, sclerema and subcutaneous fat necrosis may occur. Septicemia, hypoglycemia and disseminated intravascular coagulation (DIC) may complicate the clinical picture.

Nursing management Hypothermic baby should be immediately transferred to an incubator or open care system and slowly warmed to achieve normal skin or core temperature within 4–6 hours. Oxygen and glucose should be administered intravenously to meet the increased demands and correct hypoxia and hypoglycemia if it is present. In the event of hemorrhagic manifestestations, 0.5–1.0 mg of vitamin K is given IV. Antibiotics are given to treat associated septicemia. Exchange blood transfusion is given when disseminated intravascular coagulation (DIC) is suspected. Hydrocortisone is indicated in babies with sclerema, wherein skin becomes taut or stretched like hide of an animal.

Nursing Alert

In infants with hyperthermia due to increase in environmental temperature both trunk and extremities are warm to touch as opposed to infants with sepsis who are likely to have warm trunk and cold extremities due to vasoconstriction.

In babies with severe hypothermia and cold injury, prognosis is generally poor with a case fatality rate of 25 to 50 percent. The presence of bleeding manifestations and sclerema are associated with poor outcome.

HYPERTHERMIA

The various causes of fever in neonates include raised environmental temperature, dehydration, infections, administration of certain drugs (belladona preparation, ephedrine nose drops) and exposure of the baby to sunlight or phototherapy. However, it must be remembered that in preterm and low birth weight babies, infections more often produce hypothermia rather than fever. Iatrogenic hyperthermia may occur due to exposure to strong overhead heat source or inadvertent dislodgement of skin thermister in a baby nursed in a servo-controlled incubator or open care system.

Transient fever of the newborn During summer months when environmental temperature goes above 38.5°C, some exclusively breastfed healthy term neonates may develop fever on the second or third day of life. The baby remains active, alert and cries for feeding. It appears that raised environmental temperature in association with immaturity of heat regulatory center and inefficiency of sweating mechanism in the newborn are the most likely causative agents. The condition is benign and self-limited. The infant is best managed by cooling the environment and promotion of breastfeeding. At times, hydrotheraphy is required for prompt reduction of body temperature. *There is no therapeutic utility of antipyretic agent because there is no alteration in the setting of thermostat in the hypothalamus.*

BIBLIOGRAPHY

Hull D. The structure and function of brown adipose tissue. *Brit Med Bull* 1966, 22:92.

McCall EM, Alderdice FA, Halliday HL, et al. Interventions to prevent hypothermia at birth in preterm and/or low birth weight babies. *Cocherane Database Syst Rev* 2008, 1:CD 004210.

Scopes JW. Metabolic rate and temperature control in human baby. *Brit Med Bull* 1965, 32:88.

Silverman WA, Sinclair JC. Temperature regulation in the newborn infant. *New Engl J Med* 1966, 274:92.

Singh M, Rao G, Malhotra AK, Deorari AK. Assessment of newborn baby's temperature by human touch. A potentially useful primary care strategy. *Indian Pediatr* 1992, 29:449–452.

11

Humanized Nursing Care of Babies in the NICU

Neonatal nursing demands utmost precision in various skills which are required for optimal and rational management of high-risk and very LBW babies. There is no denying the fact that critically sick newborn babies are saved by the "mother-like" caring attitude and sophisticated skills of specially trained nurses who discharge their responsibility with dedication, commitment and compassion. *The NICU environment should be as close to the womb-like ambience as possible by reducing various external stimuli.* Despite all the technological advances, scientists have failed to fabricate an incubator with all the qualities and characteristics of the womb **(Box 12.1)**. It is preferable to assign 2–3 babies to a nurse who should provide comprehensive "customized" and developmentally supportive care to the babies under her charge so that she is able to develop a rapport with the baby and her mother.

It is a common observation that preterm and sick newborns are being looked after in an unpleasant, noisy, too bright, aggressive and invasive environment of NICU without any concern for their physiological needs and comfort. Instead they should be reared in the NICU which should simulate the ecology of the womb to ensure maximum comfort to the baby. The babies should be handled with gentle touch, love and compassion, and nurses should feel 'connected' and 'tuned' to the babies under their care.

Positioning

Preterm infant should be placed on the side or prone position and his position changed every 3 hours. It has been shown that preterm babies maintain better oxygenation, temperature control and sleep pattern when nursed in a prone or lateral position. Provide midline alignment and keep the extremities flexed. Create a soft and comfortable bed with "containment" by creating boundaries with the help of a blanket or roll of a bed sheet **(Figure 12.1)**. Place a roll of linen at the infant's feet to provide a support to the baby during stress.

Sound

The health care professionals working in the NICU should learn the art of walking gracefully and talking gently. Nurses should avoid unnecessary talking and perform their duties quietly. The door and port holes of incubator should be closed gently. The alarm of monitors and telephone rings should be replaced by blinking lights. Cover the incubator with a sound-proof thick blanket. Avoid putting any objects over the incubator and do not write notes by placing the case file over the incubator top. Restrict the entry of

---

Box 12.1   The characteristics of the womb

- Comfortable and well-cushioned aquatic abode
- Absolute thermal comfort
- Zero insensible water loss
- Shielded from light
- Protected from sound
- Effective and safe ECMO-like oxygenation
- Optimal excretion of waste products
- Isolation and asepsis
- Parenteral nutrition

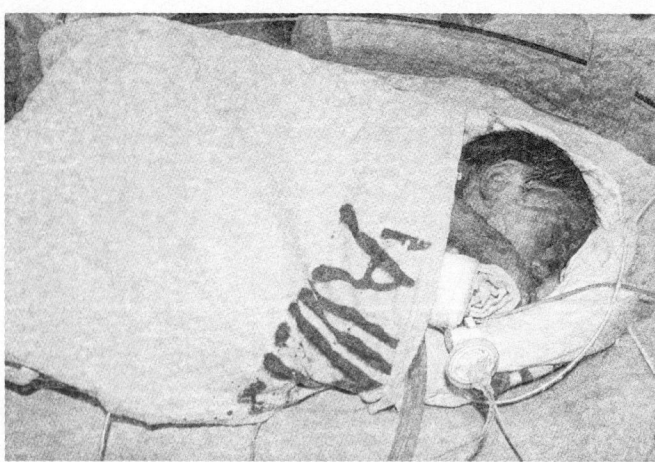

Figure 12.1 Effective nesting of baby to provide comfort

unnecessary visitors. Avoid use of noisy air compressors and ensure centralized supply of oxygen, air and suction. Play a soft and soothing music in a low volume.

Light

Avoid excessive light and dim the light further at night to simulate day and night to promote development of diurnal biorhythm. Cover the incubator with a blanket to dampen the sound and light reaching the baby **(Figure 12.2)**. The spotlight used for examination or procedure should be directed away from the baby's head and his eyes should be shielded from light. The illumination of NICU should be kept dim without compromising ease of observation. The light should be further dimmed off and on to create periods of 'quiet time' during each shift. Dim lighting has been shown to improve duration of sleep, decrease motor activity, reduce heart rate, improve tolerance of feeds and increase weight gain of stable preterm babies.

Gentle Touch

Provide a gentle and warm touch and do not disturb the baby unnecessarily. Before suddenly touching the baby, talk to her gently to awaken her. Handle the baby gently and only when absolutely necessary. The babies should not be handled as mere "objects" in a stereotyped mechanical or robotic manner. Gentle human touch (GHT) and caressing are associated with hemodynamic stability, improved sleep cycle, sucking behavior and cognition. The art of newborn care should not be sacrificed at the altar of technology.

Warmth and Humidity

The baby should be nursed in a thermoneutral environment so that there is minimal consumption of energy and oxygen by reducing the need for metabolic thermogenesis. Mother should be encouraged to provide warmth by skin-to-skin contact **(Figure 12.3)**. Ensure optimal humidity to reduce evaporative losses of water through the thin and delicate skin of preterm babies. Preterm babies should not be given a bath, but they can be cleaned gently with a wet soft napkin. Application of oil or liquid paraffin to skin reduces both heat loss and evaporative loss of water.

Developmentally Supportive Care

It is important to remember that both lack of stimulation and over stimulation are equally bad for the optimal neuropsychological development of preterm babies. After having achieved physiological stability, preemies should be provided with developmentally supportive care. It is desirable to assign one or two babies to a nurse and they should follow an individualized and flexible

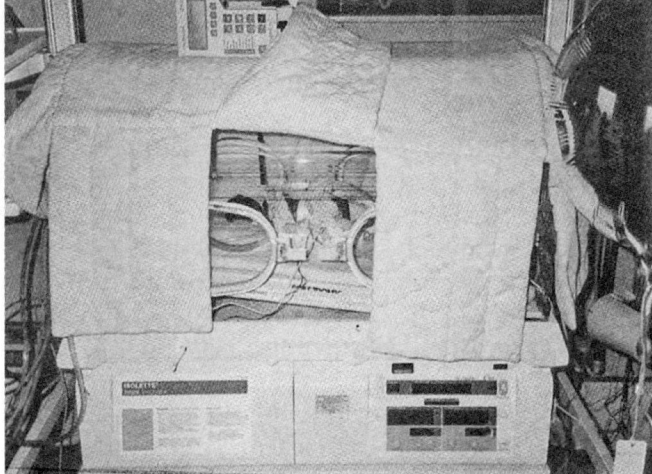

Figure 12.2 The incubator is kept covered to dampen the noise and reduce the light reaching the baby. The baby must be attached to a vital sign monitor

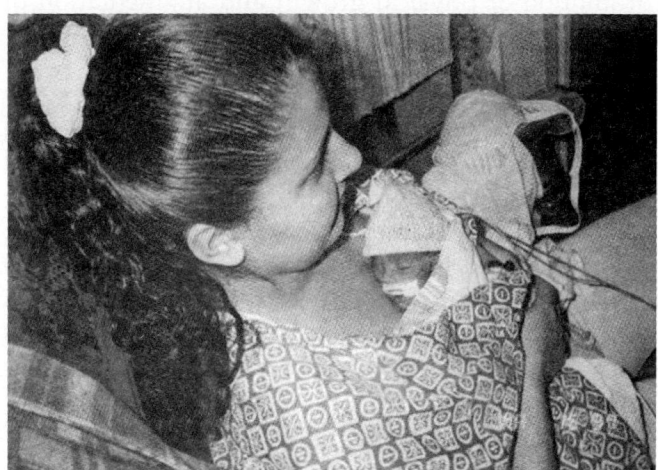

Figure 12.3 Mother providing skin-to-skin care to her baby in the NICU

approach in their care and stimulation. The nurse must feel "connected" or "tuned" with babies under her care. *Nurse must handle the baby not only with her head but also with her heart.* Brain is business like but heart brings in wholeness, harmony and healing. A variety of tactile, kinesthetic, auditory, vestibular and visual stimuli can be provided. Early and intensive family participation in the care of preterm babies is important to promote mother-infant bonding to relieve her stress and anxiety. Mother is more likely to look after her baby with devotion and compassion and thus augment the forces of healing and process of recovery.

Tactile-kinesthetic Stimulation

The nurses should provide tactile stimulation by gently touching the head or back of the baby while speaking softly in a soothing voice. The baby should be

12

positioned in such a way so that he is able to suck his fingers and is able to touch his face. The baby should be encouraged to grasp the finger of the nurse or edge of the blanket. In order to promote rooting and sucking, the angle of the mouth can be stroked with a soft brush or finger and baby given a pacifier (dummy nipple) or put on the breast before expression of milk. The mother should be encouraged to provide intermittent skin-to-skin contact to her baby. It provides comfort, warmth and 'special smell' of the mother to her baby. It improves mother infant bonding and promotes breastfeeding. During skin-to-skin contact, most babies feel comfortable, stop crying and achieve physiological stability. It reduces the risk of apneic attacks in premature babies. During skin-to-skin contact, there is a possibility of transfer of tremendous electromagnetic energy from a compassionate mother to her baby producing calmness, comfort, autonomic stability, promotion of physical growth and augmentation of healing forces.

Stimulation of Special Senses

Infants respond to auditory stimuli as early as 28 weeks of gestation. Research studies have shown that soft and soothing music to individual babies enhances their physiologic stability and improve weight gain velocity. Babies like and enjoy listening to classical or gentle instrumental music. The babies can be made to listen to the taped voice of parents and family members during their stay in the NICU. This enhances parent-infant bonding and gives family members the sense of involvement in the care of their baby. Music is credited to enhance autonomic stability, reduce stress and quietens the baby, increase oxygen saturation and reduce heart rate.

Dimlight encourages babies to open their eyes and look around. The baby should be picked up and encouraged to develop an eye-to-eye contact. Babies often turn towards a source of diffuse light. Visual stimuli can be provided with the help of bright toys and pictures. A picture of the mother or sibling with distinct facial patterns can be placed on the incubator or crib in line with the gaze of the baby.

Babies are sensitive and perceptive to the smell of the mother's milk which is useful for rooting the nipple during breastfeeding. The gauze pads or cotton balls soaked with mother's milk can be kept inside the incubator to stimulate olfactory system. Skin-to-skin contact provides pleasant and 'special' smell of the mother to her baby to promote bonding. The baby should not be exposed to strong and unpleasant or noxious odors like surgical spirit, betadine and other skin scrub antiseptics.

Feeding with Human Milk

Nothing is more humanized than feeding the baby with milk of her mother because milk is not only species specific, it is baby-specific. Extremely preterm babies cannot self feed and they are given expressed breast milk (EBM) through a nasogastric tube. Even when nutritional needs cannot be met due to physiologic instability, the baby should be provided with minimal enteral feeds to harness its trophic effects on the gastrointestinal tract.

Diaper Care

Preterm babies are worn disposable diapers made of cotton enclosed in two layers of gauze pieces. As soon as the baby voids, the diaper is removed, bottom is cleaned and dried and a new diaper is worn. Provide comfort and warmth to the baby.

Medications

Medicines should be administered with utmost care and caution. Check all medications for their expiry date and discard the drugs which have expired. It is preferable that all medications are verified by two nurses. If a medication say amikacin is being given to a number of babies in the NICU, one vial should be used for all the babies in a shift before opening another vial. The nurse shall be dealing with extremely small doses of drugs in preterm babies and there is thus an increased risk of over medication unless due care is exercised. Use 1.0 mL or insulin syringe for giving medications in the NICU to reduce the risk of over dosing. For example, vitamin K is available only in a strength of 10 mg per mL but a preterm baby is recommended to receive only 0.5 mg per dose, i.e. he should be given 0.05 mL (which is one-half of 0.1 mL). The following principles should be followed while giving medicines to babies

1. Ask for a written order by the physician but verbal instructions may be complied in an emergency situation and recorded in the case file.
2. Observe all the "five rights" for administering medications
   i. Right patient
   ii. Right medicine
   iii. Right dose
   iv. Right route
   v. Right time
   The label of the medicine should be checked at least three times:
   a. On picking the medicine vial
   b. While taking the medicine dose in the syringe
   c. Before returning the vial back

It is important to check dose of the drug with another nurse or a resident doctor before administration. This must be done when dopamine, dobutamine, doxapram, indomethacin, phenytoin, diazepam, phenobarbitone, calcium, etc. are administered. The medication must be documented in the patient's file immediately after its administration. The amount of diluent used for administration of intravenous medications should be recorded and subtracted from the recommended daily fluid requirements. A list of common and emergency drugs with their dosages and mode of administration should be available in the NICU.

BIBLIOGRAPHY

Blackburn S. Environmental impact of the NICU on developmental outcomes. *J Pediatr Nurs* 1998, 13(5): 279–289.

Charpak N, Ruis JG, de Calume ZF. Humanizing neonatal care. *Acta Paediatr* 2000, 89: 501–502.

Conde-Agudelo A, Belizan JM, Diaz-Rossello J. Kangaroo-mother care to reduce morbidity and mortality in low birth weight infants. *Cochrane Database Sys Rev* 2011, 3: CD002771.

Depaul D, Chambers S. Enviromental noise in the neonatal intensive care unit: Implications for nursing practice. *J Perinatal Neonatal Nurs* 1995, 8:71–76.

Fleisher BE, Vandenberg K. Constantinou J, et al. Individualized developmental care of very low birth weight premature infants. *Clin Pediatr* 1995, 34(10): 523–529.

Paul VK, Gupta A, Singh M, Deorari AK, Pandey RM. Effect of Indian classical music on heart rate and oxygen saturation in preterm neonates in the NICU. *Pediatr Res* 1999, 45:16A.

Ramachandran S, Dutta S. Early developmental care interventions of preterm and low birth weight infants. *Indian Pediatr* 2013, 50:765–770.

Singh M, Deorari AK. Humanized care of preterm babies. *Indian Pediatr* 2003, 40:13–20.

12

Disorders of Weight and Gestation

> *"There is no indicator in human biology, which tells us so much about the past events and the future trajectory of life, as the weight of infant at birth."*
>
> — **V. Ramalingaswami**

LOW BIRTH WEIGHT BABIES

Birth weight is the single most important marker of fetal wellbeing and perinatal outcome. Babies with a birth weight of less than 2500 g, irrespective of the period of their gestation, are called LBW babies. Around 28% newborn babies in India are LBW as opposed to only 5–7% in the developed countries. After Pakistan (32%), India has the dubious distinction of having the highest incidence of LBW babies (28%) in the south-east Asia region. About two-thirds of LBW babies in India are small-for-dates (babies with intrauterine growth retardation) and one-third are preterm (gestation of 36 weeks or less) babies. Birth weight is the single most important marker of adverse perinatal and neonatal outcome. Over 80 percent of all neonatal deaths occur among LBW babies. They are more vulnerable to suffer from common day-to-day infections during infancy and 40 percent of LBW babies are malnourished at one year of age. Babies with fetal malnutrition or intrauterine growth retardation (IUGR) are more likely to develop type 2 diabetes mellitus, hypertension and coronary artery disease later in life (Barker hypothesis).

PRETERM BABIES (IMMATURE, PREMATURE)

About 8–10 percent of babies in our country are born preterm (gestation less than 37 completed weeks). These infants are anatomically and functionally immature leading to high risk of neonatal morbidity and mortality.

Causes

Premature delivery is common in women belonging to poor socioeconomic status, undernutrition, chronic and acute systemic maternal disease, antepartum hemorrhage, cervical incompetence, emotional stress and physical exertion or trauma. Babies with congenital malformations are likely to be delivered prematurely. A history of preterm birth in the past is associated with 3 to 4 times increased risk of prematurity in subsequent pregnancies. The labor is often induced before term when there is danger to the mother or fetus, e.g. placental dysfunction, eclampsia, fetal hypoxia, maternal diabetes mellitus, antepartum hemorrhage and rhesus isoimmunization.

Clinical Features

These babies are small in size with thin, gelatinous, shiny and pink skin. Birth weight of a preterm baby is usually less than 2500 g, crown-heel length <47 cm and head circumference <33 cm but it exceeds the chest circumference by more than 3 cm. They have abundant lanugo (fine hair on skin) with very little vernix caseosa. Ear cartilage is deficient, breast nodule is small or absent and testes may be undescended in boys while labia majora are widely separated exposing labia minora and hypertrophied clitoris in girls. The salient differences between the physical characteristics of term and preterm babies are summarized in **Table 13.1**. They have poor muscle tone with sluggish automatic reflexes (Moro reflex) and slow or ineffective sucking and swallowing efforts.

Clinical Problems

They are prone to a large number of clinical disorders because of anatomical and functional immaturity of various body organs.

1. Birth asphyxia and resuscitation difficulties are common due to poor transition from fetal to neonatal physiology.
2. Hypothermia occurs due to poor quantity of brown fat which is required for metabolic thermogenesis. Biochemical abnormalities like hypoglycemia, hypocalcemia, hypoproteinemia and acidosis are common.

Table 13.1 Physical characteristics of preterm and term neonates

Physical characteristics	Preterm (<37 weeks)	Term (37–41 weeks)
■ Skin texture	Thin, shiny, oily, plethoric with plenty of lanugo and visible veins	Thick, good turgor and elasticity, scanty lanugo
■ Scalp hair	Brownish-black, wooly, fuzzy and sparse	Black, silky and abundant
■ Ear cartilage	Pinna feels soft with deficient cartilage and poor recoil	Pinna is firm with thick cartilage and instant recoil
■ Breast nodule*	Breast nodule is less than 5 mm and nipple is small or absent	Breast nodule is more than 5 mm and nipple is well formed
■ Sole creases	Faint red marks or single deep crease over anterior one-third of sole	Entire sole covered with deep sole creases
■ Genitalia		
Male	Testes may be at or above the inguinal ring, scrotum is small with few rugositis	At least one testis is in the scrotum which is deeply pigmented and has prominent rugosities
Female	Labia majora are widely separated with fully exposed labia minora and prominent clitoris	Labia majora completely cover the labia minora

* In a small-for-dates baby, the breast tissue may be deficient or absent, even when the infant is full term.

3. They have incoordinated sucking and swallowing with greater risk of gastroesophageal reflux, regurgitation and aspiration of feeds. Abdominal distension is common because of hypotonia and autonomic immaturity.

4. Respiratory distress syndrome due to hyaline membrane disease (HMD) may occur because of immaturity of lungs and deficiency of surfactant. They are prone to aspiration into the lungs due to poor cough reflex and lack of coordination between sucking and swallowing. Apneic attacks are common because of immaturity of central nervous system.

5. Septicemia may occur due to immature immune defence mechanisms and greater handling and exposure to various equipment.

6. Hyperbilirubinemia is common due to immaturity of liver, hypoxia, hypothermia, hypoglycemia and infections. Bilirubin brain damage is more likely to occur due to immature blood–brain barrier.

7. Intraventricular hemorrhage (bleeding in the lateral ventricles of brain) may occur due to increased capillary fragility and relative deficiency of vitamin K-dependent coagulation factors.

8. Retinopathy of prematurity (ROP) may occur due to oxygen toxicity because of immature vaculature of retina.

9. Patent ductus arteriosus is common in babies with hyaline membrane disease (HMD) which may lead to congestive heart failure.

10. Chronic pulmonary insufficiency may occur due to bronchopulmonary dysplasia (BPD) following prolonged assisted ventilation.

11. Necrotizing enterocolitis (NEC) may occur in preterm babies having hypoxia, acidosis and formula feedings.

Nursing Management

High-risk mother should be identified early during the course of pregnancy and referred for delivery to an appropriate health care facility which is equipped with good quality obstetrical and neonatal care facilities. When a preterm baby is delivered at home or at a peripheral health care facility, his transfer to a district hospital or NICU is associated with several hazards and poor outcome. It is, therefore, much better to transfer a high-risk mother for confinement and care of the baby after delivery because uterus is the best transport incubator.

Antenatal corticosteroids Antenatal administration of corticosteroids is one of the most cost-effective strategies to improve the survival of preterm babies. Injection betamethasone 12 mg IM every 24 hours for 2 doses or dexamethasone 6 mg IM every 12 hours for 4 doses should be administered to the mother if labor starts or is induced before 34 weeks of gestation. Betamethasone is more potent and is associated with reduced risk of side effects. It enhances the maturation of the fetus and there is reduced risk of hyaline membrane disease (HMD), intraventricular hemorrhage (IVH) and necrotizing enterocolitis (NEC).

Care at birth Effective arrangements should be made for resuscitation and care of the preterm baby at birth. Radiant warmer should be put on before the baby is born and prewarmed sheets should be used to dry

13

and cover the baby. Vitamin K 0.5 mg should be given intramuscularly. *The baby should be transferred by the nurse (not a nursing orderly!) to the NICU as soon as effective breathing is established.*

Nursing monitoring The following clinical parameters should be monitored by specially trained nurses.

1. Vital signs with the help of a multi-channel vital sign monitor.
2. Activity and behavior of the baby.
3. Color, whether it is pink, pale, grey, blue, yellow.
4. *Tissue perfusion* is considered as satisfactory if baby is warm and has pink extremities, capillary refill over upper chest is <2 seconds **(Figure 13.1)**, blood pressure is normal, urine output is at least 1.5 mL/kg/hr and there is no metabolic acidosis.
5. Record of input and output.
6. Medication chart.
7. Daily weight record.

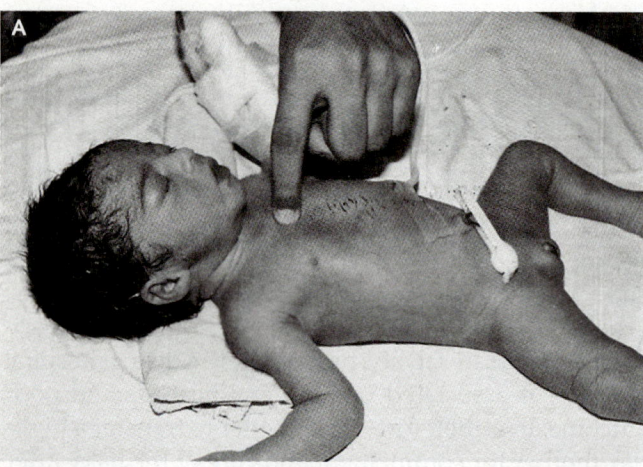

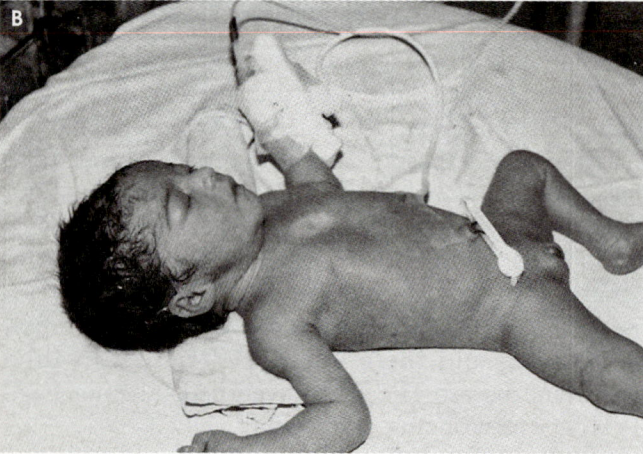

Figure 13.1 Testing for tissue perfusion. (A) Firm pressure is applied over the sternum to blanch the skin, (B) Blanching should disappear within 2 seconds in a healthy preterm baby

The Healthy Preterm Baby

The preterm baby is considered as well and healthy if vital signs are stable; baby is alert and active, his trunk is warm to touch and extremities are reasonably warm and pink, there is no respiratory distress or apneic attacks, baby is tolerating enteral feeds; and after initial two weeks, the baby is having steady weight gain of 1.0–1.5 percent (10–15 g/kg/day) of his body weight every day.

NURSING CARE

Provide Womb-like Conditions in the NICU

Uterus provides ideal ambient conditions to the baby and all attempts should be made to create uterus-like baby-friendly environment in the NICU or incubator for the care of preterm babies.

1. Create a soft, comfortable and cushioned bed.
2. Avoid excessive light, excessive sound and rough handling. Painful procedures should be performed after giving effective sedation and analgesia.
3. Provide warmth and nurse the baby in a thermo-neutral environment.
4. Ensure asepsis.
5. Prevent evaporative skin losses by effectively covering the baby, application of oil or liquid paraffin to the skin and by increasing humidity in the incubator.
6. Provide safe oxygenation.
7. Uterus is able to provide parenteral nutrition but adequate facilities for total parenteral nutrition (TPN) are not available in most NICUs in the country. Nevertheless, efforts should be made to provide at least partial parenteral nutrition along with enteral trophic feeds with expressed breast milk (EBM).

Position of the Baby

Most babies love to be placed in a prone position, they cry less and feel more comfortable. It relieves abdominal distension by passage of flatus and reduces risk of aspiration. Prone position improves ventilation, lung compliance and arterial oxygen saturation. When babies are nursed prone, they should be closely watched for apneic attacks.

Thermal Comfort

Babies below 1800 g or a gestation of less than 35 weeks should be nursed in an open care system **(Figure 13.2)**. The servo sensor of the open care system should be set to maintain skin temperature of mid-epigastric region of the baby at 36.5°C. This is called thermoneutral temperature because in this situation the baby would

13

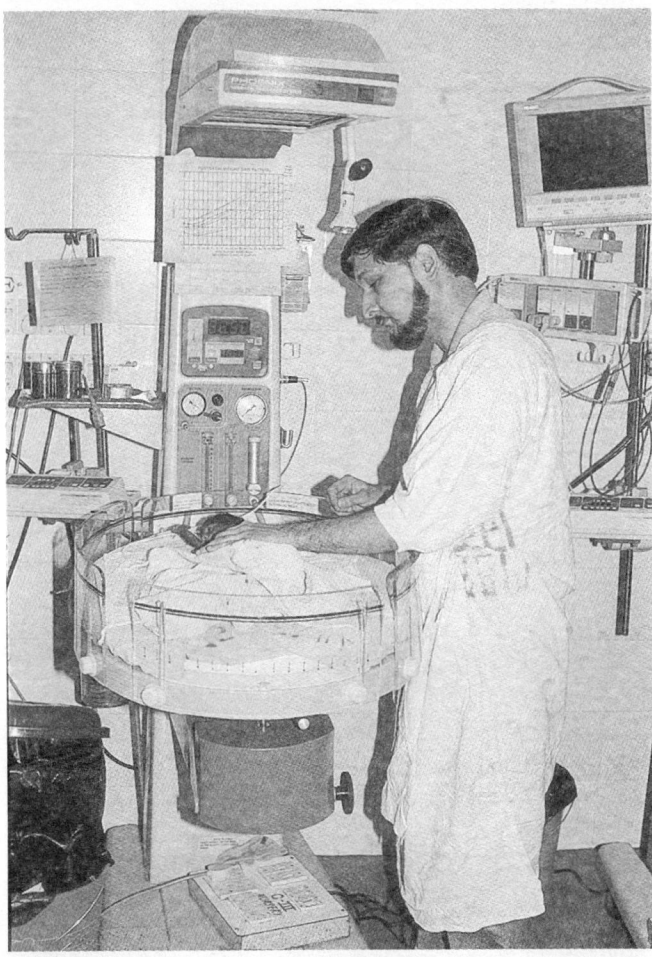

Figure 13.2 Baby being nursed in an open care system. After initial stabilization, the baby can be covered to prevent evaporative water losses

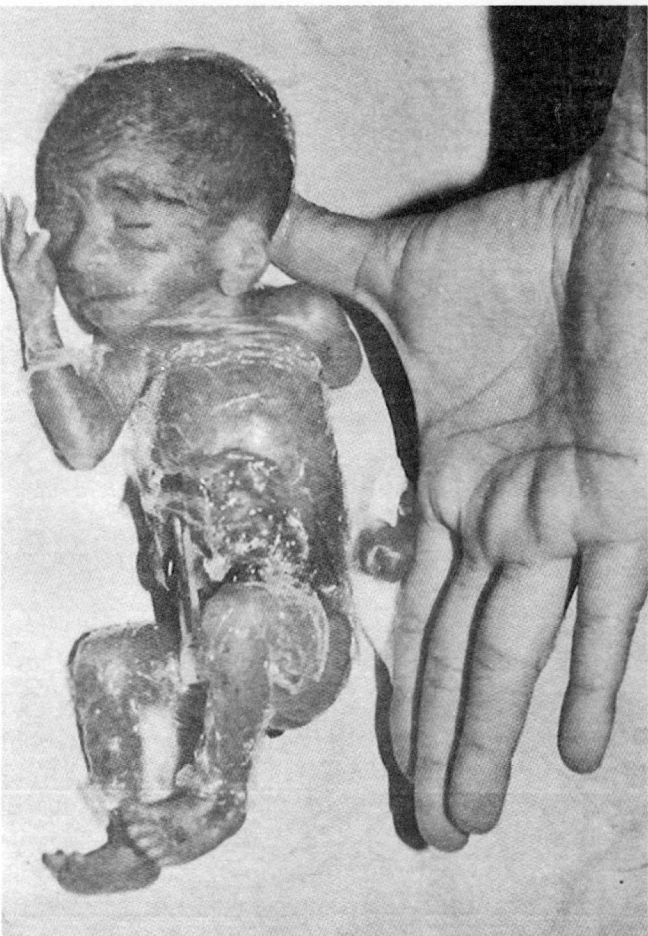

Figure 13.3 Extremely preterm baby, merely the size of a palm and weighing 650 g. The infant is covered with a cellophane to prevent evaporation and convective heat loss

have virtually no or minimal metabolic thermogenesis. The extremely LBW baby should be covered with a cellophane or thin transparent plastic sheet to prevent convective heat loss and evaporative losses of water from skin **(Figure 13.3)**. When the baby's condition is stabilized, he should be worn a frock, cap, socks and mittens. After one week or so, stable babies with a birth weight of less than 1200 g should preferably be nursed in an intensive care incubator. It is associated with reduced handling, better temperature control, reduced evaporative losses from skin and better weight gain velocity. The mother should be encouraged to visit the nursery to touch and "talk" with her baby and learn various skills to handle the baby after discharge.

Kangaroo-Mother Care (KMC)

Direct skin-to-skin contact of the baby with the mother (or any other family member) provides biologically controlled heat source to keep stable LBW babies warm. It is based on marsupial care concept of keeping the

offsprings warm in a maternal pouch, which was introduced in 1978 by Edgar Rey in Bogota, Colombia. It is a cost-effective and useful strategy to enhance the survival of LBW babies in developing countries having constraints of financial and technology resources.

Kangaroo-mother care may be continuous (round-the-clock) or more commonly it is intermittent. The procedure is most suitable for providing care to stable infants with a birth weight between 1500 and 1800 g or gestation of 32–34 weeks. A large number of physiological and clinical benefits of KMC have been documented **(Box 13.1)**. KMC is provided when baby is stable and his vital signs are maintained. Infant may be able to take the feed directly from the breast or EBM can be given with a cup and spoon or *paladay*.

The KMC Procedure

KMC is started when baby is stable and receiving oral feeds. Short-term or intermittent KMC can be started in the NICU in babies receiving intravenous or

13

Box 13.1 **Physiological and clinical benefits of KMC**

- Enhanced infant-mother bonding.
- Stimulation of all the five senses of the baby, viz. skin-to-skin contact (touch), mother's voice and heart beats (hearing), breastfeeding (taste), mother's odor (olfaction) and eye contact with mother (vision).
- Promotion of breastfeeding with improved yield of milk.
- Stability of vital signs with effective temperature control and reduced risk of apneic attacks.
- Reduced risk of nosocomial infections.
- Babies cry less, sleep better and show satisfactory neuro-behavioral development.
- Better weight gain and early discharge from NICU.
- It is a useful modality for short distance transport of stable babies.
- Mother may transmit electromagnetic vibrations of healing, love and compassion to her baby.

gastric feeds and low concentration of oxygen. Mother should be free from any infection and explained about importance of daily bath, maintenance of personal hygiene and handwashing. Mother should wear a front open gown or suitable dress which is culturally acceptable. The baby should be dressed with a front-open sleeveless shirt, cap, socks, mittens and a soakable napkin. The baby is placed between the mother's breasts by keeping the head in an upright position. The head is turned to one side and kept in a slightly extended position to keep the airway open **(Figures 13.4 and 13.5)**. The hips and arms of the baby should be kept flexed and abducted to maintain frog-like position. This enables a large surface area of the nude skin of the neonate to maintain a close contact with the chest and abdomen of the mother. The bottom of the baby should be supported with a sling or binder or a specially prepared KMC bag. The back of the baby should be covered with a woolen shawl.

Depending upon the maturity of the baby, mother can give breastfeeding or express the breast-milk and feed with a cup and spoon or *paladay*. During KMC, mother should sleep in a supine position in a semi-reclining position at an angle of 15 degrees from horizontal. A comfortable reclining chair with an adjustable back can be used to provide KMC. The mother should be given simple guidelines for monitoring the baby. During bathing or while attending to her toilet needs, the baby should be effectively covered or kept warm or provided KMC by a relative. KMC is continued till baby achieves body weight of about 2500 g or gestational maturity of 37 weeks. The baby is weamed from KMC when baby shows discomfort by

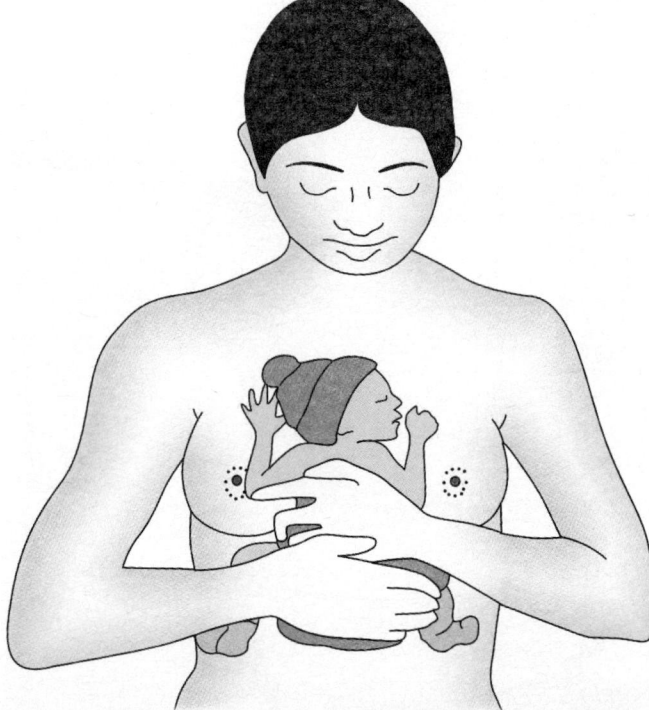

Figure 13.4 Diagrammatic depiction of positioning of the baby for effective kangaroo-mother care

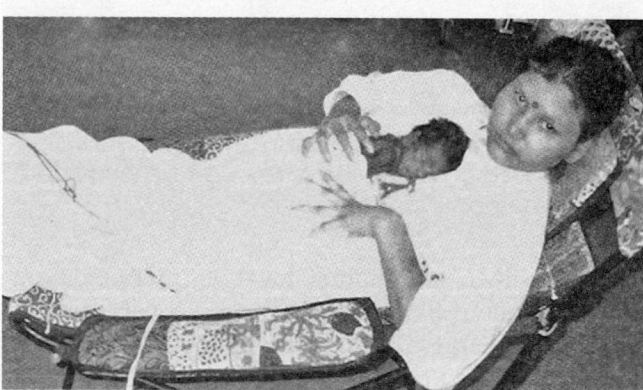

Figure 13.5 Kangaroo-mother care. It is highly cost-effective method to prevent hypothermia and promote bonding in preterm babies

crying or wriggling movements or there is sweating. It is important to remember that KMC is labor-intensive and uncomfortable to the mother (especially in hot summer months) and she needs emotional support from health care professionals (HCPs) and family members for its success.

Oxygen therapy *Oxygen should be given only when indicated and stopped as soon as its use is considered unnecessary.* The oxygen is administered with a head box when arterial oxygen saturation (SpO_2) falls below 85% and it is gradually withdrawn when SpO_2 goes above 90%. The lowest flow rate or concentration of oxygen should be used to maintain SpO$_2$ between 90 and 95% and arterial oxygen tension (PaO$_2$) between 60 and 80 mm Hg as a safeguard against development of retinopathy of prematurity (ROP).

Phototherapy Early phototherapy is needed in preterm babies to keep the serum bilirubin level within safe limits to prevent kernicterus.

Avoid unnecessary interventions In the care of preterm babies, at times greater harm is done by unnecessary therapeutic interventions which may lead to development of iatrogenic disorders. The following interventions should be avoided because they are unnecessary, useless and often associated with adverse side effects.

- Routine administration of oxygen without monitoring.
- Administration of intravenous immunoglobulins (IVIG) for prevention of neonatal sepsis.
- Prophylactic antibiotics.
- Unnecessary use of corticosteroids due to increased risk of cerebral baby.
- Prophylactic administration of indomethacin or high dose of vitamin E.
- Unnecessary blood transfusion. The definite indications for blood transfusion include hematocrit or packed cell volume of <40% in a sick neonate, <30% in a symptomatic neonate and <25% in an asymptomatic baby.
- Formula feeds instead of feeding with human milk.
- Prophylactic phototherapy.
- Avoid rough handling, exposure to bright light, loud sound, pungent odors, painful procedures without proper sedation and analgesia.

Prevention of nosocomial infections A preterm baby, who survives the initial stormy and unstable period of one week, is likely to do well if protected against development of infections and provided good nutrition. Refer to **Chapter 6** for details regarding prevention of nosocomial infections.

Feeding and Nutrition

Babies weighing less than 1200 g and sick or unstable babies (severe birth asphyxia, RDS, sepsis, seizures, apneic attacks, assisted ventilation, etc.) should be started on dextrose solution in a concentration of 10% dextrose in babies >1000 g and 5% dextrose in babies <1000 g. Trophic feeds with EBM (1–2 mL 4 times/d) through a nasogastric tube can be started in all preterm babies irrespective of their birth weight or clinical condition to enhance maturity of the gut.

When baby's condition is stabilized, enteral feeds are begun with EBM starting with a volume of 30 mL/kg/d on the first day and intravenous fluids are reduced accordingly. Depending upon the tolerance of feeds, the volume of feeds is gradually increased every day by 10–20 mL/kg/d. Feeds are given as a slow bolus by gravity every two hourly. After 10–14 days most preterm babies would receive enteral feeds at a rate of 120–150 mL/kg/d providing 150 kcal/kg/d. When baby starts gaining weight, EBM may be fortified with human milk fortifier (HMF) to increase intake of calories, protein and nutritional supplements. During nasogastric feeding, abdominal girth should be monitored and abdominal distension should be looked for as an early marker of feed intolerance and necrotizing enterocolitis.

After 2 weeks or so, when baby is gaining weight, nutritional supplements are started (when HMF is not given) to provide folic acid, vitamin E, calcium and phosphorus. Iron supplements are started after 4 weeks in a dose of 2–3 mg/kg of elemental iron per day.

Weight Record

Every baby admitted in the NICU should be weighed daily on an accurate electronic weighing scale **(Figure 13.6)**. Most preterm babies lose weight during the first 3–4 days of life and weight loss is up to maximum of 10–15% of the birth weight. The birth weight is regained by two weeks of age. After this, healthy preterm babies gain weight at a rate of 1.0 to 1.5% (10–15 g/kg/day) of their body weight per day. Excessive weight loss, delay in regaining the birth weight or slow weight gain velocity suggest that either the baby is not being fed adequately or the infant is unwell and needs immediate attention.

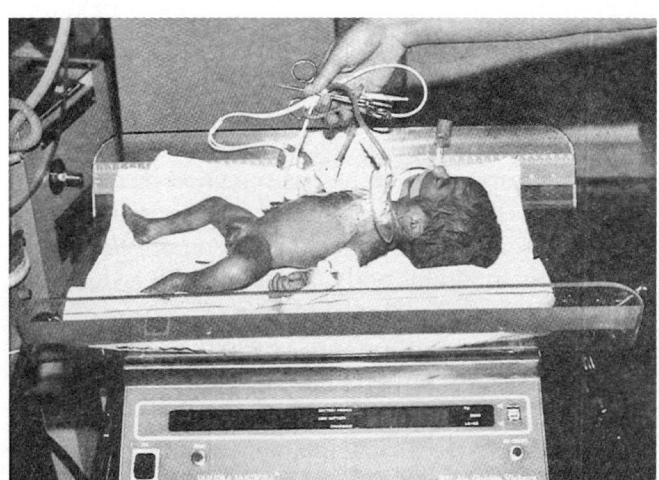

Figure 13.6 Weighing premature baby on an electronic weighing scale with a resolution of ±1.0 g

Transfer from Incubator to Cot

When a baby is tolerating the enteral feeds, is stable and reasonably active, and maintaining his body temperature, he can be transferred to the open cot. The baby should be observed for a period of 12 hours after putting the incubator off to see whether he can maintain his body temperature, before he is transferred to the open cot.

Immunizations

At the time of discharge from neonatal intensive care unit, BCG, oral polio vaccine and first dose of hepatitis B vaccine are given. Preterm babies are able to mount satisfactory immune response against various vaccines.

Nursing Support to the Family

The prolonged stay of preterm and sick newborn babies in the NICU with attendant high cost of care is associated with emotional trauma, stress, anxiety, uncertainty and lack of bonding between the family and the baby. The frightening scene of the NICU where the baby is attached to a variety of electronic machines and gadgets should be demystified and family should be constantly informed and involved in the care of their baby. The mother should be encouraged to touch and talk with her baby and provide routine care under the guidance of nurses. She should be assisted to provide intermittent kangaroo-mother-care (skin-to-skin contact) to her baby in the NICU to enhance bonding, promote breast feeding and transmit electromagnetic healing vibes to her baby. Nurse should cushion the anxiety and concern of the family by providing necessary emotional support and guidance.

Home Care

Most healthy infants with a birth weight of 1800 g or more and gestational age of 35 weeks or more can be managed at home. The preterm and sick babies discharged from NICU also need extended care at home. It is essential that the LBW baby is discharged from the hospital when he has regained birth weight and is showing a steady weight gain, is self feeding from the breast or with a cup and spoon or *paladay* and is able to maintain his body temperature. It is desirable that available physical facilities, resources and environmental conditions are assessed by a home visit by a public health nurse before the baby is discharged.

The mother should be given detailed instructions to keep the baby warm. The infant should be effectively covered and advised to wear woolen cap, socks and mittens. The baby should preferably lie next to the mother which serves as useful source of warmth. In winter, room can be warmed with a radiant heater or *angeethi*. A table lamp having a 100-watt bulb can be used to provide direct radiant heat. The use of hot water bottle should preferably be avoided. But when it is used as an emergency measure, it should be covered with a sheet and kept by the side of the baby without directly touching his skin. The mother should be trained to assess the temperature of the baby by touch. *When trunk is warm and extremities are reasonably warm and pink, it suggests that the baby is well and healthy and without any cold stress.*

Breastfeeding is ideal and should be continued if baby is able to suck. When infant is unable to suck, EBM should be given with a cup and spoon or *paladay*. When mother is unable to breast feed or provide EBM, cow's milk in 3:1 dilution or special formula for preterm babies can be used.

The baby should be kept isolated in one room and unnecessary visits by relatives should be avoided. Strict hand washing with soap and water before picking the baby or feeding the baby should be followed. The linen and clothes of the baby should be properly washed and sun-dried.

Prognosis

The prognosis depends upon the birth weight of the baby and quality of neonatal care provided to him. Most preterm babies without any neonatal complications do well and their physical growth and neuromotor development corresponds to their corrected chronological age. For example, when a baby with an expected day of delivery of August 15 is actually born on say July 1st, he should be considered as one day old on 15th August and his postnatal age should be calculated from that date. Preterm babies are prone to develop recurrent infections, nutritional disorders (poor weight gain, anemia, osteopenia), gastroesophageal reflux, reactive airway disease, hypertension and renal dysfunction. LBW babies and sick preterm babies have an increased risk of development of neuromotor disability like cerebral palsy, seizures, hydrocephalus or microcephaly, squint, blindness (due to ROP), deafness, learning disabilities and mental retardation.

SMALL-FOR-DATES BABIES (Small-for-Gestational Age, Intrauterine Growth Retardation)

Newborn babies with a birth weight of less than 10th percentile for the period of their gestation are classified as small-for-dates **(Figure 13.7)**. Around two-thirds of LBW babies are small-for-dates (SFD). These babies have suffered from intrauterine growth retardation

13

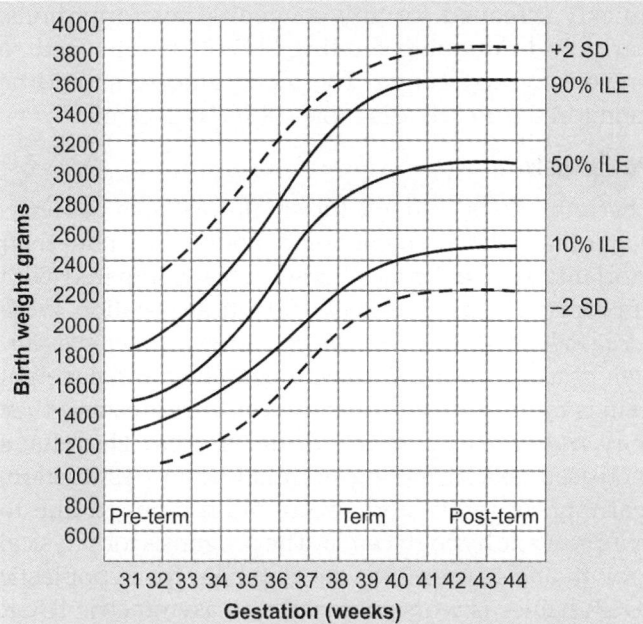

Figure 13.7 Intrauterine weight chart (AIIMS)

(IUGR) or fetal malnutrition. Depending upon their gestation, these babies may be preterm, term or post-term.

Causes

The cause of IUGR may rest with the mother, placenta or fetus. The common maternal causes of IUGR include poor health, nutrition and socioeconomic status of the mother and teenage pregnancy. *It is important to remember that growth and well being of the fetus is dependent on the health of the mother (not the father!) because she is both the seed as well as the soil where in baby is nurtured for nine months.* In our country, a large number of women are malnourished, light in weight and stunted and they are likely to produce small babies because of maternal ill health, frequent pregnancies and malnutrition. When baby happens to be a girl, she may grow up in neglect and discrimination, develop frequent infections, is fed poorly and is likely to have poor adolescent growth spurt. She is likely to grow up to become a small or undernourished poorly informed woman without any say or empowerment in society. She is likely to give birth to a small baby and perpetuate the cycle of LBW babies in the next generation **(Figure 13.8)**.

Nursing Alert

There is a mistaken cultural belief that good nutritional intake during pregnancy should be avoided because it will lead to a birth of a large baby with attendant risks of obstructed labor and birth trauma.

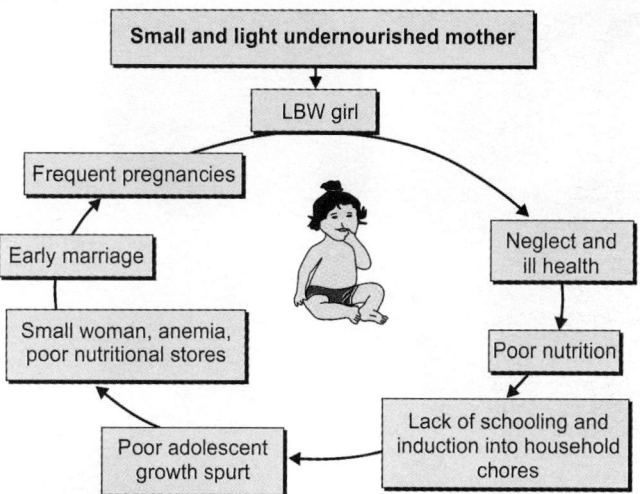

Figure 13.8 The vicious cycle of low birth weight babies in developing countries

The other causes of IUGR include placental dysfunction (due to pregnancy-induced hypertension, toxemia of pregnancy), chronic systemic disease of the mother, maternal infections during pregnancy (like malaria, urinary tract infection, tuberculosis, etc.) and drug abuse.

Fetal malformations, developmental defects, and intrauterine infections (TORCH infections) account for 10 percent cases of IUGR. They are uncommon but are associated with increased risk of neuromotor disability and poor outcome.

Clinical Features

Most babies with IUGR show features of fetal malnutrition. The baby is alert and active in accordance with his gestational age but appears long and thin with loss of subcutaneous fat over the abdomen and buttocks **(Figure 13.9)**. Abdomen is flat because internal organs especially liver and spleen are shrunken. Head appears relatively large because the brain growth is less affected compared to the physical growth. Head circumference is generally more than 3 cm bigger than the chest circumference. Because these babies have relatively normal-sized head, satisfactory length but grossly reduced body weight, they are called asymmetric IUGR babies.

When fetal growth is effected due to intrauterine infections or developmental defects of fetus, the baby is proportionately small in all the parameters, i.e. his weight, length and head size are small for the period of his gestation. These babies are called symmetric IUGR or hypoplastic babies. Some babies may have features of both asymmetric and hypoplastic babies and they are classified as mixed type of IUGR babies.

13

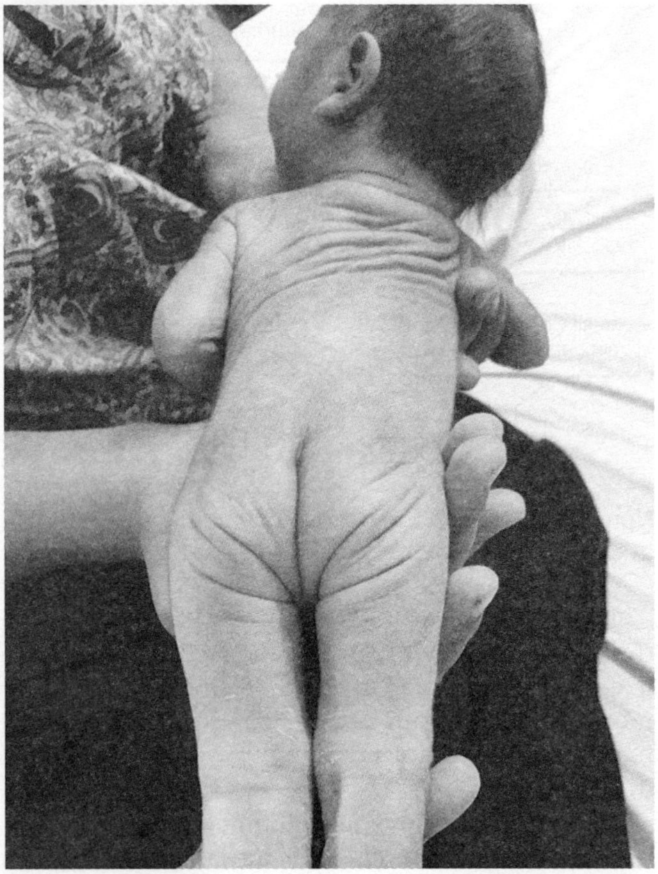

Figure 13.9 Gluteal folds in a baby with intrauterine growth retardation

Clinical Problems

These babies are at an increased risk to suffer from severe birth asphyxia due to placental dysfunction and RDS due to meconium aspiration syndrome. Hypothermia may occur due to lack of brown fat. They are extremely vulnerable to develop hypoglycemia because of disparity between the provider of glucose (low glycogen stores in the shrunken liver) and the consumer of glucose (normal sized brain). They have increased risk of having congenital malformations and poor physical growth on follow-up. There is recent evidence to suggest that asymmetric IUGR babies are at an increased risk to develop type 2 diabetes mellitus, hypertension and coronary artery disease later in adult life (Barker hypothesis). The differences between the health consequences and outcome between preterm and term small-for-dates are shown in **Table 13.2**.

Management

Early and timely delivery are important to prevent death of the baby in utero. Optimal facilities for resuscitation should be available to manage meconium-stained and asphyxiated babies. The baby should be quickly screened for any congenital malformations. Early and adequate feeding should be ensured to prevent hypoglycemia. The blood glucose should be monitored for early diagnosis of hypoglycemia.

Prognosis

The immediate outlook for small-for-dates babies is better than preterm babies of identical weight but their mortality is 2 to 3 times higher when compared with appropriately grown babies of identical gestation. *When adequately fed, these babies do not lose any weight and start gaining weight after 2 to 3 days of age.* Their initial weight gain is rapid but subsequently it slows down and they may not catch up with normal babies. They have increased risk of having minimal brain dysfunction, learning disability and severe brain damage due to symptomatic hypoglycemia. The prognosis for physical growth and neuromotor development for hypoplastic IUGR babies is worse compared to asymmetric IUGR babies.

Prevention of LBW Babies

Most neonatal deaths are limited to preterm and LBW babies. Prevention and reduction in the incidence of LBW babies is the most inportant strategy to reduce perinatal and infant mortality and improve the quality of life among those who survive. The important short- and long-term strategies for prevention of LBW babies are listed in **Box 13.2**.

LARGE-FOR-DATES BABIES (Large-for-Gestational Age or Overgrown Babies)

Infants with a birth weight of more than 90th percentile for the period of their gestation are called large-for-dates or over grown babies. Post-term infants (gestation >42 weeks) are not large because human pregnancy can sustain optimal growth of fetus up to 40–41 weeks of gestation.

Causes

1. *Genetic or constitutional.* Tall and well nourished mother is likely to produce a large baby.
2. *Maternal diabetes mellitus or prediabetes.* It is the commonest cause of large-for-dates babies. Maternal hyperglycemia leads to fetal hyperglycemia with islet-cell hyperplasia and over growth of fetus.
3. *Transposition of great vessels.*
4. *Hydrops fetalis.* The large size of the fetus is due to generalized anasarca rather than exaggerated fetal growth.
5. *Cretinisim.* Infants with congenital hypothyroidism may have higher birth weight.

Table 13.2 Differences between preterm and term small-for-dates babies		
Problems	Preterm	Term small-for-dates
▪ Intrauterine hypoxia	+	+++
▪ Respiratory difficulties		
a. Birth asphyxia	+	+++
b. Aspiration *in-utero*	+	+++
c. Hyaline membrane disease	+++	0
d. Apneic attacks	+++	0
▪ Feeding difficulties		
a. Inability to suck and swallow	+++	0
b. Aspiration of feeds	++	0
c. Functional obstruction and enterocolitis	++	+
▪ Symptomatic hypoglycemia	+	+++
▪ Hypothermia	+++	+
▪ Polycythemia	+	+++
▪ Hyperbilirubinemia	+++	+
▪ Susceptibility to infections	+++	++
▪ Congenital malformations	+	+++
▪ Hemorrhage		
a. Intraventricular	+++	0
b. Pulmonary	+	+++
▪ Prognosis		
a. Immediate	High mortality	Better prognosis but increased mortality when compared with normally grown term babies.
b. Future physical and mental development	Good if there are no perinatal complications except in extremely preterm babies.	Poor especially in hypoplastic and severe IUGR babies. There is increased risk of development of hypertension, coronary artery disease and diabetes mellitus later in life.

> **Box 13.2**   **Strategies for prevention of low birth weight babies**

- Improvement in female literacy, health status and empowerment of women in the society.
- Promotion of family life and mothercraft education among teenagers.
- Avoidance of early marriage and teenage pregnancy.
- Prepregnancy health check-up, general and nutritional guidance, and rubella vaccine.
- Ensuring interpregnancy interval of at least 3 years.
- Optimal good quality antenatal care to all pregnant women.
- Enhanced caloric and balanced protein intake with early supplements of iron, folic acid, and micronutrients during pregnancy.
- Avoidance of smoking, tobacco chewing, and drug abuse during pregnancy.
- Early recognition and management of incompetent os, placental dysfunction, pregnancy-induced hypertension, malaria, tuberculosis, urinary tract infection, and diarrhea or dysentery.
- Early and effective treatment of colonization of genital tract with mycoplasma, chlamydiae and bacterial vaginosis.
- Avoidance of physical labor, emotional stress, and sex during third trimester of pregnancy.

6. *Overgrown babies with advanced skeletal maturation.* Fetal macrosomia and advanced osseous maturation due to endocrinal or developmental causes is a rare cause of large-for-dates babies. Among these *Wiedemann-Beckwith syndrome* is well recognized. It is characterized by grooves in the ear lobes, large tongue (macroglossia), exomphalos, visceromegaly and somatic over growth. They are prone to develop hypoglycemia due to hyperplasia of islet-cells of pancreas. They are at an increased risk of development of Wilms' tumor later in life.

13

Nursing Care

There is a greater risk of birth injuries due to large size and baby should preferably be delivered by cesarean section. Early feeding with sugar-fortified feeds is recommended to reduce the risk of hypoglycemia. Hematocrit should be monitored to identify polycythemia and managed accordingly. Mothers of large babies have an increased risk to develop diabetes mellitus later in life. They should be advised to have active lifestyle and restrict the intake of simple carbohydrates and sweets to delay the onset of diabetes mellitus.

INFANTS OF DIABETIC MOTHERS (IDMs)

Diabetes mellitus is the commonest endocrinal disorder during pregnancy and it is the commonest cause of macrosomia or over grown babies (large-for-dates babies) and its consequences. Even mothers with prediabetes (genetically predisposed to develop diabetes mellitus later in life) or gestational diabetes (abnormal glucose homeostasis during pregnancy which returns back to normal after delivery) are likely to have large-for-dates babies and these mothers are at an increased risk to develop overt type 2 diabetes mellitus later in life.

Maternal hyperglycemia leads to fetal hyperglycemia (due to transplacental transfer of glucose) which causes fetal over growth and hyperplasia of fetal islet-cells in an effort to produce insulin to metabolize high levels of circulating glucose. After birth, infant no longer receives placental glucose and hypoglycemia often supervenes due to excessive release of insulin from beta-cells of pancreas. On the other hand, fetal hyperglycemia during early pregnancy or periconceptional period is an important cause of congenital malformations.

Clinical Features

1. *Macrosomia*. Infants of diabetic mother (IDM) or gestational diabetes mellitus (IGDM) are characteristically large in size, plethoric and moon faced with a hairy pinna **(Figure 13.10)**. Due to their large size, they are often delivered preterm and are at an increased risk to develop birth asphyxia, birth trauma, bruises, cephalhematoma, facial palsy, clavicular fracture and brachial plexus injury.

2. *Metabolic abnormalities*. These infants are prone to develop hypoglycemia and hypocalcemia during first 1–2 days of life. These biochemical abnormalities may contribute to excessive tremulousness, excitability and apneic attacks.

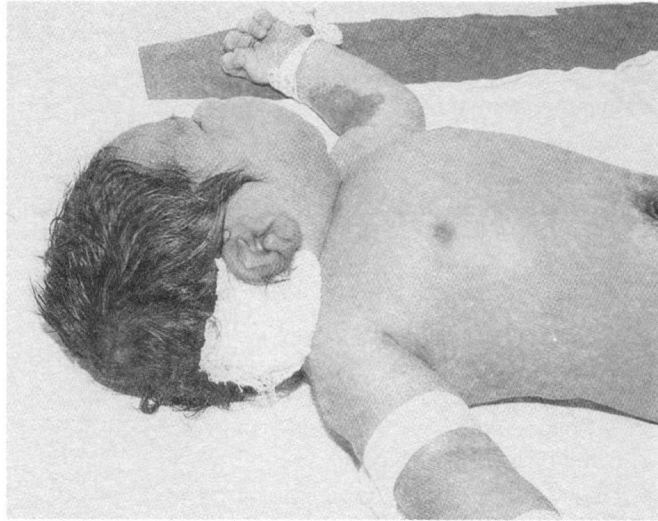

Figure 13.10 Hairy-pinna in an infant of a diabetic mother

3. *Respiratory distress syndrome*. These infants are at an increased risk to develop idiopathic respiratory distress syndrome (hyaline membrane disease) because of prematurity (they are delivered early), fetal hypoxia and raised fetal insulin levels. The increased fetal level of insulin interferes with incorporation of choline into lecithin producing deficiency of saturated phosphatidyl choline (surfactant) in the lungs and amniotic fluid.

4. *Polycythemia and hyperbilirubinemia*. These infants are likely to have polycythemia (venous hematocrit >65%), increased coagulability of blood and risk of renal vein thrombosis. Hyperbilirubinemia (severe jaundice) may occur due to number of causes like preterm birth, polycythemia, hypoglycemia, bruising and subcutaneous bleeding.

5. *Congenital malformations*. The common malformations include congenital heart disease, neural tube defects, musculoskeletal abnormalities, caudal regression syndrome and renal agenesis. Hypertrophic cardiomyopathy with asymmetric septal hypertrophy is a characteristic developmental defect in IDM.

Management and Nursing Support

1. Effective control of maternal diabetes with insulin, dietary restrictions and increased physical activity are associated with reduced fetal consequences by

Nursing Alert

Infants of diabetic mothers look deceptively healthy and pink. But these infants need specialized nursing care in keeping with their gestational maturity, biochemical abnormalities and developmental defects.

13

controlling the severity and duration of hyper-glycemia.

2. When early delivery is planned, fetal maturity should be assessed to reduce the risk of RDS. A large baby is preferably delivered by cesarean section to reduce the risk of birth trauma.

3. Baby should be screened for congenital malformations and biochemical abnormalities like polycythemia, hypoglycemia and hypocalcemia. Early and effective feeding is associated with reduced risk of hypoglycemia and polycythemia. Exchange transfusion with plasma or physiological saline is indicated for severe or symptomatic polycythemia and hyperviscosity.

4. Timely phototherapy is given to control hyper-bilirubinemia.

POSTMATURE AND POST-TERM BABIES

Infant born at a gestation of 42 weeks or more are called post-term or post-dated. Labor is often delayed in primigravida women. Infants with anencephaly fail to initiate labor at term because of failure of pelvic engagement of the head and lack of pituitay-adrenal axis.

Clinical Features

Human placenta is able to sustain the growth of fetus up to 42 weeks, beyond which it becomes senile or dysfunctional to support the growth of fetus. Post-term infants are at an increased risk to suffer from fetal hypoxia and birth axphyxia. It may lead to passage of meconium in utero with risk of development of meconium aspiration syndrome. This is maceration and desquamation of skin due to lack of vernix caseosa as pregnancy advances. Infant may look long, thin and wasted. Skin, umbilical cord and nails may be yellow stained due to passage of meconium in utero. Postmature infants look more alert and show advanced neuromotor development. These infants are more prone to develop several health hazards including congenital malformations, perinatal hypoxia, meconium aspiration syndrome, persistent pulmonary hypertension, hypoglycemia, hypocalcemia and plycythemia.

Management

When gestation goes beyond 41 weeks, placental functions should be monitored and fetus watched for any signs of hypoxia. In a depressed infant with passage of meconium in utero, thorouth oropharyngeal suction should be done as soon as the head is delivered. Early feeding is recommended to reduce the risk of hypogly-cemia and polycythemia. Child should be monitored for hypoglycemia, hypocalcemia and polycythemia and managed appropriately as per standard guidelines. Symptomatic polycythemia is managed by exchange transfusion with normal saline or plasma. Application of oil or moisturising cream is recomended to prevent dryness of skin and desquamation.

BIBLIOGRAPHY

Arora NK, Singh M, Paul VK, Bhargava VL. Etiology of fetal growth retardation in hospital born infants. *Indian J Med Res* 1987, 85:395–400.

Behrman RE. Preventing low birth weight: A pediatiric perspective. *J Pediatr* 1985, 107:842.

Kramer MS. Determinants of low birth weight. *Bull WHO* 1987, 65:663–735.

Kramer WB, Weiver CP. Management of intrauterine growth restriction. *Clin Obstet Gynecol* 1997, 40: 814–823.

Singh M, Giri SK, Ramachandran K. Intrauterine growth curves of live-born babies. *Indian Pediatr* 1974, 11:475.

13

14

Common Diseases of Newborn Babies

A large majority of newborn babies do not develop any serious difficulties and they need level 1 or minimal newborn care which can be provided by the mother under the supervision of a nurse. High-risk mothers are likely to give birth to preterm or low birth weight babies which are prone to suffer from a number of disorders. Common causes of morbidity in newborn babies include birth asphyxia, hypothermia, respiratory distress syndrome, septicemia and hyperbilirubinemia. Most neonatal disorders and deaths are limited to preterm and low birth weight babies.

RESPIRATORY DISTRESS SYNDROME

During fetal life, lungs are filled with fluid and receives only 10 to 15% cardiac output. It does not subserve any ventilatory function and gas exchange occurs entirely through the placenta. After birth, there are rapid pulmonary and hemodynamic changes and most infants make a smooth transition from dependent intrauterine to independent extrauterine life.

Respiratory difficulties are encountered in 5 to 7 percent of newborn babies. The clinical diagnosis of respiratory distress is suspected when the respiratory rate is more than 60 per minute in a quiet resting baby and there are either inspiratory intercostal recessions or expiratory grunt.

Causes

Respiratory distress in neonates is a symptom complex which can occur from a variety of etiological factors. The common causes of respiratory distress syndrome in newborn babies include pneumonia, meconium aspiration syndrome, transient tachypnea of the newborn, hyaline membrane disease and congenital malformations of the respiratory and cardiovascular systems. The infant should be assessed for degree of distress, severity of intercostal recessions, cyanosis, activity or alertness, nature of cry, feeding behavior and status of peripheral circulation.

The severity of respiratory distress can be assessed by Downe scoring system **(Table 14.1)**.

Pneumonia in a Neonate

The infant may be born with congenital pneumonia or may develop nosocomial pulmonary infection after birth. The common predisposing factors for intrauterine pneumonia include premature rupture of the membranes, multiple unclean vaginal examinations, febrile maternal illness during the peripartal period, foul smelling amniotic fluid, and difficult or prolonged labor. Pneumonia may occur during the course of septicemia or due to aspiration of feeds any time in the neonatal period. The common organisms causing congenital pneumonia include *E. coli*, Klebsiella, Enterobacter and *Listeria monocytogenes*. The postnatally acquired or nosocomial pneumonia is usually caused by Klebsiella, *E. coli*, Enterobacter, Pneumococci, *Pseudomonas aeruginosa* and *Staphylococcus aureus* and *albus*.

Clinical Features

The clinical picture is characterized by inactivity, poor feeding, respiratory distress and cyanosis. Fever and cough are uncommon in newborn babies with pneumonia. Some newborn babies may die due to pneumonia without manifesting any respiratory symptoms or signs.

Investigations

In all infants born following prolonged rupture of membranes (more than 24 hours) or those developing respiratory distress soon after birth, gastric aspirate

Nursing Alert

Newborn baby has a limited capacity to express manifestations of a disease process. Identical and often stereotyped responses are seen from a variety of disorders. Therefore, identification of associated and predisposing conditions is often crucial to make an etiological diagnosis of respiratory distress in the newborn.

Table 14.1 Downe's scoring system for assessment of severity of respiratory distress

Score	0	1	2
Respiration (rate/min)	<60	60–80	>80
Cyanosis (SpO$_2$ <80%)	None in room air	No cyanosis in 40% oxygen	Requiring more than 40% ambient oxygen
Retractions	None	Mild	Moderate to severe
Grunting	None	Audible with stethoscope	Audible without stethoscope
Air entry	Good	Decreased	Barely audible

Downe's score of 7 or more is suggestive of impending respiratory failure

should be collected in a heparinized tube and examined under the microscope after staining with Leishman's stain. The presence of more than 5 neutrophils per high power field or when their number exceeds three times the number of epithelial cells, is suggestive of intrauterine or congenital pneumonia. A bacterial culture should be obtained from liquor amnii (or cervical swab of the mother), gastric aspirate, throat and blood of the infant. Septic screen may be positive. A skiagram of the chest may show bilateral opacities and consolidation. The presence of pneumonitis in the right upper zone is highly suggestive of aspiration in a newborn baby. Esophageal atresia with tracheoesophageal fistula should be ruled out by passing an orogastric catheter.

Nursing Care

The infant should be nursed in a thermoneutral environment and given oxygen with a head box to relieve cyanosis. An intravenous line should be established to administer fluids and drugs. Intravenous fluids should be restricted to two-thirds of the maintenance requirement due to potential risk of syndrome of inappropriate antidiuretic hormone secretion (SIADH). Early and effective intravenous antibiotic therapy is mandatory to improve survival. Acid-base parameters and arterial blood gases (ABGs) should be monitored and properly managed. For administration of specific antibiotics, refer to the management of neonatal septicemia. Assisted ventilation is life saving when oxygenation cannot be maintained by administration of oxygen through the head box or T-piece. Due to excessive inflammatory exudates, frequent suctioning of endotracheal tube and chest physiotherapy is advised.

Meconium Aspiration Syndrome

Meconium is passed in utero by 10 to 15 percent of infants and it suggests that the fetus may have suffered from hypoxia in utero. The baby may be asphyxiated at birth and covered with meconium. The yellow staining of cord, skin and nails suggests that the baby had been soaked in meconium for several hours. The presence of thick particulate matter (pea-souped appearance of amniotic fluid) is associated with increased risk of meconium aspiration syndrome especially in term and post-term babies.

Pathophysiology

The pathophysiology of meconium aspiration syndrome (MAS) is extremely complex due to interplay of a number of mechanisms, like airway obstruction, chemical pneumonitis and dysfunction of surfactant. Meconium aspiration causes airway obstruction with obstructive emphysema due to ball-valve effect. The chemical constituents of meconium cause marked alveolar and parenchymal inflammation leading to edema because of leakage of proteins into the airways. There is release of inflammatory mediators or cytokines including tumor necrosis factor, and interleukins (IL-1B and IL-8). These chemical mediators directly injure the lung parenchyma causing vascular leakage thus producing an injury pattern similar to acute respiratory distress syndrome (ARDS). Meconium is known to adversely effect neutrophil functions leading to increased risk of infections. The cytotoxic effects of meconium in type II pneumocytes lead to decreased levels of surfactant with further aggravation of respiratory distress.

If the amniotic fluid is meconium-stained, thorough oropharyngeal suction should be done by the obstetrician with a thick-bored suction catheter as soon as the head is delivered (when the rest of the baby is still in the uterus). After delivery, the oral cavity and periglottic area should be thoroughly sucked under direct vision. When meconium is found deep in the hypopharynx, elective intubation is recommended to suck out any meconium which might have been aspirated into the trachea.

Clinical Features

When management of the meconium-stained baby is unsatisfactory at birth, there is a potential risk of development of meconium aspiration syndrome.

14

However, most infants with meconium-stained liquor, aspirate meconium in-utero. The baby is often asphyxiated at birth and develops progressive respiratory distress soon after birth. The course may be complicated by life-threatening persistent pulmonary hypertension (PPHN). There is marked inspiratory intercostal recessions and expiratory grunt. The chest may be overinflated or barrel-shaped due to obstructive emphysema. The X-ray chest shows bilateral coarse, irregular densities with patches of obstructive emphysema.

Treatment

The management is mostly supportive by maintaining thermoneutral environment, adequate hydration and oxygenation. There is no therapeutic utility of either prophylatic antibiotics or corticosteroids. The role of surfactant is controversial but is used in many centers. Assisted ventilation should be provided early when respiratory failure is impending as evidenced by arterial oxygen tension (PaO_2) of less than 50 mm Hg, carbon dioxide tension ($PaCO_2$) of greater than 50 mm Hg and pH of lower than 7.2 despite administration of 100% oxygen.

Transient Tachypnea of the Newborn (TTNB)

It is characterized by the development of rapid shallow breathing in a baby at birth or few hours later. The respiratory rate may vary from 60 to 100 per minute while intercostal recessions are either absent or minimal. The child remains alert and active and maintains good color. The condition is more common in babies born by cesarean section and occurs because of "wet lungs" due to failure of drainage of amniotic fluid through the lymphatics leading to reduced lung compliance. Skiagram of the chest shows linear streakings at both hila due to dilated lymphatics and presence of fluid in the interlobar fissure. The condition resolves spontaneously without any specific therapy within two to three days of life. Some infants may require administration of 40% oxygen to maintain adequate oxygenation.

HYALINE MEMBRANE DISEASE
(Idiopathic Respiratory Distress Syndrome)

Hyaline membrane disease (HMD) is the commonest cause of respiratory morbidity in preterm babies. It affects 10 to 15 percent of preterm babies in India though its incidence is relatively higher in the West. The higher incidence of placental dysfunction and fetal malnutrition in developing countries is associated with enhanced lung maturity.

Pathogenesis

The condition occurs due to lack of pulmonary surfactant because of the immaturity of the lungs. When surface-active material is deficient in the alveoli, there is alveolar collapse during expiration. Apart from prematurity, the production of surfactant may be compromised by damage to type II alveolar cells due to birth asphyxia, acidosis, hypothermia, antepartum hemorrhage, maternal diabetes mellitus, severe rhesus (Rh) isoimmunization and shock. Infants delivered by emergency cesarean section are also predisposed to develop HMD due to greater chances of perinatal hypoxia. Deficiency of surfactant leads to atelectasis or alveolar collapse leading to ineffective ventilation. The combination of end-expiratory alveolar collapse, reduced pulmonary compliance, pulmonary under-perfusion and increased capillary exudation lead to accumulation of CO_2 and reduction of PaO_2 and pH. These metabolic changes lead to constriction of pulmonary arterioles and opening up of right-to-left shunts with perpetuation of hypoxia.

Clinical Features

Hyaline membrane disease is characterized by a triad of tachypnea, expiratory grunt and inspiratory retractions in a prematurely born asphyxiated infant. The symptoms may begin at birth or within 6 hours of delivery. There is gradual worsening of retractions, grunting and cyanosis. Grunting occurs when baby breathes out against partially closed glottis. It is a compensatory mechanism on the part of a neonate to raise end-expiratory alveolar pressure during expiration. During the next 24 to 48 hours, the course of disease is relentlessly progressive and may be complicated by patent ductus arteriosus. Skiagram of the chest shows the air bronchogram extending beyond the left cardiac border followed by diffuse washed out appearance due to solid lungs **(Figure 14.1)**.

Nursing Monitoring

The infant should be attached to a vital sign monitor and pulse oximeter for continuous display of vital signs and arterial oxygen saturation (SaO_2 or SpO_2). The arterial oxygen tension (PaO_2) is maintained between 50 and 80 mm Hg and arterial oxygen saturation between 90% and 95% to reduce the risk of hypoxia and hyperoxia as evidenced by retinopathy of prematurity (ROP). The nurse should record the following clinical observations to monitor the progress of the infant.

- Continuous monitoring of vital signs with the help of a vital sign monitor and manually every 4 hourly.

14

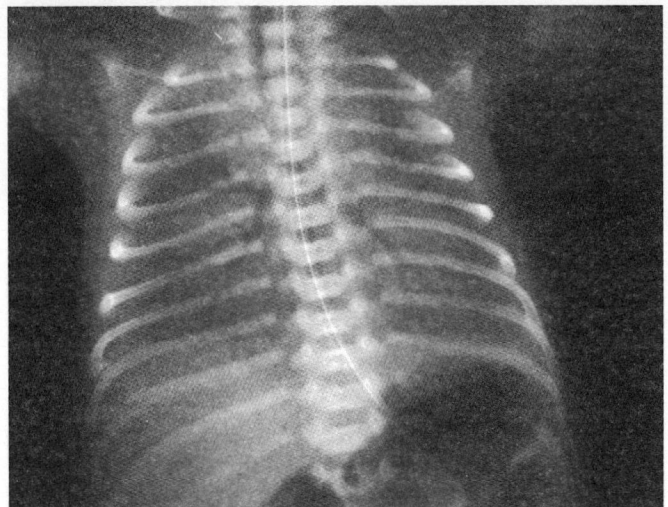

Figure 14.1 Global white out with air bronchogram in an infant with HMD

- Severity of retractions and grunting (Silverman and Andersen score)
- Status of peripheral pulses, whether extremities are warm or cold to touch and capillary refill time (CRT).
- Circumoral discoloration or pallor.
- Activity, responsiveness, abdominal girth and cry.
- Apneic episodes.
- Air entry in the lungs and any cardiac murmur.
- Urine output.

Management

When labor starts before 34 weeks of gestation, intramuscular administration of betamethasone 12 mg every 24 hr for 2 doses is associated with reduced risk of development of HMD. It is one the most cost-effective strategies to reduce the incidence and severity of HMD and associated complications like intraventricular hemorrhage and necrotizing enterocolitis.

The infant with HMD should be nursed in a thermoneutral environment and administered oxygen through a head box. An intravenous line should be established to maintain fluid and electrolyte balance, for the correction of acidosis and administration of drugs. Administration of surfactant through endotracheal tube shortens the course of disease and improves survival. Arterial oxygen saturation should be monitored with the help of a pulse oximeter. When arterial oxygen saturation cannot be maintained above 90 percent despite providing oxygen in the head box at a concentration of 60 percent, the infant should be provided continuous positive airway pressure (CPAP) through silastic nasal prongs or after endotracheal intubation. Bubble CPAP at transpulmonary pressure of 6 cm H_2O is started and gradually raised by increments of 2 cm H_2O every 15 minutes. When CPAP is also ineffective to maintain adequate oxygenation, the baby is managed by intermittent positive pressure ventilation. The acid-base parameters and blood gases should be monitored frequently to correct acidosis and hypoxia and prevent hyperoxia. *Unmonitored high concentrations of oxygen in preterm babies may lead to retinopathy of prematurity due to oxygen toxicity.* Antibiotics are administered whenever there is suspicion of superadded bacterial infection. The management of hyaline membrane disease demands excellent supportive care by trained nurses and availability of assisted ventilation facilities to manage hypoxia due to ineffective ventilation. The case fatality rate due to HMD is related to the quality of neonatal nursing care and varies between 25 and 50 percent.

Congenital Malformations

Respiratory distress in the newborn may occur due to a number of congenital malformations of pulmonary system or due to congestive heart failure because of congenital heart disease. The common respiratory malformations include choanal atresia, Pierre-Robin syndrome, esophageal atresia with tracheoesophageal fistula, diaphragmatic hernia and vascular rings.

SEPTICEMIA IN A NEONATE

Bacterial infection is one of the leading causes of mortality in newborn babies in our country. Neonatal sepsis can be divided into two sub-types depending upon whether the onset of symptoms is during the first 72 hours of life or later. Early-onset septicemia is caused by organisms prevalent in the genital tract or in the labor room and maternity operation theater. The common correlates of early-onset sepsis include febrile illness in the mother within two weeks of delivery, foul smelling or meconium stained liquor amnii, prolonged rupture of membranes (>12 hr), prolonged labor (>24 hr) single unclean or multiple vaginal examinations, birth asphyxia and difficult resuscitation. The onus for prevention of early-onset septicemia rests with the obstetricians.

Late-onset septicemia is acquired as a nosocomial infection from the nursery or lying-in-ward. The onset of symptoms is usually delayed beyond 72 hours after birth. About two-thirds cases of the neonatal septicemia are caused by Gram-negative bacilli, i.e. *Klebsiella pneumoniae,* Enterobacter, *E.coli, Pseudomonas aeruginosa,* Citrobacter and Serratia while the rest are accounted by Gram-positive organisms including *Staphylococcus aureus* and *albus.* The usual sources of infection include

14

incubators, resuscitators, ventilators, cold sterilization solutions, feeding bottles, catheters, face masks, infusion sets, etc.

Clinical Features

Nursing Alert

Sepsis should be strongly suspected when a neonate who has been active and sucking normally suddenly becomes inactive or sluggish and refuses to accept feeds.

The manifestations of neonatal septicemia are often vague and nonspecific demanding high index of suspicion for early diagnosis. Any alteration in established feeding behavior is the most characteristic early feature. The baby who had been active and sucking normally, may gradually or suddenly become lethargic, inactive, unresponsive and refuse to suck. The infant may appear pale with grayish circumoral cyanosis and a vacant look. Hypothermia is a common manifestation of septicemia in preterm babies while term babies may manifest with fever, especially in association with Gram-positive infections and meningitis. Diarrhea, vomiting and abdominal distension may occur. Jaundice and hepatosplenomegaly may be present. Episodes of apneic spells with cyanosis may be the sole manifestation of septicemia in preterm babies. The additional localising features may appear depending upon the spread of infection to different systems and organs of the baby. Meningitis occurs in one-third of babies with septicemia and should be ruled out by CSF examination. Additional clinical features may appear depending upon the development of certain complications such as shock, disseminated intravascular coagulation, osteomyelitis, arthiritis, sclerema and necrotizing enterocolitis.

Diagnosis

Septic screening should be done to support the clinical suspicion of infection before the institution of antibacterial therapy. The reliable markers of neonatal septicemia include leucopenia (less than 5000 leukocytes per cu mm), elevated band neutrophils (more than 20%), raised micro-ESR (more than 15 mm), positive C-reactive protein (more than 1.0 mg per mL) and elevation of procalcitonin (more than 2 ng/dL). Blood culture and CSF examination are mandatory before initiating specific antibacterial therapy. A skiagram of the chest must be taken even when there are no respiratory symptoms or signs. Blood should be examined for glucose, bilirubin, urea and electrolytes.

Nursing Management

The infant should be managed in a thermoneutral environment and started on intravenous infusion. Hypoglycemia, anemia and shock should be appropriately managed. Fresh blood or fresh frozen plasma is useful to improve defence mechanisms by providing opsonins, complement and polymorphonuclear leukocytes. Specific antibacterial therapy should be instituted through intravenous route. The choice of antibiotics depends upon the prevalence of bacterial flora and their sensitivity pattern against available antibiotics. In a community-acquired neonatal septicemia, a combination of ampicillin with gentamicin is appropriate. In hospital-acquired neonatal septicemia, the logical initial choice of antibiotics would be a combination of aminoglycoside such as gentamicin or amikacin with cefotaxime. When the etiologic agent is identified, the antibacterial therapy can be made highly specific. Benzyl penicillin is most suitable for the treatment of infections due to *Group B streptococci*. Septicemia due to *Pseudomonas aeruginosa* is best managed by ceftazidime. Betalactamase-resistant penicillins (cloxacillin and methicillin) are indicated for the treatment of infections caused by *Staphylococcus aureus*. Ampicillin is the drug of choice for treatment of an occasional case of listeriosis while erythromycin is specific for the topical and systemic treatment of infections due to *Chlamydia trachomatis*.

The prognosis depends upon the weight and maturity of the infant, nature of the etiologic agent and quality of specific and supportive therapy. In fulminant cases, intravenous immunoglobulins (IVIG) in a dose of 500–1000 mg/kg daily for 2–3 days has been shown to improve survival. The presence of underlying congenital malformations like meningomyelocele, tracheoesophageal fistula and surgical procedure adversely affects the outcome. The reported case fatality rate due to neonatal septicemia in various studies from India range between 20 and 50 percent. It is, therefore, essential that all efforts should be made to prevent the occurrence of bacterial infections in newborn babies by adopting strict aseptic rituals and routines.

CANDIDEMIA

Systemic candidiasis due to pathogenic yeasts is assuming greater importance in neonatal intensive care units. Most infections are caused by Candida species *Candida albicans* and *Candida parapsilosis*. Preterm babies with a birth weight below 1500 g and infants requiring prolonged ventilation, central venous catheterization and total parenteral nutrition are vulnerable to develop candidemia. Intralipids, especially when efforts are made to dispense them into small aliquots, are potent source of fungal infection.

Clinical Features

The onset of fungal infection is usually delayed beyond 2 to 8 weeks of age. There may be evidences of superficial yeast infection like oral thrush, and diaper rash due to Candida. The clinical features are nonspecific and similar to stereotyped features of neonatal sepsis. The clinical picture simulates manifestations of necrotizing enterocolitis (NEC) without any evidences of pneumatosis intestinalis. Intolerance of feed, fever, hyperglycemia and thrombocytopenia may be associated. Dissemination of infection leads to formation of microabscesses virtually in any body organ but most commonly in kidneys leading to hematuria, proteinuria and acute kidney damage.

Diagnosis

The diagnosis is suspected by finding budding yeasts or hyphae in the urine. Persistent elevation of C-reactive proteins and thrombocytopenia are useful markers of candidemia. Selective low pH culture media (Sabouraud dextrose agar) containing antibacterial agent should be used for blood culture studies. Fundus examination, ultrasonography of brain and kidneys and 3-D echocardiography may show evidences of fungal microabscesses.

Nursing Management

Systemic candidiasis is an ominous condition and demands excellent supportive nursing care and aggressive antifungal therapy. The indwelling venous catheters should be removed. The liposomal formulation of amphotericin B (5 mg/kg/d) is the drug of choice because of lower risk of toxicity, short duration of administration over 2 hours, reduced risk of thrombophlebitis and better efficacy.

In life-threatening candidemia and fungal meningitis, fluorocytosine is given orally in a dose of 100–150 mg/kg/day in 4 divided doses along with amphotericin B. The therapy should be continued for at least 6 weeks.

Nursing Alert

During administration of amphotericin B, the drug should be protected against exposure to light and serum potassium levels and kidney functions should be closely monitored.

Prevention

In view of life-threatening consequences of candidemia, all efforts should be made to prevent it. Strict aseptic protocols in NICU, restricted use of central venous line, avoidance of prophylactic antibiotics and early administration of trophic feeds with human milk are associated with reduced risk of fungal infections. The use of H_2-blockers and cephalosporins should be avoided and aliquotes of intralipids should be prepared under strict aseptic conditions by using laminar flow system. The meta-analysis of randomized controlled trials suggest that biweekly prophylactic administration of oral ketoconazole is associated with a reduced risk of candidemia but there is a potential risk of emergence of resistant strains of *C. albicans*.

TETANUS NEONATORUM

The incidence of tetanus neonatorum has drastically come down in our country but the disease still occurs when delivery is conducted at home under unsatisfactory and unsterile conditions. The disease is caused by entry of *Clostridium tetani* through the umbilical stump. The pathogenic organisms are likely to enter through the cord when it is cut with an unsterile and contaminated instrument or when umbilical stump is dressed with household remedies like mud and cow-dung. Even when a new razor blade is used for cutting the cord, it can lead to the development of tetanus neonatorum unless it is sterilized by boiling.

Clinical Features

The symptoms appear due to liberation of a neurotoxin by the organisms after an incubation period of 4–7 days. The symptoms usually occur between 5 and 10 days, never before 2 days of life or after the age of 2 weeks. There is failure to suck due to lock jaw (trismus) because of spasm of muscles of the jaw. When baby is handled or touched, he develops tetanic spasms. After 1–2 days, there is fever, marked irritability, frequent spasms of muscles, neck retraction and opisthotonos (bow-like hyperextension of trunk). The facies assume characteristic grin with clenching of jaw called risus sardonicus. Death occurs due to respiratory failure because of frequent muscular spasms and rigidity of chest muscles.

Nursing Care

The disease carries high mortality and demands intensive nursing and supportive care in an NICU. Intravenous cannula should be inserted to administer fluids and drugs. Human tetanus specific immunoglo-

14

bulins 250 i.u. are given intravenously. Penicillin and cefotaxime are given to eradicate tetanus bacilli and control intercurrent infection. The spasms are controlled by heavy sedation with diazepam, chlopromazine, and phenobarbitone. When facilities are available, assisted ventilation should be provided after paralysing the muscles. Recovery usually occurs in 5–6 days when sedative drugs are gradually tapered off. Handling should be reduced to the bare minimum and infant should not be exposed to bright light. The case fatality varies between 50% and 75% and survivors do not manifest any neurological sequelae.

Prevention

Tetanus neonatorum can be easily eradicated by simple, cheap and effective measures. Two doses of tetanus toxoid (TT) or tetanus-diphtheria toxoid (Td) must be given to every pregnant woman at an interval of 4 weeks and second dose should be given atleast 4 weeks before delivery. Delivery should be conducted with due aseptic precautions and cord should be cut with a sterile blade or knife. Disposable sterile "*Dai Kits*" are available which should be used for home deliveries. No dressing should be applied to the cord and it should be kept clean by local application of isopropyle alcohol or triple dye or betadine lotion. Application of mud or cowdung over the umbilical stump should be condemned.

NEONATAL JAUNDICE

Jaundice is a relatively common physical abnormality in a newborn baby during the first week of life. Clinical jaundice manifests as yellowness of the skin of the face when the serum bilirubin level exceeds 5 mg/dL. As the severity of jaundice increases, there is progression of yellowness of the skin from face towards trunk, limbs and finally palms and soles. When the trunk of the baby is distinctly yellow stained, the serum bilirubin level is likely to vary between 10 and 15 mg/dL. The yellow staining of the palms and soles is ominous and indicates that the serum bilirubin level has exceeded 15 mg/dL. *All newborn babies must be examined twice a day in good daylight during the first week of life to assess the onset, severity and age of disappearance of jaundice.* Transcutaneous bilirubin measurements over the sternum with a BiliChek™ is a reliable non-invasive method for assessment of severity of jaundice both in term and preterm infants.

Pathophysiology

There are several physiological handicaps that lead to increased frequency and severity of jaundice among newborn babies. Neonates have polycythemia and

shorter lifespan of red blood cells (90 days compared to 120 days in older children) releasing 0.15 g/kg of hemoglobin because 1% of blood hemolyze everyday. One gram of hemoglobin yields about 35 mg of bilirubin so that in a 3.0 kg infant about 15 mg of bilirubin is produced daily from hemoglobin sources. Additional 1.0 mg/kg bilirubin is produced from non-hemoglobin sources such as myoglobin, cytochromes and catalases, thus resulting in net daily load of about 20 mg of bilirubin to the liver in a healthy term infant **(Figure 14.2)**.

In neonates, hepatic uptake, conjugation and excretion of bilirubin are limited due to deficiency of Y and Z-acceptor proteins and UDP glucuronyl transferase enzyme. Because of paucity of bacteria in the gut of a neonate, and over activity of intestinal beta-glucuronidase enzyme, the conjugated bilirubin entering the duodenum is rapidly deconjugated and recirculated in the blood for deconjugation in the liver. The enhanced enterohepatic circulation of bilirubin further aggravates the devleopment of jaundice in neonates. The rate of bilirubin production (6–8 mg/kg/d) is at least twice in magnitude in the normal newborn population as compared to older children. These biophysiological handicaps are worse among prematurely born infants thus resulting in greater incidence and severity of jaundice among them.

> ### Practical Tip
>
> *Unlike older children in whom jaundice is most commonly due to viral hepatitis, in neonates jaundice occurs usually due to physiological handicaps and hemolytic disease of the newborn.*

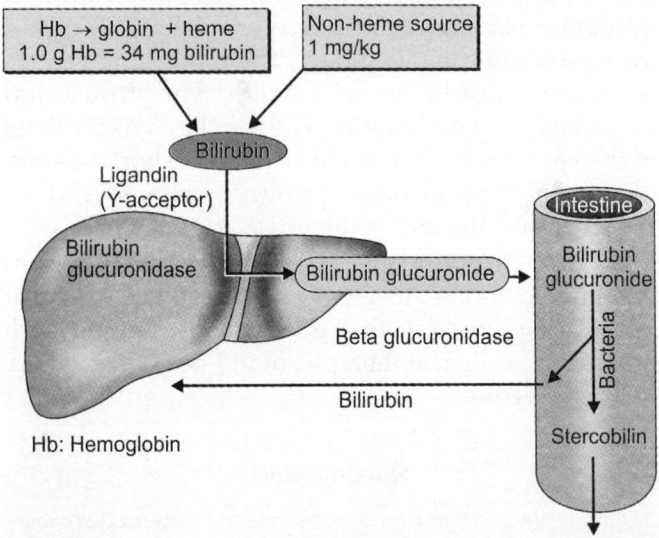

Figure 14.2 Schematic presentation of bilirubin turnover in the newborn

Causes

The important causes of pathological jaundice in newborn babies are given in **Box 14.1**. About 5 percent of newborn babies develop pathological jaundice or hyperbilirubinemia. *The onset of jaundice within 24 hours of age, its marked intensity as evidenced by yellow staining of the palms and soles and its persistence beyond two weeks of age are suggestive of pathological jaundice requiring appropriate laboratory investigations and management.*

Physiological Jaundice

About 60 to 70 percent of healthy newborn babies are likely to develop physiological jaundice which may cause undue anxiety to the parents. Physiological jaundice appears between 36 and 72 hours of age, its maximum intensity is seen on the 4th day of life and the peak serum bilirubin level does not exceed 15 mg/dL. The jaundice usually disappears between 10 and 14 days of life and does not need any specific therapy. In preterm babies the peak of physiological jaundice is seen a little later and peak bilirubin level may be higher and jaundice may take relatively longer time to disappear **(Figure 14.3)**.

The diagnosis of physiological jaundice cannot be made by examining the baby at one point of time because it depends upon a characteristic time table of jaundice, taking into consideration the time of onset of jaundice, maximal limits of intensity and age of disappearance besides the exclusion of pathological causes. Physiological jaundice occurs due to relative polycythemia with reduced lifespan of neonatal red blood cells, hepatic immaturity and exaggerated enterohepatic circulation of bilirubin. The mother must be reassured regarding the benign nature of physiological jaundice and her fears regarding infection or hepatitis should be allayed.

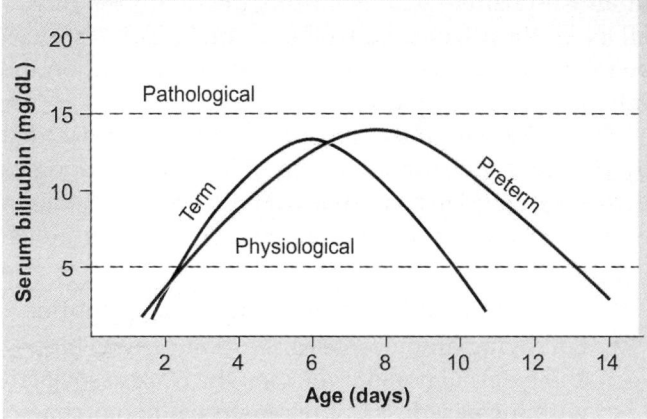

Figure 14.3 Time table of physiological jaundice

Hemolytic Disease of the Newborn (HDN)

Hemolytic disease of the newborn (HDN) due to blood group incompatibility between the mother and fetus is the commonest cause of hyperbilirubinemia in a newborn baby. The incompatibility may exist between Rhesus, ABO or minor blood group systems.

Rhesus Hemolytic Disease of the Newborn (Rh-HDN)

When an Rh-negative mother is carrying an Rh-positive fetus, the passage of fetal red blood cells into the maternal circulation may invoke an antibody response by the maternal immunological system. Enough anti-D antibodies are not produced during the first pregnancy but each subsequent pregnancy with Rh-positive fetus leads to increasing antibody production. The anti-D antibodies being IgG in type, they readily crossover to the fetus through the placenta and destroy D-positive fetal red blood cells. The Rh-isoimmunization can be suspected during antenatal period by identifying the blood group of the mother and estimating the titer of maternal anti-D antibodies by indirect Coomb's test.

There is a wide spectrum of clinical manifestations of erythroblastosis due to Rh-HDN, ranging from a normal baby to a stillborn baby with hydrops fetalis. There is increasing severity of the disease with each subsequent pregnancy. The newborn baby may be anemic at birth and has hepatosplenomegaly. Jaundice usually appears within 24 hours of age and rapidly increases in intensity. In a severely affected baby, the clinical picture is characterized by severe anemia, gross hepatosplenomegaly and generalized anasarca (hydrops fetalis) and at times the baby may die in utero.

If the mother is Rh-negative, cord blood should be collected for Rh and ABO typing, direct Coomb's test, hemoglobin, reticulocyte count, peripheral blood smear and serum bilirubin. The positive direct Coomb's test

Box 14.1 Causes of pathological jaundice

1. Idiopathic
2. Prematurity
3. ABO-hemolytic disease of the newborn (ABO-HDN)
4. Rh-isoimmunization or Rh-hemolytic disease of the newborn (Rh-HDN)
5. G-6-PD deficiency
6. Septicemia
7. Breast milk jaundice
8. Hypothyroidism
9. Neonatal hepatitis (intrauterine or TORCH infections) and biliary atresia
10. Metabolic disorders

in an Rh-positive baby confirms the diagnosis of Rh-HDN. In the affected baby, the serum bilirubin should be monitored every 6 to 12 hours depending upon the rate of rise of bilirubin.

Rhesus isoimmunization can be effectively prevented by prophylactic administration of anti-D immunoglobulins 500 µg IM in an unsensitized Rh-negative woman within 72 hours of delivery in the following situations:

1. Delivery of Rh-positive baby
2. Abortion or stillbirth of Rh-positive conception
3. Following amniocentesis, chorionic villus biopsy and external podalic version which are associated with increased risk of fetomaternal hemorrhage.

The anti-D immunoglobulin should only be given to the mother whose indirect Coomb's test is negative. In order to enhance the efficacy, it is recommended to administer 500 µg of anti-D immunoglobulins to all unsensitized Rh negative women around 28–32 weeks of gestation. If delivery occurs more than 4 weeks later and the infant is Rh positive, the mother should receive additional 500 µg anti-D immunoglobulin IM within 72 hours of delivery.

ABO Hemolytic Disease of the Newborn (ABO-HDN)

The ABO system of blood groups have preformed antibodies unlike Rh system. The ABO hemolytic disease of the newborn usually occurs when mother is O group and her baby is either A or B group. Feto-maternal ABO incompatibility exists in about 25% of these incompatible neonates. Unlike Rh-HDN, the history of increasing severity of disease in subsequent pregnancies is generally not present in ABO-HDN.

The diagnosis of ABO-HDN is suspected by early onset of jaundice in A or B group baby of an O group mother. The ABO-HDN is a relatively milder disease as compared to Rh-HDN. The anemia is usually absent or mild and there may be mild hepatosplenomegaly. The direct Coomb's test is usually negative or weakly positive. Blood examination may show reticulocytosis, microspherocytosis and increased fragility of red blood cells.

Septicemia

Jaundice is an important manifestation of bacterial infection in newborn babies and occurs due to hemolysis and hepatitis. The clinical picture is usually dominated by systemic features of septicemia and the occurrence of jaundice after the age of three days. The direct reacting or conjugated bilirubin is often elevated to 1.5 mg/dL or more and jaundice often persists beyond 10 to 14 days of life.

Glucose-6-Phosphate Dehydrogenase Deficiency

The incidence of G-6-PD deficiency varies between 5 and 20 percent among different ethnic groups in India. Deficiency is limited to male babies as the condition is inherited as X-linked recessive. The hemolysis may occur spontaneously or following exposure to certain drugs and infections. The clinical picture is characterized by the sudden and dramatic appearance of unconjugated hyperbilirubinemia requiring exchange blood transfusion.

> **Practical Tip**
>
> *When a term neonate, without any high-risk factors has prolonged physiological jaundice (>2 weeks), ask for color of his urine and poops. When urine is like water (colorless) and feces are yellow-colored, the jaundice is likely to be either breast milk jaundice or due to congenital hypothyroidism.*

Breast Milk Jaundice

Breastfed babies have greater incidence and severity of jaundice. The maximum intensity of jaundice occurs between 10 and 14 days of age and it may last for 6–10 weeks. *The child remains active, feeds well and passes yellow-colored stools and water-like urine.* The condition is diagnosed by excluding other causes of jaundice. Cretinism is also associated with prolonged physiological jaundice which should be ruled out by estimating TSH and T_4 levels. Withholding of breastfeeding for 48–72 hours may result in fall in serum bilirubin level, but inview of transient and benign nature of breast milk jaundice, there is no need or justification to stop breastfeeding.

Pathogenesis of Kernicterus

Jaundice in a newborn baby is a serious condition because unconjugated hyperbilirubinemia may cause bilirubin encephalopathy or kernicterus. The occurrence of kernicterus is related to complex interaction between the level of unconjugated bilirubin which is lipid soluble, gestational maturity of the infant and integrity of the blood–brain barrier. It is generally believed that unconjugated bilirubin level of more than 20 mg/dL due to any cause may lead to kernicterus in a newborn baby. However, it is well known that a preterm infant may develop brain damage at relatively lower serum bilirubin levels while some term babies may tolerate serum bilirubin concentration of up to 30 mg/dL without any kernicterus. Perinatal distress factors such as hypoxia, hypothermia, hypoglycemia, acidosis, birth injury and septicemia may damage the integrity of the blood–brain barrier and predispose the infant to develop bilirubin encephalopathy at a relatively lower serum bilirubin levels. Neonatal features of kernicterus include lethargy, refusal to take feeds, shrill cry, "setting sun" sign, seizures, backward arching of neck and trunk (opisthotonos). Moro reflex is sluggish or abnormal when sudden extension of arms is not followed by flexion component and is often accompanied with downward rolling of eyeballs, lid lag and a peculiar grin.

Management

Hyperbilirubinemia should be considered as a medical emergency and all attempts must be made to ensure that serum bilirubin levels are kept within safe limits. Exchange blood transfusion remains the most effective and reliable method of lowering serum bilirubin when it approaches critical levels. Several supportive and therapeutic measures are useful to prevent excessive rise of serum bilirubin.

> *"We do know how to treat hyperbilirubinemia in the newborn but we do not know when to treat it because till date there is no single test that can identify the level or type of bilirubin which is dangerous to the brain."*
> — **Meharban Singh**

Supportive measures Early feeding and maintenance of adequate hydration are useful to prevent hyperbilirubinemia. Hypoxia, hypothermia, hypoglycemia and acidosis should be prevented and if they occur they should be promptly managed. Septicemia should be treated with appropriate antibiotics. When cephalhematoma is associated with critical hyperbilirubinemia it should be aspirated or drained.

Intravenous immunoglobulins High doses of intravenous immunoglobulins (IVIG) have been shown to block FC receptors thus inhibiting hemolysis and reducing formation of bilirubin. In seriously affected Rh-isoimmunized babies, IVIG is given in a dose of 1 g/kg as slow infusion over 2 hours. When exchange blood transfusion (EBT) is given at birth, IVIG is given after EBT. The IVIG therapy has been shown to reduce the duration of phototherapy and number of EBTs.

Phototherapy Phototherapy is known to cause photoisomerization of bilirubin to more polar, water-soluble, harmless compounds which are readily excreted in the bile, feces and urine. Phototherapy units with blue or white tubes or halogen or LED lamps are useful for preventing rapid rise in serum bilirubin levels. The naked infant is exposed under phototherapy unit which is kept at a distance of about 45 cm from the baby's skin. During exposure to light, the eyes must be effectively shielded to prevent retinal damage **(Figure 14.4)**. Double phototherapy (both from above and below with over head phototherapy unit and bili blanket) and reducing the distance between light source and the baby enhances the efficacy of phototherapy. The flux of phototherapy unit should be regularly monitored with a fluxmeter and its irradiance maintained between 8 and 12 mw/cm^2/nm to ensure efficacy of phototherapy unit.

The position of the infant should be changed frequently so that the maximal area of the skin is exposed to light. The infant is kept under the light round-the-clock and taken out only for feeding or change of wet napkins. Most preterm babies are placed under phototherapy when their serum bilirubin approaches 10 to 12 mg/dL and term babies are given phototherapy when their serum bilirubin approaches 15 mg/dL. Appropriate charts are available which are based on serum bilirubin levels, postnatal age of the infant and birth weight of the child, to provide more reliable indications for phototherapy and exchange blood transfusion.

During phototherapy, the infant should be closely watched for hydration status, temperature, degree of jaundice and anemia by frequent blood examination.

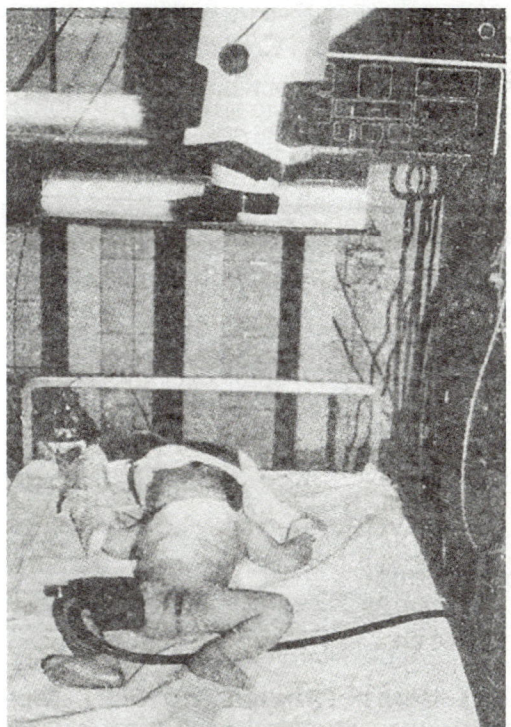

Figure 14.4 Baby under phototherapy unit. The eyes are covered effectively to protect against retinal damage

14

Phototherapy is by and large safe but may produce loose greenish stools, dehydration, hypothermia, or hyperthermia, and skin rash. During phototherapy, the clinical evaluation of the severity of jaundice becomes unreliable because the infant's skin gets bleached under light.

Sunlight It is a common practice to advise exposure of jaundiced babies to sunlight when they are discharged from the hospital. Sunlight is ineffective for purposes of phototherapy because most of the ultraviolet radiations which are effective in reducing jaundice are absorbed in the atmosphere. There is a serious risk of producing skin damage due to UV radiations and hyperthermia in summer and hypothermia in winter may occur. *Sunlight is both ineffective as well as unsafe for purposes of phototherapy and is not recommended.*

Exchange blood transfusion If despite phototherapy and other supportive measures, the bilirubin level is approaching 20 mg/dL in a term infant, exchange blood transfusion is mandatory to prevent brain damage. However, in an individual infant, the decision for exchange blood transfusion should not be based merely on the level of unconjugated serum bilirubin but other important factors like gestational maturity, postnatal age, presence or absence of perinatal distress factors and cause of jaundice should also be taken into consideration. Exchange blood transfusion is performed by cannulating the umbilical vein and a double volume (160 mL/kg blood) exchange is done. For indications and procedure of exchange blood transfusion, refer to **Chapter 49**.

METABOLIC DISORDERS

Metabolic disorders are relatively common during newborn period as compared to any other age group. Symptomatic metabolic disorders are associated with increased risk of neuromotor disability on follow up among those who survive. It is, therefore, essential that high-risk infants should be routinely screened for common metabolic disturbances such as hypoglycemia and hypocalcemia.

Hypoglycemia

Hypoglycemia is defined as a true blood glucose level of less than 40 mg/dL irrespective of period of gestation. If there are no symptoms, it should be confirmed on repeat analysis. The infant is born with a blood glucose concentration of 60–70 percent of the maternal level and it falls during first 3 days of life.

Causes

The common predisposing conditions for hypoglycemia include small-for-dates babies, large-for-dates babies, maternal diabetes mellitus and rhesus-isoimmunization. Hypoglycemia is common following severe birth asphyxia, hypothermia, septicemia and polycythemia. Hypoglycemia is known to occur in a number of life-threatening inborn errors of metabolism. Infants who are at increased risk to develop hypoglycemia should be routinely monitored for their blood glucose during first 3 days of life **(Box 14.2)**. The nurse should be able to check blood glucose level by the cotside with the help of a glucometer.

Clinical Features

Jitteriness, coarse tremors and convulsions may occur due to hypoglycemia. The infant becomes limp, apathetic and drowsy. Tachycardia and sweating may occur due to release of catecholamines. Episodes of limpness, sudden pallor, apneic attacks, tachypnea and irregular breathing may occur in preterm babies.

Management

Prevention Infant who is at an increased risk to develop hypoglycemia should be fed within one hour of birth and given supplementary sugar-fortified formula feeds in addition to breastfeeding during the first three days of life.

Treatment In symptomatic cases, therapy should be started immediately after withdrawing a blood sample for glucose estimation. The baby should be kept warm by nursing in a thermoneutral environment so that glucose is not consumed for metabolic thermogenesis. When seizures are present, give 25% dextrose 2 mL/kg IV as a bolus. When minor symptoms are present or

Box 14.2 Indications for routine monitoring of blood glucose

- Small-for-dates babies and smaller of the discordant twin
- Large-for-date babies and infants of mothers with gestational diabetes mellitus (GDM)
- Infants born before 35 weeks of gestation
- Rhesus hemolytic disease of the newborn
- Infants with perinatal hypoxia, birth asphyxia, hypothermia, polycythemia, septicemia, cardiac failure and suspected inborn error of metabolism
- Infants born to mothers receiving therapy with intravenous glucose, terbutaline, propranolol and oral hypoglycemic agent
- Infants on intravenous fluids or total parenteral nutrition
- Babies with symptoms suggestive of hypoglycemia

14

baby is asymptomatic, infant is given a minibolus of 2 mL/kg of 10% of dextrose. This is followed by continuous infusion of 10% dextrose at a rate of 8 mg/kg/min preferably with the help of an infusion pump. Glucose drip calculator as shown in **Figure 14.5** is useful for rapid estimation of rate and concentration of glucose solution needed to provide desired infusion of glucose. Dextrose infusion rate (mg/kg/min) can be calculated by the formula:

Glucose concentration (mg/mL) × fluids/kg/hr ÷ 60. The glucose infusion rate can also be directly read from **Table 14.2**.

The maximal concentration of glucose is limited to 15% to safeguard against the risk of thrombophlebitis. To prepare 14.5% solution of dextrose, add 30 mL of 25% dextrose (7.5 g dextrose) to 70 mL of 10% dextrose (7.0 g dextrose). The glucose infusion rate is gradually increased by 2 mg/kg/min every 2 hours till a maximum rate of 12 mg/kg/min is reached or the blood glucose of the infant has crossed the level of 40 mg/dL. The blood glucose level should be checked after 30 min of each change in glucose infusion rate. When blood glucose level crosses 60 mg/dL, glucose infusion rate is gradually tapered with decrements of 2 mg/kg/min every 12 hourly till glucose infusion rate comes down to 4 mg/kg/min with maintenance of blood glucose level between 60 and 100 mg/dL. Hyperglycemia should be avoided as it is also known to cause brain damage in newborn babies.

Prognosis Symptomatic hypoglycemia may cause death and those who survive are likely to develop neuromotor sequelae such as myoclonic or generalized seizures, cerebral palsy and mental retardation. In asymptomatic hypoglycemic babies of diabetic mothers, the outcome is good.

Hypocalcemia

Serum calcium level of less than 7.0 mg/dL (or ionized calcium of less than 4 mg/dL) during the first 4 weeks of life is designated as neonatal hypocalcemia. During first few days after birth, serum calcium falls while phosphorus level rises especially in preterm babies due to reduced glomerular filtration rate.

Causes

Early onset hypocalcemia (first 3 days) The common causes include prematurity, maternal diabetes mellitus and complications of delivery such as perinatal hypoxia, toxemia of pregnancy and antepartum hemorrhage.

Late-onset hypoclacemia (classical neonatal tetany) It is characterized by onset of tetany by the end of first week in healthy term babies receiving formula or cow's milk feeds. Intake of milk with high phosphate content or low calcium to phosphorus ratio (<1.5: 1.0) leads to hyperphosphatemia and hypocalcemia in the neonate. Other causes of hypocalcemia include maternal hyperparathyroidism, hypomagnesemia, hypoproteinemia, phototherapy, exchange blood transfusion, furosemide therapy and renal shut down.

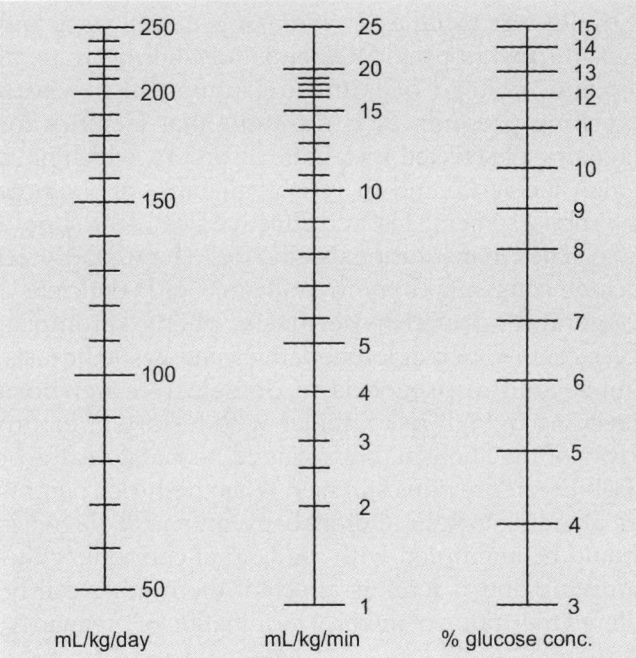

Figure 14.5 Glucose drip calculator. Use a plastic ruler to calculate interconversion of glucose infusion parameters to find out the desired infusion rate of glucose

Infusion rate mL/kg/hr (mL/kg/d)	5% dextrose	10% dextrose	15% dextrose
3 (72)	2.5	5.0	7.5
4 (96)	3.2	6.5	9.6
5 (120)	4.1	8.3	12.3
6 (144)	5.0	10.0	15.0
7 (168)	5.8	11.6	17.4

Table 14.2 Glucose infusion rates (mg/kg/min) with different infusion rates and concentration of dextrose

14

Clinical Features

There are no diagnostic features of hypocalcemia and many cases are asymptomatic and transient. Jitteriness, twitchings and convulsions or muscle spasms (tetany) may occur. The affected babies remain characteristically alert with a normal behavior. Some babies may have a high-pitched squeaky cry and stridor due to laryngospasm.

Treatment

Symptomatic babies Calcium gluconate 10% solution (2 mL/kg or 20 mg elemental calcium per kg) diluted with equal volume of distilled water is given as a slow infusion at a rate of less than 1.0 mL per minute through an established IV line. Heart rate should be continuously monitored and infusion is stopped when it falls below 100/min. Extravasation of calcium into subcutaneous tissues may lead to tissue necrosis and must be safeguarded. The maximum recommended bolus dose of 10% calcium gluconate is 10 mL for full term and 5 mL for preterm babies. After the bolus, calcium gluconate is administered as a constant infusion at a rate of 75 mg/kg/day for at least 48 hours. *Sodium bicarbonate should never be added to the infusate containing calcium gluconate, because it would lead to precipitation of calcium carbonate.* If hypocalcemia is unresponsive to calcium therapy, magnesium sulfate (0.2 mL per kg of 50% solution IM in 2 doses 12 hours apart) should be given.

Asymptomatic babies Give 2 mL/kg/dose of 10% calcium gluconate (75 mg elemental calcium/kg/day) IV every 6 hourly for 48 hours. If infant is orally fed, calcium gluconate 10% solution (2 mL/kg every 6 hourly) can be given through oral route. *Never administer calcium gluconate through IM route due to risk of tissue necrosis.*

Prevention

Infants at an increased risk to develop hypocalcemia (preterm <1500 g, severe birth asphyxia, infant of diabetic mother) should receive calcium gluconate 10% solution (elemental calcium 9 mg in each 1.0 mL) 1.0 mL/kg/dose diluted with equal volume of distilled water IV every 6 hourly or till oral feeds with supplements of calcium are started. Infants weighing less than 1500 g and receiving EBM should be given daily supplements of elemental calcium 210 mg/kg and phosphorus 100 mg/kg with a suitable oral preparation containing two parts of calcium and one part of phosphorus. The supplement should be continued till the post-conceptional maturity of 36 weeks.

Prognosis

If hypocalcemia is due to complications of labor, the prognosis is determined by the nature and severity of the underlying perinatal complications. The prognosis is excellent in infants with late-onset hypocalcemia or tetany.

NEWBORN SCREENING

There are a number of inborn errors of metabolism or genetic disorders that do not produce any obvious symptoms or signs during newborn period but may produce serious disability or life-threatening manifestations when these infants are started on oral feeding. In developed countries, routine screening is done to exclude a large number of metabolic disorders. In India as yet, universal metabolic screening is not feasible because of lack of technology and logistical difficulties because many deliveries are not taking place at health care facilities. In India, it is more logical and cost-effective to provide essential newborn care to all neonates instead of launching universal newborn screening program. It is desirable that facilities for screening of selected metabolic disorders, which have a high incidence and there is availability of a simple and robust screeing test and effective treatment, should be screened in institutional deliveries. These conditions include congenital hypothyroidism, G6PD deficiency, congenital adrenal hyperplasia, phenylketonuria, galactosemia, hemoglobinopathies and cystic fibrosis. The second approach is to do selective newborn screening in high-risk families with history of inborn errors of metabolism, unexplained neonatal deaths or disability in previous siblings. When high-risk parents are planning to have another baby, antenatal diagnosis should be attempted with the help of chorionic villus sampling and if fetus is affected, the mother can be offered the option of medical termination of pregnancy.

There is a need to gradually introduce newborn screening program in India in the institutionalized deliveries. Screening is done by measuring the presence of metabolites or enzyme activity in the whole blood samples collected on special filter papers having 'circles' for collecting blood spots. It is best to collect a blood sample between 72 hours and 7 days of life. The gestational age and birth weight should be intimated to the screening laboratory for proper interpretation of test results. When screening test is positive, the results should be reconfirmed by definitive analytical tests, like tandem mass spectrometry (TMS), combined gas-liquid chromatography and mass spectrometry (GC/MS), enzyme assays and DNA probes.

Apart from screening, it is recommended that all sick neonates, specially when diagnosis of sepsis is unlikely or ruled out, should be investigated for a metabolic disorder at the age of 7 days or later.

Neonatal Thyroid Screening

Availability of a sensitive and specific radio-immunoassay (RIA) method for T_4 and TSH has simplified the screeing program to assess thyroid status of the neonate to ensure early administration of thyroxine replacement therapy. Cord blood or preferably baby's blood collected after 3–4 postnatal days, is screened for TSH and T_4 level. TSH level of more than 50 µU/mL in cord blood is diagnositc of neonatal hypothyroidism, while T_4 may be normal or low (< 8 µg/dL). When screening is done after 72 hours, TSH level of > 20 µU/mL is suggestive of congenital hypothyroidism. It is important to remember that low levels of T_4 in association with normal levels of TSH may be seen in preterm infants due to immaturity of hypothalamic-pituitary-thyroid axis or deficiency of thyroxin binding globulin. Repeat T_4 levels after 3–4 weeks are usually normal without any replacement therapy. It is important to make an early diagnosis of congenital hypothyroidism and provide replacement therapy within two weeks of age to ensure normal physical and mental development.

BIBLIOGRAPHY

American Academy of Pediatrics. Subcommitee on hyperbiliru-binemia. Management of hyperbilirubinemia in a newbron infant 35 or more weeks of gestation. *Pediatrics* 2004, 114:297–316.

Arya VB, Senniappan S, Guemes M, Hussain K. Neonatal hypoglycemia. *Indian J Pediatr* 2014, 81(1):58–65.

Chan KN, Elliman A, Bryan E, Silverman M. Respiratory symptoms in children of low birth weight. *Arch Dis Child* 1989, 64:1294.

Cornblath M, Ichord R. Hypoglycemia in the neonate. *Semin Perinatol* 2000, 24:136–149.

Dennery PA, Seidman DS, Stevenson DK. Neonatal hyperbilirubinemia, *New Engl J Med* 2001, 344:581–590.

Diamond I. Kernicterus: Revised concepts of pathogenesis and management. *Pediatrics* 1966, 38:539.

Engle WA. American Academy of Pediatrics Committee on Fetus and Newborn. Surfactant replacement therapy for respiratory distress in the preterm and term neonate. *Pediatrics* 2008. 12:419–432.

Gartner LM, Lee K. Jaundice in breasfed infants. *Clin Perinatol* 1999, 26:431–445.

Halliday HL. Recent clinical trials of surfactant treatment for neonate. *Biol Neonate* 2006, 89(4):323–329.

Hsu HC, Levine MA. Perinatal calcium metabolism: Physiology and pathophysiology. *Semin Neonatol* 2004, 9:23–36.

Kumar A, Paul VK, Singh M. Neonatal systemic candidiasis. *Indian Pediatr* 1986, 23:643.

Murki S, Deorari AK, Vidyasagar D. Use of CPAP and surfactant therapy in newborn with respiratory distress syndrome. *Indian J Pediatr* 2014, 81(5):481–488.

Singh M, Deorari AK. Pneumonias in newborn babies. *Indian J Pediatr* 1995, 62:293–306.

Wiswell TE, Cleary GM. Meconium-stained amniotic fluid and the meconium aspiration syndrome. *Pediatr Clin North Am* 1998, 45:511–529.

Wolach B. Neonatal sepsis: pathogenesis and supportive therapy. *Semin Perinatol* 1997, 21:28–38.

Feeding and Nutrition

BREASTFEEDING

Breastfeeding is the birth right of every baby. Nature has so designed that when a baby is born, a ready-made food in the form of breast milk flows like divine nectar. Breast milk is best for all babies whether big or small and sick or healthy. Milk of different animals is specific to serve the nutritional needs of their offsprings by virtue of unique biological and biochemical composition. For example, milk of a cow or buffalo is meant for her calf, milk of mare is meant for her colt, milk of an ass is best for the pony, so on and so forth. Indeed, breast milk is not only species specific, it is baby specific. *The milk of a mother is best suited to serve the nutritional and biological needs of her baby!* Breastfeeding is natural and instinctive. Every mother wants to breastfeed her baby and she must be provided with necessary guidance, support and encouragement by her husband, family members and health care professionals. And, every mother can successfully breastfeed and provide a best start in life to her baby. *Like mother's love there is no substitute for mother's milk.*

Virtues of Breast Milk

Breastfeeding provides unique health benefits both to the baby and to her mother.

> *"The nature has designed the provision that infants be fed upon their mother's milk. They find their food and mother at the same time. It is a complete nourishment for them both for their body and soul."*
> — **Rabindranath Tagore**

Benefits to the Baby

1. Breast milk is a complete food and it provides all the nutrients a baby needs during first 6 months of life. Breast milk is more easily digestible due to presence of digestive enzymes and high quality of whey proteins. Breastfed babies do not need any supplements of vitamins and iron during first 6 months of life (except vitamin K and vitamin D).
2. Breast milk contains a number of anti-infective substances, nucleotides, protective antibodies and friendly lactobacilli, which protect the baby against development of diarrhea, respiratory illnesses (cough and cold) and other infections (especially ear infection). Breastfeeding has been shown to reduce the risk of death due to diarrhea by 14 times, acute respiratory infections by 4 times and other infections by 3 times.
3. Breastfed babies are less likely to suffer from allergic disorders like asthma and eczema. Rarely breastfed babies may develop allergic disorder if mother consumes allergenic foods like cow's milk, eggs, nuts and citrus fruits.
4. Breastfeeding provides immunological benefits to the baby for the life time. Breastfed babies have been shown to develop better protective response to various vaccines compared to bottle fed babies.
5. Breastfeeding provides emotional security and promotes close bonding between mother and her baby. Breastfeeding provides maternal warmth, physical closeness and comfort to the baby.
6. Breastfeeding stimulates all the five special senses of the baby, i.e. touch, sight, smell, hearing and taste.
7. Breastfed babies are smarter and have been shown to have 8 points higher intelligence quotient (IQ). High concentrations of two key long chain fatty acids (arachidonic acid and docosahexaenoic acid) and lactose promotes brain growth.
8. Breastfed babies are less likely to suffer from diabetes mellitus, obesity, high blood pressure, heart attacks and certain cancers during adult life.
9. There is no risk of adulteration, dilution, contamination and infection of breast milk.

Benefits to the Mother

1. During breastfeeding, there is a release of oxytocin to eject the milk. Oxytocin helps to contract the uterus

so that there is reduced risk of bleeding and anemia after delivery.

2. Breastfeeding delays ovulation and onset of menstruation which provides natural means to ensure spacing of children. Nevertheless, the protection is not fool proof and mothers who are breastfeeding must seek proper contraceptive advice.

3. Breastfeeding is convenient and less time consuming. Breast milk is readily available all the time at the desired temperature. There is no need to buy feeding bottles and animal or powdered milk and no time is wasted for sterilization of bottles and preparation of feeds.

4. There is a misconception among several women that breastfeeding spoils the figure. On the contrary, breastfeeding helps to maintain and regain the pre-pregnancy body weight earlier because energy stores laid down during pregnancy are consumed faster during lactation. As far as the shape of the breasts is concerned, there is no difference whether mother breastfeeds or gives formula feeds to her baby.

5. Mothers who breastfeed their babies have a reduced risk of development of breast and ovarian cancer and osteoporosis (brittle bones).

6. There is economic saving to the family and society because money and resources are not wasted for purchase of feeding bottles, bottle sterilizer, bottle warmer, animal milk or formula and there is reduction in medical costs because of lower incidence of various infections in breastfed babies.

Preparation for Breastfeeding

The preparation and motivation for breastfeeding should begin during antenatal visits. The cleaning of nipples, their eversion if retracted and treatment for cracked nipples must be instituted well in advance during pregnancy so that the baby does not face any difficulties while feeding. The absence of any sucking difficulties during early nursing is of great importance to establish cordial mother-child bonding and to reduce the incidence of lactation failure. There is no correlation between the size of breasts and adequacy of lactation. Breast milk is produced in the special glands in the breast which are present in good number in all women irrespective of the size of the breasts.

Physiological Basis of Lactation

Sucking is the best stimulus to enhance milk production. When baby sucks vigorously, several hormones are released to produce milk and eject it out. Sucking movements stimulate nerve fibers in the nipple. These nerve fibers transmit messages to the hypothalamus in the brain. The pituitary gland responds to these messages by release of two hormones, prolactin and oxytocin **(Figure 15.1)**. Prolactin stimulates the breast to produce more milk. Oxytocin stimulates the tiny muscles surrounding the milk ducts of the breast. The contractions of these tiny muscles squeeze the ducts and eject the milk into the reservoir under the areola. When baby sucks frequently and vigorously, the milk production is enhanced. Pain and anxiety interfere with these hormonal mechanisms leading to unsatisfactory lactation.

Promotion of Lactation

During pregnancy, breasts enlarge in size under the influence of sex hormones and become functionally mature to secrete milk when baby is born. During pregnancy mother should be motivated and emotionally prepared to breastfeed her baby. Breasts must be examined during antenatal check ups to exclude and manage any problems like cracked or retracted nipples. During lactation, mother should take plenty of liquids, extra milk and nutritious diet to provide additional 550 kcalories and 20–25 gm protein per day to meet the nutritional cost of lactation. And since breast milk is rich in calcium (300 mg/liter) and several other vital nutrients for the baby's growth, adequate intake of calcium, vitamin A, omega-3 fatty acids, DHA and other micronutrients is essential to ensure successful lactation and production of good quality of breast milk.

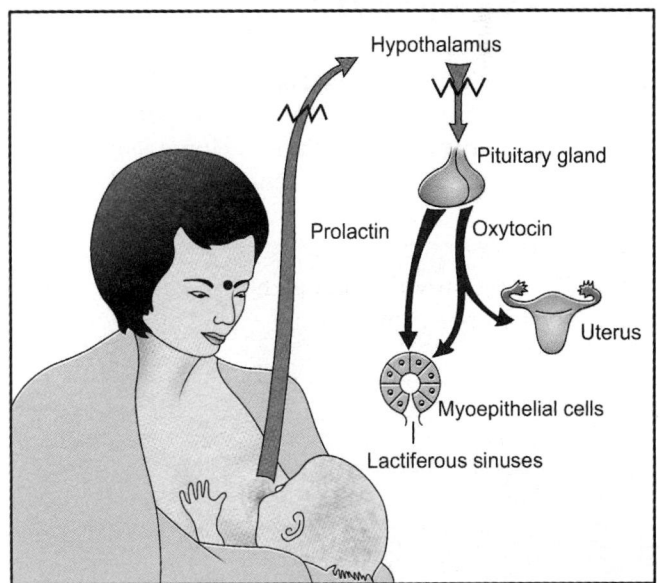

Figure 15.1 The let-down reflex. See the text for details. The release of oxytocin during sucking causes involution or contractions of uterus so that it rapidly shrinks in size to pre-pregnancy size. The release of prolactin inhibits ovulation leading to a state of relative infertility during breastfeeding

15

Healthy and normal babies should not be kept in the nursery but should lie next to the mother. Ensuring close skin-to-skin contact and eye contact with the baby enhances lactation. Early and frequent feedings are associated with increased milk production. The act of sucking is associated with release of two hormones (prolactin and oxytocin) which are known to enhance milk production and promote ejection of milk. Milk production is related to the concept of supply and demand; more vigorously and frequently a baby sucks, more milk is produced. When a mother is relaxed and confident she is likely to produce more milk. Adequate support, guidance and encouragement from family members and health care professionals are associated with enhanced milk production. Grandmother should be actively involved for providing guidance to the mother for promotion of breastfeeding **(Figure 15.2)**.

Anxiety, lack of confidence and pain (due to cracked nipples or engorged breasts) are known to adversely effect the milk yield. An anxious brain may switch off the mechanism which controls the breast milk production. Adequate rest, sleep, relaxation and frequent nursing are associated with satisfactory yield of milk. Early introduction of supplementary bottle feeds may lead to poor lactation because baby finds it easier to feed from a bottle and refuses to make efforts to breastfeed. The use of a dummy nipple or pacifier, may adversely affect the yield of breast milk.

Role of Galactagogues

The substances which are credited to enhance milk production are called galactagogues or lactagogues. In Ayurvedic system, a large number of food items are recommended to promote lactation. Home remedies for improving milk yield include fenugreek (*methi*) seeds,

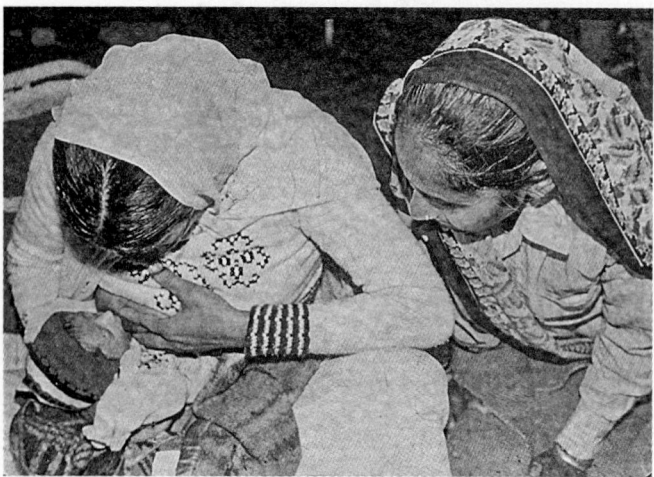

Figure 15.2 Grandmother is guiding her daughter-in-law to promote breastfeeding

tulsi seeds, pupali, fennel (*sonf*), cummin seeds (*jeera*), cinnamon (*dalchini*), poppy seeds (*khaskhas*), garlic, ajwain, ginger, gum, coriander seeds (*dhania*), alfa alfa, unripe papaya, oats, etc. virtually anything in the kitchen. The very fact that the list of galactagogues is so large, it suggests that there is no fool proof remedy and they are all based on folklore, faith and figment of imagination. The aforementioned food items are usually consumed in the form of *laddoos, kheer* or porridge, *burfi, halwa, mukhwas,* sprinklers or decoctions like herbal tea. In modern system of medicine, there is no potent or effective galactagogue. Metaclopramide (a drug used for vomiting) has been tried with a variable efficacy for promotion of lactation.

The First Feed

Baby should be put to the breast as soon as the mother has recovered from the fatigue of labor. After a normal delivery the baby can be offered the first feed within half an hour while most babies born by cesarean section can be put to the breast within 4 hours of birth. There is no need to give any other milk or drink like glucose water, tea, honey or *ghutti* and baby should be put straight to the breast without any pre-lacteal feeds.

Types of Breast Milk

The composition of breast milk varies at different stages in the postnatal period to serve the biological needs of the baby.

Colostrum The thick-yellowish milk, which is produced during the first 2–3 days, is called colostrum. It is very rich in proteins, protective antibodies and vitamin A. It must be given to the baby because of its high nutritional qualities and disease fighting capabilities. There is a cultural practice in some communities to express colostrum and discard it, which is strongly condemned. During initial few days, milk yield is low but it is enough to meet the nutritional needs of the baby. Healthy babies do have enough stores of energy and do not need any complementary feeds. The practice of introducing bottle feeds (especially to cesarean born babies), during first 1–2 days when lactation is gradually building-up, is an important cause of lactation failure. Bottle feeding leads to "nipple confusion" (because baby uses different technique to feed from rubber teat of a bottle compared to breastfeeding) and reduced hormonal stimulation to the breasts due to reduced sucking efforts.

Transitional milk It follows colostrum and is secreted in next two weeks. It is thicker than mature milk and has higher caloric content due to increased concentration of fat and lactose.

Mature milk The composition of breast milk stabilizes after the transitional phase. It becomes thinner and watery but contains all the essential nutrients (except vitamin K and vitamin D) for optimal growth of the baby.

Preterm milk The nature has profound biological wisdom. The milk of a mother who delivers prematurely contains more calories and higher concentration of fat, protein and sodium which are needed for rapid growth of her preterm baby. During next 2 to 3 weeks, the composition of milk gradually changes and becomes similar to the milk produced by mothers who deliver at term.

Fore milk The milk secreted at the start of feeding is called fore milk. It is watery and rich in protein, sugar and water. It satisfies the thirst of the baby.

Hindmilk It is released during the fag end of feeding and is richer in fat content and provides more energy and satiety to the baby. The baby should take both foremilk as well as the hindmilk to satisfy thirst and ensure optimal growth. The baby should, therefore, be allowed to empty one breast completely before being moved to the other breast.

Drip milk The milk that drips from the other breast during breastfeeding is called drip milk and can be collected to supplement the breastfeeding. It is mainly foremilk with relatively low energy and fat content.

Art and Technique of Breastfeeding

Breastfeeding is natural and instinctive and most mothers are able to breastfeed without any difficulties. There are many ways to breastfeed and every mother develops her own style to suit her baby. There are certain steps that will help the mother to breastfeed with ease and comfort. She should master the art of breast-feeding by practice, perseverance and self-confidence.

1. The mother should sit comfortably on a chair, on the bed or floor (squat) to feed her baby. It is important that she must feel comfortable and her back must be supported. She may also feed while lying down in bed if baby was born by cesarean section or she is unwell.

2. The baby is held in the arm so that his head and neck rest in the hollow of her elbow, the back along her forearm and the buttocks in her hand. If she is feeding the baby on the right breast, her right arm should be used to cradle the baby **(Figure 15.3)**.

3. The mother should bring the baby's entire body towards her so that baby's tummy touches her mother's tummy. The baby's head and neck must be comfortably supported on the hollow of mother's elbow.

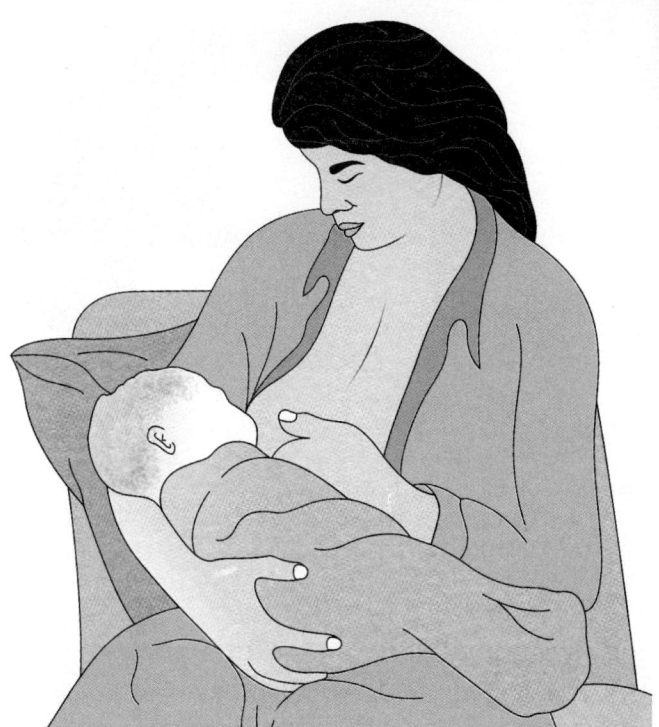

Figure 15.3 The conventional and most comfortable method of breastfeeding. The baby's head and neck are supported comfortably on the hollow of mother's elbow

4. The baby should be raised to the level of the breast to ensure that baby's mouth can easily reach the nipple and areola. Mother can place a pillow below her arm or raise her thigh to lift the baby (if she is sitting cross-legged on the floor). To bring the baby snugly close to her, at times the mother may need to tuck her baby's arm away so that it does not come in the way. Mother may use her free hand to hold her breast or to fondle her baby once baby is well "attached" or "latched" for feeding.

5. When the lips or cheek of the baby touches her breast, the baby will automatically open his mouth and "root" for the nipple. The baby should grasp the nipple and part of areola of the breast in his mouth. This is called "attachment or latchment to the breast". The lactiferous sinuses which store the milk are situated just beneath the areola. In order to effectively suckle the milk from the breast, both the nipple and areola should go into the baby's mouth. Proper "attachment" is indeed the key to successful breast-feeding. For effective sucking, the baby must form an effective seal around the nipple and areola to eject the milk from lactiferous sinuses **(Figure 15.4)**. When the baby merely grasps and sucks the nipple it leads to soreness of the nipple, poor feeding and engorgement of breasts **(Figure 15. 5)**.

15

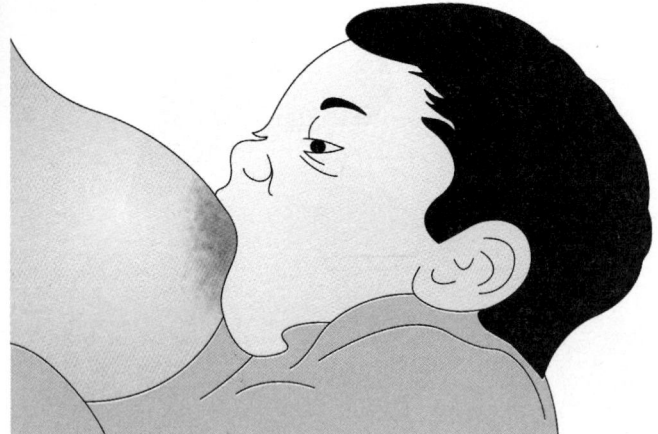

Figure 15.4 Correct technique of breastfeeding. The baby forms an effective seal around the nipple and areola to ensure "attachment" for ejection of milk from lactiferous sinuses

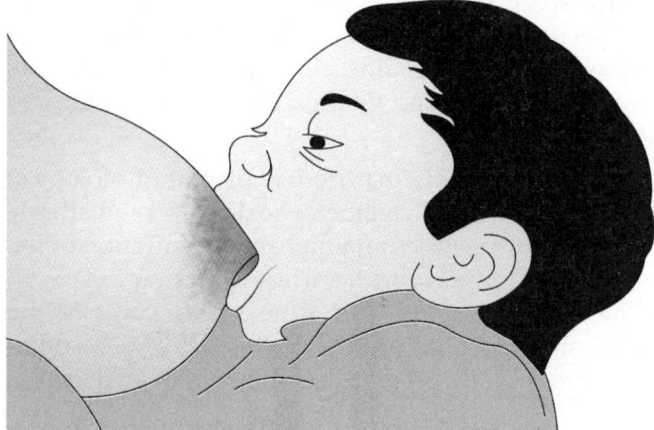

Figure 15.5 Wrong technique of breastfeeding. The baby is merely sucking at the nipple leading to soreness of nipple and poor ejection of milk with engorgement of breast

Ensuring good "attachment" at breast

The following features suggest that the baby has learnt to ensure good "attachment" or "latching" for proper feeding:

1. Baby's mouth is wide open.
2. Chin of the baby touches the breast.
3. Nipple and most of the areola are inside the baby's mouth.
4. Lower lip is turned outwards.
5. Mother feels no pain or discomfort while breastfeeding.

How to delatch the baby from the breast?

When baby is satisfied or falls asleep while feeding, he automatically releases the breast. However, when a baby has stopped sucking but is still maintaining strong suction, do not pull him off the nipple. Instead, mother should slide her index finger into the corner of the baby's mouth to break the suction and delatch the baby.

Frequency of breastfeeding

There should be no fixed timing for feeding. The baby should be fed on demand, day and night, whenever baby appears to be hungry. The more a baby sucks on the mother's breast, more milk is produced. Most babies would like to be fed every 2–3 hours. The night feeds are required for initial 6–8 weeks or even longer in healthy normal weight babies.

Duration of each breastfeed

It is variable, but most active healthy babies take 10–15 minutes to finish a feed. Many babies fall asleep after a few sucks and then demand a feed after half to one hour. Mother should play and interact with her baby while feeding by touching the ears or stroking the soles. When

baby gets lazy, she should try to partially remove her nipple; the baby will wake up again and start sucking vigorously. While feeding, mother should look at her baby intently and interact with him during the process of feeding. *Breastfeeding is an active process and mother must pay her full attention to the baby while feeding.* During breastfeeding mother provides warmth, skin-to-skin contact, love, affectionate look and tender touch and music of her heart beats to her baby thus stimulating all the five special senses of her baby! Apart from wholesome nutrition, breastfeeding provides global sensory stimulation to the baby.

The first part of milk which flows when a baby starts to breastfeed is watery and the latter part contains more fat. The baby should be allowed to completely empty one breast so that both his thirst and hunger are satisfied by taking foremilk and hindmilk. Baby should be allowed to feed as long as he wants at one breast before offering the other breast. During the next feed, the breast offered second should now be offered first, to keep up the milk supply in both the breasts.

How long to continue breastfeeding?

During initial 6 months exclusive breastfeeding is given and not even water should be given to the baby even in hot summer months. The baby will drink more milk when thirsty and would have better weight gain. *Exclusively breastfed babies do not develop diarrhea and they have adequate weight gain during first 6 months.* Breast milk is a complete food for the baby and there is no need to give any supplements of vitamins (except vitamin D) and minerals to healthy full term babies during first 6 months. There is no role of giving *janam ghutti, jaiphal* (nutmeg) and gripe water to babies. Semi-solid home-made weaning foods should be offered after 6 months of age but breastfeeding should be continued as long as feasible; at least for a minimum period of 1–2 years. Breastfeeding may be continued as long as feasible or desired but it is important to ensure that the baby gets adequate nutrition by taking enough cereals, pulses, vegetables and fruits, etc.

What is nipple confusion?

Some mothers start one or two bottle feeds along with breastfeeds with the mistaken belief that otherwise it will not be possible to wean the baby off the breast. It is unwise and strongly discouraged because firstly the mechanisms for sucking from the breast and teat of the feeding bottle are different and secondly according to current recommendations there is no place for bottle feeding in the care of babies. Bottle feeding is easier and less tiring for the baby because he can readily get the milk by pressing the soft rubber teat while in case of breastfeeding baby has to firmly take a big bite of the breast tissue under the areola and suck with a considerable effort with coordinated movements of lips, gums and tongue. Breastfeeding demands more effort and is usually tiring. Once a baby gets used to the easier option of taking milk from the bottle, he refuses to accept the breast because we are all lazy and so are the babies. More over, baby may start sucking or biting at the nipple (like he does to the rubber teat of the bottle) due to "nipple confusion" with unsatisfactory sucking efforts and development of cracked nipples. According to current recommendations, exclusive breastfeeding should be continued up to 6 months after which semi-solid complementary foods including milk products (porridge, custard, *kheer*, yoghurt, cottage cheese, etc.) are started. Breastfeeding is continued as long as feasible and liquid milk is introduced after one year, not with a feeding bottle but with a cup or a glass. *There is thus no role of introducing a feeding bottle in the care of babies.*

How to know that the baby is getting enough breast milk?

During breastfeeding when milk drips from the other breast, it suggests mother has satisfactory lactation. As a safeguard against the mess and embarassment of leaking breasts, mother can use absorbent breast pads, under the bra. When a baby is adequately fed, he is satisfied, happy and playful for 2–3 hours after a feed. Most babies pass urine after every feed. When a baby passes dilute water-like urine at least 6–8 times in a day, it suggests that baby is having enough feeds. Some babies enjoy sucking their fingers and it is not suggestive of inadequacy of breast milk. The best criterion that the baby is getting enough milk is the satisfactory weight gain. During first 4 months, most babies gain an average of 30 g weight every day (750–900 g/month). The baby must be weighed on a reliable weighing scale during each visit to the hospital for vaccination and routine check-up. "Test weighing" is unnecessary and not recommended to assess the adequacy of lactation. Excessive crying alone should not be taken as an evidence for poorfeeding because babies cry due to a variety of reasons like discomfort of wet napkins, intestinal colic, excessive wind, exposure to cold or being over clothed, insect or mosquito bites, boredom, etc.

What is the usual stool frequency during breastfeeding?

Most normal healthy breastfed babies pass 4–6 golden-yellow sticky stools. Babies fed on cow's milk or formula feeds tend to be constipated due to high casein content of the milk but are more vulnerable to develop infective diarrhea. Some babies may pass a stool during or soon after a feed because they have an overactive gastro-colic reflex. Mother should not be worried about this problem because baby would continue to have satisfactory weight gain.

Should a sick baby be given breastfeeding?

Breastfeeding is an ideal food for a sick baby. Many a times, a sick baby refuses to accept any food but continues to take breastfeeds. When a sick baby is active and able to suck, he must be given breastfeeding. A critically sick baby can be given expressed breast milk (EBM) with a nasogastric tube.

Should breastfeeding be continued when mother is ill?

Most illnesses in the mother do not contraindicate breastfeeding. The mother produces antibodies against the infective organisms and these antibodies cross over through the breast milk and protect the baby. Breast milk cannot transmit disease causing germs. The baby cannot catch cold through the breast milk but baby can get infected by close contact with her mother through hands and droplets thrown by her while talking, coughing and sneezing. When a mother is critically sick or suffering from cancer (and receiving anti-cancer medicines) or AIDS, she is advised to bottle feed her baby. Mother with jaundice can safely breastfeed her baby.

Medicines to be avoided by the nursing mother

In general what is safely tolerated by the nursing mother is safe for her suckling infant. Mother should avoid intake of sedatives because they can make her baby lazy and inactive. Intake of medicated laxative can cause diarrhea

15

in the suckling baby. It is safe for the nursing mother to take milk of magnesia, liquid paraffin and glycerin suppository for relief of constipation. Intake of antibiotics by nursing mother may cause mild diarrhea in her suckling infant. Intake of anticancer, antithyroid drugs, anticoagulants and certain antidepressant drugs contraindicate breastfeeding.

Can twins be reared on breastfeeding alone?

Many mothers can rear twin babies on exclusive breastfeeding without any complementary feeds. Many lower mammals are endowed with several breasts (and nipples) depending upon their average litter size. It would appear that two breasts should be sufficient to effectively suckle two babies before they are able to accept weaning foods. Mother can offer alternate breast for feeding each twin baby. If weight gain is unsatisfactory with exclusive breastfeeding, complementary feeds should be given alternating with breastfeeds. However, mother of twin babies must receive tremendous support, encouragement and assistance by family members because it is an herculean task to simultaneously nurture and look after two babies. She would also need additional calories, proteins and micronutrients to sustain the growth of two babies.

Diet during Lactation

It must be remembered that nutritional cost of lactation is higher than the nutritional cost of pregnancy. The nursing mother must take at least 25% additional calories and nutrients compared to her pre-pregnancy food intake. She should have a well balanced diet with sufficient proteins in the form of milk and milk products, pulses, legumes, eggs and poultry. She should have sufficient intake of fresh green leafy vegetables and seasonal fruits. It is recommended that a nursing mother should take 2.6 g omega-3 fatty acids and 300 mg DHA every day through dietary sources or nutritional supplements. Fish and sea food are excellent sources of omega-3 fatty acids and DHA The diet

> **Practical Tip**
>
> During fetal life and infancy, adequacy of nutrition is ensured entirely through transmaternal route. Adequate nutrition during pregnancy is associated with optimal fetal growth and a higher birth weight. Nursing mother must take a balanced diet with supplements of micronutrients to improve the quantity and nutritional quality of her breast milk. Adequate nutrition and health care of girl children throughout their life cycle—infancy, childhood, adolescence, pregnancy and lactation—is indeed the best investment to have healthy children and a healthy nation!

should be supplemented with commercially available micronutrients to enhance the concentration of vitamins and trace minerals in the breast milk. She should drink plenty of water and liquids to replenish the fluids lost through breast milk. Intake of nutritious balanced diet by the nursing mother is associated with improved nutritional quality of her breast milk. Healthy breastfed infants do not need any supplements of vitamins and minerals, except vitamin D.

Foods to be Avoided during Nursing

The mother who is breastfeeding should take a normal diet without too much chillies and condiments. Excessive indulgence in any particular food or fruit should be avoided. It is well known that intake of lentils with their covering, black *urad dal*, kidney beans, Bengal gram and *kabli channa* by the nursing mother may cause wind, discomfort and loose motions in her suckling infant. Cruciferous vegetables like cabbage, cauliflower, broccoli sprouts, turnips, radish, beans, mustard leaves (*sarson ka saag*) may also cause distension and gas both in the mother and her suckling infant. When a mother feels that intake of a particular food item consistently upsets her baby by causing colic or loose motions, she should avoid it or take it in moderation.

Contraindications to Breastfeeding

Most mothers can and should be encouraged to breastfeed because there are few genuine contraindications. In following situations, it is desirable to avoid breastfeeding in the interest of the baby.
- The baby is diagnosed to have galactosemia.
- Mother is receiving diagnostic or therapeutic radioactive isotopes.
- Mother is receiving antimetabbolites or chemotherapeutic agents for cancer.
- Mother is taking drugs of abuse.
- Mother has active sputum-positive untreated tuberculosis.
- Mother has active herpes simplex lesions on the breast.
- Human T-lymphotropic virus type 1 or 2 infection.
- Mother is HIV-positive. After having told the options and consequences, if an HIV-positive mother decides to breastfeed her baby, exclusive breastfeeding (without any complementary feeds) is a safer option because it is associated with reduced risk of transmission of HIV to the baby.

Breastfeeding by a Working Mother

Mother should take most of her maternity leave after the delivery of her baby. She should extend her leave as much as she can so that she can ensure exclusive breastfeeding as long as possible. If she has to get back to work, she can follow any one of the following alternatives:

1. Availability of a creche near the vicinity of work place is useful so that she can visit her baby for breastfeeding during office hours and lunch break.
2. If baby is more than 4 months old, he can be fed with a pre-cooked cereal, soft rice-*dal* gruel (*khichadi*), curd and mashed banana. Thus a working mother can introduce weaning foods earlier than the current recommendation of 6 months.
3. Mother can express her milk and store it in a container having a tight fitting lid. The milk can be safely stored for 8 hours at room temperature and upto 24 hours in a refrigerator. She can breastfeed her baby before going to work and on returning back. When she is away, expressed breast milk can be fed to the baby with a spoon. *It is desirable not to introduce bottle feeding to avoid nipple confusion and reduce the risk of infective diarrhea.*

Technique for Expression of Breast Milk

It is useful to know the proper technique to express and store the breast milk, which may be required in following situations:

1. To maintain lactation when a sick or premature baby is unable to suck from the breast.
2. To provide milk for tube feeding of a premature or sick baby.
3. To relieve engorgement of breasts.
4. When a mother plans to join her office and her baby is still on exclusive breastfeeding.

The milk can be expressed manually or with the help of a mechanical or an electrical breast pump **(Figures 15.6A, B and 15.7)**. The steps for manual expression of breast milk are summarized in **Box 15.1**.

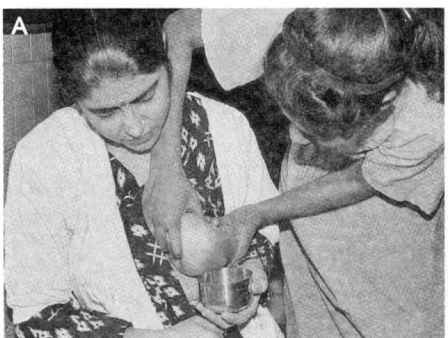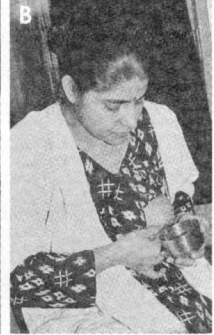

Figure 15.6 Manual expression of breast milk. (A) Breast is gently massaged with both hands from the chest towards the areola. This movement pushes the milk into the lactiferous sinuses. (B) The aerola is pinched between thumb and fingers to express the milk into a wide-mouthed container

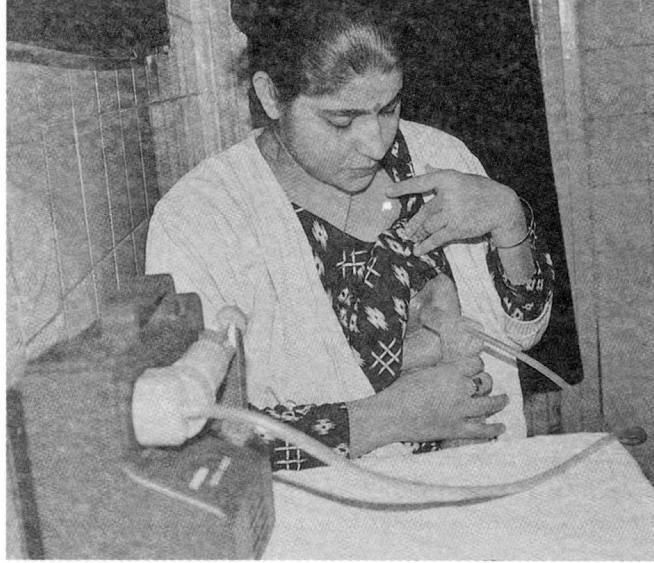

Figure 15.7 Expression of breast milk with the help of an electrical pump

Box 15.1 **Manual expression of breast milk**

- The milk can be conveniently and effectively expressed with hands or mother can use a breast pump.
- Take a wide-mouthed thoroughly washed container having a tight lid. Wash hands thoroughly with soap and water.
- Sit or stand comfortably. Place the container close to the breast and infront and below the nipple to collect the expressed milk.
- Soften the breast by gently massaging it with both hands starting from near the chest and moving forwards, towards the nipple.
- Hold the areola between the thumb and fingers and press them inwards towards chest to fill up the lactiferous sinuses.
- Compress the lactiferous sinuses by pinching the areola between your thumb and fingers to express the milk. Press and release the thumb and fingers several times until milk starts to drip out. Collect milk from one breast for at least 3–5 minutes. Rotate the thumb and fingers around the areola so that all traces of milk is removed from the lactiferous sinuses.
- Repeat the process on the other breast.

Storage of Expressed Breast Milk (EBM)

The milk should be collected in a clean container having a screw cap or a tight lid. Milk can be safely stored for 8 hours in the cool place of the room or up to 24 hours in a refrigerator. It can be stored up to 3 months in a deep freeze at –20°C. The stored milk should never be boiled or heated in the microwave oven as it will destroy the protective components of milk. It can be

15

thawed or warmed by placing the milk container in a bowl of warm water. The container should be gently shaken to recombine the separated fat globules before feeding. The EBM should be given with a spoon or *paladay*, and use of a feeding bottle should be strictly avoided **(Figure 15.8)**.

Baby Friendly Hospital Initiative

In order to encourage and promote exclusive breastfeeding to enhance child survival, the Baby Friendly Hospital Initiative (BFHI) was launched jointly by WHO and UNICEF in March, 1992. Bottle being the biggest killer of babies in developing countries, a mission approach has been launched globally to resurrect the dwindling practice of breastfeeding. Efforts are being made to improve the knowledge, attitude and practices of health care workers by providing them with information, scientific facts and skills to promote exclusive breastfeeding during first 6 months of life. Mother–baby bonding at birth, avoidance of pre-lacteal feeds, early breastfeeding and practice of keeping the mother and her baby together in the rooming-in ward are encouraged. The representatives of infant food manufactures are strictly forbidden to contact mothers or health care staff for distribution of low cost or free infant formula, feeding bottles and any literature pertaining to formula feedings. The advertisement and promotion of breast milk substitutes in media and distribution of pamphlets, calendars and growth charts, etc. is against the code of conduct and can attract penalty. The medical and nursing graduates, family physicians, pediatricians and obstetricians should be provided with adequate information, knowledge and skills during their formal training and subsequently by continuing medical education programs to ensure the sustainability of the BFHI program. Refer to **Chapter 46** for details.

Common Problems during Breastfeeding

Regurgitation Most healthy babies regurgitate some curdled milk after a feed but they continue to gain weight satisfactorily. Regurgitation is more common in bottle fed babies compared to breastfed infants. During feeding, baby swallows some air which causes distension and discomfort till baby is able to eructate. After each feed (sometimes even when only one-half the feed has been given), mother should make the baby sit in her lap or hold the baby against the shoulder to help him to eructate the swallowed air **(Figure 15.9)**. After this, the baby should be put to bed in the right lateral position with head end slightly raised.

Engorgement of breasts Some mothers develop engorgement of breasts on the third or fourth day after delivery if breastfeeding is delayed or given infrequently and baby has not learnt the art of correct "attachment". It is more common in a primigravida mother. The breasts become heavy, swollen, red, hard and painful. Mother should be asked to wear a well-fitting bra (with wide straps and no plastic lining) round-the-clock. Local application of warm packs and intake of a safe analgesic like paracetamol relieves pain and congestion. In humid climate, hair dryer can be used. At times local fomentation may aggravate engorgement due to increase in blood flow. In such a case, cold compresses (chilled cabbage leaves with a hole in the centre for nipple) may be more beneficial. At times, alternate cold and warm water compresses in-between feedings provide significant relief. The breast congestion is best relieved by expressing milk manually or with a breast pump. A healthy and hungry baby can be put to the breast after expressing some milk when breast becomes soft. When a baby cannot suck directly from the breast he can be offered EBM. Early feeding and frequent suckling by the baby prevents development of breast engorgement.

Sore or cracked nipples The most common cause of sore nipples is poor attachment to the breast. When a baby merely sucks at the nipple (instead of nipple and areola) he does not get any milk, sucks vigorously or bites the nipple damaging its delicate skin. Pulling the baby forcefully from the nipple without de-latching may also damage the nipple. Avoid frequent washing of breast with soap and water which may lead to

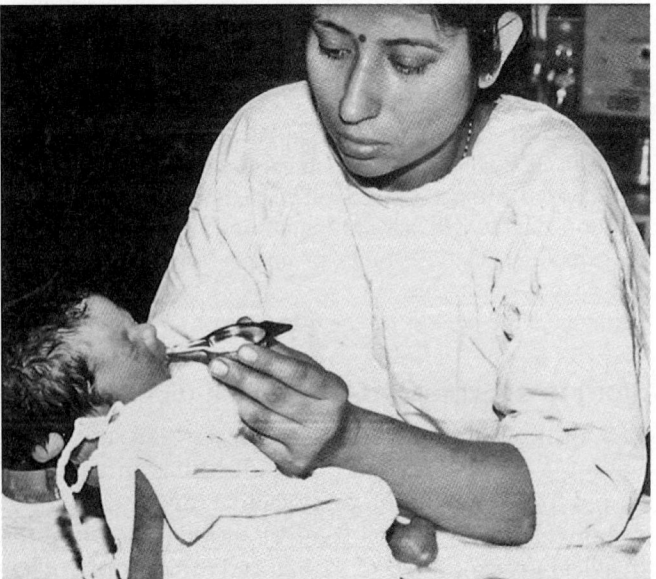

Figure 15.8 Feeding expressed breast milk to a premature baby with a *paladay*

A

B

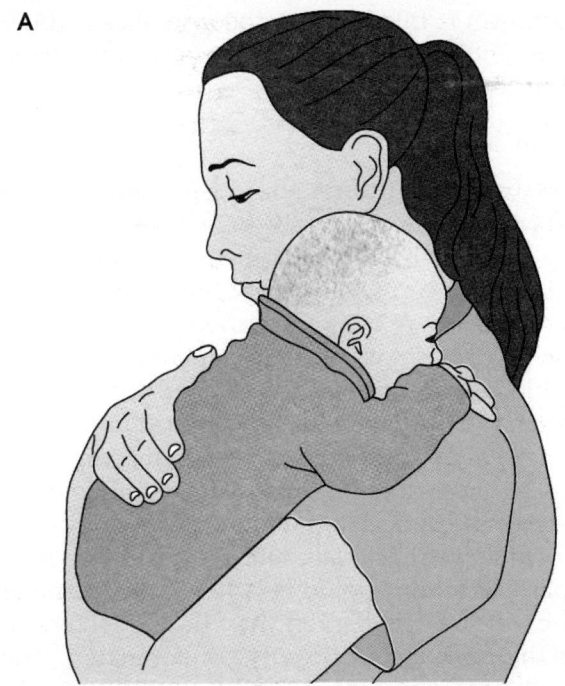
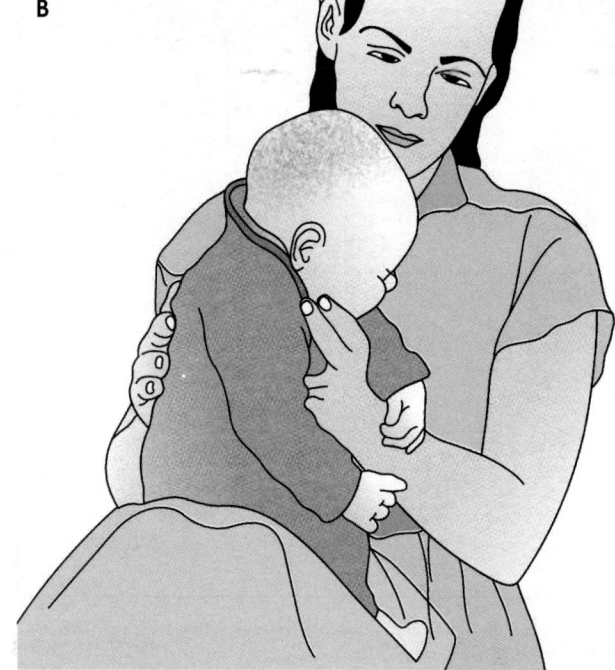

Figure 15.9 Technique for burping the baby. (A) The baby is held against the shoulder and his abdomen is gently pressed by patting his back with your right hand. (B) After feeding, the baby may be made to sit in your lap to help him to eructate the swallowed air

dryness, cracking and chaffing of nipples. Mother should wear loose clothes and avoid the use of bra to allow the cracks to heal. The plastic breast shields or plastic-lined nursing pads should not be worn because they hold the moisture. Mother can use a nursing bra with a breast shell to avoid direct pressure over the tender nipples. After nursing, express a little milk from the breasts and let it dry on the nipples to provide a protective covering which facilitates the healing process. The "hind milk" contains fats and anti-infective substances which serves as an emollient and help the process of healing. The breastfeeding should be continued and mother is asked to apply some emollient cream (ultrapurified medical grade lanolin) over the nipples in-between the feeds. If nipples are extremely sore, she can use a nipple shield for feeding.

Retracted or inverted nipples There are wide variations in the shape and size of breasts and nipples. Nipples may be small, flat or inverted. Most babies can feed from a small or flat nipple. But inverted nipples cause serious feeding difficulties leading to engorgement of breasts. The mother should be asked to pull out the flat and inverted nipple with thumb and index finger. The nipple should be rolled between thumb and index finger and pulled out before feeding. Syringe method is effective for treatment of flat nipples if above procedure fails **(Box 15.2)**.

Box 15.2 Syringe method for treatment of retracted nipples

- Take a 10 mL plastic syringe and remove its piston.
- After cutting the barrel half a centimeter from the nozzle, insert the piston from the cut end of the barrel.
- Place the other opening (smooth or non-cut side) of the barrel of the syringe around the nipple and withdraw the piston gently **(Figure 15.10)**. The nipple will slowly protrude into the barrel. After 30–60 seconds, push the piston back gently to release the hold of the syringe on the nipple.
- Repeat this procedure 5–8 times before each breastfeeding.
- As soon as the nipple becomes prominent, hold the nipple and areola in your fingers to form a teat and put the baby to the breast.
- Avoid the use of a nipple shield which is ineffective and may be harmful.
- Mother should be asked to wear a breast shell under the bra to avoid compression of nipples.

HUMAN MILK BANKING

Human milk banking is a service for screening, collecting, processing, storing and distributing donated human milk. According to a joint statement by WHO and UNICEF, when it is not possible for the biological mother to breastfeed, the first alternative, if available,

15

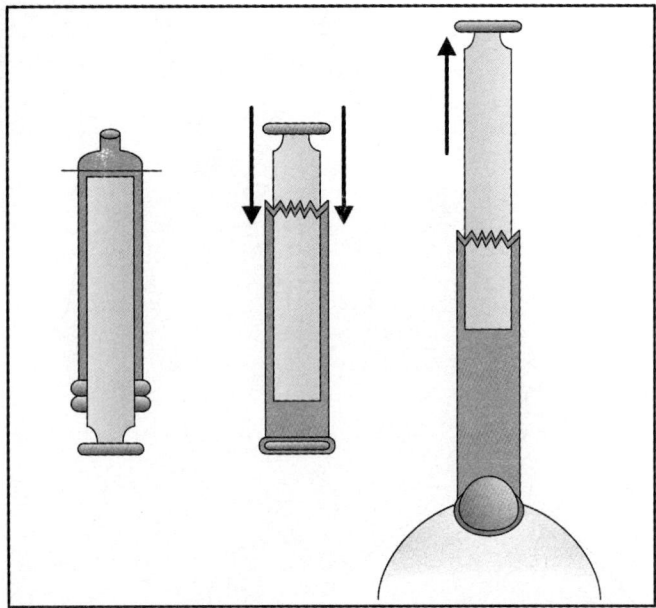

Figure 15.10 Syringe method for treatment of retracted nipples

should be to use human milk from other sources. Banked or pooled human milk is regarded as "the next best option" for feeding the babies if biological mother is unable to breastfeed. It is most suitable for feeding preterm and sick babies in the neonatal intensive care units (NICUs). The main indications for use of pasteurized donor human milk (PDHM) are given in **Box 15.3**. Other indications for use of human milk include malabsorption, short-gut syndrome, intractable diarrhea, formula intolerance, immune deficiencies (IgA), HIV-positive mother and adopted child.

Screening

One of the major issues and concerns regarding milk banking is the transmission of infections via the milk. A detailed medical history of the donor should be taken to exclude infectious diseases which can be transmitted through breast-milk. Her blood should be screened for HIV-1 and 2, HTLV-1 and 2 (potential risk for causing T-cell leukemia), CMV, hepatitis B and C and syphilis.

Box 15.3 **Indications for use of donor human milk**

- Inadequate lactation, flat or inverted nipples and mother with multiple babies.
- Abandoned or orphaned neonates.
- Sick neonates transferred to a NICU without mother.
- Infant at health risk from breast-milk of the biological mother.
- Temporary interruption of breastfeeding.

A consent form is filled by the donor mother and her doctor stating that neither the donor nor her infant will suffer if she donates her milk.

Collection

Strict aseptic precautions should be taken while collecting milk. The milk can be expressed either manually or with the help of a manual or an electric pump. Drip milk, i.e. the milk that drips from the other breast while baby is being breastfed is suitable for collection but it has lower caloric content and is more susceptible to contamination. The milk is usually pooled from 4 to 6 donors and best collected in stainless steel containers because leukocytes and macrophages may stick to the surface of glass container while poly-ethylene bags are associated with decrease in the IgA content of milk. The bacterial count of each donor's milk before pasteurization should be <103 colony-forming units because pasteurization may be ineffective to sterilize the milk if it is heavily contaminated. The pooled milk is pasteurized by heating it to 56°C for 30 minutes because most viruses and bacteria are killed at this temperature without compromising the nutritional and immunological properties of the milk. After pasteurization, the milk is again checked for bacterial growth and it should be sterile.

Storage

Fresh-raw milk or pasteurized milk can be stored at 4°C up to 72 hours after expression. Pasteurized culture-negative donor human milk in tightly sealed containers can be stored at −20°C for 3–6 months. The frozen milk is thawed by keeping the container in a water bath at a temperature not exceeding 37°C or under running lukewarm water. It should never be thawed in microwave as it results in reduction of IgA content of milk. Some centers lyophilize the milk (fresh-frozen milk is dried under vacuum) which can be stored at room temperature up to 18 months but this method is expensive and associated with inaccuracies in its reconstitution and loss of calcium and phosphorus during processing.

Funding

Most milk banks are run as non-profit voluntary organizations or funded by overall hospital budget. Most donors do not receive any payment (except incidental expenses) but recepients may have to pay a nominal charge to cover the cost of screening tests and storage. Apart from tertiary hospitals, milk banks can be established within the blood banks because they are equipped with technology and trained staff which can collect, screen, pasteurize and store the milk in a cost-effective manner.

In conclusion, WHO recommends that when a baby is unable to receive the milk of biological mother, milk of another mother is next best option compared to a formula milk or milk from another animal. Human milk is ideal to serve the nutritional and immunological needs of babies especially when a baby is preterm or sick. It has been shown that the stored and pasteurized human milk is also credited to reduce the risk of necrotizing enterocolitis (NEC). The guidelines published by North American Milk Bank (NAMB) are ideal and should be followed to reduce the risk of transmission of infections through pooled human milk. Apart from infrastructural and logistic issues there is a need to educate and motivate lactating mothers to donate breast-milk (akin to blood donation!) and explain benefits and safety of breast-milk over commercially available formulae to the parents and treating doctors. You can obtain further information on human milk banking in India at info@breast feedingindia.org and www.iycfchapteriap.org.

COMMON MYTHS REGARDING BREASTFEEDING

Myth: It is preferable to give glucose water or *ghutti* as a first feed before putting the baby to breast.

Reality: Never offer any prelacteal feeds (like glucose water, honey, tea, *ghutti*, etc.) and baby should be put straight to the breast within 1 hour of birth or as soon as mother has recovered from the fatigue of delivery. Immediate bonding and early start of breastfeeding are indeed crucial for success of breastfeeding.

Myth: Colostrum is "bad" for the baby and should be discarded.

Reality: The initial milk (first 2–3 days) which is thick and golden-yellow in color is called colostrum. It is easy to digest and is rich in proteins, vitamins, minerals and protective antibodies. *It should never be discarded and is indeed the ideal first meal for the newborn baby*. And it virtually works like a "first vaccine shot" for the baby because of its high content of protective antibodies. Colostrum coats the inner lining of baby's intestines and effectively prevents the harmful bacteria to invade the immature gut of the baby. It facilitates passage of meconim (initial stools of the baby) and promotes effective elimination of bilirubin to keep the jaundice in check.

Myth: When a baby is born by cesarean section, baby needs to be given formula feeds during initial few days.

Reality: In most cases of elective cesarean section, mother can breastfeed her baby as soon as she has recovered from general anesthesia. In case of subdural or spinal anesthesia, she can breastfeed soon after delivery. Nevertheless, when a mother has undergone cesarean section, she needs more support and encouragement to breastfeed. She needs to identify the posture of comfort and should be provided with assistance in holding or supporting the baby. During initial one or two days, she can breastfeed while lying down in bed.

However, in a case of emergeny cesarean section, when a mother is critically sick, the baby may be fed with a cup and spoon or *paladey* till she is well enough to breastfeed. Introduction of bottle feeds should be avoided because it may lead to "nipple confusion" thus causing difficulties in subsequent breastfeeding. It is important to remember, that ability to breastfeed depends upon will power and keenness or commitment to breastfeed rather than the mode of delivery or comfort level.

Myth: Breast and nipple should be washed with soap and water before each feed.

Reality: There is no need to wash the breasts and nipples with soap and water before each feed as it may lead to dryness and cracking of nipples. Daily bath and maintenance of personal hygiene is all that is needed by the nursing mother. Mother should wear nursing pads to prevent ugly patches on her clothes due to leakage of milk.

Myth: Mother should breastfeed her baby every 2 hours by clock.

Reality: Baby should be fed on demand (and not by clock) as and when baby is hungry. There is no need to unnecessarily disturb or wake up a sleeping baby to give him a feed. Whenever baby cries because of hunger (check that he is not crying because of wet diaper or discomfort) offer him a feed whether it is day or night.

Myth: Mother cannot breastfeed her baby efficiently if her breasts are small.

Reality: Just like other body attributes, breasts come in different shapes and sizes. Irrespective of the size of breasts, every woman is endowed with enough glandular tissue to effectively breastfeed her baby. Adequacy of lactation depends more on keenness, and confidence of the mother, freedom from pain or discomfort, sucking stimulation provided by an active and healthy baby rather than the size and shape of breasts or nipples. Nevertheless, there may be genetic or constitutional factors which may determine that mothers in certain families are better milk producers than in others.

15

Myth: Along with breastfeeding, mother should give one or two bottle feeds, otherwise it will be difficult for her to wean the baby off the breast.

Reality: Nothing is more deterimental to the success of breastfeeding than early introduction of bottle feeding because it leads to "nipple confusion" and the baby would be more keen to feed from the bottle rather than breast. Moreover, when a bottle is introduced, there is the potential risk of infection thus compromising the virtues of exclusive breastfeeding. According to current recommendation, breastfeeding should be continued at least up to one year or even longer. Complementary semisolid foods should be started after 6 months including milk products like yoghurt, porridge, custard, cheese, etc. But liquid milk should be started after one year directly with a glass or cup. Mother should avoid the use of a sipper because like feeding bottle, it is also difficult to clean and may serve as a source of infection with a risk of development of diarrhea.

Myth: Breastfed babies are not healthy or "chubby" unlike formula fed babies.

Reality: It is true that formula fed babies gain weight faster and look "chubby" but they are "unhealthy" and at an increased risk to develop obesity, diabetes mellitus and coronary artery disease later in life. The composition of human milk is ideal and best suited for optimal physical and mental growth of human babies. Nature has profound biological wisdom and milk of an animal is best suited to serve the biological needs of its offsprings and is not meant or is suitable to serve the nutritional needs of babies of other species.

Myth: If a mother is unable to breastfeed her first baby, she is unlikely to breastfeed her second baby.

Reality: It is untrue because if a mother has the necessary desire, motivation, will power and positive frame of mind, she can breastfeed successfully. When a mother starts thinking that she can't successfully breastfeed, it is unlikely that she would succeed.

Myth: If a breastfed baby cries frequently it means breast milk is insufficient.

Reality: Apart from hunger, the babies cry due to a variety of other reasons like discomfort because of wet napkins, wind or colic, exposure or over clothing, overstimulated or bored baby, nappy rash, insect bites, etc. When milk drips on the mere sight of the baby, baby passes urine at least 8 times or more in a day and is having satisfactory weight gain, it suggests that mother is having satisfactory lactation. Starting one or two bottle feeds on the mistaken belief that there is insufficient lactation, is the commonest cause of lactation failure and its unfortunate consequences.

Myth: Breastfeeding is more demanding and troublesome to the mother as opposed to bottle feeding.

Reality: Infact, the truth is otherwise. Bottle feeding demands more effort on the part of the mother for sterilizing the bottles, preparing the formula, ensuring right temperature of the milk before feeding, and maintaining strict asepsis; especially if all this needs to be done by mother herself without the help of husband or other family members. Breastfeeding is certainly more convenient and less bothersome especially during night.

Myth: Breastfeeding will make the breasts saggy and unattractive.

Reality: The fact is that it is not the act of breastfeeding but pregnancy per se that affects the shape, size or firmness of the breasts. During pregnancy, the breasts prepare for lactation and even if a mother decides to bottle feed, the breasts are likely to sag unless a strong support is provided with a bra. Regular exercise of chest muscles (pectoralis) maintains the shape and contour of breasts. Excessive weight gain during pregnancy, hereditary factors and increasing age are other factors which may make the breasts less globular, loose and soft. Breastfeeding should not be blamed for something which is going to happen sooner or later.

Myth: Mother should avoid breastfeeding her second baby, when breastfeeding caused jaundice in her first baby.

Reality: It is true that in some mothers breastfeeding may cause what is known as "breast milk jaundice". Jaundice may occur again in subsequent babies. However, there is nothing wrong with the mother's milk and she can safely breastfeed her subsequent babies. There is no need to interrupt breastfeedings for 2–3 days which some doctors recommend as a treatment of "breast milk jaundice". Jaundice may last 6–8 weeks and it disappears without any adverse effects to the baby. Infact it would appear that some jaundice is beneficial for the baby because bilirubin is an antioxidant and it is useful to prevent damage to various tissues due to reactive oxygen free radicals.

Myth: When a mother is having an infection or fever, she should not breastfeed.

Reality: Unless mother is critically sick, fever due to common day-to-day infections should not be considered as an indication to stop breastfeeding. There is no risk of passage of infective microbes through breast milk and instead protective antibodies produced in respone to infection will get transferred to the baby through breast milk. Mother should continue to breastfeed her baby but take strict precautions like frequent handwashing, wearing a mask (if having cough and cold), not sharing towel or handkerchief with the baby is likely to reduce the risk of transmission of infection to the baby.

Myth: Breastfeeding should be stopped when baby has cut his teeth.

Reality: Most babies cut their first tooth around 6–7 months but breastfeeding is continued till at least one year or even longer till all the milk teeth have erupted. Most babies are smart and do not bite the nipple and they know how sacred is the breast because it is their life line. An occasional angry fellow may create mischief by biting the nipple either to relieve irritation of the gums or due to frustration of not getting enough milk. Mother should not laugh or approve this prank but should firmly say "no biting" and calmly delatch the prankster from the breast and divert his attention by talking or distracting him.

Myth: Nursing mother should avoid exercise, because it may sour the milk due to elevation of lactic acid.

Reality: There is no evidence to suggest that exercise leads to souring of the milk unless exercise is indulged to the point of exhaustion. Aerobic exercises and yoga in moderation are the best. Mother should be advised to wear a firm sports bra and do the exercise immediately after having given the feed to the baby. Mother should drink extra glass of water before and after the exercise especially during summer to maintain good hydration status.

BOTTLE FEEDING

Most babies can be fed with exclusive breastfeeding up to 6 months of age. Subsequently when semisolid foods are started, breastfeeding should be continued and there is no need to start bottle or formula feeds. At a later date, generally after first birthday, when breast milk supply wanes off, milk feeds can be started directly from a cup or a glass.

Despite sincere efforts and due to certain medical or social conditions in the mother, complementary or sometimes total feeding with non-human or animal milk may be required in the following situations:

- Adopted baby
- Inadequate lactation
- Twin or triplet babies
- Mother receiving anti-cancer drugs
- Seriously or critically sick mother
- Working mother
- HIV-positive mother
- Social constraints

When for a genuine personal or medical reasons, bottle feeding needs to be given, the mother should not feel guilty or unnecessarily upset. Babies can be fed satisfactorily with formula feeds when due precautions are taken to ensure proper cleanliness and sterility of feeding utensils and bottles.

The Choice of Milk

Any liquid milk which is procured by the family for household use can be given to the baby without dilution. Children should be given full cream milk except when overweight. Dried milk powders are often preferred because of less chances of contamination and adulteration and ease of storage but they are expensive. Most infant formulas are fortified with iron and vitamins. In order to make their composition as close to human milk as possible, most baby formulas are fortified with docosahexaenoic acid (DHA) and arachidonic acid (AD) in the west. Milk powders should be reconstituted as per the instructions printed on the container. In general, one level (not heaped) measure is dissolved in one ounce (30 mL) of pre-boiled or potable warm water to obtain full-strength milk. Reconstitution of milk powder into a larger volume of water is the commonest cause of poor weight gain by the baby. The hands should be washed thoroughly with soap and water before preparing a feed. The powdered milk and water can be taken directly in the feeding bottle instead of using another container for reconstitution. It is more convenient and there is lesser risk of bacterial contamination.

Fresh liquid milk is suitable for feeding babies but it is difficult to store during summer months without an ice box or refrigerator. The milk should be warmed every time before use. During first 2 months, pure cow's or buffaloes milk may be diluted in a ratio of 3 parts of milk and one part of water to reduce protein load to the kidneys. When milk is delivered home by the milkman, the dilution should be left to him! Animal milks have greater quantity of proteins which are of different kind (casein which is difficult to digest compared to easily digestible lactalbumin or whey protein of breast milk) and are less sweet due to lower content of lactose. Sugar is added to sweeten the milk according to the baby's liking. The milk should be strained before pouring into the feeding bottle otherwise the cream may block the hole in the teat. After 2 months of age most babies can be fed with a full strength liquid milk.

Quantity of Milk

Breastfed babies regulate their feed intake depending upon their needs and mother does no need to worry about any guidelines or calculations. During bottle

15

feeding, offer 30–45 mL of milk during first week of life. Whenever baby completely empties the bottle, additional 15 mL of milk should be offered during the next feed. The volume of feeds should be gradually increased by one ounce (30 mL) after every month or so. The best guide that the baby has taken a full feed is that some milk remains in the bottle. The left over milk must be immediately discarded (or consumed by an adult) and feeding bottle should be rinsed with water to prevent bacterial growth. The maximum that baby drinks at one feed is a full bottle of 8 ounces (approximately 240 mL). After one year, baby should be given maximum of three bottles of milk feeds and rest of his nutritional requirements should be met by giving cereal-based semisolid foods, vegetables and fruits.

Technique of Bottle Feeding

A straight wide-mouthed feeding bottle should be used because of ease of cleaning. The hole in the rubber teat should be created with a red hot sewing needle. It will burn the rubber to make a hole. When a feeding bottle with milk is inverted, there should be a fine spray of milk for 1–2 seconds and then milk should flow in regular drops and not as a stream. When milk flows as a constant stream, the hole in the teat is too big and if drops fall too slowly, it is too small. In both situations the baby is likely to swallow too much air while feeding and develop colic or regurgitation of feeds. Mother can check the temperature of milk by pouring a few drops on the back of her hand to make sure it is not too hot. Use pre-boiled warm water (which can be stored in a flask) for reconstitution of milk. Feeds should be offered on self demand as in case of breastfeeding. A common sense approach should be followed instead of any strict ritual or routine. The baby should be fed when he is hungry and allowed to sleep as long he wants. After some time, baby would establish his own routine and mother can adjust her routine accordingly.

The child should preferably be taken in the lap and offered the bottle. Mother must pay full attention and interact with her baby while bottle feeding. She should provide close skin-to-skin contact and eye contact to the baby while bottle feeding. The bottle should be tilted enough so that nipple is completely filled with milk to avoid swallowing of air by the baby. The nipple may have to be removed from the baby's mouth when it gets collapsed to relieve negative pressure or vacuum in the bottle. After the feed, baby should be made to sit or put on the shoulder to eructate the swallowed air. After burping, the baby may be placed on his back or right lateral position with head end slightly raised. *It is dangerous to support the feeding bottle with a cushion or pillow and leave the baby and bottle alone for self feeding.*

There is a potential risk of choking and aspiration or the baby may suck lot of air when bottle rolls down. During bottle feeding, baby's head should be kept slightly raised, otherwise milk may enter the eustachian tube (channel between the back of nose and ear) and lead to middle ear infection. After the age of 9 months, most babies can hold the bottle and self feed without any risk of choking. After first birthday, attempts should be made to feed the baby with a cup or a glass. Use of distinctive and decorative cup or a baby glass with motifs may motivate babies to accept this method of self feeding. Most babies accept water from a cup or a glass as early as 6–9 months but refuse to take milk from a cup because they identify milk with a feeding bottle. Sipper should not be used either for drinking water or milk because of serious risk of contamination and occurrence of diarrhea.

Feeding during Sleep

It is not a good practice to offer a bottle feed during sleep. It may result in development of a bad habit and may lead to dental decay and development of caries as milk remains in contact with teeth while the baby is asleep. Feeding during sleep is also associated with the risk of development of ear infection as the milk may trickle into the eustachian tube and cause infection of the middle ear (acute otitis media). Occasional bottle feeding during sleep may be given if baby had been fussy, irritable and unwell due to teething or minor illness but it should not lead to development of a bad habit with risk of adverse consequences.

Care of Feeding Bottles and Teats

Bottle feeding is a potential source of infection (especially diarrhea) unless care is taken to maintain sterility. Mother must have at least 4 feeding bottles and enough teats. The left over milk must be discarded (or consumed by an adult) and bottle should be cleaned with a detergent or soap and water by using a brush. The left over milk is the potential breeding ground for bacteria and should never be reused. Teat should be cleaned with a small brush and common salt to remove milk curds or cream from the teat's hole. Keep a separate sauce pan or basin for boiling bottles. Bottles and teats must completely dip in water and should be boiled for a minimum of 5 minutes. After boiling and cooling, water should be drained and pan with bottles and teats should be kept covered for next use. Electrical bottle sterilizers are available and are convenient to use. The bottles and teats can be sterilized by immersing them in a solution of sodium hypochlorite (Milton). One table spoon (15 mL) of Milton is added to a liter of water and bottles are soaked for 3–4 hours. The bottles and teat should be drained and rinsed with boiled water before use. The liquid milk must be boiled before each use. The water used for reconstitution of powdered milk should be either safe bottled water, RO water or boiled for at least 5 minutes to ensure that it is sterile and safe. After taking the feed in the bottle, teat must be kept covered with a plastic lid to prevent contamination by flies unless baby is given the feed immediately. The responsibility of washing, cleaning and sterilization of feeding bottles and teats should not be given to a maid or *ayah* and mother should personally look after this most important aspect of bottle feeding.

Feeding with a Cup and Spoon or *Paladay*

Due to potential risk of infection and "nipple confusion" with bottle feeding, it is recommended to give complementary feeds to babies with a spoon or *paladay* (small cup with a rounded snout which is normally used as a *diya*). Most babies (even small babies) accept feeding with a spoon or *paladay* without any difficulty **(Figure 15.11)**. The baby should be held in the lap, head slightly raised and edge of the spoon or paladay is touched to the lips of the baby. As soon as the milk touches the lips and tongue, the baby makes swallowing efforts to drink the milk. When baby is satisfied, he will turn his head away or stop swallowing the milk which collects in the throat. The procedure is safe but time consuming. Mother needs to use lot of patience to feed the baby with a spoon or *paladay* but

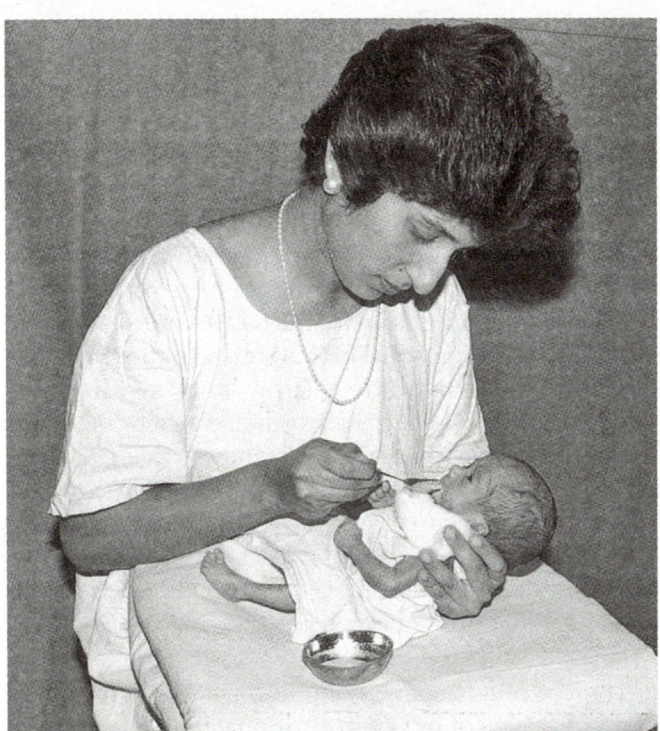

Figure 15.11 Feeding a preterm baby with a cup and spoon to avoid nipple confusion

efforts are well rewarded because risk of bacterial contamination is extremely low by this method and it is easier for the baby to accept breastfeeding concurrently or subsequently because there is no "nipple confusion". The feeding cup and spoon/*paladay* should be washed with soap and water immediately after each use and kept effectively covered.

Hazards and Benefits of Bottle Feeding

Bottle feeding is unnatural and animal milks or milk formulas are not suitable to serve the biological needs of the human babies. Bottle fed babies are more vulnerable to develop gastrointestinal infections, respiratory infections, allergic disorders, and ear infections. Due to frequent infections and over dilution of formula, the child may have poor weight gain and undernutrition. In well to do families, aggressive bottle feeding is associated with increased risk of obesity, diabetes mellitus, high blood pressure and coronary artery disease later in life.

In well off families, especially when help of a maid is available to look after and feed the baby, bottle feeding does provide greater respite, freedom and option to the mother for joining her job, better social life, lack of need for any dietary restrictions or nutritional demands and greater freedom for resumption of normal sexual activity.

THE COMPLEMENTARY OR WEANING FOODS

Health of a child depends upon genetic endowment (constitution), freedom from illness and adequacy of nutrition. Nutritional requirements of children are much higher (compared to adults) because they have to grow from an average weight of 3 kg at birth to over 50 kg at adolescence and they spend a lot of energy in their day-to-day activities. For example, daily caloric requirement during infancy is around 120 kcal/kg compared to 40 kcal/kg in adults! The requirements of proteins and micronutrients per unit body weight are also much higher in children compared to adults.

Milk is a complete food and exclusive breastfeeding is able to maintain normal growth of children during first 6 months of life. After this, infant must be gradually weaned off (changed over) to take semi-liquid or semi-solid food otherwise his weight gain will slow down and he will develop nutritional deficiencies. Prolonged milk feeding without timely introduction of weaning foods is the commonest cause of iron deficiency anemia in young children because milk is relatively deficient in iron. Weaning is the most crucial phase of child nutrition and demands considerable time, effort and ingenuity on the part of mother for its success. Efforts

15

should be made to give home-made nutritious weaning foods with utmost care by maintenance of personal hygiene to prevent risk of bacterial contamination. Hands should be washed with soap and water before preparing or serving food to her child. During weaning, child is also given water which must be safe and free from contamination. Depending upon the source of water supply, the family may have to filter the water or use RO system or boil it before use. Water can be given with a special cup that has a lid with a flat spout. The lid keeps the water from spilling and spout goes into baby's mouth. The baby can later use the cup without lid and spout. It is preferable to use a cup or a glass rather than a sipper which is difficult to clean and is an important source of infection. Unless strict hygienic precautions are taken, weaning phase may be associated with occurrence of frequent infections especially episodes of diarrhea and dysentery.

After 6 Months

After 6 months the child is offered gradually increasing amounts of semisolid or finely mashed or pureed weaning foods but breastfeeding should be continued. Offer one food item at a time and watch for acceptance and tolerance or any allergic reaction for a week or so before introducing another food. It is useful to acquire a hand blender or mixer at this stage to throughly mash and blend the semi-solid food. There is no need to offer additional animal milk to the baby but he can be given milk products like custard, curd, *kheer* and cheese, etc. Breastfeeding should be continued as long as feasible but at least for a minimum period of one year. One to two breastfeeds can be continued even up to 2 years. Start with a precooked cereal, often 2–3 teaspoonfuls in a clean bowl with a baby spoon **(Figure 15.12)**. Prepare it properly with water in a semiliquid, non sticky and smooth consistency by constantly stirring with a spoon to prevent formation of lumps. Pre-cooked cereals (wheat or rice-based) are convenient to use but are expensive. A variety of flavors are available and mother should find out what flavor/s her baby likes. Most of them are fortified with iron which often lacks in baby's diet at this age. It is preferable to give home-based weaning foods to the baby. It is recommended to use less salt and sugar so that the child develops the healthy habit of taking less salt and sugar when he grows to become an adult. Mother can prepare thin porridge or *kheer* made from cereals like *suji*, ground rice or wheat flour and milk. Offer the semi-liquid food when baby is wide awake, hungry and in good mood. The breastfeeding can be given afterwards if baby wants and accepts it. Give small amounts and gradually increase the quantity.

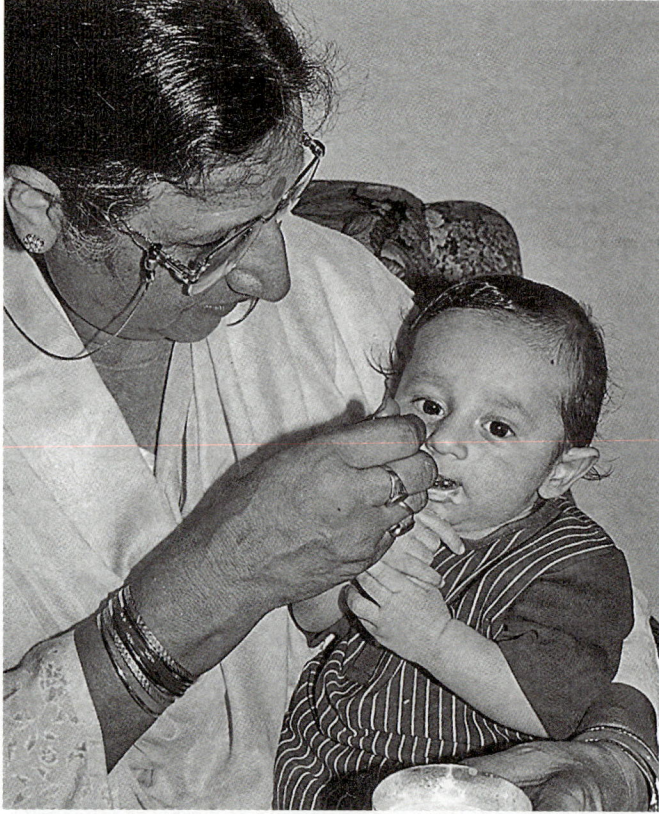

Figure 15.12 The baby is being fed with a pre-cooked cereal as a complementary food after 6 months of age

It is amazing how discriminatory and choosy many young babies are. They will first taste the new food before deciding whether to accept and swallow it or reject it. Like adults, children have likes and dislikes for various foods, some prefer sweet foods and others like saltish; some take it bland while other relish strong flavors. Initially, many babies produce usual sucking movements of the tongue (which they are used to for swallowing milk) giving the impression as if the baby is rejecting the food. Mother should have patience and perseverance, and gradually the baby would learn and start enjoying semi-solid food. Around 6 months most babies can coordinate biting and swallowing movements. Intestinal enzymes also reach adequate levels for proper digestion of starch at this stage. At this age babies love to eat a mashed banana. Mash banana with a spoon or fork in a bowl and offer it with a small spoon. Gradually increase the quantity of banana, till at the end of 2–3 weeks he is able to eat a whole banana. If the baby likes, banana can be mixed with some milk and yoghurt.

There is no virtue in giving thin watery soups or *dal ka pani* because of its poor nutritional value. It is better to make thin gravy of *dal* by mashing the *dal* in the soup. Mother can start with two semi-liquid meals (morning

15

and evening) and gradually increase the quantity and frequency. Many mothers are keen to give fruit juice to their baby. Fruit juices are time consuming to prepare, are associated with potential risk of bacterial contamination and are not cost-effective. They do not have outstanding nutritional virtues but provide sugars, vitamins, minerals and antioxidants. It is much better to offer mashed or stewed or pureed whole fruit to the child rather than fruit jucies. Tinned fruit juices and fresh fruit juice procured from the market or road-side vendors should be strictly avoided.

Multivitamin and Iron Drops

Nature has supreme biologic wisdom and human milk contains sufficient amounts of vitamins and minerals. Although human milk is relatively deficient in iron but its bio-availability is so high that exclusively breastfed babies do not develop any iron deficiency. Most powdered milks are also fortified with vitamins and iron. During first 6 months when baby is being exclusively breastfed there is no need to give any supplements of vitamins and iron to healthy full term babies except vitamin D. When baby is being fed with cow's or buffaloe's milk, vitamin C gets destroyed by boiling. After 6 months, when complementary feeds are started, the child should be given vitamin and iron supplements. Multivitamins are also needed during any prolonged illness, broad spectrum antibiotic therapy, malnutrition, food fussiness and convalescence etc. When a baby is given mutivitamin drops, it will stain the urine (and napkin) dark yellow which should not be a cause for worry. Iron supplements should be given after 6 months when complementary feeds are started. The baby needs 2–3 mg of elemental iron per kg body weight in a day and the number of drops should be calculated accordingly. Some children may not tolerate iron supplements and may develop either constipation or loose motions.

7–8 Months

A variety of foods can be started at this stage for example, rice and *dal* gruel (*khichadi*), mashed rice and *dal*, mashed vegetables, *dalia*, rice-milk, *kheer*, yoghurt, custard and boiled egg. Start one food item at a time and gradually increase the quantity and variety. Most children get bored with the same food and need a change. Offer those foods that the child likes and enjoys and don't impose your own likes or foods that you feel are good or nutritious for the child. Initially food items may have to be finely mashed and later on child would accept semi-solids or grated foods. It is a wrong belief that child must have teeth before he can accept or digest semi-solid food.

In certain conmmunities weaning is delayed until "*Anna Prasana*" ceremony is held. Green vegetables like peas, *lauki*, bottle gaurd and carrots can be cooked and mashed in *khichadi*. Vegetables can be cooked and stewed or steamed and then mashed in water in which they have been cooked. Add a pinch of salt and butter or clarified butter (*desi ghee*) to improve the flavor and taste. A variety of green vegetables can be given like peas, *tinda*, gourd, *lauki* and spinach etc. Most children love boiled and mashed potatoes. Give *dals* (*pulses or lentils*) without covering or *chhilka* to improve their digestibility. *Moong* and pigeon peas (*Ar-ar or toor ki dal*) are tolerated best. *Dal* water is useless and *dal* must be mashed in the soup with a spoon or with a hand mixie and topped with butter or *desi ghee* before offering to the child. Butter and *ghee* are liked and tolerated well by most children and are useful to increase the caloric density to provide for increased energy demands of the child. A child who has a familial tendency to be over weight or is gaining weight excessively, should not be given extra butter, oil or *ghee*. Home-made yoghurt is an excellent substitute for milk and can be given without any additive or after adding salt or sugar depending upon the liking of the child. Yoghurt is well tolerated by children who do not tolerate milk due to deficiency of an enzyme lactase in their intestines. Children who develop abdominal pain on taking milk, will tolerate yoghurt without any discomfort or bloating. Egg can be started at this stage if family is non-vegetarian. There are no nutritional virtues of giving raw egg (flipped in milk) and there is a potential risk of development of slamonella infection. Start by giving egg yolk of a full-boiled egg. Egg yolk is rich in vitamins and iron while egg white is full of high quality proteins. Egg proteins are of highest biological value and are easily digested. In some families, allergy to egg proteins may be prevalent and should be watched for. After taking an egg, if baby develops vomiting, skin rash, abdominal pain or turns pale, stop giving egg to the child. Depending upon the cultural or regional food habits, children should be offered foods of their region and liking. *Dosa, idli, sambar, upma, dhokla, suji* or *besan ka halwa*, etc. can be given as weaning foods. In north India *choori* is prepared by mashing and kneading a fried *chapati* (*parantha*) with *desi ghee* or butter and powdered *jaggery* or *shhakkar*. Before feeding the child, it is important that mother should taste the prepared food to assess its tempe-rature, flavor, salt or sweetness and freshness, etc. The cooked foods must be used within a few hours and kept covered to protect against flies, cockroaches and insects.

15

9 to 11 Months

At this stage child can accept a variety of foods and fruits 3–4 times in a day. He is able to use lips to clear a spoon, can chew and effectively move his tongue to swallow the food. The intake of breastfeeds would decrease but he should be offered milk products like yoghurt and cottage cheese (home made or white cheese). He will enjoy small bits of *chapati* or bread soaked in milk or *dal* or vegetables gravy. Most children enjoy eating fried *chapati* specially stuffed *aloo ka parantha* (*chapati* stuffed with potatoes or other vegetables). Hand-eye coordination has improved by this age and due to irritation of gums the child enjoys to have finger foods like butter toast, bread stick, cake rusk, french toast, cake piece, biscuits, apple slice, etc. Mother should stay close to her toddler when he is eating finger foods or chunky foods as a safeguard against choking.

Most children would prefer to take what other family members are eating and would accept ordinary household food items cooked with mild chillies and flavors. There is no need to mash the food at this stage as child has learnt to masticate and is usually endowed with 4–6 teeth. However, some children may accept only thoroughly mashed or semi-liquid type of foods for a prolonged period. Apart from banana the child should now be offered *cheekoo*, apple, papaya and orange. He should be given fresh de-skinned fruit without any stewing or cooking. Give seasonal fruits to the child and parents should not waste resources for purchase of non-seasonal grapes and pomegranate (*Anar bedaana*) which are popular with most mothers. Gauva (*Amrood*), a relatively affordable fruit, is rich in vitamins (especially vitamin C) and fiber. It is much better to give fresh whole fruit instead of fruit juices.

The child should not be forced fed, instead he should be encouraged to feed himself. Let the child enjoy his food and get a feeling that mother is her friend and not an "aggressive animal trainer". The child is likely create some mess and spill the food but he will soon learn to self-feed without undue fuss later in life. Mother should be totally relaxed and show utmost patience while feeding the toddler. Do not hurry the child. The child may eat a bit, play in-between and then eat again. Feed the child when he is hungry and not tired or sleepy. As far as possible, avoid using distractions or various silly pranks to make him eat. Meal times should be a pleasant experience for the child and not a tug of war between him and the rest of the family.

12 Months and above

By first birthday the child should be eating from the family pot 4–5 times in a day. He should take only 2–3 breast or milk feeds and mostly eat everyday house hold food and seasonal fruits. The child should be encouraged to self-feed. He should have his own high chair where he can sit with other family members at the height of dining table. The child should be worn a plastic bib to prevent soiling of clothes. If family is non-vegetarian they can now introduce whole egg (both white and yellow), fish and minced (*keema*) mutton or chicken. Some infants like to hold a chicken leg and enjoy licking and savoring it. He can be offered all foods and vegetables. Additional seasonal fruits like plum (*aloobukhara*), pear (*baghugosha*), mango and *litches* can be given. But, certain *dals* like kidney beans (*rajmah*), black urad, Bengal gram, chicken peas (*kabli channa*), and vegetables containing hard seeds like okra (*bhindi*) and bitter ground (*karela*) should be avoided because infants are unable to digest them.

At one year of age, although the baby weighs around 10 kg on an average, but his caloric and nutritional needs are just about one-half of an adult. This understanding gives a broad idea to the mother as how much the baby needs to eat at this stage. By 1½ year the child can eat family food and is able to use his fingers and spoon to feed himself. There is no need at this stage to cook separately for the child as the family meals can be modified in consistency and spicing to serve the taste and needs of the child.

Avoid offering soft drinks, tinned juices, chocolates and ice cream at this stage and delay their introduction to a stage where it becomes unavoidable to deny them. Avoid offering nuts, popcorn, round candies, grapes or roasted Bengal gram to a toddler due to serious risk of accidental choking and aspiration into the lungs. Almonds and other nuts can be given after soaking and mashing them or mixing them in foods like custard, *kheer* and porridge. Children should not be tickled or made to laugh while eating because of potential risk of choking. The practice of washing hands before and after feedings should be strictly followed at an early age so that it becomes a useful habit later in life. The guidelines for giving complementary or weaning foods to infants are summarized in **Table 15.1**.

Criteria for Adequate Feeding

Children have a wide range of growth and no two children look and behave alike. Depending upon their genetic or constitutional potential, some children are chubby while others are lean and less padded. Children who are over active, restless and always "on the go", are not likely to become plump. Some children gain height rapidly and appear lanky. Healthy child is active, happy, contented, palyful and "naughty". He should have satisfactory weight gain as depicted on "Road-to-

Table 15.1 Guidelines for giving complementary foods to infants

6–8 months	9–12 months	After 12 months

■ Soft, semi-liquid homogenized, gruels and soups (1–2 times/day)
  □ Pre-cooked rice-based cereals
  □ Rice and moong dal gruel (khichadi)
  □ Custard, kheer, yoghurt
  □ Mashed banana
  □ Egg yolk of a boiled egg
  □ Vegetables like potatoes, peas, gourd, carrots in the soup and topped with butter or desi ghee
  □ Moong dal and pigeon-peas (toor or ar-ar ki dal) mashed in soup and topped with butter or desi ghee
	■ A variety of semisolid and soft food items (2–3 times/day)
	  □ Wheat porridge or dalia
	  □ Chapati or bread soaked in dal or vegetable soup
	  □ Stuffed paranthas or plain parantha mashed with jaggery powder (chhakar) and desi ghee (choorie)
	  □ Rice and dal. Dosa, idli, sambar, upma, sooji ki kheer or besan ka halwa
	  □ Cottage cheese and whole egg
	  □ Finger foods like butter toast, cake rusk, biscuits etc.
	  □ Green leafy vegetables, beans, okra, lauki, pumpkin, tomatoes
	  □ Soft fruits like banana, cheekoo, papaya, melon, apple, etc.
	  □ Chicken soup, mashed and minced fish and chicken
		■ Family food without spices (4–5 times a day)

Important Messages*
1. Complementary foods should be offered when child is hungry by replacing a milk feed.
2. Offer one food item at a time and watch for its acceptance and tolerance before introducing another food item.
3. Encourage the child to self-feed and never force-feed him. Be patient and sensitive to the likes and dislikes of your child.
4. Mother must be innovative and offer a variety of food items to avoid monotony and boredom.
5. Add less sugar and salt so that it becomes a habit for him later in life.

Health" weight card. The growth curve should run parallel to the percentile curves shown on the card without any flattening or downward trend. Healthy children maintain their growth velocity close to the 50th percentile curve. The child should not suffer from frequent respiratory or gastrointestinal infections which may occur due to deficiency of certain micronutrients like vitamin A, vitamin C, iron and zinc. The child should look pink (not necessarily plump) without any evidences of nutritional anemia and any clinical deficiencies of other micronutrients.

THE FUSSY OR FINICKY EATER

There are feeding and nutritional problems in children both among the economically-deprived and illiterate families as well as the affluent and educated lot. Children belonging to poor families are keen to eat but are starving and are undernourished due to lack of food and poverty or ignorance of the parents. These children fight with each other to get a share of their family food. When you offer them a dry piece of bread or *chapati* they will grab and eat it without any fuss (**Figure 15.13**). And, on the other hand, there are fussy "black mailers"

> *"Pediatricians eat because children don't"*
> — **John Apley**

of well-to-do families who have abundant food but children refuse to eat in accordance with the wishes or to the satisfaction of their parents. The mother brings her child to the physician with the story that "my child eats nothing" or "my child eats like a bird" and says in desperation that "I have tried virtually everything to make him eat but it has been of no use." The meal times are virtual mini-wars. The battle lines are drawn. On side is the valiant, adamant and determined lone fighter and on the other side of the fence is the whole family with mother and grand parents trying to indulge in all sorts of pranks and gimmicks to make him eat. The child is coaxed, cajoled, forced and bribed to eat. He is distracted by telling a story, showing a picture book, his favourite ad on TV or a cartoon movie (**Figure 15.14A and B**). The child is running around while mother is chasing him with his food plate in her hand. The whole family revolves around the child with a fond hope that he will eat something. The meal times becomes unpleasant, emotionally surcharged and

15

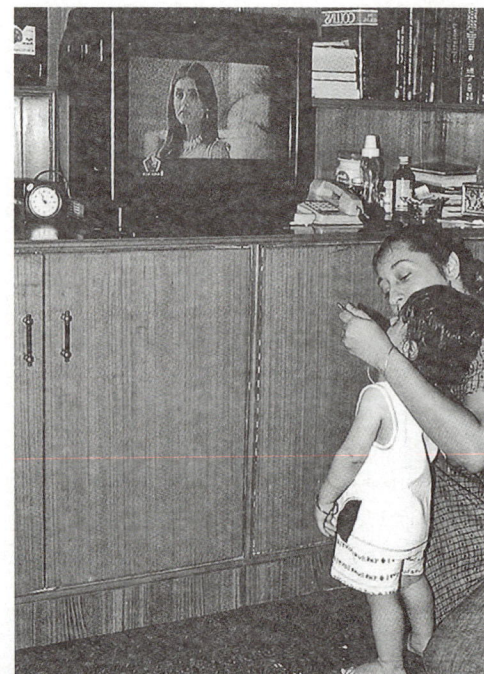

stressful both for the child and family. The morale of the child is high while the whole family is gloomy and despondent. The child is the usual winner in the end. The worst scenario is father physically restraining the child and mother literally forcing and pushing the food into the child's mouth. He may spit or vomit after the feeding brawl.

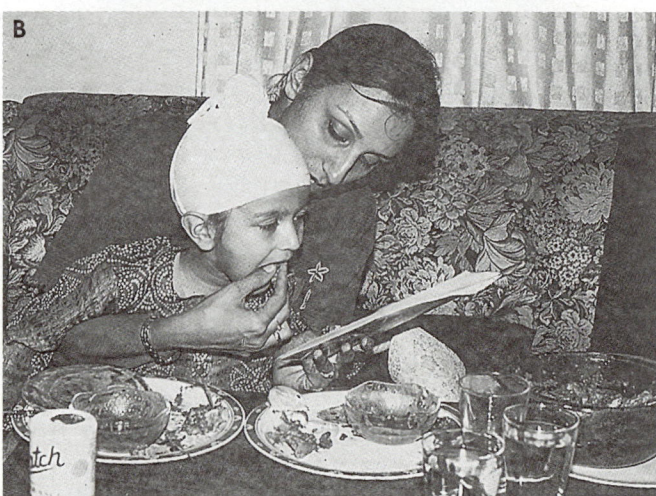

Figure 15.14 The child is being forced fed by distracting him. (A) Infront of television, (B) Showing a picture book

The child is neither having loss of appetite nor is he on "hunger strike". The more he is forced, the less he eats. He is merely rebellious and wants his own way to exercise his individuality. He has a good appetite for the foods of his liking but they are often denied by the family. The child eats well at the neighbour's house or at a birthday party (**Figure 15.15**). The child is not chubby but otherwise active, playful and wiry. The parents are worried because child is not gaining weight as he did during the first year of life. It must be remembered that weight gain velocity slows as the child grows. During 3–12 yeas of age, children gain merely 2 kg body weight during one year as compared to weight gain of 750–1000 g per month during first 4–6 months of life.

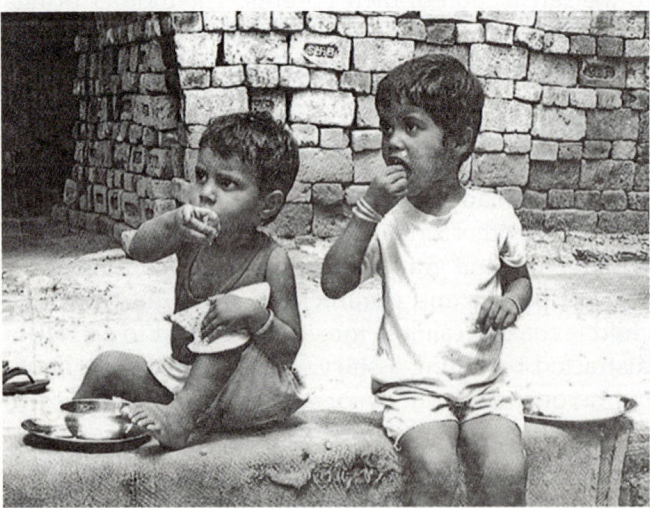

Figure 15.13 Children from a slum dwelling are enjoying their meagre meal without any fuss

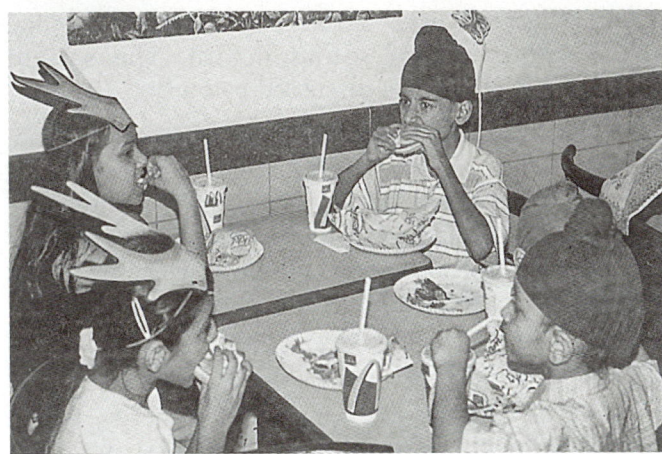

Figure 15.15 Children eating with pleasure and enthusiasm at a birthday party

Tackling the Picky Eater

The development of food fussiness should be prevented by avoiding over indulgence and not paying excessive concern and attention to the child's food. One should honor the individual likes and dislikes of the child and offer a variety of food items to break the monotony. Mother should try to prepare the food that looks good and tempting (cut into interesting shapes and funny faces) and it should be soft and delicious. The child should be given a choice between 2 and 3 food items but not an open-ended or unlimited choice. The best way to make the child eat is "not to try". Adopt a relaxed attitude at meal times and let the child enjoy what he likes to eat. There should be "intelligent neglect" of the child. Mother should pay more attention and show pleasure when child eats well and ignore him when he refuses to eat or fiddles with food. She should encourage the child to self-feed even if he creates mess (**Figure 15.16**). Most children would like to eat when other family members are eating. After giving a reasonable time, the plate should be quietly removed even if the child has not finished without showing any concern and anxiety. Children do have a rebellious attitude and many a times a negative statement that "Karan would not get his food today" may evoke a positive response. The whole family including grandparents must participate in the mission approach to change the "black mailing" tactics of the child. The family must appreciate that food fussiness is a behaviour disorder and child does not have loss of appetite or "sluggish liver". There is no role of tonics and appetizers to make him eat. One must understand the aforementioned family dynamics of food fussiness and emphasis should be placed on changing the attitude and approach in feeding the child. Tonics may be given to provide supplements of vitamins and minerals but

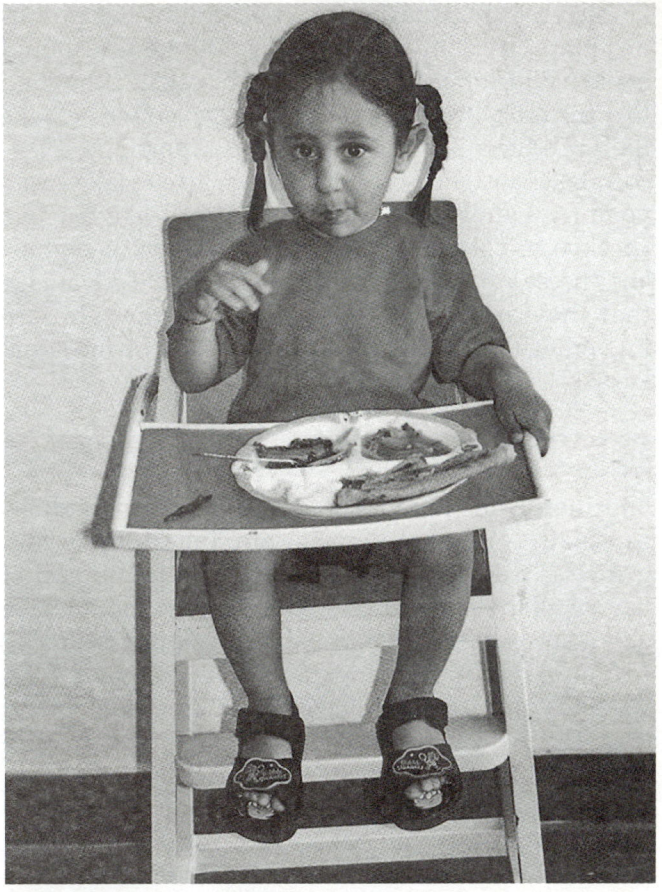

Figure 15.16 The child should be encouraged to self-feed even if he creates mess. The high dining chair-cum-table of the child can be pulled along the dining table where other family members are eating

reliance should be placed on behaviour management by adopting a relaxed and common sense approach without any sense of frustration.

Intake of Milk and Milk Products

Most children hate two things in their diet, eating green leafy vegetables and drinking milk. Milk is a balanced complete food having high quality proteins of animal origin. Infants grow wonderfully well on milk alone during first 6 months. Many school going children hate to drink milk because (i) it is insipid, unattractive and sissy, (ii) it may cause tummy ache and flatulence in some children, (iii) there are catchy, bold and aggressive advertisements in TV by soft drinks lobby and, (iv) because of over concern of parents that their child must drink milk. When parents are more concerned about a food item, children are least interested and they virtually blackmail their parents. There are several options to make children milk-friendly. Milk can be offered by adding a flavor or chocolate, and other brownies like Bournvita, Maltova, Boost or Junior

15

Horlicks, etc. Milk can be dispensed in attractive cartons or tetrapacks with catchy motifs. The family should avoid having unnecessary "fights" by cajoling the child to drink milk. Instead, he should be encouraged to take milk products like yoghurt, custard, porridge, *kheer*, cornflakes and cheese. Most children love to take sweet yoghurt with small pieces of soft fruits like banana, cheekoo and grapes. The nutritional virtues of yoghurt and cheese are similar to milk with the added advantage that they are well tolerated by children who are intolerant to milk because of deficiency of intestinal lactase.

THE BALANCED DIET

Nutrition is the foundation of health. All individuals especially pregnant women, nursing mothers and growing children need a balanced nutritious diet having all the essential nutrients. The diet should have adequate proportion and balance of body-building proteins, energy-giving carbohydrates and fats, vitamins and minerals like calcium, iron, iodine and zinc. The diet gets balanced if you take a good mixture of cereals like wheat or rice, lentils (*dals*), legumes, fresh green vegetables, fruits, milk and milk products. The non-vegetarians can take eggs, mutton, poultry products and seafood. Lean meat (poultry products and fish) are preferred over mutton because latter contains more saturated fat and is not very heart-friendly. Soft drinks and fizzy colas merely provide empty calories and their excessive intake should be condemned.

Table 15.2 gives a list of 42 nutrients which are essential for maintenance of sound health. The salient components of diet are discussed below:

Water Water is second only to oxygen as an essential requirement to sustain life and it constitutes 60 percent of total body weight in adults (70 – 75% in infants). Life is not possible without oxygen beyond few minutes, without water beyond few days and without food beyond a few weeks. Water is required for many biological processes and for excretion of waste products to keep the life going.

Calories Calories are a measure of energy, which is required for growth and physical activity. Carbohydrates and fats are the main sources of energy or heat to the body. Of the total caloric requirements, approximately 50% should be supplied by carbohydrates, 35% by fats and 15% by proteins. The energy value of food is measured in calories or more correctly in kilocalories (kcal). Infants need 120 calories per kg body weight per day which is at least four times compared to an adult (40 calories kg/day). At one year, healthy infant needs 1000 calories per day and additional 100 calories are required for every year of age. For example, a five-year-old child would need 1400 calories per day. *By his first birth day, an infant needs to eat about half of the food that his mother eats.* This gives a rough estimate to the mother as to how much food needs to be given to the restless toddler. The young child cannot eat too much quantity of food at a time, so he must be fed more frequently and given calorie-dense

Table 15.2 List of essential nutrients*		
Macronutrients	*Vitamins*	*Minerals*
Water	Thiamine (B1)	Sodium
Carbohydrates	Riboflavin (B2)	Potassium
Fats	Niacin (B3)	Chloride
Linoleic acid	Pantothenic	Iron
Linolenic acid	acid (B5)	Calcium
Proteins (essential amino acids)	Pyridoxine (B6)	Phosphorus
Histidine	Cobalamine (B12)	Magnesium
Isoleucine	Biotin	Manganese
Leucine	Folic acid	Iodine
Lysine	Vitamin C	Flouride
Methionine	Vitamin A	Cobalt
Phenylalanine	Vitamin D	Molybdenum
Taurine	Vitamin E	Selenium
Threonine	Vitamin K	Sulfur
Tryptophane		Zinc
Valine		

* Carbohydrates, proteins and fats are called macronutrients while vitamins and minerals are called as micronutrients because they are required in extremely small quantities.

food. On an average, a child should be given at least 5 meals in a day at the age of one year. The energy density of the food should be increased by adding butter, oil or *desi-ghee*. Children tolerate fats well and long chain polyunsaturated fatty acids are needed for brain growth.

Carbohydrates The main sources of carbohydrates are cereals (wheat, rice, barley, *bajra*, corn etc.) and refined sugars. Cereals are a good source of energy and fiber in the diet. Many tuberous or root vegetables like potatoes, *arbi*, sweet potato and beet root are good sources of complex carbohydrates. Fruits are excellent source of glucose, fructose, sucrose, vitamins, minerals and antioxidant agents.

Proteins Proteins provide amino acids which are the building blocks of the body. When sufficient calories (through carbohydrates and fats) are not consumed, proteins are wasted for supply of energy rather than for body building, growth or repair of body tissues. A one-year old child needs about 15 g of protein, the demand increases to 20–25 g around 5 years and 40–45 g between 10 and 12 years. Animal proteins (eggs, milk and milk products, meat, fish etc) are biologically of a very high quality. Eggs are relished by most children and are a good source of high quality protein and micronutrients (**Box 15.4**) Proteins of vegetable sources are relatively of poor quality. But when a child is given a judicious mixture of wheat, rice, *dal*, lentils and vegetables along with milk and milk products, the biological quality of proteins become acceptable. For vegetarians, legumes and *dals* are a rich source of proteins providing 20–25 percent protein. Soybeans contain 40 percent protein content but most people do not like its taste. Newer methods of processing have improved its taste and it can be mixed with other cereals or foods to increase its acceptability. Cereals are also good source of protein, varying from 7 percent in rice to about 12 percent in wheat. When a child is taking enough of the balanced food, his requirements for proteins are adequately met. He does not need any special protein-rich foods or supplements available in the market. However, dietary supplements of proteins and micronutrients may be given to children with food fussiness or those convalescing from a serious or a chronic disease.

Fats These are derived from animal (butter, *ghee*) or plant sources (vegetable oils) and provide a rich source of energy. One gram of fat provides 9 calories compared to 4 calories per gram of carbohydrates and proteins. Children do need extra intake of fat to sustain their growth and activity. Fats provide high concentration of fat soluble vitamins. Preschool children should be given whole milk and not skimmed or toned milk. Excessive intake of fat is an important cause of obesity and should be avoided if there is a familial predisposition to develop obesity.

DHA in the diet Polyunsaturated fatty acids (PUFAs), i.e. omega-3 and omega-6 fatty acids are essential for health and wellbeing. Docoxahexaenoic acid (DHA), a long chain metabolite of omega-3 fatty acids, is the predominant structural fatty acid in the brain and retina. During pregnancy, fetus is completely dependent on the maternal dietary intake of omega-3 fatty acids and DHA and after birth breast milk is a rich source of DHA. The DHA content of breast milk is 30 times more than cow's milk. But as the child is weaned off the breast, his requirements of omega-3 fatty acids and DHA must be met from dietary sources like vegetable oils (flaxseed, linseed, soy, peanut), green leafy vegetables, broccoli, kidney beans, nuts (almonds, walnuts, peanuts), avocados, quinoa and above all oily fish, seafood and seaweed. Unfortunately an average vegetarian Indian diet does not provide adequate quantities of omega-3 fatty acids and DHA during preschool years. Apart from nutritious balanced diet, nutritional supplements fortified with DHA should be provided to preschool children.

The Hazards of Junk Food

There is a growing craze to eat junk food from the ever burgeoning self-service jaunts by children belonging to well-to-do families. The intake of unbalanced starchy and fatty junk food (without fresh green vegetables and

▌ **Box 15.4** **Composition of one standard egg (60 g)**	
Calories	100 kcal
Carbohydrates	Nil
Proteins	7 g
Fats	7 g
Cholesterol	300 mg

Most vitamins and minerals are present except vitamin C and vitamin K.

Practical Tip

Almost 70% of brain growth occurs during fetal life and around 15% during infancy. DHA accounts for a major anatomical component of CNS and retina. According to WHO, pregnant and nursing mothers should take 2.6 g of omega-3 fatty acids and 300 mg DHA daily to sustain the rapid growth and maturation of brain and retina during fetal life and infancy.

15

fruits) is associated with the risk of development of obesity and its consequences. Excessive intake of soft drinks, tinned juices, potatoe chips/crisps, french fries, pizzas, humburgers, hot dogs, snacky munchings in-between meals, puddings, ice cream, chocolates and sweets etc. should be avoided especially by children who have a familial tendency to become overweight. There are a number of Indian junk foods which are loaded with unhealthy transfats, i.e. *samosas, kachoris, pakoras, poories, bhathuras, mathies, namkeen*, etc. and they should be avoided or taken in moderation. Soft drinks provide empty calories without any essential nutrients and their excessive intake is associated with loss of appetite, restlessness and irritability (due to caffein) and dental decay and caries (due to sugar). The manufacturers of soft drinks should be asked to put a statutory warning on the bottle that "excessive intake of soft drinks may be hazardous to the health of children." Even canned juices are loaded with empty calories and should be avoided or taken after dilution. The tips for healthy eating and avoidance of junk food are summarized in **Box 15.5**.

Vegetarian versus Non-vegetarian Diet

Human beings by virtue of their evolution and nature of their teeth are vegetarian. Unlike animals, human beings never like to take raw meat. Non-vegetarian foods have a high salt, fat and cholesterol content and a low fiber content. There is an increasing scientific evidence that individuals who take non-vegetarian diet are more likely to have increased incidence of high blood pressure, heart disease, cerebrovascular strokes, cancer, gout and reduced lifespan. What we eat has a profound effect on our thoughts and emotions. Eating of meat and meat products is likely to be associated with greater aggression, passion, anger and cruelty.

There is an increasing trend to adopt a vegetarian food style in many countries of the world. Albert Einstein was a staunch vegetarian and he said *"nothing will benefit human health and increase the chances of survival of life on earth as much as the evolution to a vegetarian diet"*. There is such a variety of plants, cereals, vegetables and fruits to choose for our daily diet. There is no doubt that vegetarians can be as muscular and athletic as non-vegetarians. There is enough scientific evidence to suggest that intake of vegetarian diet is more health-friendly and is associated with lower incidence of

> *"You become what you eat! Food we eat influences our memory, comprehension, thinking, judgement, intellect and emotions."*

> **Box 15.5 Tips for healthy eating***
> - Except in preschool children, give fat-free milk and dairy products made from it.
> - Avoid junk food or give it sparingly. Avoid foods containing colors and preservatives. Give an occasional cocoa-based chocolate.
> - Avoid fried and roasted foods, instead give steamed, grilled, baked or boiled items.
> - Give plenty of fresh seasonal fruits and green vegetables— and use them as healthy snacks instead of potato chips, crisps and french fries.
> - Give foods rich in omega-3 fatty acids and DHA like green leafy vegetables, broccoli, kidney beans, flaxseed or soy oil, fish and sea food, dry fruits especially almonds and walnuts
> - Water and butter milk (chhaj) are the best drinks, avoid cola drinks and tinned fruit juices
> - Salt and sugar should be used in moderation or sparingly
>
> * Healthy eating habits in childhood lay a sound foundation for a healthy lifestyle later in life.

various diseases. Fresh fruits and vegetables are replete with antioxidants, which provide protection against various degenerative diseases including cancer. Vegetarian individuals are more likely to have greater poise, peace of mind, serenity and spirituality in their life. They are likely to have better control of their emotions and common vices of mankind such as lust, anger, greed, possessiveness and arrogance. Vegetarian diet provides all the essential nutrients except vitamin B_{12}. Most vegetarians, however, do take milk and milk products (and sometimes eggs) which are rich sources of vitamins B_{12}. Children should be encouraged to adopt vegetarian diet style by informing about its virtues but they should never be forced or cajoled to become pure vegetarian against their wishes.

MINERALS AND VITAMINS

Calcium Calcium is required for formation of bones and teeth. Children need relatively more calcium compared to adults. Milk and milk products are excellent sources of calcium. The other dietary sources of calcium include millet, *ragi, bajra*, and green vegetables like *cholai, methi* and drumsticks.

Iron Iron is required for formation of hemoglobin and its deficiency leads to anemia. Iron deficiency is extremely common among infants and adolescent children in our country. Iron deficiency may lead to poor growth, perverted taste (pica or eating mud), lethargy, fatigability and sluggish neuromotor development. Good dietary sources of iron are meat, liver, egg yolk, green vegetables, lentils, fruits, jaggery and cereals particularly wheat, bajra and ragi. Milk is a poor source of iron and children fed mainly on milk for a prolonged period are likely to develop anemia.

Iodine It is an essential trace element, which is necessary for production of thyroid hormone. Its deficiency is an important cause of slow physical growth, mental dullness and deafness. When a pregnant woman has deficient intake of iodine, her baby may develop brain damage due to deficiency of thyroid hormone. People living in hilly areas develop swelling of thyroid gland (goiter) in the neck due to low content of iodine in soil and water. The good dietary sources of iodine include fish, meat, green vegetables (especially spinach), cereals, milk and milk products. Common salt fortified with iodine should be consumed.

Zinc Its deficiency can cause poor weight gain, frequent infections, delayed wound healing, poor sexual development and skin disorders. Zinc intake is credited to promote recovery from diarrhea. The good sources of zinc are wheat, breast milk, nuts, eggs, cheese, grains and meat products.

VITAMINS

Vitamins are essential for the maintenance of good health and their deficiency can produce several health problems. Vitamins should be taken in the recommended daily amount because excessive intake may lead to side effects. Large doses of vitamins A and D can be dangerous because these vitamins are stored in the body. Excessive intake of vitamins B and C are merely excreted in the urine. It has become fashionable to take vitamins with breakfast, which has doubtful therapeutic benefit unless there are specific indications for their intake. Vitamins are broadly divided into two classes, fat soluble and water soluble. Salient clinical features of deficiency of vitamins are summarized in **Table 15.3**.

Fat-Soluble Vitamins

They are present in fatty food and their absorption is facilitated by fats.

Vitamin A

Vitamin A is needed for healthy eyes and has anti-infective and anti-oxidant role to prevent occurrence of respiratory and gastrointestinal infections. Night

Table 15.3 Salient clinical features of deficiency of vitamins	
Vitamins	*Features of deficiency state*
Vitamin A	Night blindness, dryness of cornea (xerophthalmia), bitot spots, phylectenular conjunctivitis, keratomalacia, phrynodermia (toad skin), keratinization of mucous membranes, retarded growth, defective tooth enamel, impaired immunity
Vitamin B complex	
B_1 or thiamine	Beriberi leading to polyneuritis and cardiac abnormalities with cogestive heart failure
B_2 or riboflavin	Photophobia, blurred vision, itching of eyes, circum-corneal vascularization, angular stomatitis (cheilosis), poor growth
B_3 or niacin	Pellagra characterized by diarrhea, dementia and dermatitis
B_5 or pantothenic acid	Burning sensations in hands and feet, gastro-intestinal disturbances, muscle cramps, fatigue, tiredness and hypoglycemia
B_6 or pyridoxine	Hypochromic anemia, irritability, seizures, peripheral neuritis
B_{12} or cyanocobalamin	Juvenile pernicious anemia, malabsorption, thrombocytopenia
Biotin	Circumoral skin rash, brittle hair, seborrheic dermatitis, anemia, anorexia and lassitude
Folic acid	Megaloblastic anemia, glossitis, pharyngeal ulcers, impaired immunity
Vitamin C or ascorbic acid	Scurvy characterized by marked irritability, anemia, bleeding gums, scorbutic rosary (due to posterior dislocation of sternum), epiphyseal bleeding with painful pseudoparalysis of a limb, poor wound healing, impaired immunity
Vitamin D	Rickets characterized by widening of wrists and ankles, knock knees, prominent costochondral junctions (rickety rosary), Harrison's sulcus, bossing of skull, wide anterior fontanel (with delayed closure), spinal deformities, delayed dentition, slow growth, stunting and tetany
Vitamin E	Hemolytic anemia of prematurity, neuromyopathy, paralysis of extrinsic ocular muscles
Vitamin K	Hemorrhagic disease of the newborn, impaired bone growth

15

blindness (inability to see in the dark) is the earliest manifestation of vitamin A deficiency. The rich dietary sources of vitamin A are butter, *ghee*, cod liver oil, vegetable oil, green leafy vegetables, yellow vegetables (especially carrots), egg yolk and dairy products. Fruits like papaya, mango and apricot are also good sources of vitamin A.

Vitamin D

Vitamin D is essential for growth of healthy teeth and bones. Its deficiency may lead to development of rickets with various deformities in the bones. The non-skeletal health benefits of vitamin D include modulation of immunity and enhanced neuropsychiatric functioning. There is reduced risk of autoimmune disorder, coronary artery disease, malignant disorders and better control of type 2 diabetes mellitus in adults. Vitamin D is formed in the body by the action of sunlight on the skin. It is important for children to play in the open for adequate exposure to sunlight. The dietary sources of vitamin D are butter, *ghee*, margarine, fish, liver, egg yolk and fortified dairy products. Breast milk is relatively deficient in Vitamin D. Vitamin D is stable to heat and does not leach out of foods cooked in water.

Vitamin E

Its exact role is uncertain. It is an antioxidant, improves fertility, memory and muscular activity. The good sources of vitamin E include wheat, vegetable oils, green leafy vegetebles, dairy products, eggs, liver and nuts.

Vitamin K

Vitamin K is required for production of prothrombin in the liver which is needed for normal clotting of blood to stop bleeding. Vitamin K is produced in the intestines by the effect of friendly bacteria in the gut. The dietary sources are milk and milk products, cabbage, cauliflower, spinach, beans, peas, potatoes, carrots and liver. It is not destroyed by cooking. Breast milk is relatively deficient in vitamin K. All newborn babies are given one dose of vitamin K soon after birth to prevent hemorrhagic disease of the newborn.

Water-Soluble Vitamins
Vitamin B complex

There are at least eight vitamins grouped together under vitamin B complex, i.e. thiamine (B_1), riboflavin (B_2), niacin (B_3), folic acid, pyridoxine (B_6), cobalamin (B_{12}), biotin and pantothenic acid (B_5). They are necessary for normal functioning and protection of central nervous system, lining of oral cavity and gut.

Good dietary sources of vitamins B complex include milk and milk products, wheat, parboiled or unpolished rice, green leafy vegetables, meat, fish and nuts. Strict vegetarians get their quota of vitamin B_{12} from dairy products. Sprouted *dals* and legumes are extremely rich in vitamin B complex. Avoid cooking the food too long as it destroys its vitamin B content and do not throw away the water in which vegetables are cooked. The B complex vitamins are also produced endogenously by friendly bacteria or probiotics in the gut.

Vitamin C

Vitamin C is necessary for development of bones, teeth, blood vessels and healing of wounds. It helps in the absorption of iron from gut. Its deficiency may lead to development of scurvy (bleeding gums, bone pains and anemia). Regular intake of vitamin C is essential because it is not stored in the body and is easily destroyed by heating. Good sources of vitamin C include citrus fruits (orange, sweet lemon, *keenoo*, grape fruit), *amla*, guava, tomatoes, potatoes and dark green vegetables, etc. Most fruits and vegetables, which have a sour and stringent taste are rich in vitamin C. Breast milk provides sufficient quantities of vitamin C but bottle fed babies are likely to have poor intake of vitamin C because it gets destroyed by boiling.

Recommended dietary allowances (RDAs) of various nutrients in children of different age groups are shown in **Table 15.4**. The requirements of various nutrients are calculated on the basis of the ideal body weight and becomes less per unit body weight in older children due to reduced growth velocity.

Preservation of Nutrients during Cooking

When vegetables are cut into small bits and kept soaked in water for a long duration, it is likely to lose several nutrients. It is best to cut the vegetables just before cooking and they should be washed to get rid of residues of insecticides and chemical fertilizers before they are chopped. Whenever feasible vegetables and fruits should be eaten with peel because it is rich in nutrients. Cooking kills bacteria and parasites in the food, improves digestibility, taste and flavor. But prolonged cooking especially boiling and steaming are associated with loss of nutrients. Frying is associated with relatively less loss of nutrients. The use of baking powder while cooking aggravates nutrient loss while use of tamarind tends to preserve vitamins. The longer the food is cooked, greater is the loss in nutrients especially vitamins C and B complex. Water used for cooking should never be thrown away as it is rich in nutrients. Rice should be cooked with a lesser quantity

Table 15.4 Recommended daily dietary allowances of nutrients

Nutrient	Under 1 year	1–10 years	Over 10 years
Water (mL/kg)	120–150	100–120	50–100
Calories (per kg)	100–120	80–100	50–80
Proteins (g/kg)	2.5–3.5	2.0–2.5	1.0–2.0
Iron (mg)	10.0	15.0	20.0
Iodine (μg)	50	100	150
Zinc (mg)	5.0	7.5	10.0
Calcium (g)	0.5	0.75	1.0
Vitamin A (i.u)	1500	2500	5000
Vitamin D (i.u)*	200	400	600
Vitamin C (mg)	30	40	50
Thiamine (mg)	0.5	1.0	1.5
Riboflavin (mg)	0.5	1.0	1.5
Nicotinic acid (mg)	6.0	12.0	18.0
Pyridoxine (mg)	0.5	1.0	1.5
Vitamin B12 (mg)	0.2	0.5	1.0
Folic acid (mg)	25	50	100

* 400 i.u. vitamin D = 10 mg

of water so that no water is decanted off. Cooking in a pot with a lid on preserves nutrients better. A pressure cooker is useful for cooking as not only it saves the fuel and time but it also tends to preserve the nutrients.

Traditional Beliefs about Foods

There are many age-old beliefs regarding various foods and their attributes and effects in different people. In Ayurveda, different foods are recommended for different people depending upon their basic body type or *dosha*. All foods are classified into alkaline and acidic and cold and hot. For example, cucumber, okra, potatoes, banana, grapes and dairy products are considered as cold foods while garlic, ginger, onion, tomato, pepper, mango, orange, dry fruits, meat, eggs, tea, coffee etc are believed to be hot foods. Cold foods are best taken during summer while hot foods should be consumed in winter. Banana, rice, curd and milk are believed to produce cough and phlegm and best avoided by asthmatics. Some mothers stop giving orange juice to the baby if he develops cold with the mistaken belief that orange juice aggravates cold. At times orange juice is warmed up before giving it to the child with cold. It should never be done because it destroys vitamin C and makes it acidic. Mango is a "hot" food but becomes "cool" when it is soaked in water for some time. Cereals are supposed to be bad for liver. There is such a variety of food items that if one food item is prohibited it can be easily replaced by another. In winter, for example, extra milk, *kheer* and cheese can be taken instead of yoghurt. In modern

system of medicine there are much less dietary restrictions in various disease states. Nature has profound biological wisdom and if you consume seasonal vegetables and fruits, you cannot go wrong. The major emphasis should be placed on giving a balanced nutritious food to the child both during health and whenever he falls sick.

PARENTERAL NUTRITION

Intravenous alimentation or total parenteral nutrition (TPN) is considered in the treatment of critically sick or tiny newborn babies when it is impossible to provide nutrition through enteral route due to immaturity of the gut or clinical condition of the baby. The technique is, however, handicapped by lack of easy availability of satisfactory infusates which are rather expensive and there is relatively high incidence of side effects and complications. Satisfactory growth velocity, comparable to intrauterine growth pattern, can be achieved by parenteral alimentation. Adequacy of nutrition is crucial to enhance linear growth, neuromotor development and ensure optimal functioning of various body organs.

Indications

1. Birth weight less than 1000 g or gestation <28 weeks.
2. Sick LBW babies requiring prolonged intravenous infusion exceeding 4–5 days, e.g. RDS, apneic attacks, sepsis, seizures, bronchopulmonary dysplasia, and necrotizing enterocolitis.

3. Chronic intractable diarrhea
4. Neonates born with major anomalies of gastrointestinal tract requiring extensive surgical procedures. They include gastroschisis, omphalocele, tracheoesophageal fistula, intestinal atresia, meconium ileus, malrotation of gut and short bowel syndrome.
5. Partial parenteral nutrition to supplement gavage feeding is recommended in infants weighing less than 1,200 g.

Contraindications

1. Hypoxia, acidemia and shock.
2. Hyperbilirubinemia (serum bilirubin >12 mg/dL).
3. Azotemia (blood urea >48 mg/dL).
4. Thrombocytopenia.

The Composition of Infusates

Energy

Preterm infants should not be starved as they have low energy reserves because of poor fat content as well as low reserves of glycogen. The parenterally nourished infants need about 100–120 kcal/kg/day (as opposed to 120–150 kcal/kg/day for enterally fed) for satisfactory weight gain because there are no losses due to digestion, specific dynamic action of food or wastage in stools. The ideal distribution for availability of calories from different sources include 50–55% from carbohydrates, 10–15% from proteins and 30–35% from fats.

Carbohydrates Glucose is the most suitable source of carbohydrate because of its immediate bioavailability to the central nervous system. Due to its osmolarity (18 mg/dL of glucose contributes osmolarity of about 1.0 mOsm/L) and sclerosing effect, concentrations in excess of 12.5% (125 mg glucose per mL) should not be infused through a peripheral vein. Higher concentrations up to a maximum of 20% may be infused through a silastic or silicone catheter placed in a central vein. To reduce intolerance, it is recommended that dextrose infusion should be started at a rate of 6 mg/kg/minute and gradually increased to a maximum of 12–14 mg/kg per minute in increments of 2 mg/kg/minute everyday over next couple of days. Insulin is given (0.05 units/kg/hr) to manage hyperglycemia (>120 mg/dL) when despite lowering glucose infusion rate to 4–6 mg/kg/min is unable to achieve it.

Proteins Protein requirements are inversely related to gestational age or birth weight because of rapid growth velocity and greater protein losses in ELBW babies. Solutions containing crystalline amino acids are satisfactory to provide nitrogen during parenteral nutrition. Protein hydrolysates carry greater risk of infection and hyperammonemia. In addition to eight amino acids which are essential in the older infants, histidine, cysteine, tyrosine, glutamine, arginine, proline, glycine are also essential for premature and possibly full term infants. The commonly used formulations include Aminoven Infant 6% and 10% (Fresinus Kabi India Pvt Ltd) and Primene 10% (Baxter Healthcare). Amino acid solutions are administered in a starting dose of 0.5 g protein equivalent per kilogram per day and increased daily by 0.5 g/kg and maintained between 3.0 and 3.5 g/kg per day. To prevent hyperchloremic acidosis, amino acid mixture should be buffered with sodium bicarbonate or hydrochloride salts of arginine, lysine and histidine should be replaced by acetate equivalents.

Fats In order to provide sufficient calories without enhancing osmolar load, availability and administration of fat emulsions is mandatory. Apart from high energy density, they are required for supply of essential fatty acids and delivery of fat soluble vitamins. Intralipid (10% or 20% emulsion of soya bean oil stabilized with 1–2% egg phospholipid) and Liposyn (derived from safflower oil) are commercially available and provide all the essential fatty acids. Intralipid is infused in a dose of 1.0 g/kg day which is gradually increased by 0.5–1.0 g/kg evey day till maximum of 3.0 g/kg/day is achieved. The daily requirement of essential fatty acid can be met by infusion of 0.5–1.0 g/kg of intralipid per day. Higher quantities of intralipid can be infused by slow infusion spread over a period of 24 hours with an infusion pump. The rate of intralipid infusion should be maintained below 0.25 g/kg per hour and a concentration of 10–20% can be used in the newborn.

Lipids do not impose any osmolar load. The use of 20% intralipid emulsion is preferred due to lower risk of hypertriglyceridemia, hypercholesterolemia and hyperphospholipidemia. Lipids should be infused through a separate infusion syringe which can be used as a vehicle for administration of vitamins to prevent their photodegradation and adhesion to the infusion tubing. When lipids are exposed to light, they can form potentially toxic lipid hydroperoxides. Photoprotection of PN solution reduces the peroxide load and is credited to reduce the risk of BPD. Therefore, the lipid syringe and tubing should be wrapped with an aluminum foil. Lipids should be avoided or used with caution in low doses in critically sick ELBW babies on assisted ventilation, disseminated intravascular coagulation, hyperbilirubinemia and thrombocytopenia. Lipids can adversely affect the gas exchange. Lipids and free fatty acids compete with binding sites in the albumin and thus predispose to development of bilirubin encephalopathy at lower serum bilirubin levels. A free fatty acid to albumin ratio (FFA: albumin) should be kept below 6:1 in high risk situations. Lipids are administered in minimum doses to meet the nutritional needs of essential fatty acids.

Minerals and Vitamins

Prolonged and exclusive intravenous alimentation must be supplemented with electrolytes, minerals, trace elements and vitamins. Daily sodium and potassium needs of the newborn baby are 2–3 mEq/kg. Preterm babies especially those below 1500 g require higher sodium intake of 4–6 mEq/kg/day. The estimated intravenous requirements of both elemental calcium and phosphorus are 20–40 mg/kg/day. Magnesium should be supplemented in a dose of 0.25–0.50 mEq/kg/day. Except phosphates all the minerals are available for intravenous use. The precise parenteral requirements of trace elements are uncertain. Zinc (150–400 µg/kg/d) should be started from day one of TPN while other trace elements are gradually introduced. MVI adult is the most suitable preparation for providing daily requirements of vitamins to newborn babies on TPN. Daily administration of 0.5 ml/kg of intravenous multivitamin preparation is satisfactory though it provides higher than recommended concentrations of certain vitamin. Folic acid (100 µg), vitamin B_{12} (100 µg) and vitamin K (500 µg) should be administered weekly through intramuscular route. Carnitine is a conditionally essential nutrient for neonates as it facilitates beta oxidation of long chain fatty acids. It should be supplemented in a dose of 5 mg/kg/d in infants receiving TPN. The available PN solutions in Indian market are shown in **Table 15.5**.

Fluids

Fluids serve as the carrying medium for parenteral nutrients. They are started at a rate of 60–80 mL/kg/d and gradually increased by 10–20 mL/kg/d to maximum of 150 mL/kg/d by the end of first week of life. Fluid therapy is fine tuned by monitoring hydration status of the infant by daily weight changes, urine output, serum sodium/osmolality and urinary specific gravity and osmolality. A computer software is available which can be used for calculation of various components of PN solution because manual calculation is time consuming and cumbersome.

Technique of Administration

It is preferable to use a peripheral vein by inserting a medi-cathether. Thorough asepsis must be ensured during the procedure. Intralipid emulsion with

Table 15.5 Available parenteral solutions in Indian market

Component	Source	Concentration
Glucose	Dextrose	5%, 10%, 25%, 50%
Protein	Aminoven	6% and 10%
	Primene[a]	10%
Lipids	Intralipids[b] Linoleic[c]	10%, 10% PLR, 20% PLR, i.e. phospholipids reduced 20%
Sodium and chloride	NaCl	0.9% and 3%
Potassium and chloride	KCl	15%
Calcium	Calcium gluconate	10%
Magnesium	Magnesium sulfate	50%
Multivitamins	Adult MVI	—
Trace elements	Celecel[d] 4, 5 TMA	—

[a]Fresinus Kabi India Pvt Ltd.
[b]Baxter Healthcare Ltd.
[c]Drugs and Pharmaceuticals Pvt Ltd.
[d]Claris Lifesciences Ltd.

vitamins on one hand and protein–carbohydrate mixture with electrolytes and trace elements on the other, are suspended through separate infusion sets and connected with a Y-connector just proximal to the catheter or micropore filter **(Figure 15.17)**. It is also feasible to administer TPN solution through a single bottle. A short term and partial PN can be provided through a peripheral venous line by restricting dextrose concentration up to 12.5%. When prolonged PN is anticipated it should be delivered through peripherally inserted central catheter (PICC). Single lumen catheter is inserted to ensure that its tip lies in the superior or inferior vena cava which should be confirmed by an ultrasound or X-ray examination. In neonates, a central line can be established through umbilical vein. Silicone or polyvinyl catheter should be used to establish central venous line. Carbohydrates and amino acid solutions are mixed first. Fat emulsion is added subsequently by gently shaking the bottle during mixing. Mixed TPN solution must contain heparin (1 unit/mL) and is stable up to 36 hours. The amino acid and lipid solutions should be protected against light to reduce the risk of peroxide load to the baby.

It is essential that precise infusion rate is maintained by regulating its flow through a constant infusion pump. It is desirable to use bacterial filters (0.2 microns)

15

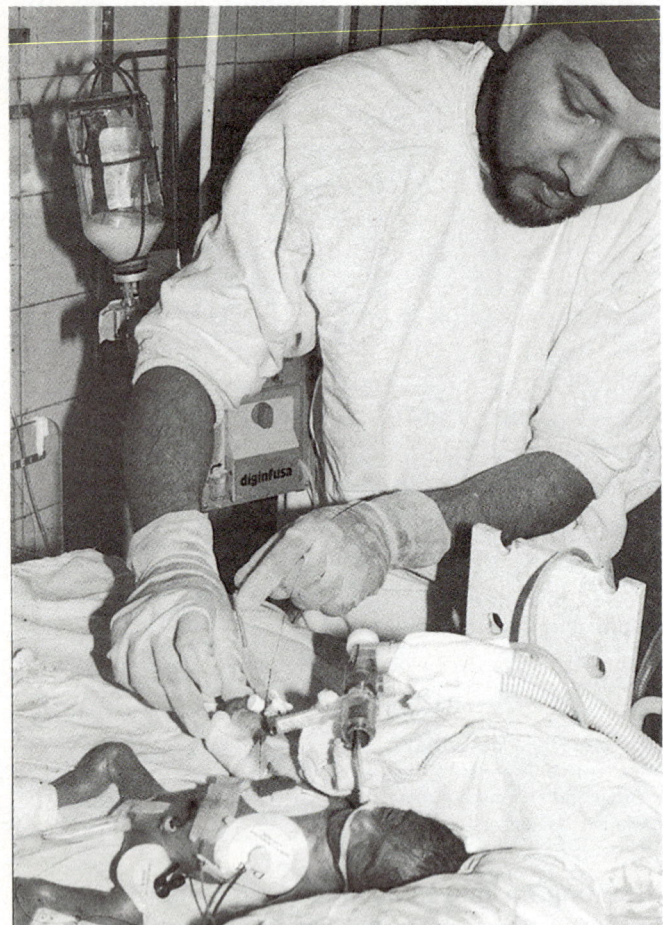

Figure 15.17 Setting up 3-way stopcock for administration of TPN with strict aseptic precautions

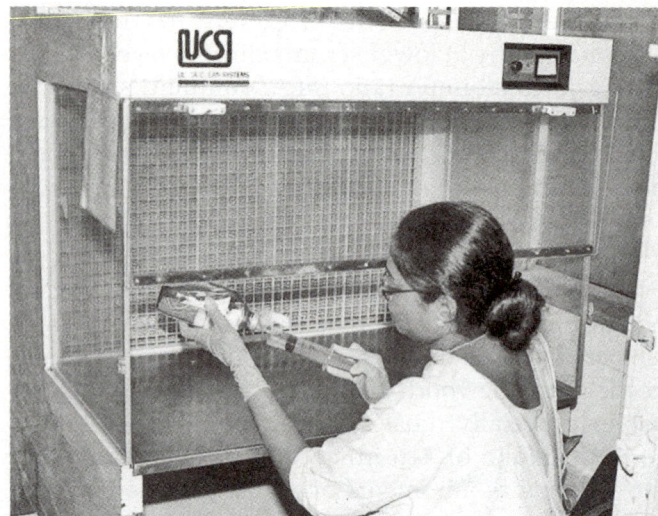

Figure 15.18 The preparation of TPN solution under laminar flow

Monitoring by Nurse

A flowchart should be maintained by nurse to record daily changes in weight, status of hydration, urine output and intake of fluids, calories and its sources. Serum electrolytes, BUN, glucose, hematocrit, blood pH, plasma and urinary osmolality should be checked daily. Plasma osmolality should be maintained between 285 and 300 mOsm/L. Plasma should be inspected daily to look for turbidity due to fat emulsion. Liver function tests, serum proteins and fatty acids should be checked once every week **(Table 15.6)**. An accurate record of amount of blood removed for biochemical monitoring should be maintained.

Complications

They may be related to the catheter or to the infusate. Inflammation and sloughing of skin at infusion site is alarming. Hospital-acquired infection (HAI) especially candidemia is a common life-threatening complication and should be prevented by use of effective aseptic precautions like use of laminar flow for mixing of PN solutions, use of bacterial filter in amino acid-glucose line and daily change of infusion sets. The metabolic complications include competitive displacement of albumin-bound bilirubin by free fatty acids, and alterations in the concentration of a variety of blood constituents such as glucose, acid–base status, sodium, potassium, chloride, calcium, magnesium, phosphorous, BUN, essential amino acids, vitamins and trace elements. Hyperglycemia with osmotic diuresis and dehydration can occur among ELBW babies receiving hyperosmolar infusates. A constant clinical and chemical monitoring with the aid of a micro chemistry

which are now available in India. Infusion bottles and sets must be changed everyday to reduce chances of contamination. Infusion site should be promptly changed at the first sign of reddening or devitalization of the skin. Strict asepsis and local application of antimicrobial cream at the site of exit wound of catheter are essential to prevent septic complications. Most infusates are marketed in large-volume packs entailing considerable wastage unless mini-bagged. The formulation or sub-packing of commercial infusates into small packs should be undertaken under a laminar flow with meticulous aseptic precautions by using sterile plastic bags **(Figure 15.18)**. The osmolarity of various infusates should be restricted to 300–900 mOsm/L when PN is administered through a peripheral venous line. The volume and concentration of various nutrients should be increased gradually. The venous access used for PN should not be exploited for administration of antibiotics and medications. As soon as clinical condition of the patient permits, oral feeding should be started and infant gradually weaned off from intravenous feeding over a period of 3 to 4 days.

Table 15.6 Monitoring schedule for neonates receiving parenteral nutrition

Parameter	Frequency
Anthropometry*	
Weight (g)	Daily (same time each day)
Length (cm)	weekly
Head circumference (cm)	Weekly
Biochemistry	
Urine glucose and specific gravity	8 hourly first week, then once daily
Inspection of plasma sample for lipemia	Once daily
Blood glucose	6 hourly initially, 12 hourly when glucose infusion rate is static
Serum sodium and potassium	Daily initial 3–4 days, then twice weekly
BUN, creatinine	Daily initial 3–4 days, then twice weekly once protein intake becomes static
Blood pH	Daily initial 3–4 days, then twice a week once protein intake becomes static
Hemogram	Weekly
Serum calcium, phosphorus, magnesium, proteins, triglycerides, liver function tests	Weekly

*The target anthropometric gains during TPN include weight gain 15–18 g/d (1.0% of body weight/d), length gain 0.75–1.0 cm/week, and head circumference gain 0.75 cm/week.

Note: Daily intake of fluids (mL/kg/d), urine output (mL/kg/hr), energy intake (kcal/kg/d), glucose infusion rate (mg/kg/min), protein intake (g/kg/d) and lipids (g/kg/d) should be recorded. Catheter-related complications including hospital acquired infection (HAI) should be looked for. Eosinophilia is a useful marker of allergy to intralipid. Blood transfusion is mandatory as soon as 10% of blood volume has been removed by sampling.

laboratory support is essential for early diagnosis and prompt management of metabolic alterations.

Hepatomegaly with cholestasis and jaundice is a frequent complication of TPN in very LBW babies. TPN-associated hepatic dysfunction is possibly related to disorder in bile secretion due to toxic effect of certain amino acids, deficiency of essential fatty acids or associated sepsis. The deficiency of essential fatty acids is managed by cutaneous application of sunflower oil, oral administration of sunflower oil 2.5–5.0 mL/day and intermittent plasma transfusion. Intralipid administration is contraindicated in infants with jaundice and bleeding manifestations. Rapid infusion of intralipid in tiny preterm babies may cause reduction in pulmonary diffusion capacity producing dyspnea and cyanosis. Thrombocytopenia and hypercoagulability of blood are rare complications.

BIBLIOGRAPHY

Agarwal R, Deorari AK, Paul VK (Ed). Parenteral nutrition. In: AIIMS Protocols in Neonatology. *New Delhi, CBS Publishers and Distributors Pvt Ltd* 2015, pp 336–347.

American Academy of Pediatrics Working Group on Breastfeeding. Breastfeeding and use of human milk. *Pediatrics* 2005, 115(2):496–506.

Atkins SA. Human milk feeding of the micropremies. *Clin Perinatol* 2000, 27:235–247.

Bharadva K, Tiwari S, Mishra S, et al. Human milk banking guideliens: Infant and Young Child Feeding Chapter, Indian Academy of Pediatrics. *Indian Pediatr* 2014, 51:469–474.

Lang S, Lawrence CJ, Orme RLE. Cup feeding: an alternative method of infant feeding. *Arch Dis Child* 1994, 71:365–369.

Singh M. Breastfeeding. In: Art and Science of Baby and Child Care. CBS Publishers and Distributors Pvt. Ltd., New Delhi, 4th edition 2015, p 78–94.

Ziegler E., Carlson S. Early nutrition of VLBW infants. *J Maternal-Fetal Neonat Med* 2009, 22:191–197.

Nutritional Disorders

Physical growth and mental development of children depends upon the interaction between nature (genetic potential and constitution) and nurture (nutrition, health care, safe and stimulating environment). Children must receive a well balanced diet and optimal nutrition to enable them to achieve their full genetic potential.

Over the years, the deficiency of macronutrients (carbohydrates, fats and proteins) have decreased with reduced incidence of frank cases of severe protein-energy malnutrition and kwashiorkor due to greater food availability, awareness and improvement in the socioeconomic status. Even severe deficiency states of single micronutrients (vitamins and minerals) producing scurvy (vitamin C deficiency), rickets (vitamin D deficiency), beri-beri (vitamin B_1 deficiency), pellagra (nicotinic acid deficiency), keratomalacia (vitamin A deficiency) have become rare. However, there is still wide spread prevalence of diseases of public health importance due to deficiencies of single micronutrients like iron deficiency anemia, iodine deficiency disorders and milder forms of vitamin A deficiency.

It is being increasingly realized that there is a wide spread prevalence of subclinical or biochemical deficiencies of certain micronutrients which is being referred to as "Hidden hunger". The child survival has improved due to control of severe cases of protein-energy malnutrition but the quality of life and human resource development have not improved **(Figure 16.1)**. The studies conducted at the National Institute of Nutrition, Hyderabad have shown that over 50 percent apparently healthy school going children have subclinical deficiencies of vitamin A, vitamins B_2, B_6, folate, vitamin C and vitamin D. Children with deficiencies of micronutrients are more vulnerable to develop a variety of common day-to-day infections. Infective illnesses are known to further aggravate nutritional deficiencies by causing loss of appetite, tissue catabolism, enhanced utilization and increased losses of micronutrients. Acute infections thus adversely affect the nutritional status which makes an individual more vulnerable to contract infection, thus setting-up a vicious cycle of undernutrition and recurrent infections.

Etiopathogenesis

Children are more vulnerable to develop nutritional disorders compared to adults. Nutritional disorders are most prevalent during fetal life, preschool years and adolescence. The increased susceptibility of children to develop nutritional disorders is accounted for by the following factors.

1. During fetal life and early infancy (exclusive breastfeeding for 6 months), nutrition is entirely transmaternal. The general neglect of girl children (future mothers) particularly their health care, nutrition and education is an important cause of poor health and well-being of children in India.

2. Children are dependent and at the mercy of their parents and care takers to look after their nutritional and healthcare needs. Because most parents are ignorant and socially disadvantaged, their children are likely to be undernourished and have suboptimal physical growth (stunting) and mental development.

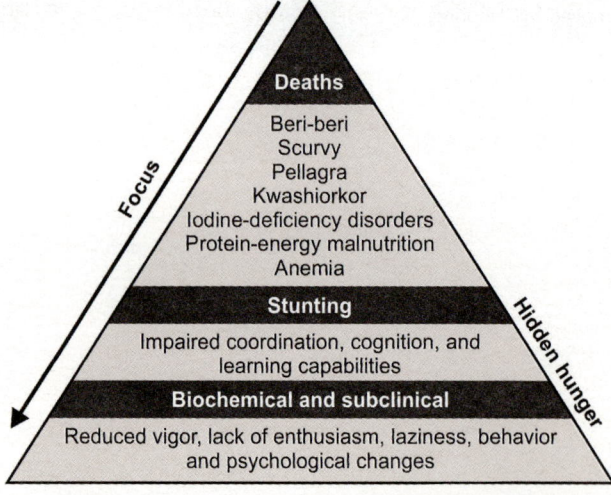

Figure 16.1 Pyramid of nutritional disorders

3. In order to sustain high growth velocity (1.0 kg neonate becomes .50 kg adolescent) and maintain high level of physical activity, children need high intake of energy and essential nutrients. For example, the caloric needs of neonates and infants (120 kcal/kg/d) is about three times that of adults (40 kcal/kg/d).

4. Other causes of undernutrition in developing countries include poor socioeconomic status, high incidence of low birth weight babies, denial or short duration of breastfeeding, delayed weaning, denial of food during illness, emphasis on fruit juices and watery soups rather than nutrition dense home-cooked weaning foods. These harmful child rearing practices further compromise the nutritional status of children.

5. Children have high incidence of gastrointestinal and respiratory infections and a various cycle of interaction between under-nutrition and infections makes matter worse.

FAILURE TO THRIVE

The weight and height of under-5 children should be recorded and monitored on Road-to-Health cards during their visits to the physician for immunizations.

The diagnosis of failure to thrive (FTT) cannot be made on the basis of a single weight record. It should be diagnosed when a child shows unsatisfactory physical growth over a period of time. Children with poor genetic potential for growth may not grow along the 50th percentile line but some where between 10th and 50th percentile in a consistent pattern without showing any dips or drops in their growth velocity. On the other hand, the weight curve of the child with FTT shows flattening or a downward trend and it may drop below two major percentile lines. The diagnosis of FTT can also be suspected if the weight-for-height of the child is less than 5th percentile. The common causes of FTT are listed in **Table 16.1**. Apart from poor nutritional intake, lack of love and emotional support by maladjusted parents is an important cause of FTT. A large number of systemic diseases are associated with FTT and should be ruled out by a detailed history, physical examination and relevant investigations.

PROTEIN-ENERGY MALNUTRITION (PEM)

Protein-energy malnutrition (PEM) occurs either due to dietary inadequacy or chronic systemic disease and recurrent infections. The child is considered as

---

Table 16.1 Causes of failure to thrive

1. **Psychosocial deprivation, neglect and child abuse**

2. **Faulty feeding practices**
   Failure to breast feed, feeding of diluted milk/formula, delayed and unsatisfactory weaning practices

3. **Infections**
   Intrauterine infections, recurrent bacterial infections, tuberculosis, malaria, kala azar, worm infestations, HIV infection, etc.

4. **Systemic diseases**
   Gastrointestinal disorders
   Recurrent or persistent diarrhea, gastroesophageal reflux disease, milk allergy and lactose-intolerance, celiac disease, protein-losing enteropathy, and inflammatory bowel disease
   Respiratory disorders
   Recurrent respiratory infections, bronchial asthma, bronchiectasis, and cystic fibrosis
   Cardiovascular disorders
   Congenital and acquired heart diseases
   Renal disorders
   Recurrent urinary tract infections, nephrotic syndrome, renal tubular acidosis, and chronic renal failure
   Hematologic disorders
   Nutritional anemia, thalassemia major, and sickle cell anemia
   Neurologic disorders
   Cerebral palsy, mental retardation, and diencephalic tumor
   Endocrinal disorders
   Diabetes mellitus, diabetes inspidus, hypothyroidism, hyperthyroidism, and congenital adrenal hyperplasia
   Immunologic disorders
   Primary immune deficiency disorders, and collagen vascular diseases

5. **Developmental disorders**
   Preterm or extremely LBW babies, severe IUGR babies, congenital malformations, developmental disorders, chromosomal disorders, genetic or metabolic disorders.

16

underweight when his weight is less than 2SD from the median weight-for-age of NCHS or WHO reference standards. Stunting is diagnosed when height-for-age of the child is below 2SD of the expected (median height-for-age of NCHS or WHO reference standards). By this criterion around 48 percent under-5 children are stunted in India. Wasting is defined as weight-for-height of the child as less than 2SD of the expected (median weight-for-height of NCHS or WHO refrence standards). When PEM is acute in onset, body weight is affected more than height. In chronic cases of PEM both body weight and height are affected. In severe malnutrition even brain growth may be affected with reduced size of head circumference. According to Indian Academy of Pediatrics, PEM is graded as follows:

Grade I Body weight between 71% and 80% of the expected weight-for-age.

Grade II Body weight between 61% and 70% of the expected weight-for-age.

Grade III Body weight between 51% and 60% of the expected weight-for-age.

Grade IV Body weight up to 50% or less of the expected weight for age.

Stunting and wasting may occur due to deficient intake of calories and proteins or due to an underlying systemic disorder but more recently it is being recognized that deficiency of micronutrients (vitamins and trace minerals) are important cause of growth failure and recurrent infections. The extreme forms of nutritional disorders called as marasmus and kwashiorkor are relatively uncommon these days.

Causes

Protein-energy malnutrition may be primary due to lack of food and interplay of infections and dietary intake or it may be secondary because of underlying systemic disorder such as chronic disease of gastrointestinal tract, kidneys, liver and cardiovascular system. There may be underlying chronic infection (tuberculosis, HIV-infection) or autoimmune disorder. The immediate or precipitating causes of PEM include inadequate intake of food and occurrence of acute diarrhea and pneumonia or it may follow an attack of measles or whooping cough with activation of latent tuberculosis. The root causes of PEM include poor socioeconomic status, lack of housing, over crowding, lack of environmental sanitation, unsafe drinking water, lack of awareness of health and nutrition, gender inequality and poor status of women in the society.

MARASMUS

There is gross wasting of muscles and subcutaneous tissues resulting in emaciation and stunting. The loose folds of skin are seen over the buttocks and inner side of thighs. The buccal pad of fat is the last to disappear. Skin is thin, loose, dry, inelastic and wrinkled **(Figure 16.2)**. The abdomen is distended due to wasting and hypotonia of muscles of abdominal wall. The bony points including ribs stand out prominently because of loss of subcutaneous fat and muscles. The baby appears alert, may be irritable but has good appetite unless complicated by intercurrent infection. When a child with marasmus develops edema due to intercurrent infection and aggravation of protein deficiency, the condition is called as marasmic kwashiorkor.

KWASHIORKOR

It is a severe form of dietary protein deficiency when a child is weaned from breast feeding with starchy gruel following the birth of another sibling. Kwashiorkor in Ga language of West Africa means "The disease of the displaced child".

Kwashiorkor has become rare due to better socio-economic status and availability of food. The classical features include growth retardation, psychomotor changes, generalized edema, skin changes (flaky paint or mosaic dermatosis due to exposed raw skin areas with pigmentation and hypopigmentation), hair changes (thin, dry, brown and brittle hair), enlargement of liver due to fatty infiltration and mental changes (lethargy, listlessness and apathy). The child looks miserable and has loss of appetite. Stunting is present but body weight may be normal due to generalized edema **(Figure 16.3)**. There may be associated deficiency of micronutrients especially iron, folic acid, zinc and vitamin A and vitamin B complex.

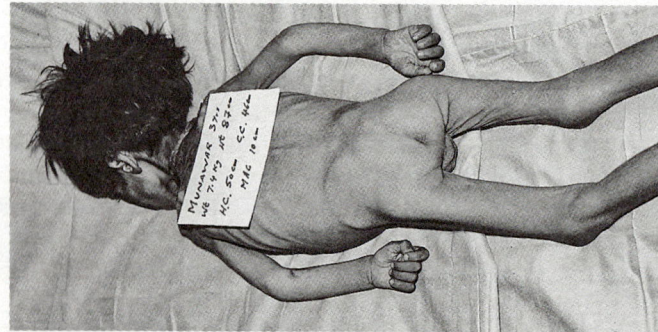

Figure 16.2 A 3-year-old boy with marasmus. Note wasted extremities, poor muscle mass, loss of subcutaneous fat (skin hangs in folds over buttocks and thighs) and visible bony prominences

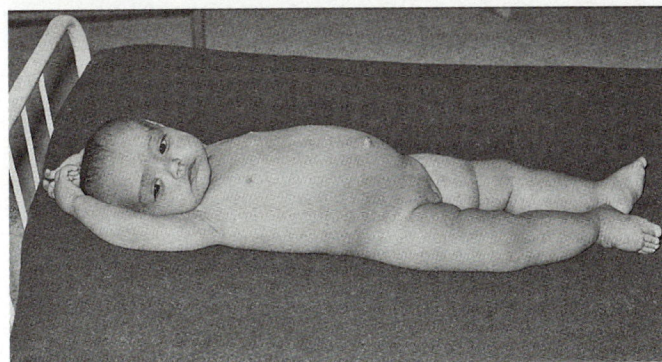

Figure 16.3 One and half year old girl with kwashiorkor. Note apathy, growth retardation, generalized edema, sparse hair, and crazy-pavement dermatosis over legs. There was hepatomegaly due to fatty infiltration of liver

Complications

Children with severe PEM are prone to suffer from acute intercurrent infections, oral thrush, septicemia and tuberculosis. They are unable to maintain body temperature and may develop severe hypothermia, hypoglycemia and electrolyte disturbances. It is difficult to assess the severity of dehydration in malnourished children because skin is loose and inelastic due to loss of subcutaneous fat. There may be associated deficiencies of other micronutrients especially nutritional anemia. Rickets is uncommon in malnourished children because rickets is a disease of growing bones.

Nursing Management

Nutritional rehabilitation is a slow process and demands health education to the family. It must be explained to parents that PEM is not a disease but child is suffering from lack of food. The following principles of management should be followed and explained to parents.

1. Keep the child warm and protected against nosocomial infections.
2. Identify intercurrent infections and treat them promptly with an appropriate antibiotic.
3. Look for associated metabolic disturbances like dehydration, hypoglycemia and dyselectrolytemia and treat them appropriately through intravenous route. In children with persistent diarrhea, lactose intolerance should be ruled out. Potassium supplements are required in all malnourished children.
4. Provide increasing quantities of well balanced liquid and semisolid food depending upon the appetite and acceptability of the child. When child refuses to accept oral feeds due to severe anorexia, nasogastric feeding is recommended. The calculation of the calories and proteins are based on the current or actual weight of the child. Start with 80 kcal/kg/d of energy and 0.7 g/kg of protein. The food intake is gradually increased, depending upon the tolerance of feeds, to 150 kcal/kg/d with 2–3 g proteins/kg/d over next 7–10 days. Milk based diet fortified with vegetable or coconut oil with additional commercially available protein supplements or egg is suitable. Availability of ready-to-use therapeutic food (RUTF) has simplified the management of PEM. In children with lactose intolerance, lactose-free milk is recommended. Supplements of micronutrients including potassium and magnesium should be provided. Iron should preferably be given through parenteral route. When hemoglobin is below 6 g/dL, packed cells transfusion or whole blood can be given slowly after administration of a diuretic.
5. Nutrition education and health education must be provided to the family to prevent the recurrence of malnutrition.

SEVERE ACUTE MALNUTRITION (SAM)

Severe acute malnutrition (SAM) is a major public health problem affecting over 8 million under-5 children in India. In view of the fact that malnutrition is the core health problem in children, SAM is an important component of Integrated Management of Neonatal and Childhood Illnesses (IMNCI) at the community level. In children between the ages of 6 and 59 months, severe acute malnutrition is diagnosed by the presence of any one of the following clinical criteria.

 i. Weight-for-length/height of < −3SD of WHO reference standard.
 ii. Presence of severe wasting.
 iii. Pitting edema of both feet due to malnutrition.
 iv. Mid-upper arm circumference (MUAC) of < 11.5 cm.

Most children with SAM can be managed on an ambulatory or OPD basis if there are no complications and child has a good appetite. The appetite of the child can be assessed by a "trial of feeding" test at home or health center **(Table 16.2)**.

Table 16.2 Criteria for passing appetite test	
Body weight (kg)	*Minimum amount of RUTF to be consumed for passing the appetite test (mL or g)*
< 4	15
4 – 6.9	25
7 – 9.9	35
10 – 14.9	50

RUTF; ready to use therapeutic food.

16

Appetite and weight gain of the child should be assessed during each home visit or visit of the child to the health care facility. When appetite is good and child is gaining weight at a rate of >5g/kg/day (after disappearance of edema), ambulatory care should be continued. The indications for referral and hospital management of children with SAM are listed below:

1. Age below 6 months.
2. Presence of edema of both feet.
3. Reduced appetite (failed appetite test).
4. Presence of one or more complications.

A detailed assessment of the child should be done and management provided as per algorithm **(Figure 16.4)**. The care taker or mother should be counseled about breast feeding, optimal intake of complementary feeds, importance of personal hygiene, immunizations and appropriate health promotional activities.

OBESITY

Overnutrition and obesity is being increasingly recognized in children belonging to the affluent families of our society. Over one-third of adolescent children attending private schools are obese. School going and adolescent children are crazy to take calorie-dense unhealthy and ill balanced snacks and junk foods like soft drinks, burgers, pizzas, chocolates, desserts, etc. A weight-for-height of greater than 85th and 95th percentile of NCHS or WHO reference standards is suggestive of over weight and obesity, respectively. According to WHO body mass index [weight in kg/ (height in meters)^2] of greater than 2SD of BMI-for-age, reference standard is considered as a more reliable criterion for making the diagnosis of obesity. Obese children are usually likely to be tall for their age if obesity is due to constitutional causes or overeating. The bone age is usually advanced. It is important to

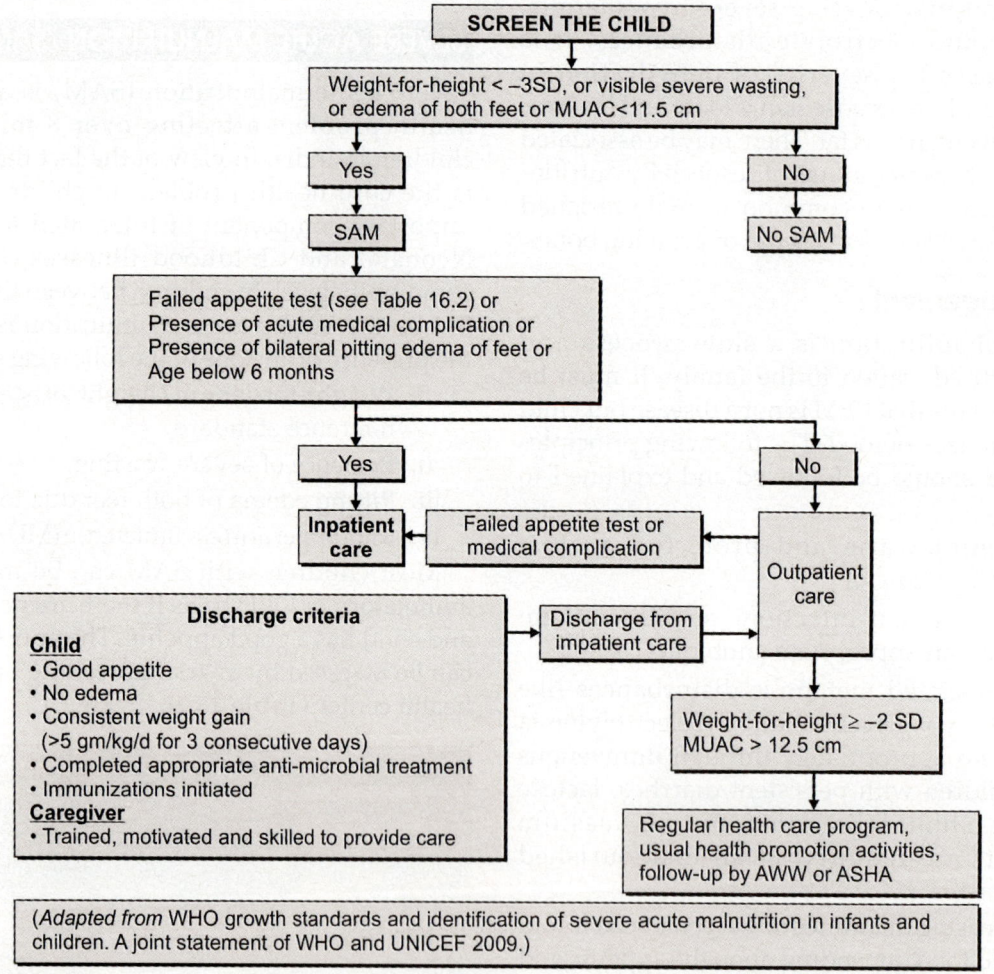

Figure 16.4 Identification and management of children with severe acute malnutrition (SAM)
ASHA, accredited social health activist; AWW, *anganwadi* worker; MUAC, mid-upper arm circumference; SAM, severe acute malnutrition

remember that obese adolescent children are likely to become obese adults later in life with all the attendant health hazards like hypertension, type 2 diabetes mellitus and coronary artery disease. Obese children are likely to have low self-esteem and emotional problems leading to isolation, laziness and excessive intake of food. Obesity due to hormonal imbalance is uncommon. It occurs at a younger age and is usually associated with additional manifestations like hypertension, short stature and mental retardation **(Figure 16.5)**. Other features of secondary or endogenous obesity include excessive oppetite, central obesity with "buffalo-hump", and hypogonadism.

Causes

Obesity occurs due to imbalance between energy or food intake and energy expended by physical activity. Intake of excessively fatty energy-dense junk food and

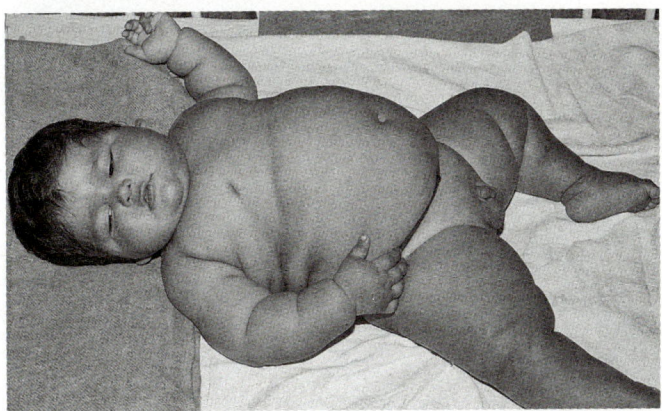

Figure 16.5 One and half year old boy with obesity and hypogonadism

munching of snacks in-between meals are important risk factors. Sedentary life style, lack of participation in outdoor games, excessive viewing of television and playing video games for prolonged periods of time further aggravates the situation because the food consumed is not utilized and extra calories are laid down in the fat depots like abdomen, buttocks and limbs. The risk of obesity is high if there is family predisposition to develop obesity. There is increasing incidence of hypertension, metabolic syndrome X and type 2 diabetes mellitus among obese adolescent children. Endogenous or secondary obesity is rare and account for less than 1% cases and occurs because of genetic and endocrinal causes. The salient differences between constitutional and pathological or endogenous obesity are shown in **Table 16.3**.

Nursing Management

1. The whole family should be advised to change the life style. It is impossible to change the routine and habits of the child unless every body in the family cooperates and participates.
2. The child should be asked to maintain a record of all foods eaten over a 24-hour period over a period of 1–2 weeks. Healthy food habits should be practiced by taking plenty of green leafy vegetables, salads, and seasonal fruits. Food should be prepared in minimum oil or fat. Energy dense foods like soft drinks, junk food, crisps and french fries, fried items (poories, samosas, kachoris, mathies, namkeen, etc.), desserts, dry fruits, and chocolates, etc. should be restricted. Double-toned or fat-free milk should be used for drinking and for making curd, cheese and

Table 16.3 Salient differences between constitutional (familial) and pathological or endocrinal obesity		
Feature	*Constitutional obesity*	*Pathological obesity*
■ Family history	Common	Absent
■ Eating behavior and lifestyle	Excessive eating, faulty eating habit, sedentary lifestyle	Eating normal or excessive, activity is affected after onset of obesity
■ Distribution of fat	Generalized	Central obesity with "buffalo hump" with greater deposition of fat on the face and upper back
■ Height and bone age	Usually increased with advanced bone age	Usually stunted with retarded bone age
■ Blood pressure	Usually normal	May be raised
■ Endocrinal features	None	Acne, hirsutism, amenorrhea or menstural irregularities, metablic syndrome X and type 2 diabetes mellitus.
■ Hypogonadism	None but penis may be embedded in the pubic pad of fat	May be associated in several syndromes
■ Central nervous system manifestations	None, laziness and inactivity may be the cause or consequence of obesity	Excessive sleep, hydrocephalus with visual field defects, papilledema or retinal degeneration and mental retardation.

16

other milk products. Before eating the meals, salads and water can be taken to fill the stomach. Missing of meals and "dieting" are strongly condemned. The use of drugs to reduce appetite is not recommended

3. The child should be encouraged to take part in outdoor activities and sports like running, jogging, skipping, cycling, and swimming. He should be encouraged to play outdoor games like badminton, tennis, football or cricket depending upon his interest. Aerobic exercises and dancing with music are extremely useful and health-friendly activities. Television viewing should be restricted to maximum of one hour and no snacks should be allowed while viewing the television.

4. The goal for weight reduction should be realistic, slow and sustainable. Motivation and will power are required to stick to the weight reduction program. It is reasonable to target a weight reduction of about 0.5–1.0 kg every 2 to 4 weeks.

5. Treatment of secondary or endogenous obesity is symptomatic and depends on the underlying cause.

BIBLIOGRAPHY

Jolley CD, Failure to thrive. *Curr Prob Pediatr Adosesc Health* 2003, 33(6): 183–206.

Lodha R. Nutritional rehabilitation of children with severe acute malnutrition. *Indian J Pediatr* 2016, 83(1):1–2.

Maggioni A, Lifshitz F. Nutritional management of failure to thrive. *Pediatr Clin North Am* 1995, 42(4): 791–810.

Menon PSN. Childhood obesity, metabolic syndrome and pentraxin-3. *Indian J Pediatr* 2015, 82(1):3–4.

17

Immunity and Allergy

IMMUNE DEFENSE MECHANISMS

Our body is equipped with an efficient immune system that protects us from the onslaught of various antigens and disease-causing pathogens. Disease is caused by an interaction between the load or virulence of the pathogens and the status and strength of the host defenses to contain or eliminate the disease-producing microbes. As children grow and develp from fetal life, through infancy, and childhood, their immune system gradually matures and becomes competent and efficient. Children (especially newborns and infants) are more vulnerable to develop infections, which are likely to take a serious course, because it is their first or nascent contact with the microbes. At this stage, children lack any specific antibodies to ward off the infections and their immune system is not primed to elicit an enhanced cell-mediated or humoral response to eliminate disease-causing microbes. To boost their defense capabilities and ward off common life-threatening or disabling infections, children are given vaccines. Active immunization by administration of vaccines is the most cost-effective and safe strategy to build specific immune capabilities of children to improve their survival. The immune system also protects against autuimmune diseases and malignancy.

Natural or Innate Host Defense Mechanisms

The human body is equipped with several innate protective mechanisms to ward off infections. The salient innate defense mechanisms are discussed below.

Skin Barrier

Bacteria cannot penetrate intact skin, which is made up of four layers. The outer layer or epidermis is constantly shed and does not allow bacteria to settle or penetrate. The sweat is anti-infective because of high salt content, low pH (sebum), and the presence of lysozyme and lactobacilli. Skin cells also secrete antimicrobial peptides such as cathelicidins, defensins, and dermicidins. Some of the non-pathogenic bacteria colonizing the skin secrete proteins toxic to other species, which are known as bacteriocins. The protective cells of the innate immune system (Langerhans cells and mast cells) and the acquired immune cells (lymphocytes) are also found in the dermis to tackle bacteria that are able to penetrate through the broken epidermis.

Mucous Membranes

Internal body surfaces that are exposed to the environment can be broadly classified into respiratory tract, gastrointestinal tract (GI), and urogenital tract. These organs are provided with protective mucous membranes that prevent the entry of allergens and pathogens from various body orifices such as nostrils, mouth, urethra, vagina and anal orifice.

The secretions of mucous membranes such as tears, saliva, and gastric juices have a washing effect and are replete with anti-infective agents. Cilia in the respiratory tract and cough mechanism try to expel pathogens trapped in the viscous mucus. The respiratory epithelium secretes several antibacterial agents including lysozyme, transferrin, α-1-antitrypsin, opsonins and interferon.

In contrast to the respiratory tract where potential pathogens are swept retrograde or proximally, the bacteria are moved forward by peristalsis and expelled distally (except through vomiting because of gastritis) in case of the GI tract. Most bacteria are killed in the stomach because of acidic pH and those entering the small intestine are tackled by bile and pancreatic secretions. The intestinal wall is protected by mucins, lysozyme, and immunoglobulins, which are secreted on the surface of epithelial cells. The gut is not sterile but is loaded with a host of friendly probiotics or non-pathogenic bacteria (such as lactobacilli, bifidobacteria, and bacteroides), which keep the pathogenic bacteria at bay by blocking the adhesion site, competing for nutrients, secretion of bacteriocins, and modulation of immune functions in the gut. They are also useful for synthesis of vitamin K and vitamin B_{12} in the gut.

The close proximity of introitus to the anal orifice is a risk factor for development of ascending urinary tract infection in girls. They should be taught to wash the bottom from front backward to prevent entry of fecal pathogens into the vagina and urethra. The flow of urine washes the microorganisms away from the urogenital tract. The host factors that may predispose to the development of urinary tract infection include defective hydrokinetic mechanism, increased density of receptor sites for bacteria, decreased secretory IgA and as a consequence of septicemia.

Non-Specific Defense Mechanisms

There are several innate or non-specific immune mechanisms, both humoral and cell-mediated, which prevent occurence of infection. The acute-phase proteins that are produced in response to inflammation (C-reactive protein, α-1-antitrypsin, ferritin, and mannose-binding lectin) bind with complement to cause lysis of bacteria. Several natural antibacterial agents such as lysozyme, defensin, lactoferrin, and myeloperoxidase help inactivate the invading pathogens. Defensins are a group of molecules produced by epithelal cells that cause lysis of various bacteria and fungi. They are produced in abundance in the oral cavity and perianal region. Despite high concentration of bacteria at these sites, clinically manifest infections are relatively uncommon due to protective role of defensins.

The circulating white blood cells, tissue phagocytes, mast cells, and natural killer (NK) cells serve as useful defense sentinels, which are ready to fight with invading pathogens. Neutrophils, monocytes and macrophages engulf the opsonized (coated with antibody or complement) bacteria and kill them in the phagosome by oxidative burst mechanism with the help of oxygen-free radicals, hydrogen peroxide, and hydroxyl ions. Eosinophils and basophils mostly provide a defense role against parasitic infections. The mast cells, which develop from pluripotent stem cells, migrate to the tissues to control allergic manifestations of disease by elaboration of peptide mediators such as substance P, endothelin, and lgE. They release several disease-fighting chemicals such as histamine, neutrophil chemotactic factor, inflammatory proteases, heparin, and preformed inflammatory mediators. Natural killer cells are large lymphocytes that recognize and kill cells that are infected with viruses or intracellular pathogens, as well as tumor cells.

ACQUIRED IMMUNITY

The acquired or adaptive immune response is of two types, humoral and cell-mediated.

Humoral Immunity

Immunoglobulins mediate antibody responses and they are found in blood, secretions, tissues and cell membranes. They combine with antigens to form immune complexes and can opsonize bacteria, fix complement, and neutralize viruses. There are five classes of immunoglobulins:

1. **Immunoglobulin G (IgG) antibodies** These are present in abundance and they activate complement via classical pathway, opsonize organisms, and mediate antibody-dependent cytotoxic responses.

2. **Immunoglobulin M (IgM) antibodies** These are the first antibodies to be elaborated in response to an infection. They are important for clearing bacteria from the blood stream by agglutination and opsonization. They are the most efficient fixer of complement via the classical pathway.

3. **Immunoglobulin A (IgA) antibodies** These are the secretory or surface antibodies and exert antiviral and antibacterial activity on the mucosal surfaces. They can fix complement via the alternate pathway and exert bactericidal activity on combining with lysozyme and complement.

4. **Immunoglobulin D (lgD) antibodies** These are mostly bound to B cell membranes and serve as antigen receptors to initiate the development of B cell responses.

5. **Immunoglobulin E (lgE) antibodies** These are known to trigger immediate hypersensitivity reaction and are useful for providing defense against parasitic infections.

Immunoglobulins are produced by the bone marrow-derived B cells. The IgD-coated B cells bind the antigen and with the help of T cells (helper T cells, Th cells), the B cells proliferate and evolve into plasma cells to produce IgM antibodies. The antigen coated or primed B cells become memory cells. When they are exposed to the same antigen again, they evolve into mature plasma cells and produce IgG antibodies as a booster response. In case of polysaccharide antigens (surrounding encapsulated organism), the B-cell response occurs without the help of T cells and it is limited to the production of mainly IgM antibodies without any B cell memory component. The development of IgG-producing plasma cells and T-independent responses are delayed up to 2 years of age. Infants are therefore more susceptible to suffer from infections because of encapsulated organisms having polysaccharide antigens such as pneumococcus, *Neisseria meningitides,* and *Haemophilus influenzae.*

Cell-mediated Immunity

Pluripotent hematopoietic stem cells evolve into lymphoid stem cells, which differentiate into T, B, and NK cells. Their further differentiation takes place in both the primary lymphoid organs (thymus and bone marrow) and the secondary lymphoid organs such as spleen, lymph nodes, tonsils, Peyer patches, and lamina propria.

Thymus and T Cells

During early fetal life, immature lymphocytes enter the thymus and evolve into thousands of T cells with different receptors. Those T cells that recognize "foreign antigens" bound to major histocompatibility complex (MHC) are preserved while those that recognize "self-antigens" are eliminated, reducing the risk for development of autoimmune disorders. During the process of phagocytosis and elimination of the organisms in the phagosome, a portion of the bacterial or viral antigen is presented to the T cell receptor sites that are associated with MAC molecules. Apart from macrophages, dendritic cells and B cells also capture antigen and present to the specially evolved T cells. During the maturation process, T cells acquire the surface markers CD_3, CD_4, and CD_5 (CD refers to *clusters of differentiation*), and differentiate into T-helper and cytotoxic or suppressor cells. T cell numbers are greater in infancy than in older children or adults but majority of them are naive and not primed to proliferate rapidly following their exposure to an antigen.

T-Helper Cells

T-helper cells have CD_4 marker and recognize antigen associated with MHC class II. They are classified into two types of T-helper cells. *T-helper* 1 (*Th1*) *cells* are credited to release interleukin 2 (IL 2), interferon gamma (lFN-γ), and tumor necrosis factor (TNF). They provide cell-mediated immune response including development of delayed tissue hyper-sensitivity (DTH). *T-helper* 2 (*Th2*) *cells* possess CD_{40} ligand and bind to CD_{40} to prime B cells into memory cells with an ability to provide an enhanced immune response. Th2 cells produce IL 4, IL 5, IL 6, IL 13, and IgE antibodies, which mediate immediate hypersensitivity response with allergic manifestations.

Cytotoxic or T-Suppressor Cells

T-cytotoxic cells (Tc) are characterized by CD_s marker and they bind to MHC class 1 receptors. They are responsible for killing virus-infected cells with the help of perforins and proteases.

Nutrition and Immunity

The association between undernutrition and increased susceptibility to respiratory and GI infections is well known. Apart from a higher incidence of infections, malnourished children are likely to have more severe infections with poor outcome. It is important to keep in mind that conditions leading to undernutrition are also associated with overcrowding, lack of sanitation or access to safe water, and poor vaccine coverage. The recurrent episodes of infections increase metabolic demands for nutrients, decrease the appetite with poor intake of food, thus setting up a vicious cycle of undernutrition–infection–undernutrition.

The immune cells have an extremely short half-life (half-life of polymorphs is merely 36 hours!) and therefore our immune system needs a constant supply of essential nutrients for its regeneration. *It is well known that immunological dysfunction is the earliest marker of a nutritional deficiency state.* Protein-energy malnutrition adversely affects T cell responses with atrophy of thymus and depletion of germinal centers in the lymph nodes. There may be lymphopenia with decreased CD_4:CD_8 ratio and reduced or delayed hypersensitivity response with occurrence of frequent viral, fungal, and opportunistic infections. The innate barrier or "frontline" defenses may be compromised by atrophy of skin and mucous membranes. Phagocytic functions are compromised with impaired bacterial killing (despite increased production of reactive oxygen-free radicals) because of reduced functioning of NK cells. Undernutrition is also associated with poor production of lysozyme and interferon, while levels of complement, CD_3, and CD_4 are raised. The level of leptin, which is credited to promote Th1 responses, may be reduced. The serum immuonoglobulin levels are usually well maintained or may be raised because of frequent infections. A large number of micronutrients are credited to be immunoprotective. The optimal intake of certain vitamins (especially vitamins A, C, D, E, B_6, and folic

Key Message
Promotion of exclusive breastfeeding, optimal nutrition and timely immunizations are the most cost effective strategies to prevent common day-to-day infections and promote health of children.

17

acid) and trace minerals such as iron, zinc, selenium, and copper are essential for optimal functioning of the immune system.

Breastfeeding

Exclusive breastfeeding during the first 6 months of life is the most cost-effective strategy to improve infant nutrition, prevent occurrence of day-to-day infections, and enhance child survival in developing countries. Human milk contains a large number of anti-infective agents such as immunoglobulins (especially secretory IgA), cellular elements (lymphoid cells, macrophages, and plasma cells), and non-specific humoral factors such as lysozyme, lactoferrin, opsonins, lactoperoxidase, and oligosaccharides. The highest concentration of secretory IgA in any body fluid is found in colostrum. Human milk contains friendly bacteria or probiotics such as lactobacilli and bifidobacteria, and their growth factor. By virtue of its anti-infective properties and virtual freedom from risk of contamination, the breastfed babies have a low incidence of infective diarrhea, respiratory infections, acute otitis media, and necrotizing enterocolitis. Breastfed babies have also been shown to have better humoral and cellular responses to oral and parenteral vaccines.

Correlates of Immune Deficiency Disorders

In developing countries, there is a high incidence of infections that occurs due to increased exposure to environmental pathogens because of poor environmental sanitation, lack of personal hygiene, contaminated water supply, overcrowding, denial of breastfeeding, and lack of effective immunization coverage. There are higher opportunities and greater risk of catching infections for a period of about 6 months when a child is sent to a creche or play school. Children with chronic medical conditions such as protein-energy malnutrition, nephrotic syndrome, severe burns, lymphoreticular malignancy, cystic fibrosis, atopic disorders, sickle cell disease, foreign bodies, and splenectomy are more vulnerable to suffer from infections. Immune dysfunction may occur because of administration of immuno-suppressive agents (steroids and chemotherapy) and following certain viral infections such as human immuno-deficiency virus, measles, and Epstein-Barr virus.

Congenital or primary immunodeficiency disorder is suspected when a child is having frequent episodes of infections in the absence of above-mentioned risk factors. Recurrent infections may occur by a particular type of pathogens (such as encapsulated organisms, namely pneumococcus, meningococcus, and *H.*

influenzae type b) with severe manifestations and a prolonged course. The infections may occur by opportunistic organisms (which are not usually pathogenic) such as candida, *Pneumocystis carinii*, cytomegalovirus, atypical mycobacteria, and crypto-sporidiosis. Recurrent abscesses are suggestive of chronic granulomatous disease (CGD). Immune deficiency is suspected when there are features of a syndrome that is known to be associated with immune disorders such as DiGeorge syndrome, ataxia telangiectasia, and Wiskott-Aldrich syndrome. The presence of neutropenia or lymphopenia on a routine blood test is a useful clue for further laboratory work-up. When there is severe local reaction or dissemination following BCG vaccine, it is suggestive of T cell deficiency and dysfunction of IFN-γ or IL 12. Family history of early child deaths or recurrent infections provides a supportive clue.

ALLERGY

The term *allergy* was coined by von Pirquet in 1906 to describe the "altered state of reactivity" to common environmental antigens or allergens. *Atopy* refers to a familial tendency to manifest IgE-mediated allergic disorders such as eczematous dermatitis, urticaria, hay fever, and bronchial asthma alone or in combination with atopic dermatitis.

Our body's immune system is designed to recognize and eliminate any foreign particle or protein (antigen) that enters our body. It has a remarkable ability to distinguish between "self" and "non-self" cells or antigens. There are many antigens that enter our body and our immune system views them as harmless. However, when a person has genetic susceptibility for allergy, the immune system reacts to these harmless substances (antigens or allergens) as a potential threat and starts reacting. Lymphocytes play a key role for both production of immunity as well as allergy. There are two types of lymphocytes, T and B lymphocytes. T lymphocytes are classified as killer-T and helper-T cells. The Th cells are again of two types; T and B lymphocytes. T lymphocytes are classified as killer-T and helper-T cells. The Th cells are again of two types; Th1 (infection fighters) and Th2 (allergy promoters). Dendritic cells, Langerhans cells, monocytes, and macrophages are called as antigen-presenting cells (APCs) as they play an important role in induction of allergic inflammation by presenting allergens to Th cells. When an atopic individual is exposed to an allergen, he or she responds by brisk proliferation of Th2 cells that secrete cytokines IL 4 and IL 13, which promote synthesis and development of eosinophils and basophils and prime the plasma cells to produce IgE antibodies. The binding of IgE antibodies to human mast cells and basophils sensitize these cells for subsequent antigen-specific activation or enhanced response. Mast cells reside in tissues. while basophils circulate in the blood. Each of these cells has more than 100,000 receptor sites for binding IgE antibodies. When a sensitized person is reexposed to the same allergen, it leads to enhanced production of specific IgE antibodies, which bind to sensitized basophils and eosinophils. which in turn are activated to release several chemicals that produce the symptoms of allergy. The most important chemical mediator is histamine, which gets attached to H1 receptors on the blood vessels, mucous glands, and bronchi to produce allergic manifestations. Other mediators that are released from mast cells induced leukotriene D_4 and prostaglandin D_2, which are credited to cause inflammation of airways of lungs.

Nursing Alert

When infections are controlled in a community, there is an increased risk of allergic disorders. Nature is supreme to maintain a balance in life.

When microbial pathogens enter the body, their products or toxins are carried by APCs to Th1 cells, which secrete cytokines including IFN-γ, which then prime plasma cells (B lymphocytes) to produce IgG and IgM antibodies. Th1 cytokines also activate phagocytes, produce opsonizing and complement-fixing antibodies to neutralize toxins and eliminate disease-causing microbes. There is evidence to suggest that proliferation of disease-fighting Thl cells inhibits the growth of allergy-mediating Th2 cells. In the past four decades, there has been remarkable increase in the prevalence of allergic diseases as a consequence of better sanitation facilities and control of infectious diseases. *It seems there is an inverse relationship between infections and allergic disorders in the community.* The developed countries are thus facing an epidemic of allergic disorders after having achieved some control over infectious diseases.

Atopy

Atopy is genetic or familial tendency for development of allergic or hypersensitivity disorders such as eczema, atopic dermatitis, hay fever, and bronchial asthma. The atopic individual readily becomes sensitized to common protein allergens at normal levels of exposure. Atopy is an immediate hypersensitivity disorder that is mediated through immunoglobulin IgE and atopic individuals usually have high levels of circulating IgE.

Familial predisposition to atopy has been linked to a gene on chromosome 11q which is located in close proximity to interleukin 4 (IL 4) gene on chromosome 5q.

Pseudoallergy

Pseudoallergy is a poorly undestood entity, which produces clinical manifestaions that are identical to an allergic reaction. Pseudoallergic reactions are usually associated with intake of certain medications and foods. In contrast to allergic reactions, the abnormal response may be triggered on first exposure (without any earlier sensitization) to the substance and there is no elevation of specific IgE antibodies. Drugs that are commonly implicated in pesudoallergic reactions include non-steroidal anti-inflammatory drugs, salicylates, angiotensin-converting enzyme inhibitors, contrast materials, plasma expanders, morphine, muscle relaxants, various anticonvulsants and antibiotics. A variety of foods can trigger pseudoallergic reactions, especially those rich in biogenic amines (histamine, serotonin, tyramine). Foods that are likely to trigger pseudoallergic reactions include nuts, cheese, red wine, and certain food additives such as preservatives and taste modifiers.

Idiosyncrasy

This is an inborn non-immunological reaction to a foreign substance in a susceptible individual. The symptoms are dose-related and appear with first exposure to the substance. The abnormal reaction is initiated through an enzyme defect such as lactose intolerance, acute hemolysis due to G6PD deficiency and hepatotoxicity to various drugs such as paracetamol and nimesulide.

Common Allergic Disorders

The common allergic disorders include anaphylaxis, angioedema, food intolerance or allergy, nasobronchial allergy (allergic rhinitis and bronchial asthma), skin allergy (atopic dermatitis, eczema, urticaria, and contact dermatitis), allergic conjunctivitis, insect-mediated allergy (mosquitoes, wasps, dust mites, cockroaches, and animal dander), drug allergy, and serum sickness.

ANAPHYLAXIS

Anaphylaxis is an immediate or type 1 hypersensitivity reaction that may be life-threatening. The allergen (protein, drug, or hapten) forms a complex with a specific IgE, which is then bound to the surface of effector cells such as mast cells and basophils. This leads to the release of chemical mediators (histamine,

17

leukotrienes, and proteases such as tryptase) because of mast cell degranulation that causes various clinical manifestations such as vasodilatation, capillary leaks, bronchoconstriction, laryngeal obstruction, and increased intestinal peristalsis and circulatory collapse. This mechanism is also operative in causation of symptoms of peanut allergy, milk allergy, drug reactions, allergic rhinitis, and bronchial asthma.

Adolescent children (especially girls) are prone to get vasovagal attack or syncope following a vaccine shot. There is sudden pallor, dizziness, lightheadedness, bradycardia, or feeble pulse. There is no bronchospasm or respiratory obstruction. The child with syncope should be placed flat on the bed, legs should be elevated, and provided with emotional support and reassurance. Syncope is usually transient and recovers spontaneously within a couple of minutes without any medications.

Management

Every nurse should have the know-how and should be adequately equipped to handle anaphylaxis in her practice. Adrenaline 0.01 mL/kg (1:1000 solution) should be given deep intramuscularly and can be repeated after 5 to 10-minute intervals. Subcutaneous administration is not recommended because subcutaneous tissues have only α-receptors leading to local vasoconstriction that inhibits absorption of adrenaline. Gastrointestinal and skin manifestations usually respond to administration of diphenhydramine or chlorpheniramine maleate 1 to 2 mg/kg intramuscular or intravenous. Administration of corticosteroids has a limited therapeutic utility because of its delayed onset of action. Methylprednisolone (1 to 2 mg/kg) or hydrocortisone (5 to 10 mg/kg) can be administered IM or IV if a child is prone to have asthmatic attacks. When ventilation is unsatisfactory, bag and mask resuscitation should be provided. Shock is managed by administration of normal saline or Ringer lactate 20 ml/kg IV bolus.

BIBLIOGRAPHY

Atkins D. Food allergy principles and practices. *Medical Scientific Update* 2008; 24(2):4–13.

Braide DH. Molecular and cellular mechanism of allergic disease. *J Allergy Clin Immunol* 2001; 108 (2 suppl 2):S65–S71.

Brownell J, Casale TB. Anti-IgE therapy. *Immunol Allergy Clin North Am* 2004, 24(4): 551–568.

Buckley RH, Schiff RI. The use of intravenous immune globulin in immunodeficiency diseases. *N Engl J Med* 1991; 325(2):110–117.

MacDonald SM, Vonakis BM. Emerging therapies for allergic diseases. *Immunol Allergy Clin North Am* 2004;24(4):551–752.

Sampson HA. Anaphylaxis and emergency treatment. *Pediatrics* 2003; 111(6 Pt 3):1601–1608.

Savage JH, Matsui EC, Skripak JM, Wood RA. The natural history of egg allergy. *J Allergy Clin Immunol* 2007; 120(6):1413–1417.

Vaccine-Preventable Diseases

A number of deadly and disabling infectious diseases can be prevented by timely administration of vaccines. When a child is effectively immunized at the recommended age, most of these diseases are either entirely prevented or at least modified so that child suffers from a mild disease without any disability. The most amazing success stories of modern medicine include global eradication of smallpox in December, 1979 and paralytic poliomyelitis in 2014 following universal immunization program.

Modes of Spread of Infections

Communicable diseases are transmitted from an infected person to a susceptible host either directly or through an intermediate living host or vector and non-living objects (fomites). The common modes of spread of infection are given below:

1. *Direct contact* Infected person transmits infection directly by close contact, i.e. skin infections and sexually transmitted diseases.

2. *Air-borne and droplet infections* Air-borne transmission occurs by infected droplets of dust particles that remain suspended in the air for a variable period. The infected air particles remain viable and are dispersed by air currents for a variable distance. They get inhaled or deposited on the susceptible person leading to infection. The classical example of air-borne infection is pulmonary tuberculosis due to *Mycobacterium tuberculosis*. In case of droplet infection, the infected person transmits infection to close contacts through bouts of coughing, sneezing and by talking. The infected droplets are infectious for a brief period and are transmitted for a short distance thus requiring a close contact. Viral infections like common cold, exanthematous diseases, pertussis, streptococcal throat infection and influenza are transmitted through droplet infection.

3. *Food and water-borne diseases* Contaminated water and food are important sources of infection causing episodes of food poisoning, diarrhea, dysentery, cholera, typhoid fever, viral hepatitis (HAV, HEV infections) and worm infestations, etc.

4. *Living subjects* may serve as intermediate hosts or vectors of infection.

   Mosquitoes : Malaria, dengue fever, chikungunya, filaria, yellow fever, zika and Japanese encephalitis

   Sandflies : Kala-azar

   Dogs : Rabies, hydatid disease, visceral larva migrans

   Cats : Toxoplasmosis, visceral larva migrans, rabies, cat scratch disease

   Chicken : Bird flu, severe acute respiratory syndrome (SARS)

   Pigs : Japanese encephalitis, swine flu, *T. solium*, cysticercosis, trichinosis

   Cattle : Anthrax, leptospirosis, atypical mycobacteria, brucellosis, *T. saginata*, Creutzfeldt-Jakob disease

   Rats : Rat bite fever, plague, tularemia, leptospirosis

   The infectious diseases transmitted from vertebrate animals to human beings are called zoonosis.

5. *Non-living objects* (*fomites*) Direct contact with infected clothes (handkerchief, towel, sheet, bedding, etc.), medical and surgical instruments, and appliances, books, toys and utencils can transmit several viral and bacterial infections.

6. *Blood-borne infections* Infection may be transmitted through contaminated needles (abscess, HBV, HCV, HIV), transfusion of infected blood or blood products (malaria, HBV, HCV, HIV, CMV), homo- or heterosexual activity (HIV, HBV).

7. *Placenta* Maternal infections may be transmitted to the fetus (mother-to-fetus vertical trsansmission)

18

during pregnancy, labor and delivery (TORCH infections, HBV, HIV).

A brief description of vaccine-preventable diseases is given below. Children with vaccine-preventable diseases are generally so sick that they need to be admitted in the hospital for management.

TUBERCULOSIS

It is caused by *Mycobacterium tuberculosis* and remains a public health problem despite the availability of a vaccine. Infection occurs at any age through droplets disseminated by breathing and coughing by an adult patient who discharges bacilli in the sputum. Children account for 10% of all cases of tuberculosis. Most cases occur during 1–4 years of age and adolescents. Among adolescents, fibrocaseous tuberculosis is three to four times more common in girls because of high incidence of nutritional disorders and stress of menstruation.

Pathogenesis

The tubercular bacilli are inhaled through droplet infection during close contact with an adult patient who is sputum positive. The usual incubation period is 4–6 weeks but it may take up to 3 months for development of delayed skin hypersensitivity to tuberculosis or positivity of Mantoux test. During primary infection, the bacilli lodge in the peripheral region of middle and lower lobes of the lungs. The bacilli spread through lymphathics to involve hilar or mediastinal lymph nodes. *The classical triad of pulmonary focus in the lungs with lymphangitis and enlarged hilar lymph nodes is called primary complex.* The host develops both protective cell-mediated immunity against future infection, and reactive tissue hysensitivity or delayed type hypersensitivity (DTH) response which may cause caseation and necrosis, especially during subsequent reinfection or reactivation of dormant bacilli during adolescence and adult life. It seems that cell-mediated immunity is a favourable immunologic response, whereas DTH is an adverse immunological reaction against various antigens of tubercular bacilli. The symptoms appear depending upon the virulence of the organisms, nutritional status of the host, the level of specific protective cell-mediated immunity against tubercle bacilli and the extent of reactive DTH response. In most primary infections, there are no symptoms because the body is able to eliminate or control the multiplication of bacilli. The recovery occurs by calcification, but the bacilli may remain dormant and get reactivated when the body's resistance falls because of adverse factors such as malnutrition, viral infections (measles, HIV) intake of corticosteroids and chemotherapy.

Clinical Features

Tuberculosis most commonly affects lungs causing a low grade fever, cough, loss of appetite, night sweats, easy fatigue and weight loss. Tuberculosis can virtually affect any organ of the body including lymph glands, brain, heart, liver, kidneys, intestines, bones, joints, and skin. The disease manifests when body defences are weakened by undernutrition and viral infections like measles and HIV. *The diagnosis of tuberculosis should be seriously considered when any child has prolonged fever (>2 weeks), failure to thrive, irritability, poor weight gain or weight loss with or without cough.*

> **Nursing Alert**
>
> *Tuberculosis may occur at any age group, can infect any organ of the body, produce any symptom complex and must be considered in the differential diagnosis of each and every disease process.*

The classical anatomical features of tuberculosis at the site of entry of tubercular bacilli are designated as *Primary complex*. There is a parenchymal focus of infection in the lung with involvement of draining lymphatics and inflammation and enlargement of regional lymph nodes in the hilum. In a healthy or immune host, there may be spontaneous recovery or disease may remain localized. But when child is malnourished or immunocompromised, the disease may spread locally (causing pleural, pericardial and peritoneal effusion, progressive primary complex, bronchopneumonic tuberculosis, abdominal tuberculosis, cervical lymphadenitis, etc.) or there may be hematogenous spread leading to miliary tuberculosis, tubercular meningitis, tubercular osteomyelitis or arthritis and genitourinary tuberculosis.

Diagnosis

The diagnosis is suspected on the basis of suggestive clinical features and history of contact with an adult patient of tuberculosis. Despite introduction of several newer diagnostic tests, the diagnosis of tuberculosis is usually based on conventional tests like tuberculin test, charactersitic evidences of tuberculosis in the chest, bones, joints and various body organs by imaging studies and isolation of AFB on smear and culture studies.

Mantoux test (tuberculin skin test) by intradermal injection of 0.1 mL 2 TU purified protein derivative (PPD) RT-23 or 5TU PPD-s over anterior or volar surface of left forearm. The test site is inspected for size of induration (not erythema) after 48 to 72 hours. Induration of 10 mm or more suggests that either the child had tuberculosis in the past or is currently having active disease. If Mantoux test is positive in a children less than 3 years of age, they are treated for tuberculosis. Tuberculin test may show minimal or no response in an immunocompromised child or in a child with disseminated or life-threatening disease. There may be radiological evidences of tuberculosis on imaging studies of chest, bones, joints and other body organs.

Identification and isolation of AFB on smear and culture remains the gold standard for definitive diagnosis of tuberculosis. In children, most cases are paucibacillary and concerted efforts are required to isolate the bacteria. In adolescents with fibrocaseous tuberculosis, two samples of sputum should be collected for Ziehl-Neelsen (ZN) stain and culture. GeneXpert MTB/RIF cartridge based assay detect DNA sequences specific for *M. tuberculosis* and resistances to rifampicin (RIF) by nucleic acid amplification test (NAAT). The test is done on sputum sample or body fluid, it can be processed with little technical training and result is available in 90 minutes.

In young children, induced sputum can be collected following nebulization with a bronchodilator and hypertonic saline (sodium chloride 3% or 5% solution). Alternatively, gastric aspirate can be examined for isolation of tubercular bacilli because young children swallow the sputum. Nasogastric tube is inserted at night and 20 to 50 mL gastric aspirate is collected early in the morning without disturbing the child. The sample is neutralized with sodium bicarbonate after collection because acidic pH of aspirate may kill the bacilli. When procedure is done diligently and three consecutive morning samples of gastric aspirate are processed, the isolation rate of tubercular bacilli varies between 40% and 70%.

Efforts can be made to isolate the pathogens from bronchoscopic lavage, CSF (at least 15 mL sample), pleural, pericardial and peritoneal aspirate, cold abscess and urine by smear and culture studies. Aspiration material or biopsy from lymph node, liver and bone marrow may yield the bacilli specially in children with AIDS.

Culture studies on conventional agar-based or Lowenstein-Jensen medium usually takes 2 to 4 weeks. The automated liquid culture techniques, such as TB-BACTEC radiometric method and mycobacterium growth indicator tube (MGIT) 960 system gives the results within 7 to 12 days. Apart from definitive diagnosis, culture studies are useful to study the sensitivity pattern of bacilli to various antitubercular drugs.

The diagnosis can also be confirmed by histopathological features on fine needle aspiration cystology (FNAC) of lymph node and liver biopsy. A large number of serological tests are being promoted for the diagnosis of tuberculosis but WHO has issued specific guidelines that serological tests are unreliable and should not be used for the diagnosis of tuberculosis. Interferon-gamma release assay (Quantiferon-TB gold test) is a "glorified" Mantoux test with the advantage that the result is not affected by previous BCG vaccination.

Treatment

Adequate rest, good nursing care, exposure to sunshine, nutritious balanced diet with adequate intake of calories and proteins is recommended. The source of infection should be identified and managed appropriately. The family should be screened to identify all infected subjects. A combination of antitubercular drugs is used to prevent emergence of resistant strains of tubercular bacilli. The drugs are given as a single dose on empty stomach. The first line antitubercular drugs include isoniazid or INH (H), rifampicin (R), ethambutol (E), streptomycin (S) and pyrazinamide (Z). Pyrazinamide is given for initial 2 months while total duration of therapy varies between 6 months and 9 months, depending upon the extent and severity of disease process as follows:

Pulmonary primary complex, fibrocaseous tuberculosis, pleural effusion, cervical adenitis: 2 HRZ + 4 HR, i.e. 2 months of isoniazid, rifampicin and pyrizinamide followed by additional 4 months of isoniazid and rifampicin.

Progressive pulmonary tuberculosis, miliary tuberculosis, tubercular meningitis, skeletal tuberculosis, abdominal tuberculosis, genitourinary tuberculosis: 2 HRZE + 7 HR.

The daily doses of first-line antitubercular drugs are given below:

Rifampicin 10 mg/kg (max 600 mg/d), isoniazid or INH 10 mg/kg (max 600 mg/d), ethambutol 20–25 mg/kg (max 1500 mg/d), pyrazinamide or PZA 30–35 mg/kg (max 2000 mg/d) and streptomycin sulfate 15 mg/kg (max 1.0 g/d). It is desirable to have rational combination of antitubercular drugs in a dispersible format for ease of administration.

Corticosteroids are used in children with tuberculous meningitis, serosal tuberculosis (pericarditis, pleuritis, peritonitis), miliary tuberculosis and terminally ill children.

In order to ensure compliance and reduce the duration of antitubercular therapy to 6 months, Government of India has launched DOTS (directly observed therapy schedule) wherein health worker administers medicines to the patients 3 times in a week under her direct supervision. Based on six weight

18

groups (6–8, 9–12, 13–16, 17–20, 21–24 and 25–30 kg), the health worker keeps the medicines in patient-wise boxes (PWBs). In DOTS program, four drugs (HRZE) are given for 2 months in all types of ambulatory cases of tuberculosis. The DOT centers are provided with pestle and mortar for crushing the tablets.

Multidrug resistant (MDR) tuberculosis is emerging as a major public health problem when infection occurs from an adult having MDR-tuberculosis and when irregular or suboptimal treatment is given especially in immuno-compromised children. The WHO sponsored new molecular test known as "line probe assay" and GeneXpert MTB/RIF assay can diagnose MDR-tuberculosis in less than two hours. The Revised National Tuberculosis Control Programme (RNTP) is designed to provide an effective treatment against drug resistant cases of tuberculosis. These patients are classified into MDR-tuberculosis (resistant to both INH and rifampicin) and extensively-resistant tuberculosis when tubercular bacilli are resistant to INH, rifampicin, fluoroquinolone, aminoglycosides, bedaquiniline and delamanid.

> *"The World tuberculosis day is commemorated on march 24 to highlight the global efforts in eradicating the disease."*

Prevention

Bacille-Calmette-Guerin (BCG) is a live (attenuated or weakened bacilli) vaccine and given intradermally (inside the skin) with a special 26 G needle and syringe on the top of left shoulder. The vaccine is given soon after birth (within 4 weeks of age) in a 0.1 mL single dose. There is no need for any boosters. It is not very effective vaccine but does prevent occurrence of severe and disseminated disease so that vaccinated child suffers from a mild and localized disease. INH chemoprophylaxis (10 mg/kg/d) is recommended for 6 months to (i) asymptomatic contacts (<5 years) of a smear positive case, (ii) HIV-positive children with history of contact with an infectious case of TB or those with positive Mantoux test (>5 mm) and (iii) all Mantoux positive children receiving immunosuppressive drugs.

LEPROSY (Hansen Disease)

Leprosy is a chronic granulomatous disease caused by acid-fast rod-shaped bacilli called *Mycobacterium leprae*. Leprosy is among the world's oldest and most dreaded diseases because of the stigma and development of hideous physical deformities. The disease primarily affects skin, peripheral nerves, skeletal muscles, upper respiratory tract and eyes. India is the home for the largest number of leprosy patients, which are distributed in over 700 leper colonies. According to WHO, over 35% new cases of leprosy occur in India. The current prevalence of leprosy in India has dropped to 0.68 per 10,000 population. Most infections occur during childhood and require close contact with an infectious patient over several months. The leprosy causing bacilli multiply very slowly with an average incubation period of about 5–7 years. Leprosy is called *Kusht rog* in Hindi and a large number of humantarian organisations including *Hindu Khusht Nivaran Sangh* (Indian Leprosy Association 1981) have provided yeoman's service to eradicate leprosy. World anti-leprosy day is celebrated on January 31 to create awareness against leprosy.

Epidemiology

The disease is caused by extremely slow growing pathogens *Mycobacterium leprae*. The infection occurs through air-borne droplets discharged from upper airway passages by sneezing, nose blowing or coughing. Rarely, baclli are discharged from ulcerated or broken skin lesions. The infection usually occurs due to prolonged household contact with an infectious patient living in overcrowded, poor hygienic and unsatisfactory socioeconomic conditions. The disease is characterized by a large number of psychosocial characterisitcs like fear, guilt, social stigma and wrong belief about lack of effective treatment or incurability of the disease.

Clinical Features

It is a relatively 'silent' or slow evolving disease, which demands high index of suspicion for an early diagnosis. It is an important cause of development of acquired hideous deformities, disfigurements and disabilities. Based on the morphology of skin manifestations, the disease is classified into five clinical subtypes.

1. *Indeterminate type* It is characterised by one or two well defined hypopigmented macules which have reduced sensations or no sensations (anesthetic). There is atrophy of skin with localized loss of sweating and hair over the involved site. The skin lesions are smear negative.

2. *Tuberculoid type* The skin lesions are flat or raised or nodular, hypopigmented, erythematous and anesthetic. Skin lesions are smear negative.

3. *Borderline type* This variant may overlap or merge either with tuberculoid or lepromatous leprosy. There are at least four or more skin lesions which

may be flat or raised, well defined or ill defined, hypopigmented, erythematous with sensory impairment or complete sensory loss. Skin lesions may or may not be smear positive.

4. *Lepromatous type* These patients are characterized by numerous skin lesions which are flat or raised, poorly defined, shiny or smooth, and symmetrically distributed. Nasal smears and skin lesions are usually smear positive.

5. *Neuritic type* These patients demonstrate predominant involvement of peripheral nerves which are thickened and cause progressive peripheral neuropathy with sensory-motor disturbances.

In advanced cases of leprosy, the diagnosis is obvious on the basis of ugly deformities like saddle nose, disfigured nodule-ridden face, loss of eyebrows and eyelashes, clawed hand and toes, foot drop, intractable plantar ulcers due to glove and stocking anesthesia and ocular complications. Recurrent episodes of reactivation of disease, due to Arthus phenomenon or lepra reactions because of administration of sulfone drugs are characterised by episodes of high grade fever, arthralgias, lymph node enlargement, erythema nodosum, iridocyclitis, glaucoma and orchitis.

In view of emerging multidrug therapy protocols, leprosy may be classified into two major types. Paucibacillary leprosy account for 60% cases and it includes smear-negative cases of indeterminate, tuberculoid, borderline or pure neuritic type of leprosy. The other major variant is multibacillary leprosy which include smear-positive cases of borderline or lepromatous leprosy.

Laboratory Diagnosis

Skin smear, nasal smear or scrapings should be examined for *M. leprae*. A punch biopsy from the edge of skin lesion or nasal lesion is confirmatory. A delayed skin hypersensitivity (akin to tuberculin test) or lepromin test can be performed. The extract of inactivated leprosy bacilli is injected under the skin of anterior left forearm. Induration of more than 10 mm after 48 hr or a nodule of >5 mm after 21 days is suggestive of a positive lepromin test. The test is positive in all forms of leprosy except in the most severe or contagious lepromatous leprosy. A dipstick assay test can detect *M. leprae* specific phenolic glycolipid 1 (PGL-1) antibodies within 10 minutes with a sensitivity

of 90–97%. In multibacillary lepromatous leprosy, the availability of one-step reverse transcriptase PCR assay is a sensitive test to detect bacilli in slit smears and skin biopsy specimens.

Treatment

In view of social stigma attached to the disease, the patient needs compassionate and humanized care both in hospitalized and home-based care. The principles of nursing care include isolation, healthy and hygienic environment, nutritious diet, prevention of injuries and aseptic care of wounds. A number of drugs are available for eradication of *M. leprae*.

WHO provides blister packs of antileprosy drugs free of charge to ensure compliance. A single lesion paucibacillary disease (PB) is treated by administration of a single dose of rifampicin 600 mg, ofloxacin 400 mg and minocycline 100 mg. Patients of paucibacillary disease (Indeterminate, tuberculoid or borderline disease) with multiple skin lesions are treated with rifampicin 600 mg over a month, and dapsone 100 mg daily for 6 months. Multibacillary (MB) patients with lepromatous leprosy are managed with rifampicin 600 mg over a month, dapsone 100 mg daily and clofazimine 300 mg once a month and 50 mg daily are administered for 12 months or till patient is smear-negative for *M. leprae*. Children between 5 and 14 years are administered one-half of the adult dose. Anti-leprosy drugs are contraindicated in children below 5 years and pregnant women.

During treatment with sulfone drugs, acute allergic lepra reactions can be managed by short course of corticosteroids. In advanced cases, correction of deformities, cosmetic surgery and rehabilitation are integral part of management.

Prevention

Multibacillary cases of leprosy should receive early multidrug therapy along with nasal instillation of rifampicin drops or spray. Health education and public health measures are essential to prevent infection to family contacts. There is some evidence that BCG vaccination and administration of dapsone for chemoprophylaxis to close contacts, are useful preventive measures. Avoidance of overcrowding and intake of nutritious diet are associated with reduced risk of transmission of the disease.

18

> *"Leprosy work is not merely medical relief, it is transforming frustration of life into joy of dedication, personal sacrifice and selfless service of humanity"*
> — **Mahatma Gandhi**

POLIOMYELITIS

Poliomyelitis is caused by 3 serotypes of viruses (polio 1, 2, 3) and usually affect children below 5 years of age. The virus enters the body by taking contaminated water and food (orofecal route). The virus is shed in the stools of a polio patient for 2–4 weeks. This contaminates sewage water, which in turn contaminates drinking water and food when sanitation conditions are unsatisfactory. The initial symptoms are fever, vomiting, diarrhea and cough. Most cases recover like any other viral infection without any paralysis. It is important to remember that for one case of paralytic polio there are at least 100–1000 children who develop non-paralytic polio and recover without any paralysis. Intramuscular injections in these asymptomatic patients can lead to development of paralytic polio. In some children, disease progresses to cause pain and soreness in muscles, stiffness of neck and back followed 2–3 days later by weakness or paralysis of a group of muscles in the lower limbs, upper limbs and muscles of breathing. Transistory urinary retention and constipation may occur due to autonomic involvemet. The paralysis of vagus nerve causes weakness of soft palate, pharynx and vocal cords leading to nasal voice and nasal regurgitation. The paralysis is flaccid, asymmetrical (unequal on two sides) and patchy. Apart from severe disability due to paralysis, death can occur due to involvement of brainstem and paralysis of muscles of breathing. About 5–10% of patients develop bulbar or respiratory paralysis. Other conditions which are known to cause acute flaccid paralysis include infective polyneuritis (Guillain-Barre syndrome), post-diphtheritic paralysis, transverse myelitis and severe hypokalemia.

Treatment

Management is primarily symptomatic and supportive. Muscle pain and spasms are relieved by application of moist hot packs and administration of paracetamol. Ensure strict bed rest and give mild sedation to relieve anxiety. *Avoid intramuscular injections.*

Good nursing care and nutritious diet is essential for recovery. Intermittent oral suction is done to clear pooled secretions from pharynx. Child should be nursed in a prone position with head turned to one side to prevent aspiration. When respiratory failure supervenes, following paralysis of respiratory muscles, assisted breathing is provided with a mechanical ventilator. Physiotherapy is started as soon as muscle pain and spasm are relieved. Limbs are placed in a neutral position with soft splints and supports to prevent deformities. Passive movements and active exercises are started to promote development of muscle power in the non-paralyzed muscles. Emotional and psychological support should be provided to the child and family for better adjustment in life.

Prevention

Oral polio vaccine (OPV) 2 drops are given at birth (along with BCG), 6–8 weeks, 10–12 weeks, 14–16 weeks (with DTP), 15–18 months (with DTP booster) and 4½ years (with DTP booster). Vaccine can lose its potency unless stored under strict cold chain conditions or a refrigerator. In addition, all children below the age of 5 years, should receive additional doses of OPV which are given on predesignated sundays after every 2 weeks by public health authorities under the Pulse Polio Immunization Program. These doses are inaddition to six doses of OPV received during the routine immuniza-tion schedule. Inactivated polio vaccine (IPV) subcutaneously alone or in combination with OPV can be given to reduce the risk of vaccine-associated paraly-sis in immunocompromised children and as a part of strategy during eradication of poliomyelitis. India introduced bivalent OPV (containing polio viruses 1 and 3) on 24th April, 2016 to maintain protective efficacy of the vaccine and reduce the risk of vaccine associated paralytic poliomyelitis (VAPP). Proper environmental sanitation (effective and safe disposal of sewage) and personal hygiene (safe drinking water, hand washing with soap and water) are essential to prevent infection. Intramuscular injections should be avoided in children unless they are mandatory because paralysis of injected muscles may occur during an epidemic of polio. Following concerted public health measures and pulse polio immunization programme, India was declared polio free on 13 January, 2014.

HEPATITIS B

Hepatitis can occur due to a large number of viruses (Hepatitis A, B, C, D, E, G, etc). Hepatitis B infection occurs through blood (like HIV) from mother to her baby (during pregnancy and delivery), use of infected needles and syringes, administration of infected blood and blood products and through unsafe sex. The prevalence of hepatitis B (HBsAg-positive) in India varies between 3 to 5%. Hepatitis B is more contagious than HIV infection or AIDS. After incubation period of 1–3 months (time taken from the time of entry of virus into the body and development of symptoms of disease), the patient develops fever, loss of appetite, nausea, vomiting, pain over upper abdomen (due to enlargement of liver), high colored urine and jaundice (yellowness of eyes). Hepatitis is often prolonged and intractable and may lead to death due to liver failure. Some patients may develop extrahepatic manifestations like skin rash, arthritis, aplastic anemia, glomerulo-nephritis and myocarditis. Rarely a patient may develop cancer of liver after several years of infection with hepatitis B virus. Hepatitis B surface antigen (HBsAg or Austraila antigen) is positive in blood.

Laboratory Diagnosis

Urine examination is a useful screening test to find presence of urobilin, bile pigments and bile salts. Liver function tests are deranged with elevation of total and direct or conjugated bilirubin, elevation of hepatic transaminases and prothrombin time. Serological tests are useful for making an etiological diagnosis of hepatitis. Acute hepatitis is characterized by elevated hepatits B core IgM antibodies, while carriers are positive for hepatitis B surface antigen (HBsAg) and hepatitis e antigen (HBeAg). Hepatitis e antigen positivity is associated with rapid multiplication of hepatitis B virus with greater risk of transmission of infection.

Treatment

Treatment is supportive and symptomatic with high carbohydrate, normal protein and low fat diet. Fruit juices and sweet drinks are recommended. Several hepatoprotective drugs are available (L-ornithine, L-aspartate, silymarin) but their therapeutic utility is doubtful. Vitamin B complex is useful for providing nonspecific protection to the liver. There is no specific antiviral therapy.

Prevention

Hepatitis B vaccine (HBV) is given in three doses at 0 (at birth), 1 month and 6 months of age. A booster dose may be given after the age of 5 years. It is given subcutaneously over the outer side of mid-thigh. The baby born to a known hepatitis B carrier mother should receive 0.5 mL hepatitis B immune globulin (HBIG) along with a dose of HBV (at two different sites) within 12 hours of birth. The other preventive strategies are the same as recommended for prevention of AIDS.

DIPHTHERIA (Khunak)

It is caused by an infection by *C. diphtheriae*. Infection occurs through droplets spread by coughing, sneezing, talking or crying of an infected child. The incubation period is 2 to 5 days. There is moderate fever, sore throat and marked swelling of neck due to enlargement of lymph nodes. The child looks sick and toxic due to exotoxins produced by the bacteria. There is breathing difficulty as the air passages are blocked by thick whitish-grey pseudomembrane over the throat and larynx (voice box). There may be hoarseness of voice and stridor (noisy breathing) and chest retractions. The elaboration of toxins may cause post-diphtheritic palatal paralysis (inability to swallow with nasal regurgitation, nasal twang in the voice due to paralysis of palate), polyneuritis and myocarditis (swelling and weakness of heart). Death may occur due to suffocation (blockage of upper airways by diphtheritic membranes) and myocarditis.

Laboratory Diagnosis

Diphtheria-specific IgM antibodies are elevated. The diagnosis is confirmed by identification of *C. diphtheriae* on Albert stain of throat swab taken from beneath the membrane. Smear findings should be confirmed by doing culture studies, which can provide results within 8 hours.

Treatment

Penicillin or erythromycin is given for a duration of 14 days to eradicate bacteria from throat. Antidiphtheritic antitoxin 20,000–80,000 units is given IM or IV after skin sensitivity testing. Bedrest is advised to reduce cardiac decompensation. Easily digestible high-calorie diet is given. Supportive therapy includes administration of antipyretics and sedatives.

Complications should be looked for and appropriately managed. There is characteristic time table of occurrence of complications. Upper airwary obstruction occurs during initial 2 to 4 days of illness. Myocarditis usually occurs by the end of first week, followed by palatal paralysis (2 weeks), loss of accomodation (3 weeks) and polyneuritis (between 3 and 6 weeks). Humidifed oxygen is given for treatment of hypoxia due to respiratory obstruction. Severe airway obstruction is managed with timely tracheostomy. Children with palatal paralysis are fed with a nasogastric tube. Myocarditis is treated by bed rest, fluid and salt restriction, and diuretics.

Prevention

Triple antigen (DTwP or DTaP) contains antigens against 3 diseases; diphtheria, tetanus and pertussis (whooping cough). Three primary doses are given at 6–8 weeks, 10–12 weeks and 14–16 weeks followed by boosters at 15–18 months, 4½ years and 10 years. The Td (tetanus and low-dose diphtheria) vaccine is now available, which can be given whenever tetanus boosters are required to reduce the risk of diphtheria in adolescents and young adults. The vaccine is given intramuscularly over outer side of mid-thigh region or deltoid region. *It should never be given in the buttocks due to poor immune response and risk of injury to the sciatic nerve.*

18

18

PERTUSSIS (Whooping cough, *Kali khansi*)

Whooping cough is caused by *B. pertussis*. Infection occurs through droplets coughed out by the patient. The incubation period varies between 7 to 14 days. Initial symptoms are like cough and cold, i.e. fever, watery discharge from nose and cough. After 5–6 days there are bouts of severe paroxysmal cough. The cough is intense and spasmodic with face becoming red or blue and is usually followed by vomiting. At the end of bout of coughing, the child may take a deep breath which produces a typical sound of a "whoop". Whoop is produced by the rush of air during inspiration through the partially open glottis. The paroxymal bouts of cough may lead to development of hernia, rectal prolapse and subconjunctival hemorrhage. The child is unable to feed properly due to frequent bouts of coughing and vomiting. The bouts of spasmodic cough may last for 2–4 weeks. Whooping cough is a serious disease in young infants leading to development of pneumonia, subcutaneous emphysema, pneumothorax, bronchiectasis, tuberculosis and swelling or bleeding in the brain (encephalopathy). The convalescence may be prolonged with development of pulmonary complications and malnutrition.

Treatment

Disease is life-threatening in infants below 6 months and they should be managed after hospitalization. Humidification of air reduces viscosity of mucus and facilitates expectoration. Erythromycin (40–50 mg/kg/d) is given for 10–14 days to reduce period of infectivity and shorten the course of disease. Nebulization with salbutamol or oral bronchodilators may reduce the bouts of coughing. Provide good nursing care and ensure intake of nutritious diet. It is best to feed the child immediately after the bout of cough. In intractable cases, corticosteroids may be tried. Cough suppressants and antihistaminics are contraindicated.

Prevention

Triple antigen (DTP) as per schedule mentioned under diphtheria provides protection against pertussis. Acellular pertussis vaccine (DTaP) is preferred if whole cell pertussis vaccine (DTwP) produce serious side effects. However, acellular pertussis vaccine is less immunogenic and breakthrough infections are common despite effective immunization.

TETANUS (*Lock Jaw*)

It is caused by spore bearing bacilli *C. tetani* which reside in the soil contaminated by the excreta of animals. The organisms produce a neurotoxin called

tetanospasmin which produce muscle spasms. Tetanus can occur in a newborn baby when umbilical cord is cut with a dirty knife or blade and mother is not immunized and lacks protective antibodies against tetanus. In older children, infection occurs by roadside injury, sports accidents, cuts by sharp objects, nail piercing through the sole and suppurative otitis media (infection of the ear with pus discharge). Tetanus is characterized by lock jaw (inability to open the mouth), inability to feed, spasms of muscles when child is touched or handled, stiffness of whole body and breathing difficulty. Patient is not contagious to others. Tetanus is a life-threatening disease with a mortality risk of 50 to 80% in newborn babies and 20–30% in older children.

Treatment

Neonatal tetanus is a life-threatening disease and is managed in the NICU (refer to **Chapter 14** for details). Excellent nursing and supportive care is life-saving. Patient is nursed in a quiet and dark room. All kinds of visual, acoustic and physical stimuli should be avoided. Human tetanus immune globulins (250 units) is administered IM and intrathecally. Diazepam and chlorpromazine are given through intravenous route in high doses to control muscle spasms. Crystalline penicillin is administered IV for 10 days for elimination of *C. tetani*. Mechanical ventilation and tracheostomy may be required in some cases.

Prevention

Tetanus in a newborn baby is prevented by vaccination of mother during pregnancy by giving two doses of tetanus toxoid (TT) or tetanus-diphtheria toxoid (Td) 4 weeks apart (second dose should be at least 4 weeks before delivery). Cord should be cut by a sterile blade or knife (even a new blade should be boiled for at least 5 minutes before use), by following aseptic precautions and leaving the cord open without any dressing or application of any home antiseptics. Triple antigen (DTP) should be given to children as per the recommended schedule to provide protection against tetanus. After completing DTP schedule, TT or Td should be given every 10 years.

H. INFLUENZAE TYPE B INFECTION

H. influenzae type b is a bacterium which can cause life-threatening pneumonia, bone infection, meningitis and sepsis in infants during first 2 years of life. Treatment depends upon the site of infection. Pneumonia and osteomyelitis are treated with amoxycilin-clavulanic acid or cefuroxime axetil while meningitis is best treated with a third generation cephalosporin like cefotaxime or ceftriaxone.

Prevention

H. influenzae type b (Hib) vaccine is given along with 3 primary doses of DTP and its first booster. A combined vaccine containing DTP + Hib is available which is convenient to administer.

SWINE FLU

Swine flu is also known as influenza A (H_1N_1) or H_1N_1 influenza 09. Droplet or air-borne infection may occur through contact with infected humans or by handling of infected pigs in the piggeries. The infection does not occur through intake of food products or by eating pork.

Clinical Features

There may be history of travel to an epidemic area or contact with a patient diagnosed to have swine flu. The incubation period varies between 4 and 6 days. The disease is more common in preschool children and children with underlying chronic disease or compromised body defences. The symptoms are similar to seasonal flu and characterized by high grade fever, chills, headache, coryza (running or watering nose) and cough. There may be bimodal course of the disease, i.e. a brief period of recovery may be followed by return of worse symptoms of fever, cough and toxemia. Some children may develop severe life-threatening manifestations like toxemia, rapid or labored breathing, blood-tinged sputum, irritability or drowsiness, inability to feed, cyanosis or arterial oxygen saturation (SaO_2 or SpO_2) of less than 90°

Laboratory Diagnosis

The diagnosis can be confirmed by examining nasopharyngeal swab or aspirate for swine flu antigen by real-time reverse transcriptase polymerase chain reaction (rRT-PCR). A fourfold or greater rise in H1N1-specific neutralizing antibodies is also diagnostic.

Treatment

Most patients can be managed on ambulatory basis by good nursing care, and symptomatic therapy with paracetamol, fluids, nutritious soups and antibiotics to control superadded bacterial infection. Patients with toxemia, respiratory distress, debilitating underlying disease and hypoxia should be admitted to the hospital. The therapeutic utility of antiviral agents is controversial but they reduce the period of infectivity to three days or less. Osletmivir (Tamiflu) or Zanamivir (Relenza) is given orally in a dose calculated on the basis of body weight, <15 kg: 30 mg every 12 hours, 15–23 kg: 45 mg every 12 hours, 23–40 kg: 60 mg every 12 hours, and >40 kg: 75 mg every 12 hours, for 5 days. The same dose is given, once a day, for 7 to 10 days to close contacts for prophylaxis.

Prevention

Effective preventive measures include avoidance of close contact with an infected person, frequent handwashing, blowing and rinsing of nose, refraining from touching or picking the nose and liberal use of paper napkins for wiping the nose. The combined seasonal flu (H_3N_2) and swin flu (H_1N_1) vaccines (Vaxigrip, Vaxiflu, Fluarix) are available, but their efficacy against swine flu is doubtful. Two doses of vaccine are given at 4-week interval, 0.25 mL during 6 months–3 years or 0.5 mL in children above 3 years through intramuscular route. In children above 9 years, a single primary dose is given. Boosters are given once a year after the rainy season, with a vaccine which is formulated every year depending upon the circulating strain of the virus. Pandemrix and Celvapan are specific swine flu vaccines but they are not currently available in India.

MEASLES (*Khasra, Gobari, Mata*)

Measles is caused by a virus belonging to paramyxo-virus family. Infection occurs by dissemination of droplets on coughing by the patient. Every year infection is more common during the period November to March.

Clinical Features

After incubation period of 8–10 days, the prodromal feature of fever, running nose, red eyes, and cough appear. After 2 to 3 days of febrile illness, Koplik spots, which are pathognomonic of measles, appear inside the cheeks. These appear as discrete red lesions with bluish white spots in the center like grains of sago, over the buccal mucosa at the level of premolars. After 3–4 days, there is sudden rise of fever and appearance of diffuse tiny pink spots over the skin. Skin rash appears on the face and behind the ears and spreads downwards to the neck, chest, abdomen, arms and thighs. It takes 48 hours for skin rash to spread from face to feet. Fever settles within 1–2 days of appearance of skin rash unless child develops superadded bacterial infection. After recovery, there is brownish or coppery discoloration of skin with desquamation or exfoliation. Measles is known to suppress cell-mediated immunity for several weeks. Common complications include pneumonia, tuberculosis, ear infection, diarrhea, malnutrition and

18

encephalitis (inflammation of the brain). Measles is most contagious during the phase of "cough and cold" and remains contagious up to 5 days after the onset of skin rash.

Treatment

Paracetamol is given for control of fever and discomfort. Humidification relieves irritating cough. Administration of vitamin A (200,000 units daily for 2 days) reduces the severity of complications of measles. Appropriate antibiotics are given for control of superadded bacterial infection. Child should be given plenty of fluids and nourishing diet. Daily bath should be given and oro-dental hygiene maintained.

Prevention

Measles vaccine (single shot subcutaneously over the outer side of mid-thigh), or according to current recommendation by Indian Academy of Pediatrics, first dose of MMR vaccine is given at the age of 7–9 months. The second dose of MMR vaccine, which is given at the age of 15 months, further boosts the protection against measles. The unvaccinated sibling, who comes in contact with a case of measles, can be given pooled human gamma globulins (0.25 mL/kg IM) which may prevent or modify the disease. The vaccine can be administered 3 months later.

MUMPS (*Kan pedey*)

Mumps is caused by a virus belonging to paramyxovirus family. Infection occurs through oro-nasal droplets spread by the patient. The incubation period varies between 14 to 21 days. The initial symptoms are fever, cough and running nose. After 2–3 days of fever, child develops a painful swelling (of parotid gland) on the side of cheek infront and below the ear. The ear lobe is pushed upwards and laterally. After 2–3 days, a similar swelling may appear on the other side. The child may have difficulty and pain on chewing and intake of sour food or lemon drink. The common complications of mumps include inflammation of testis (orchitis), pancreas (leading to diabetes mellitus), myocarditis and aseptic meningitis and encephalitis (edema of brain). The child is contagious during the phase of "cough and cold" and as long as the parotid swelling lasts (usually for about 7 days).

Diagnosis

The diagnosis is based on clinical fundings and aggravation of pain on intake of lemon. Serum amylase may be elevated even in the absence of pancreatitis. The complement fixation, neutralization and hemagglutination inhibition tests or enzyme-linked immunosorbent assay (ELISA) may be used for identification of mumps-specific IgM and IgG antibodies.

Treatment

Paracetamol or ibuprofen is given for symptomatic relief of pain and discomfort. The child should be given soft food without any spices and lemon juice to avoid pain in the parotid gland. Warm compresses over the swollen gland provides relief. Orodental hygiene should be maintained. Orchitis is treated by bed rest and local support to testes.

Prevention

MMR (Measles, mumps and rubella) vaccine is given subcutaneously over outer mid-thigh region around 9 months of age. A booster dose of MMR is recommended during 15–18 months. Recently, a combined MMR + varicella vaccine (Priorix Tetra) is available, which can be given at this stage.

RUBELLA (*German measles*)

It is a viral infection, which is spread through oro-nasal droplets. It generally causes a mild disease, which may go undetected. But, German measles during first 10–12 weeks of pregnancy, can cause serious congenital malformations in the fetus (Congenital rubella syndrome). The pregnant woman may develop fever for 1–2 days with cough and cold followed by mild skin rash on the trunk and enlarged painful lymphnodes in the back of neck. Infants with cogenital rubella syndrome are small in size with microcephaly (small head size) and may have cataracts, deafness, heart defect (patent ductus arteriosus) and neuromotor retardation. These infants may shed the virus for up to 1 year posing serious threat to pregnant women. The diagnosis can be confirmed by elevation of rubella-specific IgM antibodies, reverse transcriptase polymerase chain reaction (PCR) test and viral culture from pharyngeal secretions.

Treatment

Rubella is a mild self-limiting disease. Paracetamol may be given for symptomatic relief of fever and discomfort.

Prevention

MMR vaccine is given as per the schedule described under mumps.

CHICKENPOX OR VARICELLA (*Chhotti mata*)

It is caused by varicella-zoster virus (VZV) which is spread through droplets from cough or direct contact with a patient.

Clinical Features

After 2–3 weeks of exposure to a patient, child develops mild fever, cough and cold. After 3–4 days, skin rash appears in crops mostly on the trunk and proximal parts of limbs. Skin rash has all types of lesions at the same time, i.e. red macules, papules, and vesicles (like dewdrops). Itching is usually present.

Enanthem (rash on mucosa) in the form of vesicles or ulcers over the oral mucosa, pharynx and genital mucosa may occur. The common complications include secondary infection of skin lesions, pneumonia, cerebellar ataxia (difficulty in walking due to lack of balance which usually recovers) and rarely encephalitis and Reye syndrome. Chickenpox is usually a mild disease in healthy children but can be serious in adolescents and adults and children receiving immunosuppressive drugs or suffering from malignancy or immunodeficiency disorder. Patient is contagious during the phase of "cough and cold" (2 days before the onset of rash) and remains contagious till all the scabs have dried.

Treatment

Patient should be treated with paracetamol and an antihistaminic (to relieve itching) and given plenty of fluids and normal diet. *Aspirin should never be given to a child with chickenpox due to potential risk of development of Reye syndrome*. Bath can be given by adding antiseptic (savlon) in water. Local application of a soothing calamine lotion provides relief from itching. The nails should be kept trimmed and clean to prevent scratching.

Prevention

A single dose of chickenpox vaccine is given subcutaneously over the outer side of upper arm (deltoid region) or mid-thigh. The vaccine can be given anytime after the age of one year in children who had not suffered from the natural infection. A booster dose is recommended after the age of 5 years. In children above the age of 12 years, two doses of vaccine are given at an interval of 4–6 weeks. Vaccinated children are also protected against development of herpes zoster later in life.

HEPATITIS A

Hepatitis A is caused by a virus that spreads through contaminated water or food by orofecal route. The incubation period varies between 15 to 45 days. The common symptoms include fever, nausea, vomiting, loss of appetite, high-colored urine, pain upper abdomen (due to enlargement of liver), and jaundice (yellowness of eyes). The jaundice may become intense with marked itching of skin. Most children recover but there is a potential risk of acute liver failure. At times hepatitis may occur simultaneously by two water-borne viruses, i.e. hepatitis A and E causing life-threatening hepatitis. Hepatitis E more often produces features of cholangitis, cholestasis and cholesystits. It may be associated with passage of clay-colored stools and marked itching. Liver is usually enlarged and tender. Spleen is palpable in about 10% patients. Hepatitis A more often causes acute liver failure in children compared to hepatitis B.

Laboratory Diagnosis

Urine examination is a useful screening test to find presence of urobilin, bile pigments and bile salts. Liver function tests are deranged with elevation of serum bilirubin, serum glutamic pyruvic transaminase (SGPT), r-glutamyl transpeptidase, alkaline phosphatase and prothrombin time are elevated. The elevation of anti-HAV IgM antibodies is diagnostic.

Treatment

There is no specific therapy and disease is self-limiting. Physical activity should be restricted till the transaminase levels remain high. Good nutritious diet rich in carbohydrates with adequate proteins should be given. Intake of fats may be restricted but not necessarily eliminated.

Prevention

Hepatitis A vaccine (HAV) can be given anytime after the age of one year. Two doses (6 months–1 year apart) of vaccine are given subcutaneously over the deltoid region or lateral side of mid-thigh. Drinking of safe water and ensuring high standard of personal hygiene can reduce the risk of infection.

TYPHOID FEVER (*Enteric fever*)

Typhoid fever is caused by *S. typhi*. It can occur at any age but is relatively uncommon below 2 years. It is a water-borne bacterial disease and infection occurs through orofecal route by taking contaminated food and water.

Clinical Features

The average incubation period varies between 10 and 14 days. It is characterized by prolonged high-grade fever, chills, headache, constipation or diarrhea,

18

abdominal distension, enlargement of spleen and toxemia. Fever starts with a mild to moderate severity and gradually becomes high grade after 3–4 days (stepladder type of fever) There are no symptoms of cough and cold or difficulty in passing urine. *Whenever high-grade fever persists for more than 5 days and there are no specific symptoms, typhoid fever should be seriously considered.* The common physical findings include toxemia, coated tongue, abdominal distension and mild splenomegaly. The characteristic rose-spots are uncommon in dark-skinned individuals. The common complications include bleeding from intestines, circulatory collapse (shock) and encephalopathy. At times two water-borne diseases like typhoid fever and hepatitis A may occur simultaneously causing difficulties in the diagnosis and management.

Laboratory Investigations

The complete blood count (CBC) usually shows normal or low leukocyte count, lymphopenia and absence of eosinophils. Typhidot IgM may be positive after 3–4 days of illness. The Widal test is usually positive after one week of illness. The 'H' titer or flagellar agglutinins may be positive because of previous infection or vaccination but elevation of 'O' titer in a dilution of 1/160 is suggestive of typhoid fever. Blood culture is the gold standard for making the diagnosis and is usually positive during first week of illness. At least 5 mL of blood sample should be collected into 25 to 50 mL broth and incubated in an automated blood culture system for faster isolation of bacteria.

Treatment

Paracetamol is a useful and safe antipyretic agent. Patient should be given plenty of fluids and nutritious diet. The child with fever should never be starved. There is no virtue to give fruit juices but seasonal fruits can be given. The patients can be given normal diet except vegetables which have hard seeds (okra, bitter gourd) and dals with hard covering (like kidney beans, Bengal gram, *kabli channa*, etc.). The antibiotics of choice include azithromycin, third generation cephalosporins (cefixime, ceftibuten and ceftriaxone) and fluoro-quinolones (ciprofloxacin and ofloxacin). The dose of antibiotics used in typhoid fever is usually double of that used for other indications. Despite effective antibiotic therapy, it may take 3 to 4 days for fever to settle down. The antibiotic therapy should be continued for 4–5 days after resolution of fever to prevent risk of relapse. Corticosteroids are given for treatment of shock and encephalopathy. Vitamin supplements are given during antibiotic therapy and convalescence.

Prevention

Typhoid vaccine is given as a single primary dose after the age of 2 years. The vaccine is given intramuscularly or subcutaneously over the deltoid or mid-thigh region. Booster doses are needed after every 3 years to maintain protection. Purified vi-capsular polysaccharide *S. typhi* Ty_2 conjugated to tetanus toxoid (Typbar TCV™) is credited to provide life long protection. It is administered intramuscularly to infants above 6 months of age followed by a booster dose at 18 months. The protective efficacy of available vaccines is only 60–70%. Typhoid fever may occur despite intake of typhoid vaccine but the disease will be mild and without any complications. Drinking safe potable water and maintenance of strict standards of personal hygiene are important to reduce the risk of infection.

RABIES

Rabies is a viral infection caused by the bite of a rabid dog, cat, monkey, mongoose and jackal. Rodents like rats, mice, bandicoots and squirrels have not been shown to transmit rabies. The incubation period varies between 20 and 90 days. Initial symptoms are fever, muscle pains, headache and change in mood. This is followed by changes in behavior, agitation, tingling sensation around the site of bite, excessive tears and saliva. *Paresthesias, tingling sensation, and fasciulations at the site of bite at this stage is highly suggestive of impending rabies.* The most characteristic feature is hydrophobia (fear of water). When shown a glass of water, patient develops violent spasms of muscles of swallowing. A drought of air over the face may cause similar symptoms (aerophobia). Rabies is invariably fatal. Patient should be isolated and managed in a separate room, with good supportive and nursing care.

Prevention

Domestic pets should be effectively protected against rabies by proper vaccination. Stray animals and dogs should be controlled compassionately by public health authorities. The bite should be cleaned thoroughly with soap and water. Do not apply any turmeric, chilly powder or oil over the wound. Local application of betadine, alcohol or savlon is recommended. The wound should be kept open.

Sheep brain vaccine, which is available in most government hospitals is associated with high incidence of various side effects on the central nervous system. Tissue culture vaccines are safe but expensive. The standard schedule consists of giving 4 doses by intramuscular route for post-exposure prophylaxis on days 0, 3, 7, 14 and an optional dose on day 28 in an immunocompromised child. Day 0 refers to the day on which the first dose of vaccine is given and not the day of bite. In case of wounds on the face, multiple bites, and bites associated with oozing of blood, rabies immune globulin (RIG) should also be given along with first dose of rabies vaccine. RIG is infiltrated around the site of wound but if there is any left over RIG, it is given intramuscularly. When a victim reports after 24 hours of bite, total RIG is administered intramuscularly. If the animal survives 10 days period of observation, further vaccine doses may be omitted. When a fully immunized person is bitten by a potentially rabid animal, it is recommended to give him only two doses (days 0 and 3) of vaccine. There is no need to administer RIG in these subjects. Pre-exposure prophylaxis is recommended to high-risk individuals like veterinary doctors, laboratory workers, animal handlers, wildlife officers, postmen and health personnel. Indian Academy of Peridatrics has recommended that pre-exposure prophylaxis may be given to children having pets and hostelers. Three primary doses of 1.0 mL each are given intramuscularly on day 0, 7 and 21 or 28. A booster dose is given after one year, followed by booster every 5 years to maintain serum rabies virus-neutralizing antibodies above 0.5 iu/mL.

BIBLIOGRAPHY

Acharya SK, Madan K, Dattagupta S. Panda SK. Viral hepatitis in India. *Natl Med J India* 2006, 19(4):203–217.

Barrett AD, Higgs S. Yellow fever: A disease that has yet to be conquered. *Annu Rev Entomol* 2007. 52:209–229.

Chauhan LS, Arora VK. Management of pediatric tuberculosis under the Revised National Tuberculosis Control Program (RNTCP). *Indian Pediatr* 2004, 41(9):901–905.

Dogra S, Narang T, Kumar B. Leprosy—evaluation of the path to eradication. *Indian J Med Res* 2013, 137:15–35.

Halsey NA. Measles in developing countries. *BMJ* 2006, 333 (7581):1234.

Heininger U, Seward JF. Varicella. *Lancet* 2006, 368 (9544):1365–1376.

Helb D, Jones M, Story E, et al. Rapid detection of *Mycobacterium tuberculosis* and rifampin resistance by use of on-demand near-patient technology. *J Clin Microbiol* 2010, 48(1): 229–237.

Kimberlin DW. Antiviral therapies in children: Has their time arrived? *Pediatr Clin North Amer* 2005, 52(3): 837–867.

Kumar A, Gupta D, Nagaraja SA, et al. Updated national guidelines for pediatric tuberculosis in India 2012. *Indian Pediatr* 2013; 50:301–306.

Kunder R., Ganguli N. Ghosh TK, et. al. IAP Task Force Report. Management of typhoid fever in children. *Indian J Pediatr* 2006, 43:884–887.

Peeling RW, Mabey D. Point-of-care tests for diagnosing infections in the developing world. *Clin Microbiol Infect* 2010, 16(8):1062–1069.

Rapid detection of *Mycobacterium tuberculosis* and rifampin resistance by use of on-demand, near-patient technology. *J Clin Microbial* 2010, 48(1):229–237.

Small PM, Pai M. Tuberculosis diagnosis—time for game change. *New Engl J Med* 2010, 363:1070–1071.

Tolle MA, Mosquito-borne diseases. *Curr Prob Pediatr Adolesc Health Care* 2009, 39(4): 97–140.

Working group on Tuberculosis, Indian Academy of Pediatrics. Consensus statement on childhood tuberculosis. *Indian Pediatr* 2010, 47(1):41–55.

18

Mosquito-borne Diseases

In tropical countries, a large number of viral diseases are transmitted to humans and intermediate hosts through mosquito bites. In India, two parasitic infections, malaria (female *Anopheles*) and filaria (*Culex fatigans, Anopheles*, and *Aedes* sp.), are transmitted through the mosquito bites. Four viral diseases, dengue fever, chikungunya, yellow fever (*Aedes aegypti* and *Aedes albopictus*), and Japanese encephalitis (*Culex* species), occur as epidemics of life-threatening and disabling diseases in various regions of our country. Environmental sanitation and stringent mosquito control measures can prevent occurrence and spread of these five mosquito-borne diseases of public health importance in our country.

MALARIA

Malaria (mal: bad, aria: air) is the leading cause of morbidity and mortality in developing countries. Nearly 2.48 million malaria cases are reported annually from South Asia, of which 75% cases are contributed by India alone. Recently, there has been an increase in the falciparum cases, and they account for 50% of all cases. Almost one-half of falciparum cases have become resistant to chloroquine, and some have become multidrug resistant especially in the Northeast region. The disease is transmitted by the female Anopheles mosquitoes and caused by protozoan parasites in the red blood cells (RBCs), which include *Plasmodium vivax, Plasmodium falciparum, Plasmodium ovale*, and *Plasmodium malariae*. A fifth species, *Plasmodium knowlesi*, has recently been recognized that causes malaria in macaques and can also infect humans. The parasites have two cycles of existence: the sexual in the body of the mosquito and asexual in the humans.

Life Cycle of Malarial Parasite

When an infected female Anopheles mosquito bites, it inoculates sporozoites into the subcutaneous capillaries of the victim.

Pre-erythrocytic schizogony or hepatic phase

Sporozoites multiply in the hepatocytes and within 6 to 15 days produce thousands of merozoites. The swollen hepatocyte finally ruptures releasing the merozoites into blood stream. These merozoites invade erythrocytes but can reinfect the hepatocytes to start fresh cycle of preerythrocytic schizogony. In *P. vivax* and *P. ovale* infections, the merozoites may remain dormant for several weeks or months and can restart the cycle unless radical cure is achieved by administration of primaquine. In *P. falciparum* and *P. malariae* infections, there is no dormant or persistent pre-erythrocytic phase and therefore no risk of relapses. But some merozoites can lie dormant in RBCs for some period with occasional risk of recrudescence.

Erythrocytic schizogony

The merozoites in RBCs are called trophozoites. In *P. falciparum* malaria, the degree of parasitemia is markedly high because merozoites invade both mature and immature RBCs. During the early phase of asexual development, trophozoites appear as "ring form," which further develops to form schizonts. After 36 hours of invasion of RBCs, the infected erythrocytes burst to release daughter merozoites, which may invade uninfected erythrocytes to repeat the cycle or get eliminated by natural immunity of the host or antimalarial drugs (Figure 19.1). The paroxysms of fever occur when merozoites are released after the completion of erythrocytic cycle, which is every 48 hours (tertian) in *P. vivax, P. ovale*, and *P. falciparum* and 72 hours (quartan) in *P. malariae* infections. After a variable period of erythrocytic schizogony, some parasites differentiate into sexual forms known as microgametocytes (male) and macrogametocytes (female). They usually appear within 3 to 15 days of illness and are not associated with any symptoms. The further development of sexual forms of parasites takes place in the mosquito.

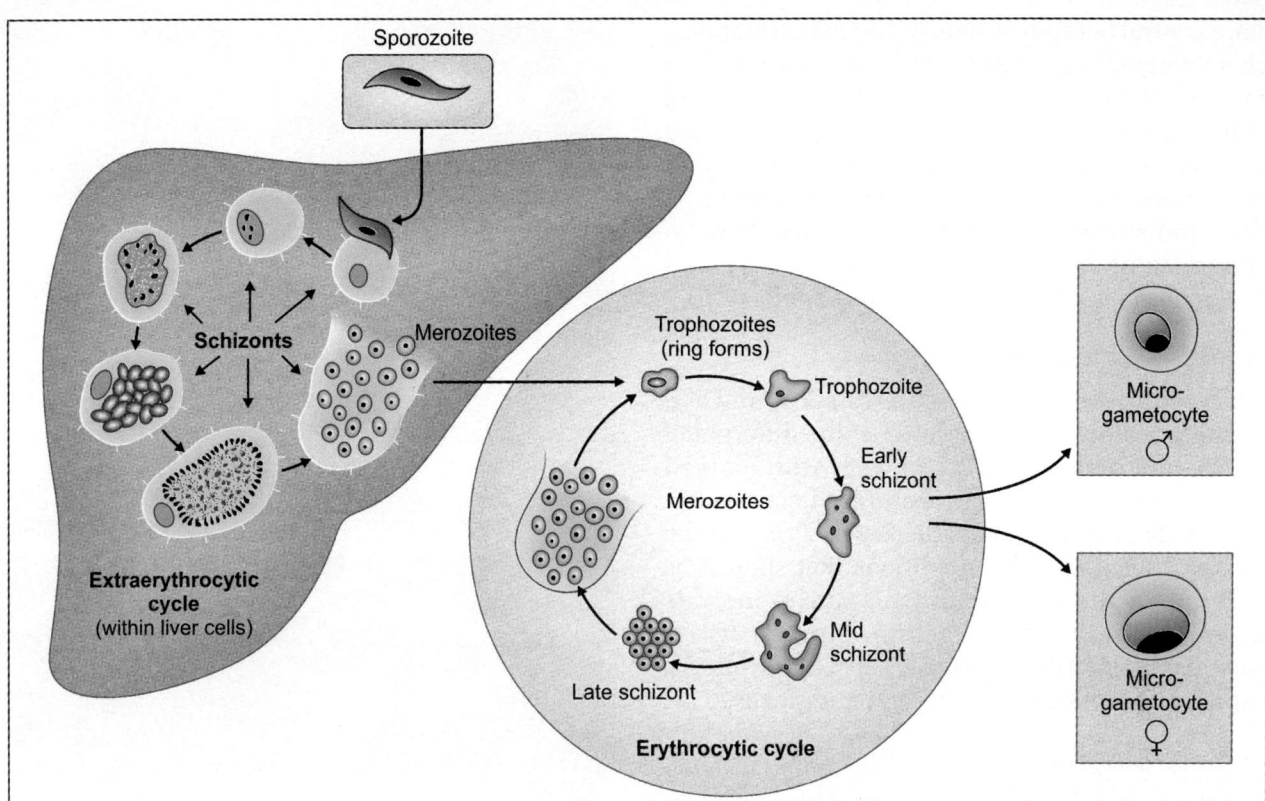

Figure 19.1 Life cycle of *Plasmodium* in humans

Sexual development

When a female mosquito bites the infected person, gametocytes are ingested, which undergo further development in the midgut of the mosquito. The fusion of male and female microgametes forms a zygote, which develops into motile ookinete within 18 to 24 hours. Ookinete penetrates the stomach wall and lies dormant beneath the outer surface as oocyst. The oocyst rapidly proliferates to form numerous sporozoites. The oocyst finally ruptures, releasing thousands of motile sporozoites into the coelomic cavity from where they migrate to the salivary glands of the mosquito. The phase of development of the parasite in the mosquito is called sporogony. The female mosquito is now infective and ready to transmit the infection to humans at the next bite.

Clinical Features

After a variable incubation period of 9 to 40 days, the patient develops characteristic febrile paroxysms of highgrade fever with marked chills and rigors, which is associated with headache, myalgias, and fatigue There is marked sweating and prostration when fever settles. The fever is typically intermittent occurring on every second day (tertian) in case of P. *vivax* and P. *ovale* and every 3rd day (quartan) in patients with P.

malariae infections. Paroxysms of fever coincide with rupture of schizonts, which occur every 48 hours with P. *vivax* and 72 hours in P. *malariae*. The fever may be continuous in children infected with P. *falciparum* or mixed infections and is atypical in infants. There is usually a drop in hemoglobin with splenomegaly. In chronic cases with recurrent episodes of malaria, there may be massive enlargement of spleen (tropical splenomegaly).

In severe malaria because of heavy parasitemia with P. *falciparum*, there is marked toxicity, prostration, anorexia, vomiting, diarrhea, and shock with high mortality (algid or cold malaria). Severe anemia, jaundice, and gross hemoglobinuria may occur because of hemolysis and is aggravated if the child is glucose-6-phosphate dehydrogenase (G-6-PD) deficient (black water fever). Hemorrhagic manifestations may occur. If treatment is delayed, multiorgan dysfunction may set in.

Cerebral malaria occurs when P. *falciparum* parasites are sequestered in the blood vessels of the brain, and paradoxically peripheral blood smear may not show malarial parasites. Sequestration of parasites occurs because of cytoadherence with endothelium of blood vessels and adherence of parasites with each other (rossetting). Early during the course of illness, patient develops central nervous system (CNS) manifestations. It is characterized by seizures, which may be subtle like intermittent nystagmus, irregular breathing, salivation, and facial twitchings. There may be generalized seizures with opisthotonos. The progressive alteration in consciousness leads to coma. Hypoglycemia is common and may get aggravated by quinine therapy. There are significant differences in the severe and cerebral malaria in children and adults (Table 19.1).

Differential Diagnosis

Infective conditions with acute-onset and CNS abnormalities should be considered in the differential diagnosis. Intermitted episodes of fever with marked chills and rigors are diagnostic features of malaria but may be absent in infants and patients with *P. falciparum* and mixed infections. The conditions that should be considered in the differential diagnosis include influenza, urinary tract infection, typhoid fever, invasive gastroenteritis, hepatitis, sepsis, brucellosis, leptospirosis, aseptic meningitis, and encephalitis.

Laboratory Diagnosis

Examination of thick and thin peripheral blood smears remain as the "gold standard" for diagnosis. They are cost-effective, simple, and highly sensitive if examined by an experienced technician with diligence and sincerity. But the procedure is time consuming and demands at least 30 minutes for reliable screening purposes. Thick smears are useful for screening, whereas thin smears are used to identify the morphological characteristics of parasites (Figures 19.2 A to C).

> "In P. falciparum ring forms, crescent-shaped gametocytes and multiple parasites in a single RBC are characteristic. In other species, all stages of the parasites are seen but density or severity of parasitemia is low."

Table 19.1 Differences between severe malaria in children and adults

Symptoms/signs	Children	Adults
Duration of illness (d)	1–2	5–7
Cough and diarrhea	May occur	Rare
Jaundice	Uncommon	Common
Hypoglycemia	Common	Uncommon
Convulsions	Very common	Common
Pulmonary edema	Rare	Common
Renal failure	Uncommon	Common
Lactic acidosis	Common	Uncommon
Brainstem abnormalities	Common	Rare
Neurological sequelae (%)	>10	<5

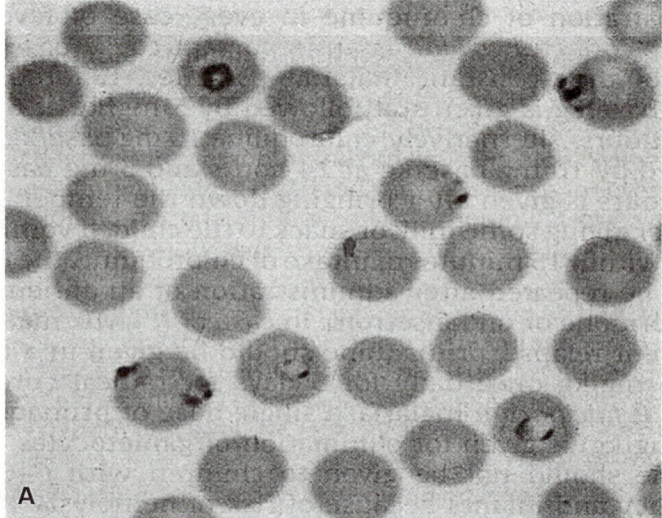

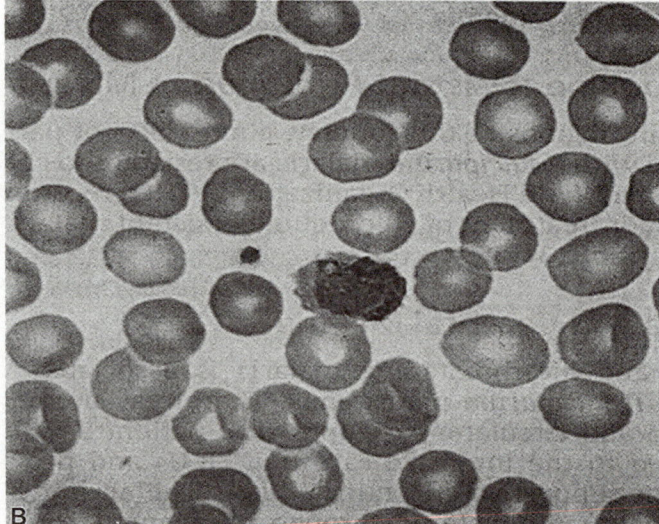

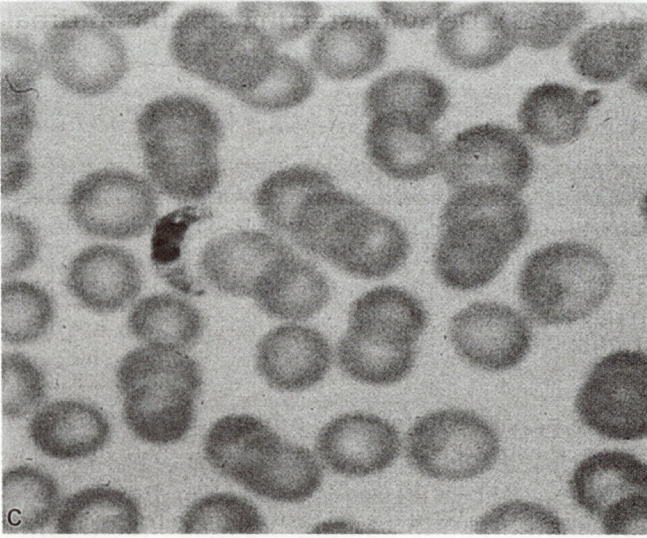

Figures 19.2 A to C Blood smears of patients with malaria. (A) Erythrocytes with trophozoites (ring forms). (B) Erythrocytes with schizont (*Plasmodium vivax*). (C) Gametocyte (*Plasmodium falciparum*)

If peripheral blood smears are negative, they should be repeated after every 12 hours for 48 hours. In patients with severe anemia, parasites may not be seen in the RBCs, but presence of malarial pigments (hemozoin) in the RBCs, polymorphonuclear leukocytes, and monocytes may provide clue to the diagnosis.

Rapid diagnostic tests (RDTs) based on immunochromatographic enzyme-linked immunosorbent assay (ELISA) techniques are available for detection of malarial antigens with the help of monoclonal antibodies. The metabolic enzyme, parasite lactic dehydrogenase, is produced by the viable parasites of all the four species, whereas histidine rich protein II (HRPII) is produced by P. *falciparum*. Rapid diagnostic tests are reliable kit-based tests, less time-consuming, and do not require the services of a skilled technician. They are useful for the diagnosis of cerebral malaria even when parasites are sequestered in the vascular compartment of the brain.

Treatment

Supportive management is provided, and the fever is brought down with paracetamol or ibuprofen and hydrotherapy. Intake of fluids and nutritious diet are encouragecl without any restrictions. Specific therapy should be given when diagnosis is confirmed on peripheral blood smear examination or detection of malarial antigen. *Administration of chloroquine in every case of fever is strongly condemned and is an important cause of emergence of drug-resistant malarial parasites.* Chloroquine 10 mg base/kg is given stat followed by 5

> "Malaria should not be treated on empirical basis. And when treatment for malaria is initiated, the full course of treatment should be completed."

mg/kg at 6, 24, and 48 hours. Alternatively, chloroquine 10 mg base/kg stat followed by 10 mg base/kg at 24 hours and 5 mg base/kg at 48 hours is given after bringing down the temperature and after giving some milk or snack to the child. If vomiting occurs within 15 minutes of intake of chloroquine, the dose should be repeated after administration of an antiemetic (domperidone or ondansetron). In case of P. *vivax* malaria, to prevent relapse, primaquine should be given in a dose of 0.25 mg/kg once daily for 5 days for radical cure. In case of P. *faliciparum* malaria, a single dose of primaquine (0.75 mg/kg) is given for elimination of gametocytes. Primaquine should not be given to children with G-6-PD deficiency and infants because of risk of hemolysis. After recovery, supplements of iron and folic acid should be given to correct anemia.

Chloroquine-resistant P. falciparum Malaria

In certain regions of the country, almost 50% of patients infected with P. *falciparum* malaria are resistant to chloroquine. The World Health Organization (WHO) recommendations for treatment of chloroquine-resistant malaria are given in **Table 19.2**.

Severe and Cerebral Malaria

Severe and life-threatening malaria is associated with intense P. *falciparum* parasitemia. There may be marked toxemia and circulatory collapse. The patient should be admitted to the intensive care unit (ICU) and provided excellent supportive and nursing care. The antimalarials are initially administered through intravenous route till the patient is stable and well enough to take oral medications **(Table 19.3)**. Delay in starting specific antimalarial therapy is the leading

Table 19.2 Treatment of drug-resistant *Plasmodium falciparum* malaria	
Chloroquine-resistant cases	*Multidrug-resistant cases*
Artesunate 4 mg/kg once daily for 3 d plus a single dose of sulfadoxine-pyrimethamine (sulfadoxine 25 mg/kg + pyrimethamine 1.25 mg/kg) on day 1 or mefloquine 15 mg/kg in two divided doses on day 2 and 10 mg/kg on day 3 of artesunate administration.	Oral quinine plus doxycycline or tetracycline (older than 8 y) or clindamycin. Quinine sulfate 10 mg salt/kg per dose three times daily for 7 d. If symptoms of cinchonism appear. It is stopped after 3–5 d. Children tolerate quinine better than adults.
Or	Doxycycline 3.5 mg/kg once a day for 7 d or tetracycline 4 mg/kg/dose for every 6 h for 7 d or clindamycin 20 mg/kg/d two divided doses for 7 d. It can be given in children younger than 8 y.
Coformulated tablet containing 20 mg artemether and 120 mg lumefantrine. It is used as a six-dose regimen by giving two doses daily for 3 d.	
5–14 kg: 1 tablet Starting dose followed by a 15–24 kg: 2 tablets dose after 8 h on day 1 and 25–35 kg: 3 tablets then 2 doses daily on day 2 > 35 kg: 4 tablets and 3	

19

Table 19.3 Antimalarial therapy of choice for severe and cerebral malaria

Chloroquine-resistant cases	Multidrug-resistant cases
1. **Quinine dihydrochloride** (12 mg of salt is equivalent to 10 mg base). Available as 300 mg salt/mL.	20 mg salt/kg (loading dose) is diluted in 10 mL/kg isotonic fluid and given by IV infusion over 4 h. After 12 h of loading dose, maintenance dose of 10 mg/kg (concentration 1 mg/mL) is given over 2 h and repeated after every 8 h from beginning of the previous infusion. When patient becomes conscious, oral quinine sulfate in a dose of 10 mg salt/kg is given for every 8 h to complete 7 d course of treatment (including both parenteral and oral therapy) . Doxycycline or tetracycline or clindamycin is also started and continued for 7 d as soon as a patient is able to swallow. When controlled IV infusion cannot be maintained, quinine can be administered by deep IM injection in anterolateral aspect of thigh (avoid buttock and never give it subcutaneously). Quinine is diluted in normal saline to a concentration of 60–100 mg salt/mL. The dose is divided into two halves, and each half is given on either thigh. The dosage schedule is the same as for IV therapy. Oral therapy is started when patient can swallow. Doxycycline or tetracycline or clindamycin is given *vide supra*. *Caution: Watch for hypotension, hypoglycemia and cinchonism while giving quinine.*
Or	
2. **Artesunate** Available as 60 mg vial, which is diluted with 0.6 mL of 7.5% sodium bicarbonate and made up to 5 mL with 5% dextrose.	Administer 2.4 mg/kg IV bolus stat 12 h, 24 h and then once a day for total of 7 d. When patient is able to swallow, oral medications are started along with doxycycline or tetracycline or or clindamycin *vide supra*.
Or	
3. **Artemether** Available as 80 mg/mL ampoule in peanut oil.	Administer 3.2 mg/kg loading dose through 1M route (do not administer through IV route) followed by 1.6 mg/kg daily for 6 d. When patient is able to swallow, artemether is given orally along with doxycycline or tetracycline or clindamycin *vide supra*.

1. Loading dose of quinine should not be given if the patient has received quinine, quinidine, or mefloquine within the preceding 12 h.
2. Quinine should never be given by bolus or push injection and infusion rate should not exceed 5 mg salt/h.
3. If there is no improvement after 48 h of parenteral therapy or patient develops acute renal failure, the dose of quinine should be reduced to one-third or one-half.
4. Artesunate and artemether should be avoided in immunocompromised and G-6-PD deficient children.

Abbreviations: d. day(s); G-6-PD. glucose-6-phosphate dehydrogenase; h. hour(s); 1M. intramuscular; IV. intravenous.

cause of high mortality. The management steps are summarized below:
1. Vital signs, level of consciousness, input-output, and blood smears for parasite load are monitored.
2. Airways, breathing, and circulation (ABC) are maintained.
3. Fever is controlled with oral or rectal paracetamol and body sponging with tap water.
4. Establish IV line to administer fluids and electrolytes and for administration of drugs.
5. Convulsions are treated with IV lorazepam (0.1 mg/kg) or diazepam (0.2 mg/kg).
6. Hypoglycemia should be treated by administration of 5 mL/kg of 10% dextrose followed by infusion of 5% N/5 glucose saline solution.
7. Metabolic and lactic acidosis are treated by administration of sodium bicarbonate.
8. Circulatory collapse is managed with dopamine or dobutamine. There is no role of corticosteroids and hypertonic mannitol. Shock may occur because of

associated septicemia, which should be diagnosed and managed with an appropriate antibiotic.

9. Blood or packed cell transfusion is given if hemoglobin level is less than 5 g/dL. In severe malaria with parasitemia involving more than 5% RBCs, exchange blood transfusion is recommended in infants and preschool children to improve survival.

10. The comatose child should be provided with excellent nursing care by proper positioning, and care of the eyes, bowels, bladder and back.

Prognosis

Malaria is a life-threatening infection with frequent reinfections and relapses unless radical cure is achieved by administration of primaquine and steps are taken to prevent mosquito bites. The clinical and laboratory parameters that are associated with poor outcome are listed in **Table 19.4**. Among survivors of cerebral of malaria, 10% develop neuromotor sequelae, such as hemiparesis, cortical blindness, and cranial nerve palsies.

Prevention

The strategies for control of mosquitoes and individual protection against mosquito bites are discussed on p 187. Chemoprophylaxis is recommended for travelers visiting endemic areas of the country. Prophylaxis is begun 1 week before the visit and continued for 4 weeks after leaving the endemic area. In chloroquine-sensitive areas, chloroquine is given in a dose of 5 mg base/kg once a week; and in other areas, mefloquine is advised in a dose of 3.5 mg base/kg once in a week Despite concerted research efforts for several decades, no antimalarial vaccine is available as yet.

Table 19.4 Poor prognostic correlates of severe malaria

Clinical indicators	Laboratory indicators
▪ Delay in therapy	▪ Hyperparasitemia (>5% RBCs)
▪ Age younger than 3 y	▪ Gross hemoglobinuria
▪ Multiorgan dysfunction	▪ Hematocrit <15% or hemoglobin <5 g/dL
▪ Spontaneous bleeding and DIC	▪ Blood glucose <40 mg/dL
▪ Circulatory collapse	▪ Deranged renal and liver functions
▪ Deep coma, absent brainstem reflexes, and decorticate rigidity	▪ Raised tumor necrosis factor

Abbreviations: DIC, disseminated intravascular coagulation; RBCs, red blood cells; y, year(s).

DENGUE FEVER

Dengue fever is an acute viral infection caused by anyone of the four serotypes of flaviviruses (DEN-1, -2, -3, and -4), which is transmitted through the bite of female A. *aegypti* or A. *albopictus*. The epidemics of dengue fever have been occurring in the Southeast Asia region for several decades. The last major epidemic of dengue fever occurred in Delhi during 1996. Every year. sporadic cases of dengue fever occur during or after monsoon. The epidemic usually abates after the onset of winter.

The incubation period from the time of mosquito bite to onset of fever varies between 5 and 8 days. Primary dengue infection leads to a self-limited dengue fever with development of neutralizing antibodies and inflammatory mediators that eliminate the virus. But reinfection with DEN-2 in a subject who has subneutralizing or enhancing antibodies because of previous exposure to other dengue viruses leads to the development of life-threatening dengue hemorrhagic fever (DHF) and dengue shock syndrome (DSS) through a series of ill-understood pathogenetic mechanisms. The clinical subtypes of dengue infections include dengue fever, dengue fever with hemorrhages, DHF, and DSS. Recently, the terms DHF and DSS have been replaced by severe dengue infection.

Clinical Features

Dengue fever is characterized by fever with chills, flushed face, headache, retro-orbital pain, body aches especially back ache (break bone fever), scarlatiniform or maculopapular skin rash, epistaxis, and occasionally bleeding from mouth in some cases. Coryza and cough are usually absent. The clinical features of dengue fever in children are not very characteristic, and it is difficult to diagnose it during non-epidemic situations.

> "Primary dengue infection is a self-limited disease, which settles within 4 to 5 days with symptomatic treatment without any complications."

Dengue hemorrhagic fever is characterized by fever, which is followed after 2 to 3 days by petechiae over the face and extremities and frank bleeding from different sites especially gastrointestinal tract.

Practical Point

"The patient with dengue fever should be closely monitored when fever seems to be settling down. The features of severe dengue fever such as capillary leakage and hemoconcentration set in during defervescence and subsequent 48 hours."

19

Vomiting, upper abdominal pain, generalized lymphadenopathy, and hepatomegaly are the common features. During defervescence of fever, the patient develops features of capillary leakage in the form of puffiness, swelling of hands and feet, ascites, and pleural effusion especially on the right side. Because of profound leakage of plasma through the capillaries, it leads to hypovolemia, resulting in shock-related symptoms in the form of restlessness, cold and clammy extremities, rapid thready pulse, low blood pressure with narrow pulse pressure (less than 20 mm Hg), poor tissue perfusion (delayed capillary refill), and oliguria. The WHO classification of DHF/DSS is shown in the Box 19.1. During recovery, some children demonstrate desquamation of skin with marked itching in extremities, palms, and soles.

Diagnosis and Laboratory Investigations

Dengue fever in children does not have any characteristic or diagnostic clinical features and is difficult to diagnose except during an epidemic. The criteria for the diagnosis of DHF include history of

Nursing Alert

"Early and rapid elevation of dengue-specific IgG antibodies is a reliable marker of secondary infection with dengue virus and is associated with an increased risk of DHF/DSS."

fever, positive tourniquet test, thrombocytopenia ($<100,000/mm^3$ or less than 1 to 2 platelets/oil immersion), and rise in hematocrit. Rising hematocrit or a single hematocrit value of more than 40% or retrospectively when peak hematocrit is more than 20% of the hematocrit at the time of recovery are suggestive of hemoconcentration because of widespread capillary leakage. Capillary exudation in the serosal cavities can be identified early by an ultrasound examination. A rising hematocrit due to selective leakage of plasma into pleural and abdominal cavities is a unique feature of DHF. Hypotension and narrow pulse pressure (<20 mm Hg) are suggestive of DSS. Leukocyte count is usually normal or low with relative lymphocytosis and atypical lymphocytes. In critically sick children, serum

Box 19.1 — WHO classification of dengue hemorrhagic fever/dengue shock syndrome

- **Grade I** Fever, positive tourniquet test, thrombocytopenia, and hemoconcentration.
- **Grade II** Spontaneous bleeds but no hypotension.
- **Grade III** Hypotension (pulse pressure less than 20 mm Hg).
- **Grade IV** Blood pressure not recordable.

electrolytes, liver function tests, coagulogram, blood gases, and acid-base parameters should be monitored. Hepatic transaminases especially serum glutamic oxaloacetic transaminase (SGOT) is often elevated. Activation of complement system leads to profound depression of C_3 and C_5 levels. Virus isolation and serological tests are performed for a specific etiological diagnosis and for epidemiological surveillance. Estimation of dengue-specific immunoglobulin M (IgM) antibodies on day 5 of fever on a single sample of blood by IgM antibody capture (MAC)-ELISA technique can be used for making serological diagnosis of dengue fever. Early elevation of dengue-specific IgG antibodies is suggestive of secondary dengue infection with increased risk of DHF/DSS.

A relatively new test that has become popular for early diagnosis of dengue fever is identification of dengue NS1 antigen. NS1 antigen is a highly conserved glycoprotein that is essential for virus replication, although its precise function is unclear. This protein is produced in abundance and secreted by the dengue virus-infected cells. It can be detected by an antigen-capture ELISA test even on the first day of fever thus preceding the appearance of IgM antibody. The sensitivity of this test is reported to be nearly 94% with a specificity of 100%.

Management

Dengue fever is treated symptomatically with a safe antipyretic drug such as paracetamol given in a dose of 15 mg/kg every 4 to 6 hours. Aspirin and other non-steroidal anti-inflammatory drugs (NSAIDs) should be avoided because of potential risk of aggravating

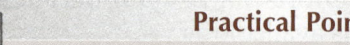

Practical Point

"During an epidemic of dengue fever, every febrile episode should preferably be treated with paracetamol. NSAIDs and aspirin should be avoided because of potential risk of aggravating bleeding manifestations."

bleeding manifestations. During an epidemic, every patient with fever should be considered a potential case of dengue fever; and symptomatic relief should preferably be provided with paracetamol alone. The child should be kept in a cool well-ventilated room. The temperature should be kept below 38°C by tepid water sponging. The child should be encouraged to drink plenty of fluids and take nutritious balanced diet. There is no specific therapy or any role of antibiotics.

Baseline hematocrit, platelet count, and tourniquet test should be evaluated. They should be rechecked during convalescence from fever when patient is most likely to manifest clinical evidences of DHF. A rise in hematocrit by 20% or more from baseline (e.g. increase from 35 to 42%) reflects significant plasma leakage and indicates the need for IV fluid therapy.

The patients with DH F/DSS demand utmost skill and precision in evaluation and management of fluid and electrolyte therapy. In mild to moderate cases (grades I and II DHF), IV fluids may be given for a period of 12 to 24 hours at an outpatient clinic. Patients who continue to have elevated hematocrit, platelet count below 50,000/mm³, develop bleeding manifestations other than petechiae, and fall in blood pressure should be hospitalized.

Dengue hemorrhagic fever

It is characterized by rising hematocrit, thrombocytopenia, and bleeding manifestations but without any hypotension. The child is started on IV normal saline w ith 5% dextrose or Ringer lactate. The fluids are administered in accordance with the guidelines shown in the **Table 19.5**. The rate of administration of fluids is adjusted according to the leakage of plasma, which is reflected by the hematocrit level, vital signs, and urine output. During recovery, infusion rate is reduced at the rate of 2 mL/kg/h. The IV fluids are continued till the child remains stable for 24 hours. The recovery is heralded by return of appetite, onset of diuresis, and fall in hematocrit.

Dengue shock syndrome

Dengue shock syndrome is managed more aggressively with vigorous fluid replacement therapy during the initial 12 hours. Serum electrolytes, acid-base parameters, and disseminated intravascular coagulation (DIC) indices should be closely monitored. There is no role of antibiotics and corticosteroids in the management

Nursing Alert

"The management of DHF/DSS demands high levels of expertise and skills for administration of fluids and electrolytes to correct hypovolemia because of leakage of serum from capillaries into the extravascular compartment."

of DHF/DSS. Vasopressors and inotropic agents are indicated if there is no improvement in blood pressure despite normal or raised central venous pressure (CVP). In refractory shock, infusion of desmopressin in doses of 0.3 mg/kg over 30 minutes daily for 3 to 4 days has shown benefit.

Administer 10 to 20 mL/kg 5% dextrose in normal saline or 5% dextrose in Ringer lactate as two or three boluses, followed by 10 to 20 mL/kg/h. If shock persists despite adequate administration of crystalloid fluids for 2 hours, give colloidal fluids, that is, dextran 40 in normal saline or plasma. During recovery, the infusion volume is gradually reduced at the rate of 2 mL/kg/h. Blood transfusion (10 mL/kg) is indicated when shock persists despite declining hematocrit values (which are indicative of adequate fluid replacement) because of overt or internal hemorrhage. Invasive procedures such as gastric intubation for checking concealed bleeding or for cold lavage are dangerous and not recommended. Intravenous fluids are continued for a period of 24 to 48 hours, and their rate of administration is guided by close monitoring of hematocrit, vital signs, and urine output **(Figure 19.3)**. Hematocrit is initially monitored every 1 hour for 4 hours and then every 4 hourly till stable **(Box 19.2)**.

In critically sick children, CVP and accurate urine output with an indwelling urinary catheter should be monitored. Ascites and pleural effusion are tapped if they compromise breathing. In critically sick children with CVP monitoring, broad-spectrum antibiotics are administered. The role of fresh frozen plasma, platelet concentrate, and cryoprecipitate is controversial and reserved for critically sick children with platelet count lower than 20,000/mm³ or those with evidences of bleeding and DIC. Critically sick children with unusual complications such as hepatic encephalopathy (Reye-like syndrome) or acute renal failure are managed with exchange blood transfusion and hemodialysis, respectively.

Intravenous fluid therapy is usually required up to 48 hours period. Fluid therapy is stopped when hematocrit drops to approximately 40% and vital signs are stable. The return of appetite and diuresis herald the onset of recovery. During the next 24 to 48 hours, extravasated plasma from serous cavities is reabsorbed, which may lead to hypervolemia, heart failure, and pulmonary edema with further fall in hematocrit.

Table 19.5 Fluid requirements for a 2-year-old, 10-kg child with grade II DHF

Calculate fluid requirements as for mild to moderate "dehydration" (because of capillary leakage), that is, 5 to 8% deficit + maintenance fluid needs.

Maintenance fluid needs	= 100 × 10 = 1000 mL
For 5% deficit	= 50 × 10 = 500 mL
24 hour requirement	= 1500 mL
Volume per hour	= 63 mL
Rate of infusion	= 20 drops/min (i.e. volume/ hour divided by 3)

Give 5% dextrose in normal saline or 5% dextrose in Ringer lacate.

The rate of administration of IV fluids should be adjusted according to the rate of plasma leakage, which is reflected by hematocrit level, vital signs, and urine output.

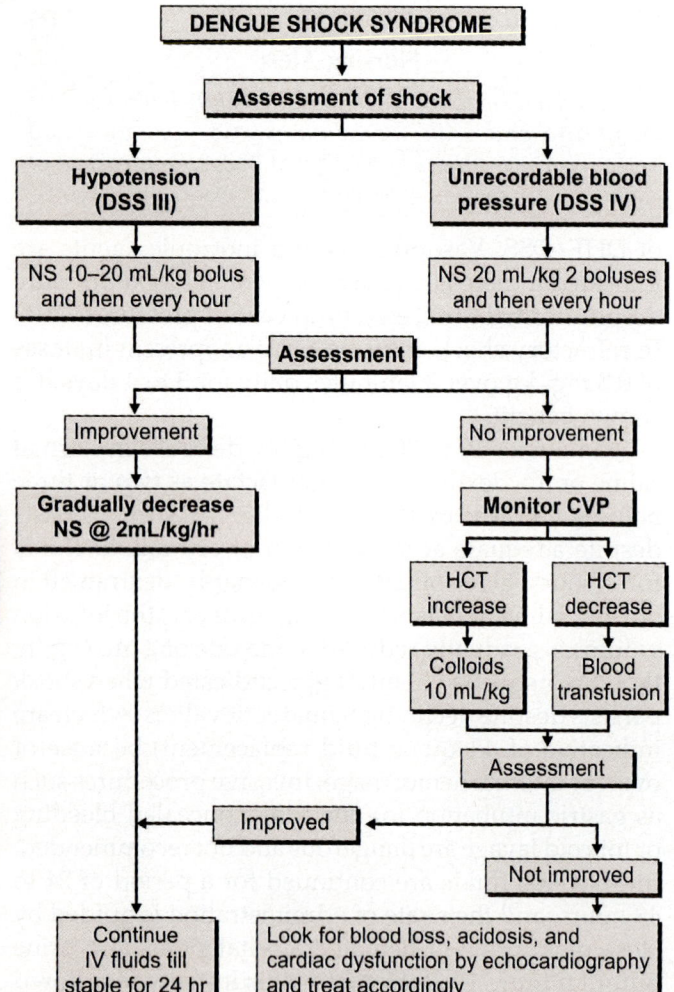

Figure 19.3 Algorithm for the management of a child with dengue shock syndrome. CVP, central venous pressure; DSS, dengue shock syndrome; HCT, hematocrit; IV, intravenous; NS, normal saline

---

| Box 19.2 | **Monitoring of critically sick children with DHF/DSS** |

1. Vital signs every 30 minutes till stable.
2. Hematocrit every 1 hour for 4 hours, and then every 4 hours for 24 hours. Monitor for every 12 hours during recovery.
3. Fluid balance sheet: Type of fluid , amount, rate, and so on.
4. Accurate urine output.
5. Platelet count, serum electrolytes, blood gases, and acid-base parameters every 12 to 24 hours.
6. DIC profile, and liver and kidney function tests as and when indicated.
7. Body weight every 12 hours.

Abbreviations: DHF, dengue hemorrhagic fever; DIC, disseminated intravascular coagulation; DSS, dengue shock syndrome.

During this stage, patient needs to be closely watched and effectively managed to prevent cardiac decompensation and pulmonary edema. It should not be confused with internal hemorrhage.

Outcome

Dengue fever because of primary infection is a self-limited condition and recovery occurs spontaneously. Early and effective fluid management and supportive care of children with DHF/DSS is associated with a case fatality rate of less than 2%. The important correlates of poor outcome include delay in seeking medical care, stage IV disease, severe thrombocytopenia, abnormal prothrombin time, and metabolic acidosis. Massive capillary leakage as evidenced by hypovolemic shock and massive ascites/pleural effusion is associated with poor outcome. During recovery, overinfusion and reabsorption of extravasated plasma may lead to hypervolemia, congestive heart failure, and pulmonary edema with poor outcome. Education of parents for rational management of febrile children with adequate fluids, use of a safe antipyretic such as paracetamol, and early recognition of danger signs of DHF or evidences of shock would go a long way to improve their survival.

Prevention

Public health measures to control breeding of *A. aegypti* mosquitoes and personal measures to safeguard against bites of mosquitoes are described on p 187. A live attenuated quadruple vaccine has been developed from primary dog kidney cells and is undergoing phase 3 clinical trials in Thailand.

CHIKUNGUNYA

Chikungunya is a viral disease caused by chikungunya virus that belongs to the family Togaviridae (single-stranded ribonucleic acid alphaviruses) and has three distinct genotypes, that is, East African, West African, and Asian. The virus is transmitted to humans by the bites of mosquitoes of the species *A. aegypti* and *A. albopictus*. The word chikungunya has its origin from kungunyala, a word from Makonde language of Tanzania. which means the "bended walker" because a severely affected patient assumes a stooped posture owing to arthritis of the spine **(Figure 19.4)**. The disease has nothing to do with chickens!

Epidemiology

In India, first outbreak of chikungunya occurred in 1964 in South India (Puducherry, Chennai, and Vellore) followed by another epidemic in Central India (Nagpur

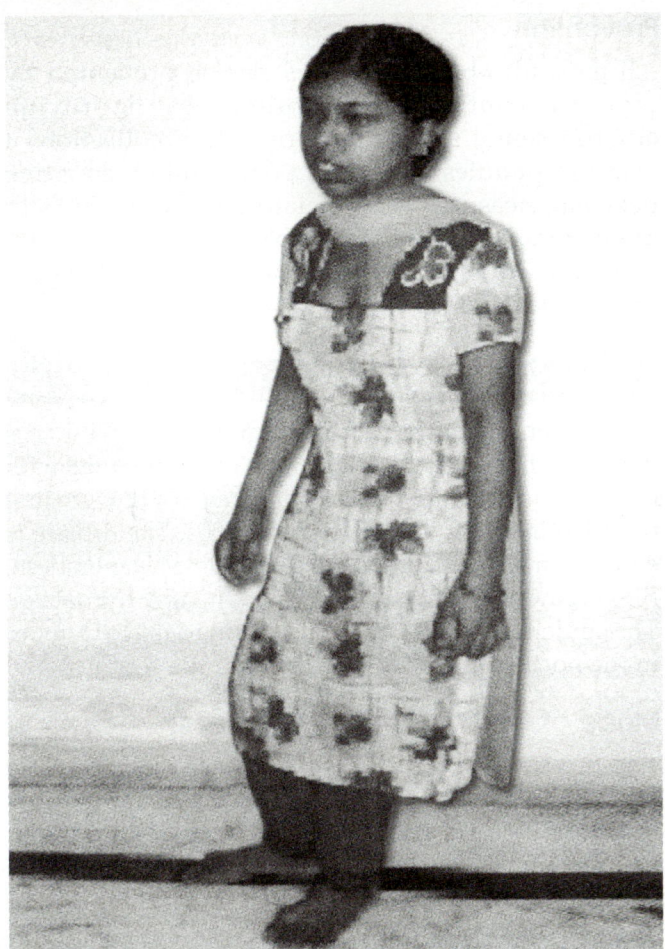

Figure 19.4 Typical stance because of bent knees and back due to chikungunya in a tribal girl

and Barsi). In 2006, the disease reemerged after 32 years and affected 1.38 million people, of whom almost half were from Karnataka and a quarter from Maharashtra. Sporadic cases have been reported from several other states, including Andhra Pradesh, Gujarat, Kerala, Tamil Nadu, Madhya Pradesh, Rajasthan, Andaman and Nicobar, Puducherry, Delhi, and Goa. A large proportion of chikungunya cases from India belong to areas with high prevalence of filarial infections, suggesting that filarial parasitic infections may be modulating the reemergence of chikungunya. The past outbreaks of chikungunya in India were caused by Asian strain of chikungunya virus; but during 2006 epidemic, most cases were confirmed to be caused by an East African strain, which apparently arrived in India 8 years ago.

Vectors of Chikungunya

Mosquitoes of the genus *A. aegypti* and *A. albopictus* transmit the chikungunya virus. *Aedes aegypti* is the most common vector, prefers to live close to people,

and bites painlessly mostly during the daytime. The mosquito is well adapted to survive in urban settings and mostly breeds in clean puddles of standing water and collection of water in artificial containers, such as tin cans, pots, plastic containers, buckets, and discarded tires. *Aedes aegypti* can fly only for few metres and the disease is thus spread to large geographical areas or globally through human travels, tourists, and trade. Aedes species are known to lay their eggs in puddles of water collected in discarded tires. And because discarded tires are transported widely across countries, they can also spread the infected Aedes sp. and their eggs worldwide.

Clinical Features

The infection may affect any age group but is most common in adults. The incubation period usually ranges between 2 and 10 days. The disease is characterized by acute onset of fever, headache, nausea, abdominal pain, photophobia, redness of eyes, skin rash, and disabling arthralgias. Papular or maculopapular and vesiculobullous skin rash occurs on the arms and abdomen after 2 to 3 days of onset of fever. There may be enlarged and tender lymph nodes in the neck. Joint involvement is widespread and most disabling. Typically, wrists, hands, ankles and feet become intensely painful, but any joint may be affected. Involvement of spine leads to severe pain in the back, and the patient may assume a stooped posture. Because of incapacitating pain, the motor disability may be wrongly considered neurological in origin. The joint pains are intractable and may recur or linger on for several months and even as long as 3 years.

Differential Diagnosis

During an epidemic, the triad of fever, skin rash, and arthritis is highly suggestive of chikungunya. Dengue fever is not only transmitted by the same vectors, that is, *A. aegypti and A. albopictus* but also has several identical clinical manifestations, such as fever, skin rash, and myalgias. Bleeding manifestations, hemo-concentration, and thrombocytopenia are characteristic features of severe dengue fever. Acute febrile illnesses that should be differentiated from chikungunya include acute rheumatic fever, viral hepatitis, human immuno-deficiency virus infection, malaria, typhoid fever, juvenile chronic arthritis, mycoplasmal infections, rickettsiosis, and relapsing fever. Acute onset of fever, conjunctival injection, and cervical lymphadenopathy may be confused with Kawasaki disease. In central India, acute vaso-occlusive crises of sickle cell anemia presenting with fever and polyarthritis should be considered in the differential diagnosis. In infants, the triad of fever, skin rash, and dactylitis caused by

19

chikungunya should be differentiated from congenital syphilis, tuberculosis, rheumatoid arthritis, and acute lymphoblastic leukemia.

Complications

Fever in chikungunya is self-limiting and resolves in 3 to 4 days, but joint pains are severe and may cause protracted disability. There have been reports of cases of chikungunya associated with meningoencephalitis, acute inflammatory demyelinating neuropathy, optic neuritis, encephalopathy, myocarditis, hepatitis, and Burkitt lymphoma. Mother-to-fetus transmission of chikungunya virus with abortions have been documented. Case fatalities are rare and are mostly limited to elderly subjects with comorbidities.

Diagnosis

Chikungunya is associated with non-specific laboratory findings, such as leukopenia, anemia and elevation of aminotransferase enzymes. In an epidemic situation, diagnosis is based on clinical features. The specific diagnosis of chikungunya and identification of the causative virus is based on serological tests, molecular methods, or viral cultures. Elevation of anti-CHIK antibodies (cut off level IgM > 0.15 and IgG > 0.10) using MAC-ELISA is diagnostic. However, anti-CHIK IgM antibodies appear only after 4 to 5 days of fever. After an epidemic of chikungunya, sero positivity (IgG anti-CHIK antibodies) is seen in more than 75% population because of asymptomatic infections and cross-reactivity with other viruses. Molecular diagnosis of chikungunya by using reverse transcriptase polymerase chain reaction (PCR) and facilities for viral culture are available only at the specialized centers such as National Institute of Virology, Pune, and National Institute of Communicable Diseases, New Delhi. However, viremia in chikungunya is short-lived and lasts up to 6 days providing a narrow window for a definitive diagnosis.

Treatment

The treatment is supportive and symptomatic to provide relief and comfort against unbearable and disabling joint pains. Paracetamol (15 mg/kg/dose) is the analgesic of first choice by virtue of its safety profile especially when it is required to be used for a prolonged period of time. When pain is severe or intractable, a short course of a safe NSAID (such as ibuprofen and aceclofenac) can be given. Aspirin should be avoided. There is no therapeutic utility of broad-spectrum antibiotics and corticosteroids. There is no established antiviral therapy for chikungunya. In cases of persistent, recurrent, or chronic joint pains, chloroquine therapy has been used with variable results.

Prevention

All mosquito-borne diseases can be prevented by effective control of mosquitoes by improving environmental sanitation; preventing collection of water in puddles, pots, and pools; and by adopting personal measures to safeguard against the bites of mosquitoes. No vaccine is available against chikungunya, and efforts to produce a vaccine are at a preliminary stage of development.

JAPANESE ENCEPHALITIS

Japanese encephalitis (JE) is a mosquito-borne flavivirus disease, which is the leading cause of encephalitis with high mortality and sequelae. Epidemics of JE were first reported in Japan during the late 1800s. The disease is endemic in several states of India, including Uttar Pradesh, Bihar, Andhra Pradesh, Tamil Nadu, and Karnataka. The epidemics occur after rains, during May to October in the north and July to December in the south.

Mode of Transmission

The JE vector in India is *Culex tritaeniorhynchus.* The intermediate host where the virus actively multiplies is chiefly pigs and some birds. Humans are considered the dead-end hosts and have brief periods of viremia with low titers of virus. Man-to-man transmission of JE virus has not been reported.

Clinical Features

The incubation period varies from 4 to 14 days. Most cases are asymptomatic; for one symptomatic case, there are at least 250 asymptomatic cases. More than 90% cases occur in children between 1 and 15 years. There is a sudden onset of high-grade fever with mild rigors, headache, nausea, and vomiting. After 3 to 5 days of fever, severe CNS manifestations in the form of raised intracranial tension, convulsions, altered sensorium, hemiparesis, hypertonia, and decorticate or decerebrate posturing are seen. Extrapyramidal features in the form of mask-like face, abnormal movements, dystonia, and muscular rigidity are common because of the involvement of basal ganglia. Common complications include GI hemorrhage, pulmonary edema, and superadded bacterial infection.

Laboratory Diagnosis

Cerebrospinal fluid (CSF) examination shows pleocytosis, mildly raised protein, and normal glucose. Electroencephalographic changes are non-specific and generalized unlike herpes encephalitis. Computed tomography or magnetic resonance imaging scan of brain shows diffuse cerebral edema, bilateral thalamic lesions, and hypodensity in the region of basal ganglia (Panda sign). Neuroimaging techniques are useful to rule out herpes encephalitis, which shows characteristic involvement of frontotemporal areas of cerebral cortex. Japanese encephalitis virus specific MAC-ELISA both in blood and CSF are diagnostic. Japanese encephalitis virus antigen in blood or body fluids can be detected by PCR or by isolation of virus.

Treatment

There is no specific antiviral therapy, and the child is managed by providing excellent supportive and nursing care in the pediatric ICU. The airways, breathing, and circulation should be maintained. Fever should be controlled by administration of paracetamol and hydrotherapy. Intravenous line is establish to

> ### Practical Point
> *"In the management of any encephalitis, herpes encephalitis should be ruled out or confirmed because it has a specific antiviral therapy (Acyclovir)."*

administer fluids, electrolytes, and drugs. Seizures should be controlled with diazepam or lorazepam. Elevation of head by 30 degrees, administration of furosemide (1.0 mg/kg IV), and 20% mannitol (1.0 g/kg over 30 minutes) are useful to control raised intracranial pressure. In children with brainstem involvement, ventilatory support is required.

Prognosis

The reported case fatality rate varies between 10% and 70%. The poor prognostic correlates include younger age, brain stem involvement, coma, shock, GI bleeding, and pulmonary edema. There is high incidence of neuromotor sequelae among the survivors. Common neurological sequelae include speech defects, aphasia, paralysis of upper limbs, muscular rigidity, and intellectual deficits.

Prevention

The breeding of mosquitoes should be controlled, and strategies to prevent mosquito bites should be followed. Stray pigs should not be allowed to enter residential areas, and piggeries should be located far away from human dwellings. Vaccination of pigs can reduce viral amplification, but it is very expensive.

Vaccination is recommended to children living in endemic areas and travelers who are likely to stay in the endemic area for more than 30 days. Mouse brain-derived inactivated JE vaccine is given through subcutaneous route (0.5 mL in children aged 1 to 3 years and 1.0 mL in older children) as three primary doses on day 0, 7, and 30. Booster dose is recommended after 1 year followed by boosters every 3 years. Recently, more effective and safe live attenuated SA-14-14-2 JE Vero cell culture vaccine has been introduced in China. It is given to children aged 1 to 15 years in two doses (0.5 mL subcutaneous) 6 to 8 weeks apart. There is no need for boosters.

FILARIASIS

Refer to **Chapter 20** on Helmenthic and Protozoal Diseases for details.

YELLOW FEVER

It is an acute viral disease caused by an RNA virus of the genus *Flaviviridae*. The disease is primarily spread by infected female *Aedes aegypti* mosquitoes. The disease is endemic in the tropical areas of South America and Africa, while it is rare in Asia. It is a life-threatening disease that belongs to the group of hemorrhagic fevers.

Clinical Features

The incubation period varies between 3 to 6 days. Most cases are mild and characterized by fever with chills, headache, back pain, fatigue, muscle pain, nausea, vomiting and loss of appetite. The disease is self-limiting and recovery occurs within three to four days. In about 15% cases, the patient develops toxic or second phase of the disease which is characterized by pain abdomen, severe liver damage with bleeding manifestations from mouth, eyes and gastrointestinal tract. About 20% patients develop liver damage and account for overall case fatality rate of 3%. Survivors do not manifest any sequelae and develop lifelong immunity. The diagnosis is made on epidemiological and clinical criteria. It can be confirmed by elevation of disease specific IgM or fourfold increase in IgG-titer on enzyme-linked immunosorbent assay. The serological tests may cross react with other flaviviruses like dengue fever. The virus can be isolated from blood until 6 to 10 days after the onset of illness by reverse transcriptase polymerase chain reaction.

Treatment

Most cases respond to symptomatic therapy. Patients with severe liver damage are managed as per acute hepatic failure protocol and avoidance of hepatotoxic drugs. There is no specific antiviral therapy.

Prevention

In endemic areas, vector control and immunization are crucial to control the disease. It is a mandatory travel advisory for people visiting endemic countries to

19

19

receive the vaccine at least 10 days before the journey. A single shot of live attenuated vaccine is given to subjects above 9 months of age. The validity of the certificate lasts for 10 years. Pregnant women can be issued an exemption certificate, but they have to be extremely careful to avoid the risk of contracting the disease by following strict regimen for prevention of mosquito bites.

CONTROL OF MOSQUITO-BORNE DISEASES

All mosquito-borne diseases can be prevented through effective control of mosquitoes by improving environmental sanitation and preventing collection of water in puddles. pots, and tires. There should be no opportunity for stagnation of water in the bathroom, kitchen. terrace, lawn, and other places. All drains and sources of stored water should be kept covered. Cooperation from every house owner and public establishment is crucial for the success of vector control program. The youth force in schools and colleges and residential welfare associations should be effectively harnessed to strengthen vector control measures. Special drives should be launched during and soon after the rainy season. Malathion sprays/fogging twice at an interval of 7 to 10 days during the transmission season provides protection for a period of 3 to 4 months. The water in the coolers should be frequently changed and treated with larvicidal chemicals. Window curtains should be treated with insecticides to prevent entry of mosquitoes in the dwellings. The hospital wards admitting patients with malaria and dengue fever should be made mosquito free. A strong motivation and commitment on the part of government and its employees are fundamental prerequisites for the success of control measures. In Vietnam, shell fish mesocyclops have been effectively used in the ponds and pools of water collection because they are credited to eat larvae of *A. aegypti*. A pheromone (C_{21} attracticide) and insect growth regulator have been successfully used to attract and kill mosquitoes in ponds through studies conducted by Defence Research and Development Establishment, Lucknow. India. Recently, a novel low-cost sustainable strategy has been developed in Australia for dengue control by infecting *A. aegypti* with a bacterium *Wolbachia pipientis*. The presence of *Wolbachia* in the infected mosquitoes, blocks the ability of dengue viruses to grow in them.

The importance of personal protective measures against mosquito bites, for example, the use of nets or repellant fumes and creams, should be promoted through the media. During night, mosquito nets are most effective compared with mosquito sprays, electrical vaporizers, and mats. *Aedes aegypti* thrive in collections of clean water and usually bite during daytime, whereas *Anopheles* mostly reside in dirty or drain water and usually bite from dusk to dawn. Insect repellent creams containing 30% DEET (*N*, N-methyl-meta-toluamide) are effective against mosquito bites for an average of 5 to 6 hours. Children should be encouraged to wear full sleeved shirt and full pants and use mosquito-repellent cream over the exposed skin during outdoor activities. The efficacy of medicated bands and patches is doubtful. The school authorities should slacken their rules during an epidemic of dengue fever and allow children to wear an appropriate dress (and gloves and socks) to safeguard against mosquito bites.

BIBLIOGRAPHY

Dondorp AM. Pathophysiology. Clinical presentation and treatment of cerebral malaria. *Neurology Asia* 2005; 10:67–77.

Gupta P, Khare V, Tripathi S, et al. Assessment of World Health Organization definition of dengue hemorrhagic fever in North India. *Infect Dev Countr* 2010; 4(3):429–441.

Houwen B. Blood film preparation and staining procedure. *Lab Hematol* 2000;6:1–7.

Kabra SK, Lodha R. Singhal T. Dengue fever and severe dengue infection. In: Singh M, (ed.) Medical Emergencies in Children. Revised 5th edition, *New Delhi, CBS Publishers and Distributors Pvt Ltd.*, 2016, p437–446.

Kalantri SP, Joshi R, Riley LW. Chikungunya epidemic: an Indian perspective. *Natl Med J India* 2006; 19(6):315–322.

Kumarasamy V, Wahab AH, Chua SK, et al. Evaluation of a commercial dengue NS1 antigen-capture ELISA for laboratory diagnosis of acute dengue virus infection. *J. Virol Methods* 2007; 140(1–2):75–79.

Kundu R. Ganguly N. Ghosh TK; Infectious Diseases Chapter. Indian Academy of Pediatrics. Management of malaria in chidren: update 2008. *Indian Pediatr* 2008;45(9):731–735.

Mourya DT, Mishra AC. Chikungunya fever. *Lancet* 2006:368(9531):186–187.

Nimmannitya S. Management of DF/DHF: Monograph on Dengue/DHF. *WHO Regional Publication,* 1993;SEARO, 22:48–61.

Sebastian MR, Lodha R. Kabra SK. Chikungunya infection in children. *Indian J Pediatr* 2009; 76(2):185–189.

Singh M. Diagnosis and management of dengue infections in children. *Indian J Pract Pediatr* 1999; 1: 161–165.

Wang SM, Sekaran SD. Evaluation of a commercial SD dengue virus NS1 antigen capture enzyme-linked immunosorbent assay kit for early diagnosis of dengue virus infection. *J. Clin Microbiol* 2010;48(8): 2793–2797.

World Health Organisation. Outbreak and spread of chikungunya. *Wkly Epidemiol Rep* 2007; 82(47):409–415.

World Health Organization. Treatment of uncomplicated *P. falciparum* malaria. Guidelines for the treatment of malaria, *Geneva, World Health Organization* 2006. 16–40.

Helminthic and Protozoal Diseases

Mode of Infestation

The eggs of worms are passed in feces contaminating the soil and the growing vegetables. Infection occurs through fecal-oral route. Worm infestations are extremely common in children living in poor environmental sanitation conditions and having poor sense of personal hygiene. Eating of mud (pica) is a common mode of infection. Infection can also occur by taking raw vegetables without proper washing or peeling. Larvae of some worms like hookworm enter the body by piercing through skin in children who walk bare feet. Eating infected pork and beef (without proper cooking) may lead to infection by tapeworms. Drinking contaminated water and taking infected food lead to acute amebic dysentery and giardiasis. **Box 20.1** outlines the preventive measures to protect children against infestation with worms.

Diagnosis

The specific clinical features of various infestations are given under individual worms. Adult worm may be seen on naked eye examination of stools. Eggs of worms may be seen in the stools especially when examined by concentration method. At least three consecutive stool samples should be examined by concentration method in a reliable laboratory. Due to their allergic propensity there may be slight elevation of eosinophils in the peripheral blood smear.

Pinworms (Threadworms, enterobius vermicularis)

These worms are most common. They are white in color, small in size and thin like a thread (about 10 mm long). Pregnant female worms wriggle out of anus at night and cause perianal itching and sleeplessness. It is usually believed that excessive intake of sweets aggravates itching though there is no scientific basis for it. In girls, the worms may enter the vaginal orifice causing the child to suddenly wake up at night with unexplained episodes of shrieking. Mother may be able

> **Box 20.1** **Measures to prevent worm infestations**
>
> - Daily bath and strict personal cleanliness should be maintained. The under clothes should be clean and changed daily.
> - Children should be taught the habit of washing hands with soap and water after defecation and before taking food.
> - Nails should be kept trimmed and clean.
> - Children need supervision to prevent eating of mud. Toys should be kept washed and clean.
> - Wear tight underwear at night so that child has no direct access to anus for itching.
> - Salads and raw vegetables should be thoroughly washed in running water and taken after peeling.
> - Children should wear shoes while playing outdoors.
> - The water used for drinking should be clean and protected against contamination with excreta.
> - Avoid taking raw pork which should be properly cooked before eating.

to see the wriggling thread worms by examining the stretched and exposed anal orifice under bright light at night. The eggs of pinworms are not seen in stools but may be picked up from bottom by affixing a scotch tape at the anal region at night and examining it in the morning under a microscope. These worms are a source of nuisance but do not cause any serious health hazards.

Treatment Itching can be relieved by local application of a soothing cream or bland oil (avoid mustard oil which is highly irritant). It is preferable to treat all the members of the family simultaneously to prevent cross infection. A number of medications are available like albendazole, pyrantil pamoate and mebendazole. The course of medication must be repeated after 2 weeks to break the cycle of re-infection. Autoinfection can be prevented by wearing a tight underwear at night (so that anus is not directly accessible for itching) and by keeping the nails trimmed and clean.

20

Roundworms (Ascaris lumbricoides)

These worms may not produce any symptoms or may cause attacks of abdominal pain. The appetite may be increased as if the worms are eating away the food taken by the child. Despite good appetite, the child may look pale and may not have satisfactory growth. The larvae of worms may travel into the lungs producing wheezing and asthma-like symptoms. Teeth grinding at night is not due to worm infestation although it is commonly believed so by the parents. The adult worms may be passed in the stools (male worm 15–20 cm long and female worm 25–35 cm long) or at times vomited out when infestation is excessive. Heavy infestation may lead to intestinal obstruction due to formation of a ball of worms.

Treatment Effective single or multiple-dose medicines (albendazole 400 mg single dose, pyrantel pamoate 11 mg/kg single dose, and mebendazole 100 mg twice a day for 3 days) are available. Preventive measures should be followed to prevent re-infection. In susceptible children, regular deworming can be advised every 6 months.

Hookworms (Ancylostoma duodenale)

These are tiny dark-pink worms which are not visible in the stools on naked eye examination (male worm is 8 mm and female 12 mm in size). The infection occurs by penetration of larvae through feet. These worms are attached to the gut and suck blood. The child looks pale, sickly and puffy. There may be vague upper abdominal discomfort and loss of appetite.

Treatment Anemia should be treated by administration of iron and intake of iron-rich foods. Specific antiworm medications (levamisole, albendazole) are advised.

Tapeworms (Taenia solium (pork), Taenia saginata (beef))

These are extremely long (2–3 meters) and flat worms. Most infestations do not produce any symptoms. Infection occurs by taking improperly cooked or processed pork or beef. Intake of unwashed raw vegetables contaminated with eggs of tape worms may lead to development of cysticercosis (nodules in the muscles or brain causing convulsions). The diagnosis can be made by looking for eggs or segments of tapeworms in the stools. Cysticercosis is diagnosed by CT scan or MRI of brain and muscle biopsy.

Treatment Adult tapeworm is treated by niclosamide and quinacrine. Cysticercosis of brain is treated with anticonvulsants and specific medications like albendazole and praziquantel.

Giardiasis

Giardiasis is a common infestation in children caused by *Giardia lamblia*. The infection occurs by drinking contaminated water. It is an important cause of recurrent abdominal pain with flatulence. The child often passes semiloose, large, bulky and frothy stools. There may be loss of appetite and failure to thrive. The diagnosis is made by isolation of cysts or vegetative foms of *G. lamblia* in the stools. Elisa can be used to detect fecal *Giardia* antigens.

Treatment A number of drugs (metronidazole, albendazole, quinacrine, nitazoxanide, ornidazole, secnidazole and tinidazole) are available but cure rates are not satisfactory and re-infection or persistence of infection are common. The other family members should be investigated and appropriately treated.

Amebiasis

Amebiasis is caused by *Entamoeba histolytica*. The infection occurs by taking food and water contaminated by *E. histolytica*. Acute infection causes loose motions with blood and mucus in stools (dysentery), abdominal cramps, flatulence and tenesmus (frequent urge to pass stools). In chronic amebiasis, there are episodes of recurrent diarrhea, constipation and abdominal pain. Amebic abscess may form at any site in the body but is most common in the liver. A fresh specimen of stools should be examined for identification of cysts and vegetative forms of *E. histolytica*. Skiagram of chest in a case of liver abscess may show elevated dome of diaphragm and pleural effusion on right side. Amebic serology may be positive by ELISA test, which is most sensitive.

Treatment Amebic dysentery is treated with a combination of metronidazole 35–50 mg/kg/d in three divided doses or tinidazole 50–60 mg/kg once daily for 3 days along with a luminal agent like diloxanide furoate 20 mg/kg/d in three divided doses for 10 days. Liver abscess should be aspirated under ultrasonographic guidance to confirm the diagnosis and drain the abscess to prevent rupture. Metronidazole is the drug of choice and given in a dose of 35–50 mg/kg/d in three divided doses for 10 days. Alternatively, dehydroemetine dihydrochloride 1.5 mg/kg/d can be given in a single daily dose SC or IM for 10 days. It should be followed by administration of a luminal agent such as diloxanide furoate for 10 days.

KALA-AZAR (Visceral Leishmaniasis)

Visceral leishmaniasis (VL) is caused by parasites *Leishmania donovani*, which are transmitted by female sandflies of the genus Phlebotomus. The Indian name kala-azar (black sickness) is derived from the fact that there is marked hyperpigmentation of skin during advanced stage of the disease. In India, it is mostly prevalent in Bihar (90% cases), Eastern UP, West Bengal and North-Eastern states.

Clinical Features

After an incubation period of 2–6 months, the onset of disease is insidious or slow. The common features include fever, abdominal discomfort, pallor with progressive weight loss despite good appetite, and enlargement of spleen. Spleen becomes large by the end of first month of illness and grows at the rate of 2–3 cm/month leading to massive splenomegaly. There may be mild to moderate enlargement of liver. Hyperpigmentation of face, hands and trunk occur during later stage of the disease.

Diagnosis

Routine examination of blood shows pancytopenia, i.e. low hemoglobin, leukopenia and thrombocytopenia. There is marked elevation of globulins with reversal of albumin to globulin ratio. Napier aldehyde test and dipstick ELISA using recombinant K39 antigen (rK39) are positive. Identification of amastigotes or LD bodies on bone marrow examination or splenic aspirate is the gold standard for confirmation of the diagnosis.

Treatment

The patient should be given good nutritious diet with supplements of micronutrients. Severe anemia may require transfusion of packed red blood cells. Antibiotics are given to treat intercurrent infections. Patient should be admitted to the hospital for parenteral administration of specific therapy. Many patients with kala azar have become resistant to first line drugs like sodium antimony gluconate and pentamidine isothionate. Liposomal amphotericin B is the drug of choice for treatment of antimony-resistant patients. Miltefosine (2.5 mg/kg/d in one or two divided doses orally for 4–6 weeks) is the first oral drug that is effective against kala azar and has few side effects. Patient should be followed up for about one year because relapses are common.

LYMPHATIC FILARIASIS

Lymphatic filariasis is endemic is several states in India, for example, Bihar, Eastern Uttar Pradesh, Andhra Pradesh, Odisha, Tamil Nadu and Kerala. There are eight different types of thread-like nematodes that cause filariasis, of which three are known to cause lymphatic filariasis. Most cases of filariasis in India are caused by *Wuchereria bancrofti*, while *Brugia malayi* and *Brugia timori* are reported from Kerala. *W. bancrofti* are transmitted through bites of female *Culex quinquefasciatus* mosquitoes and no animal reservoirs have been identified. Mosquitoes serve as intermediate hosts, where in microfilariae develop into infective stage. When infected mosquito bites a person, infective larvae are deposited in the skin and wriggle their way into the lymphatic system. The larvae develop into thread-like adult worms over a period of 4–6 months and circulate in the lymphatic system of the host. The adult female worm produce microfilariae that circulate in the blood stream. The life cycle of parasite is completed when female mosquitoes of the specified genres, ingest the microfilariae during a blood meal and complete the life cycle.

Clinical Features

The microfilariae may remain dormant or asymptomatic for a long period of time. The symptoms may appear after a long incubation period of 8 to 16 months. The disease is characterised by recurrent episodes of fever, associated with inflammation of lymphatics (lymphangitis) and enlargement of regional lymph nodes. The episodes of fever may occur after an interval of 4–6 weeks and subside spontaneously over 7 to 10 days. The disease involves predominantly the lymphatic system with special predilection for lower limbs and genitals. In chronic cases, there is progressive development of hydrocele, chyluria, lymphedema with progressive increase in the girth of lower limbs like an elephant (elephantiasis). By the time these manifestations appear, the infected child has already become an adult!

In some patients with filariasis, microfilariae cause an allergic and inflammatory response when they are rapidly cleared from blood stream by immune mechanism. The condition is called tropical pulmonary eosinophilia and is characterized by episodes of paroxysmal nocturnal cough with dyspnea and wheezing, fever, weight loss and easy fatigability. There may be lymphadenopathy and hepatosplenomegaly. Skiagram of chest may show increased bronchovascular markings, discrete opacities or diffuse miliary mottling. The diagnosis is suggested by marked eosinophilia (>2000/mm^3), elevated IgE levels (>1000 iu/mL) and high titers of microfilarial antibodies.

Diagnosis

Microfilariae can be detected in blood, urine, hydrocele fluid and lymphoid tissues. Blood sample should be collected at night or during the bout of fever, both thin and thick blood smears examined after Giemsa staining.

Polymerase chain reaction (PCR) and antigenic assays are more sensitive.

Treatment

It is a chronic disabling and intractable or life long disease which should be prevented by administration of large scale chemotherapy and control of vectors in endemic areas. Albendazole 400 mg and either ivermectin 200 µg/kg or diethylcarbamazine (DEC) 6 mg/kg single dose is administered once a year. The same regimen is followed for treatment of acute febrile illness due to circulating microfilariae. Diethylcarbamazine 6 mg/kg per day in 3 divided doses for 4 weeks along with doxycycline 100 mg daily for 8 weeks can be given. The drugs have no role in eliminating adult worms but eliminate the risk of transmission of the disease by killing microfilariae. Pulmonary eosinophilia is managed by administration of diethylcarbamazine 10 mg/kg per day in 3 divided doses for one month. In long-standing cases of lymphatic filariasis, supportive nursing care is required to prevent and treat bacterial and fungal infections in lower limbs, drainage of hydrocele and cosmetic surgery.

HYDATID DISEASE (Echinococcosis)

Hydatid disease is caused by the larval stage of cestodes *Echinococcus granulosis* or *Echinococcus multilocularis*. The definitive host for adult worms is dog while cattle and goats (*E. multilocularis*) act as intermediate hosts. Larvae are hatched in the intestines, penetrate mucosa, and get disseminated through bloodstream to various organs of the body. Cysts may develop in any organ of the body but are most common in the lungs and liver. They grow slowly at the rate of 1 cm per year.

Clinical Features

The clinical symptoms occur because of the mass effect of the cyst. Hydatid disease should be considered whenever a cyst is suspected in any organ or region of the body. The percussion over the hydatid cyst may elicit classical "hydatid thrill" because of movements of the hydatid sand and tiny daughter cysts. Rapture or leakage from a hydatid cyst may cause fever, itching, skin rash, anaphylaxis, and eosinophilia.

Laboratory Investigations

Ultrasonography (USG) or computed tomography (CT) scan reveals double-walled cyst with floating echogenic material (hydatid sand and daughter cysts within the parent cyst). There may be unilocular or multiseptated cyst showing "rosette-like" or "honeycomb" appearance. There may be "snow-flaked" sign because of free-floating protoscolices within the cyst. Casoni skin test may be positive. Echinococcal antibodies may be detected on ELISA test.

Treatment

Surgical removal of the cyst, when it is single and accessible, is the treatment of choice. Recently, USG or CT-guided percutaneous aspiration and instillation of hypertonic saline and reaspiration (PAIR) has been tried with success. This procedure must be conducted with due care because leakage of hydatid fluid may cause anaphylaxis. The risk of anaphylaxis can be reduced by starting medical therapy before PAIR and continuing it after the procedure for one month. Medical therapy includes albendazole 15 mg/kg/d every 12 hour for 2 weeks. Several courses (5 to 15 depending upon the size of cyst) are administered after every 2 weeks of drug-free interval. The common side effects of prolonged albendazole therapy include headache, pain abdomen, alopecia, and elevation of hepatic enzymes. The response to therapy is monitored by serial USG. During recovery, the cyst shrinks, becomes more echogenic, and the cyst membrane gets dislodged from the capsule and floats in the cyst fluid (water lily sign).

BIBLIOGRAPHY

Ali SA, Hill DR. Giardia intestinalis. *Curr Opin Infect Dis* 2003, 16(5): 453–460.

Bhattacharya SK, Sur D, Karbwang J. Childhood visceral leishmaniasis. *Indian J Med Res* 2006, 123(3): 353–356.

Eziefula AC, Brown M. Intestinal nematodes: disease burden, deworming and potential importance of co-infection. *Curr Opin Infect Dis* 2008, 21(5): 516–522.

Haque R, Huston CD, Hughes M, Houpt E, Petri WA Jr. Amebiasis. *New Engl J Med* 2003, 348(16): 1565–1573.

Keiser J, Utzinger J. The drugs we have and the drugs we need against major helminth infections. *Adv Parasitol* 2010, 73: 197–223.

Lockwood DNJ, Sundar S. Serological tests for visceral leishmaniasis. *BMJ* 2006, 333(7571): 711–712.

Murray HW, Berman JD, Davies CR, Saravia NG. Advances in leishmaniasis. *Lancet* 2005, 365(9496): 1561–1577.

21

Immunizations

A large number of infectious diseases which can cause disability or death can be prevented by timely administration of safe and effective vaccines. Vaccines are the greatest boon of modern medicine. The dream of Jenner was realized in the year December 1979 when smallpox was declared as eradicated from the universe. Paralytic poliomyelitis has been eradicated from India on January 13, 2014 following the success of Pulse Polio Immunization Program. It is a moral obligation on the part of all parents to cooperate with the public health authorities to ensure that their children receive all the vaccines in accordance with the recommended national schedule and under the guidance and supervision of their pediatrician or family physician. Most of the mandatory or essential vaccines are available free of cost in various health posts and government hospitals.

ACTIVE AND PASSIVE IMMUNITY

The immunity or protection against a disease may be natural or innate, or acquired through active or passive means. Passive protection is provided to the fetus or newborn by transplacental passage of antibodies from the mother to her baby and subsequently through breast feeding. The preformed antibodies or immunoglobulins, specific or non-specific, from either animal or human source, can be administered before or soon after exposure to prevent development of the disease. The passive protection is immediate but short lived because the half-life of immunoglobulins is 3 to 4 weeks.

In active immunity, the immunological defense mechanisms of the baby (both humoral and cell mediated) are activated or stimulated by administration of a vaccine when a child is healthy and before exposure to infectious agents. The active immunity provides robust and long-lasting protection against the disease, which gets boosted by any subsequent exposure to the natural infection or by virtue of booster doses of

vaccine. The vaccine is developed when there are following characteristics or correlates of the disease:

1. The disease should be of frequent occurrence and associated with significant morbidity, mortality or disability on survival.
2. The disease should be caused by a single microbe having limited number of serotypes. It is not possible to develop a vaccine against cough and cold because it is caused by over 200 viruses.
3. When patient recovers from natural infection, the disease should produce a prolonged protection against reinfection.

Immunization and Immunity

When a disease-causing microbe (bacterium or virus) enters the body, the body tries to launch a protective response by producing antibodies to neutralize and destroy the infectious agent. When the microbes are wild, tough and virulent, they overpower the immune system of the body and cause the disease, which may at times lead to disability or death. The vaccines are prepared by either killing the microbes or by taming the microbes to a milder non-virulent form by various techniques. At times the toxins of the microbes are extracted and used for immunization. The vaccines would thus be either live vaccines, killed vaccines or toxoids and antigen-based vaccines prepared by modern genetic engineering (recombinant) technology like Hepatitis B vaccine. When a vaccine is administered, it stimulates the immunologic system to produce protective antibodies and sensitize the protective cells of the body to mount a good fight when body is invaded by the disease-causing microbes. The subsequent or booster doses of the vaccine provide a heightened or enhanced antibody response. When a child who has been effectively protected by a vaccine, is exposed to the wild microbes through natural infection, he is able to fight the assault by enhanced production of specific antibodies with complete success or may manifest mild or modified disease without any serious illness or disability. Vaccines thus provide safe and reliable means to build up body defences to effectively fight against the wild and virulent microbes.

An ideal vaccine should provide prolonged or life long protection by producing adequate titers of antibodies, should be easy to administer, effective, safe and affordable.

TYPES OF VACCINES

There are different kinds of vaccines which are described below:

Killed Vaccines

The whole organism is killed (formaline or acetone-killed) and formulated into a suitable vaccine. The examples are whole-cell pertussis vaccine, typhoid vaccine, cholera vaccine and inactivated polio vaccine (IPV or Salk vaccine). In general, killed vaccines are poorly immunogenic (produce less protection) but more reactogenic, i.e. more likely to produce serious side effects.

Live-attenuated Vaccines

The microorganisms are subjected to certain processes or passages to attenuate or reduce their disease-causing capabilities while retaining the immunologic properties. The administration of a live vaccine produces an immunologic response which is similar to the natural infection. The examples of live vaccines include BCG, measles, mumps and rubella (MMR), chickenpox, yellow fever, oral polio vaccine (OPV or Sabin vaccine), oral typhoid vaccine and rotavirus vaccine. In general, live vaccines are more immunogenic and produce better and prolonged protection. They need strict cold-chain requirements to ensure the viability of attenuated pathogens. There is a potential risk of producing the disease (paralytic poliomyelitis by administration of OPV) if attenuation of the pathogen is unsatisfactory or recipient is immunocompromised.

Toxoids

Toxoids are suitably detoxified exotoxins of bacteria, which have the capability to stimulate formation of antitoxins in the recipient, for example, tetanus toxoid (TT) and combined tetanus and diphtheria toxoid (Td). These are low-technology vaccines, easier to prepare, highly immunogenic and cost-effective.

Subunit Vaccines

A part of the microorganisms that has the capability to generate the immune response is utilized for production of the vaccine, for example, acellular pertussis and vi-antigen typhoid vaccine.

Conjugated Subunit Vaccines

Polysaccharide vaccines produce only B cell-mediated immunological response (by producing antibodies alone) and they do not provide protection to children below 2 years of age. They can be modified to produce T cell response (cell-mediated immunity) by a process of conjugation with a protein carrier (usually tetanus toxoid) which a associated with a satisfactory immunological response below the age of 2 years. This technique has been used to produce pneumococcal, meningococcal, *Haemophilus influenzae type b* (Hib) and typhoid vaccines.

Recombinant and Deoxyribonucleic Acid (DNA) Vaccines

The immunological components of the pathogenic organisms are synthesized and tagged to a carrier non-pathogenic organism and an adjuvant system such as aluminium hydroxide, ASO_4 and virosomes, for example, hepatitis A and B vaccines and human papillomavirus and meningococcal vaccine.

THE VACCINATION SCHEDULE

Every country has its own immunization schedule depending upon the spectrum of diseases, need of the community and financial resources. The Government of India provides essential vaccines to all under-5 children under Universal Immunization Program (UIP). The vaccines administered under this program include BCG, DTwP, OPV and measles. Two doses of TT or DT are provided to pregnant women. In some states, hepatitis B (HBV), *H. influenzae type b* (Hib), one dose of IPV and Rotavac vaccine are provided with the help of Global Alliance for Vaccines and Immunization (GAVI). However, all the latest vaccines are available in India but they are expensive and dispensed in private hospitals and ambulatory clinics of practicing pediatricians. The Indian Academy of Pediatrics has recommended a schedule of immunization which includes essential (mandatory) and optional (additional) vaccines after one-to-one discussion with parents and selected vaccines for administration to high risk children or during special situations (Table 21.1).

The vaccines should be taken as per the recommendation of a pediatrician or family physician. It is mandatory that primary doses of vaccines and their boosters are taken in accordance with the recommended schedule. However, when a shot is missed, the previously administered dose(s) of a vaccine remains valid and there is no need to restart the vaccination schedule. The vaccine must be stored properly by the

Table 21.1 Recommended vaccination schedule

Age	Vaccine	Dose
	Essential Vaccines	
Birth to 2 wk	BCG	Single dose
	OPV[a]	1st dose
	HBV	1st dose
6–8 wk	DTwP or DTaP + Hib + IPV	1st dose
	OPV	2nd dose
	HBV	2nd dose
10–12 wk	DTwP or DTaP + Hib + IPV	2nd dose
	OPV	3rd dose
14–16 wk	DTwP or DTaP + Hib + IPV	3rd dose
	OPV	4th dose
6–9 mo	HBV	3rd dose (may be given along with 3rd dose of DTP)
	MMR vaccine	1st dose
15–18 mo	MMR or MMR + varicella	2nd dose
	DTwP or DTaP + Hib + IPV	Ist booster
	OPV	5th dose
After 2 y	Typhoid vaccine[b]	Boosters every 3 y
4.5–5 y	DTwP or DTaP	2nd booster
	OPV	6th dose[b]
	MMR or MMR + varicella booster (optional)	
	HBV booster	
10 y	Tdap or Td or TT booster[c]	Every 10 y
	Optional Vaccines after One-to-One Discussion with Parents who can Afford	
6–8 wk	Rotavirus vaccine + pneumococcal vaccine (PCV 13)	1st dose
10–12 wk	Rotavirus vaccine + pneumococcal vaccine	2nd dose
14–16 wk	Rotavirus vaccine pneumococcal vaccine	3rd dose
12 mo	HAV	Two doses at an interval of 6 mo – 1 y.
15 mo	Pneumococcal vaccine	Booster
	Varicella vaccine	Single dose up to 12 y, subsequently two doses 4–8 wk apart, a booster dose is being recommended after the age of 5 y
10–12 y	HPV	Two doses at 0, and 6 mo during 9–14 years. After 14 years, three doses are given at 0, 1 or 2 and 6 months

Vaccines during Special Situations

- IPV (injectable or inactivated polio vaccine) is given to immunocompromised or HIV-positive children. It is being administered routinely as a part of post-polio-eradication policy.
- Meningococcal vaccine (during an epidemic, Haj pilgrims, sickle cell disease and CSF rhinorrhea). Polysaccharide vaccine is given in a single dose after 2 years of age or maximum of two doses.
- Pneumococcal polysaccharide vaccine, namely, PPV 23 (chronic lung and heart disease, sickle cell disease, splenectomy, nephrotic syndrome and immunocompromised child) is given as a single dose or maximum of 2 doses.
- Influenza vaccine (bronchial asthma, congestive heart failure and immunocompromised child). Initially two doses (single dose is given in children >9 y) are given 4 wk apart after the age of 6 mo, followed by yearly boosters at the onset of rainy season.
- Antirabies "pre-exposure" prophylaxis is given to high risk populations, i.e. children with pets, hostelers, postmen, veterinary doctors, wild life handlers and technicians. Three primary doses 1.0 mL IM are given on day 0, 7 and 21 or 28, followed by a booster, after one year. In immunized subjects, for 'post-exposure' protection only two doses are given on days 0 and 3. In these subjects, no rabies immunoglobulins (RIG) are needed.
- Cholera vaccine (to control epidemics, visitors to *kumbh mela*, Haj pilgrims).

21

(Contd.)

Table 21.1 Recommended vaccination schedule *(contd.)*

- Japanese B encephalitis vaccine (endemic areas, during epidemics) is administered (0.5 mL 1–3 y, 1.0 mL 3–10 y SC) in two primary doses 4 weeks apart to children above one year of age. The need for boosters is still undermined.
- Yellow fever (travelers to South Africa). Vaccine is given as a single dose (>6 mo age) followed by boosters every 10 y). Avoid during pregnancy.

BCG, bacillus Calmette-Guerin; CSF, cerebrospinal fluid; d, day(s); DTaP, diphtheria, tetanus and acellular pertussis; DTP, diphtheris tetanus and pertussis (whooping cough); DTwP, diphtheria-tetanus-whole-cell pertussis; HAV, hepatitis A vaccine; HBV, hepatitis B vaccine; Hib *H. influenzae type b*; IPV, inactivated polio vaccine; MMR, measles, mumps and rubella; mo, month(s); OPV, oral polio vaccine; PCV 13, 13-valent pneumococcal conjugated vaccine; PPV 23, 23-valent pneumococcal polysaccharide vaccine; TT, tetanus toxoid; Td, tetanus–diphtheria dual vaccine with low dose diphtheria antigen (5 Lf or 2 Lf) which can be safely given to adults; Tdap, tetanus toxoid with low-dose diphtheria and pertussis; wk, week(s); y, year(s).

[a]Additional doses of oral polio vaccine given under pulse immunization program must be taken by all children below the age of 5 years.
[b]vi capsular polysaccharide *S. typhi* Type 2 conjugated to tetanus toxoid (Typbar–TCV) is given in two doses at an interval of one year. The first dose is given during 9–12 months of age.
[c]Pregnant woman must receive two doses of TT or Td at 4 weeks interval. The second dose should be taken at least 4 weeks before delivery.

1. The suggested schedule may be modified by the consultant pediatrician as per the local needs.
2. Breastfeeding can be given after oral polio vaccine and it does not interfere with development of satisfactory immunity.
3. Most immunizations can be given in the presence of a minor illness. Paracetamol can be given following a vaccination for relief of local pain and fever, but it may reduce immunogenicity of the vaccine.
4. There is no need to give Hib vaccine (*Haemophilus influenzae* type b vaccine) if it has not been taken by the age of 1½ years.
5. The need and cost-effectiveness of optional vaccines must be explained to the parents before they are recommended.
6. Live vaccines should be avoided in immunocompromised children and symptomatic HIV-positive infants.
7. A number of vaccines can be administered together simultaneously at two different sites or as a combo formulation without interfering with development of protection against different antigens. A live vaccine can be administered after an inactivated vaccine (or *vice versa*) without any minimum recommended interval. However, a minimum interval of 4 weeks is recommended between administration of two live vaccines.
8. When a dose of a vaccine is missed, the remaining doses should be administered at the earliest opportunity while keeping in mind that the vaccine dose already given is valid.
9. Before giving the next dose of vaccine, ask the mother if the child had any significant reaction to the last dose of the vaccine.
10. OPV-related paralytic poliomyelitis is being increasingly reported from developed countries. These countries have changed their strategy and are giving IPV (injectable or inactivated or killed polio vaccine).

nurse in a satisfactory cold chain system. They must be administered with due aseptic precautions with a disposable syringe and needle. In infants, vaccines are usually administered into the outer side of mid-thigh region while in school going children they can be given into the outer side of upper arm (deltoid region). *The vaccines should never be injected into the gluteal region due to poor absorption because of pad of fat and potential risk of causing damage to the sciatic nerve.* BCG vaccine is given inside the skin (intradermal) over the top of the left shoulder. The side effects, if any encountered by the child with the previous dose of the vaccine, must be asked by the physician or nurse before giving the next shot. It is important that parents must be asked to keep the vaccination record of their children in a safe custody. It is an important document for the doctor and school health authorities.

Optional vaccines are not available through government health channels and are not included in the national immunization schedule. Nevertheless, they are effective and safe vaccines and have become essential or mandatory in several developed countries. However, most of them are expensive at this stage and may be taken if parents can afford. Chickenpox among healthy children is not a serious disease and provides life long protection. However, chickenpox in adolescents and adults is more severe with greater risk of complications. If a child does not suffer from natural chickenpox by the age of 12 years, he can be given a single shot of chickenpox vaccine to prevent the occurrence of disease in adult life. Chickenpox vaccine also provides protection against herpes zoster. Hepatitis A, typhoid, poliomyelitis, rotavirus diarrhea and cholera are water-borne diseases and can be prevented by drinking safe potable water and avoiding intake of fruit juices and foods from road side stalls and *dhabas*.

COMPOSITION OF AVAILABLE VACCINES

Bacillus Calmette-Guerin (BCG) Vaccine

BCG vaccine is derived from bovine strain of tubercular bacilli and was developed in 1921 by a French microbiologist, Albert Calmette and the veterinary doctor, Camille Guerin. The two common strains of tubercular bacilli used for production of vaccine include Copenhagen and Pasteur, of which the former was produced in India at the BCG Laboratories, Guindy, Tamil Nadu. BCG induces cell-mediated immunity and its protective efficacy is limited. It does not provide absolute protection against tuberculosis but reduces the risk of development of disseminated tuberculosis, like miliary and meningeal tuberculosis. There is a need to have a new, improved and potent vaccine against tuberculosis.

BCG is available as a lyophilized (freeze-dried) formulation dispensed in vacuum sealed, multi-dose, dark colored vials along with 2 mL ampoules of normal saline as diluent. The lyophilized vaccine can be stored at 2 to 8°C for upto 12 months. The reconstituted vaccine should be stored in the frige between 2 to 8°C, protected from light and consumed within 4–6 hours of reconstitution.

BCG is administered intradermal over top of the left shoulder by using tuberculin syringe and 26 G needle. The site for administration should not be cleaned with surgical spirit or antiseptic. The skin is stretched and 0.1 mL of vaccine is administered intradermally to produce a wheal of 5 mm. Care should be taken to avoid subcutaneous administration of vaccine, which is associated with an increased risk of discharging ulcer and BCG adenitis. The vaccine site shows no visible change for several days. After 4–5 weeks, a papule develops which may ulcerate and take 6–12 weeks to heal by formation of a scar.

BCG is given at birth before mother is discharged from the hospital or within one month of age. If BCG vaccine is missed, a catch up vaccine may be given till the age of 5 years. There is no need for routine tuberculin testing prior to catch up vaccination. If there is no local reaction up to 8 weeks of administration of BCG vaccine, a repeat dose may be given without tuberculin testing. However, there is evidence to suggest that even when there is no local reaction, the child may develop cell-mediated immunity.

BCG should not be given to immunocompromised children especially those with cellular immunodefi-ciency and active HIV disease (AIDS) but can be given at birth to non-symptomatic infants born to HIV-positive mothers. BCG may be given along with other vaccines at the same time or at any interval with the exception of measles and MMR vaccines, when a gap of 4 weeks between two vaccines is recommended. In some infants, whether due to immunodeficiency, excessive dose or subcutaneous administration, the infant may develop severe or persistent local reaction with formation of cold abscess and enlargement of regional lymphnodes in the axilla or neck. It may respond to administration of erythromycin if there is

secondary bacterial infection. In persistent cases, repeated needle aspiration of abscess and surgial excision of enlarged lymph node is the treatment of choice. The role of antitubercular therapy for treatment of exaggerated BCG-adenitis is controversial.

POLIO VACCINES

The availability of two effective vaccines against poliomyelitis has ensured remarkable decline in the global burden of disease. The vaccines was developed in USA during 1950s, first the inactivated polio vaccine (IPV) by Jonas Salk and later the live oral polio vaccine (OPV) by Albert Sabin. The Global Polio Eradication initiative was launched in 1988 using oral polio vaccine as the eradication tool by employing four-pronged strategy comprising, (i) improved coverage of routine immunization, (ii) supplementary immunization activities or pulse immunization program, (iii) AFP surveillance and (iv) Mop-up immunization drives. The initiative has been rewarded with huge success with global eradication of poliomyelitis since January 13, 2014 except some endemic cases from Pakistan, Afghanistan and Nigeria.

Oral Polio Vaccine (OPV)

OPV is a trivalent (tOPV) vaccine consisting of suspension of attenuated poliovirus types 1, 2 and 3 grown in monkey kidney cell cultures and stabilized with magnesium chloride. It is dispensed in dropper vials as a buffered salt solution, with light pink color indicating the desired pH. It is a heat-sensitive vaccine and should be carried to the out reach facility in ice packs and can be stored in the refrigerator between 2°C and 8°C for a period of 6 months. The dose is 2 drops, zeor dose is administered at birth followed by booster doses along with DTP or triple antigen. To improve the immunogenicity and efficacy of OPV, the Government of India has replace tOPV with bOPV (bivalent OPV containing polio 1 and 3 viruses) on 24th April, 2016. There are two reasons to make the shift, firstly polio 2 strain has been eradicated way back 1999, secondly bOPV behaves like monovalent polio vaccine and provides enhanced immunogenicity and protection.

Oral polio vaccine is usually safe but there is a potential risk of development of vaccine associated paralytic poliomyelitis (VAPP) and emergence of vaccine derived polio viruses (VDPVs). OPV is contraindicated in children with humoral immuno-deficiency state and should not be administered even to their healthy household contacts due to risk of cross-infection.

21

Inactivated Polio Vaccine

It is currently recommended that along with OPV additional IPV should be given. It is expected that the switch to IPV will be inevitable during the post-polio-eradication era to reduce the risk of vaccine-associated polio paralysis (VAPP). It is expected that after eradication of polio, the use of OPV will be stopped or replaced by monovalent or bivalent vaccine but vaccine protection will continue by administration of IPV.

It is suggested that OPV should continue at this stage, but IPV should be introduced in the schedule gradually in families who can afford. The currently available IPV vaccines are enhanced potency IPV (eIPV) that contains 40, 8 and 32 D antigen units of types 1, 2 and 3 respectively. The vaccine is highly immunogenic and safe. It produces excellent local pharyngeal and systemic immunity and some intestinal protection. The studies in developed countries have shown that it has excellent herd effect.

Inactivated polio vaccine may be administered as an isolated or a single vaccine (0.5 mL) or as a combination vaccine with diphtheria, tetanus, and acellular pertusis (DTaP) plus Hib. The currently recommended schedule includes OPV at birth; OPV + IPV at 6, 10, 14 weeks and at 15 to 18 months; and OPV at 4.5 to 5 years. The additional doses of OPV during national and subnational immunization days must be taken. There is evidence to suggest that sequential administration of IPV, two or more doses followed by OPV, two or more doses (at an interval of 4 to 8 weeks) provides effective immunological protection against polioviruses without any risk of VAPP.

A child who has completed primary schedule of OPV can be offered IPV if younger than 5 years. Inactivated polio vaccine is given in three doses: the first two doses at 2 months interval followed by the third dose at 6 months after the first dose. In immunodeficient children or their close contacts, IPV is the preferred vaccine because OPV is associated with an increased risk of VAPP. In addition to three primary doses, boosters of IPV should be given at 1.5 and 5 years of age. The Ministry of Health and Family Welfare, Government of India has introduced single dose of IPV in certain states of the country w.e.f. November 2015.

According to current guidelines by Indian Academy of Pediatrics, it is recommended to give 'zero dose' of OPV at birth, three primary doses of IPV at 6, 10, 14 weeks, followed by two doses of OPV at 6 and 9 months. Additional booster dose of IPV can be given at 15–18 months and a dose of OPV at 5 years. Alternatively two doses of IPV can be given at 8 weeks and 16 weeks of age. If IPV has been missed, catch-up vaccination is recommended by administration of two doses at an interval of two months followed by a booster after 6 months.

Hepatitis B Vaccine

Hepatitis B virus (HBV) is the most important cause of chronic hepatitis, cirrhosis of liver and hepatocellular carcinoma. In India, 2–4% of individual are carriers of HBV. The plasma-derived hepatitis B vaccine is no longer available. The currently available vaccine containing the surface antigen of hepatitis B is produced by recombinant technology in yeast and adjuvanted with aluminium salts. It is available as single or multidose vials and should be stored at 2°C–8°C. The vaccine is also available as a combination vaccine with DTaP or DTwP. The dose in children below 18 years is 0.5 mL/10 µg and in those 18 years and older 1.0 mL/20 µg. It is administered intramuscularly in the anterolateral thigh or deltoid region. The classical schedule of hepatitis B vaccine is 0 (monovalent vaccine only), 1 and 6 months but greater flexibility can be used when combination vaccine is used. A booster dose after the age of 5 years is optional. If mother is HBsAg positive (especially when HBeAg positive), the baby should be given hepatitis B vaccine and hepatitis B immunoglobulins (HBIG 0.5 mL) as early as possible but preferably within 12 hours of birth, using two separate syringes and separate sites for administration. HBIG may be given up to 7 days of birth but its protective efficacy is doubtful when it is administered after 48 hours. All infants born to HBsAg positive mothers should be tested for HBsAg and anti-HBsAg antibodies at the age of 9–15 months to identify carriers or non-responders. Catch-up vaccination can be done at any age by using 0, 1, 6 months schedule. Hepatitis B vaccine should be routinely offered to all individuals but is considered as mandatory in high-risk settings that include health care professionals and workers, laboratory technicians, public safety personnel and workers in other allied health professions.

Diphtheria, Tetanus and Pertussis (DTP) Vaccines

Triple antigen or DTP vaccines are available either as whole cell pertussis (DTwP) or acellular pertussis (DTaP) vaccines. The whole cell vaccines are more reactogenic and immunogenic providing better protection while acellular vaccines are less reactogenic (often believed as "painless" by parents) but provide relatively lower immunity and protection.

DTwP Vaccines

The vaccine is composed to tetanus (5–25 Lf) and diphtheria (20–30 Lf) toxoids as well as killed whole cell pertussis bacilli adsorbed on insoluble aluminium salts which act as adjuvants. The protective efficacy varies between 60 and 90% but immunity gradually wanes off unless it is maintained by regular boosters. Most adverse effects of DTwP are because of pertussis component and consist of local pain, swelling and redness, fever, irritability and anorexia. Serious adverse effects include high grade fever, inconsolable crying, hypotonic hyporesponsive episodes (HHE), seizures and developmental retardation due to encephalopathy. When serious side effects occur with the first dose of DTwP, the vaccination schedule should be completed with dual antigen (DT vaccine) by avoiding pertussis component. In view of increased protective efficacy of DTwP, many countries are shifting back to use whole cell pertussis vaccine. There is a need to develop less reactogenic and safer whole cell pertussis vaccines.

DTaP Vaccines

In view of serious adverse effects of whole cell pertussis vaccine, acellular pertussis (DTaP) vaccine was first introduced in Japan and subsequently licensed in US in 1996. Acellular vaccines have much better safety profile because of use of purified antigens and removal of lipopolysaccharide (LPS) and other parts of bacterial cell wall. Acellular vaccines are safer with less risk of adverse reactions but there are some concerns regarding relatively lower efficacy and protection. DTwP and DTaP combination vaccines with hepatitis B and H. influenzae b antigens are available to reduce the number of vaccination shots. Pentavalent (DTwP + Hib + HBV + IPV) and quadrivalent (DTwP or DTaP + Hib + HBV) formulations are available.

Triple antigen is administered in three primary doses at 6, 10 and 14 weeks, followed by boosters at 15–18 months and 4½ years. The dose is 0.5 mL intramuscularly over anterolateral aspect of thigh. The standard strength DTwP and DTaP vaccines should not be given to children above 7 years of age due to increased reactogenicity. A booster dose of standard strength tetanus and reduced strength diphtheria and acellular pertussis vaccine (Tdap or boosterix) is recommended at 10 years for boosting immunity among adolescents.

Tetanus Toxoid (TT)

Tetanus toxoid containing 5 Lf toxoid is available as one of the most heat stable and immunogenic vaccines with least adverse effects. It is being increasingly replaced by normal strength tetanus (5 Lf) and low strength diphtheria, (2 Lf) Td or dual vaccine. The dual vaccine can be used in all situations where TT was used. During pregnancy, when mother is unimmunized, two doses of TT (or preferably Td) are administered so that protective antibodies in adequate titers are transferred to the fetus to prevent neonatal tetanus. The first dose should be given at the time of first contact or as early as possible and second dose after 4 weeks but preferably atleast 2 weeks before delivery. When a woman is effectively immunized, one dose of TT or Td during first pregnancy is enough to cover future pregnancies. The protective efficacy of tetanus toxoid is believed to last for 10 years and there is no need to administer booster dose if wound is minor and clean. However, when there are extensive wounds with contamination, automobile accident and burns, local cleaning and debridement of wound should be followed by administration of TT or Td and tetanus immunoglobulins (TIG 250–500 iu IM).

Hemophilus Influenzae Type B (Hib) Conjugate Vaccines

Hemophilus influenzae type b (Hib) is an invasive Gram-negative pathogen which is known to cause bacteremia, pneumonia, meningitis, osteomyelitis, arthritis and epiglottitis in children during first 2 years of life. All Hib vaccines are conjugated vaccines where Hib capsular polysaccharide is conjugated with a protein carrier to provide protection in early years of life. Isolated Hib vaccine is available but it is mostly administered as a quadrivalent or pentavalent combination vaccine with DTaP or DTwP, Hib and hepatitis B with or without IPV.

Isolated Hib vaccine is given in 3 doses when initiated below 6 months, 2 doses between 6 and 12 months and or a single dose between 12 and 15 months, followed by a booster at 15 and 18 months. The combination vaccine is administered as per schedule of triple antigen. The vaccine is stored between 2°C and 8°C and administered intramuscularly.

Measles, Mumps and Rubella (MMR) Vaccines

Measles vaccine is formulated from Edmonston-Zagreb strain grown on human diploid cells or purified chick embryo cells. It is available as freeze-dried single dose or multidose vials with distilled water as a diluent. Instead of single dose measles vaccine at 9 months of age, Indian Academy of Pediatrics, has replaced it with administration of first dose of MMR followed by a booster dose at 15 months. Most countries use MMR vaccine instead of monovalent measles vaccine.

Rubella vaccine is derived from RA 27/3 strain and mumps vaccine is prepared from Leningrad-Zagreb, Leningrad-3, Jeryl Lynn, RIT 4385 or Urabe AM9 strain grown in chick embryo or human diploid cells. MMR vaccine contains live attenuated viruses of measles, mumps and rubella. It is available in a lyophilized form, which should be kept frozen for long term storage or 2°C–8°C in the clinic. The reconstituted vaccine should be protected from light and used within 4–6 hours of reconstitution. It is administered in a dose of 0.5 mL subcutaneously at 9 and 15 months of age. The vaccine can be given along with all other childhood vaccines except BCG.

The vaccine can be safely given to children with history of egg allergy. There is no evidence for causal relationship between MMR vaccine and autism spectrum disorder. Recently, combined MMR plus chickenpox vaccine (Priorix Tetra) has been introduced.

Rotavirus Vaccines

Rotavirus is an important cause of diarrhea-related morbidity and mortality. Epidemiological studies in India indicate that 20% of all childhood diarrheas that need hospitalization are because of rotavirus. The mortality because of rotavirus diarrhea is higher among the poor and malnourished children living in developing countries. India accounts for 22% of all global deaths because of rotavirus diarrhea. Rotavirus is an icosahedral ribonucleic acid virus and seven serogroups (A to G) have been described. Currently, three live oral vaccines are licensed and marketed worldwide; Rotarix (GlaxoSmithKline Biologicals SA, Rixensart, Belgium) and RotaTeq (Merck Sharp and Dohme, Ambler, PA) and Rotavac (Bharat Biotech).

Rotarix is a monovalent attenuated human rotavirus vaccine derived from rotavirus strain 89–12 and contains GIPIA(8) strain. It is administered orally in a two-dose schedule after an interval of 4 to 8 weeks. It is available as a lyophilized vaccine, which is reconstituted with a diluent before administration.

RotaTeq is a pentavalent human-bovine reassortant vaccine and consists of five reassortants between bovine WC 23 strain and human G1, G2, G3, G4 and PIA(8) rotavirus strains. The vaccine is available as a liquid formulation with a buffer and no previous reconstitution is required. Three oral doses are given: the first dose is administered between 6 and 12 weeks followed by subsequent doses at intervals of 4 to 8 weeks. Rotavirus vaccine is not recommended for administration after the age of 6 months because of lower efficacy or need and potentially higher risk in intussusception as a side effect.

Rotavac is a monovalent live attenuated vaccine containing 116E human-bovine reassortant Indian strain (G9P) prepared in vero cells. The vaccine strain

was isolated in 1985 from asymptomatic neonates admitted in the NICU of All India Institute of Medical Sciences, New Delhi. In liquid form, vaccine is usually pink in color and 0.5 mL of vaccine is administered orally in three doses along with DTP. It is recommended that when a particular rotavirus vaccine is administered, the schedule should be completed with the same vaccine without interchanging with other vaccine formulation.

Pneumococcal Vaccines

Streptococcus pneumoniae is an important cause of community-acquired pneumonia, acute otitis media, and bacterial meningitis. Ninety serotypes of *S. pneumoniae* have been identified, but only serotypes 14, 6, 19, 18, 9, 23 and 7 are responsible for 85% cases of invasive pneumococcal disease in the developed countries. In India, the limited studies available suggest that serotypes 6, 1, 19, 14, 4, 5, 45, 12, 7 and 23 are most prevalent with serotypes 1 and 5 accounting for 30% of invasive pneumococcal disease.

Three vaccines are available; one unconjugated polysaccharide vaccine and two conjugated vaccines. *The unconjugated polysaccharide vaccine* is a 23-valent vaccine (pneumococcal polysaccharide vaccine (PPV23) which is a T-cell independent vaccine that is poorly immunogenic below the age of 2 years. It is administered to "high risk" children after the age of 2 years or elderly subjects in a single dose or maximum of two doses.

The 13-valent PCV (Prevenar or Synflorix) is given to healthy children 0.5 mL intramuscularly in three primary doses at 6, 10 and 14 weeks and one booster dose at 15 to 18 months (along with diphtheria, tetanus and pertussis (DTP) vaccine but at a different site). When pneumococcal vaccine is missed before 6 months of age, a catch-up vaccination is provided with lesser number of shots: 6 to 12 months, two doses 4 to 8 weeks apart and a booster at 15 to 18 months; 12 to 23 months, two doses 4 to 8 weeks apart; and 24 to 59 months, a single dose.

In *high-risk* children, PCV 13 or Synflorix should be given as per the aforementioned schedule up to the age of 9 years if the family can affort it. In children above 2 years, PPV 23 should be given in a single intramuscular dose of 0.5 mL. *Only one repeat dose of PPV 23 is recommended after 3 to 5 years if the child is younger than 10 years of age and after 5 years if the child is older than 10 years of age.* When a child has received PCV 13 or Synflorix earlier, a gap of 2 months must be maintained between PCV and subsequent administration of PPV 23.

Tetanus Toxid with Low-Dose Diphtheria (Td) and Tetanus Toxoid with Low-Dose Diphtheria Plus Acellular Pertussis (TdaP) Vaccines

There is a recent evidence to suggest that immunity following full course of diphtheria-tetanus-whole cell pertussis (DTwP) or diphtheria-tetanus-acellular pertussis (DTaP) wanes off gradually by the age of 10 to 12 years. In general, DTwP vaccines have greater efficacy and longer duration of protection than DTaP vaccines but are more reactogenic with higher incidence of adverse effects. There is a need to develop DTwP vaccine with detoxified lipopolysaccharide which is the main cause of reactogenicity of whole-cell vaccines. There are reports of development of diphtheria and pertussis in adolescent children who had received full course of DTaP. It is not possible to boost the protection against diphtheria or pertussis with standard strength or conventional DTP vaccine because of severe reactions in children above the age of 6 years.

Instead of isolated TT, it is currently recommended to use a combination of TT and a low-dose (2Lf) diphtheria toxoid (Td) whenever there is a need for boosting tetanus protection (every 10 years, pregnancy, trauma, and animal bites). it is safe, can be given at any age, and is useful to prevent occurrence of breakthrough diphtheria in adolescents and adults.

In low-dose triple antigen containing TT(5Lf), diphtheria toxoid (2Lf), and the acellular pertussis components, namely, pertussis toxoid 8 μg, filamentous agglutinin 8 μg, and pertactin 2.5 μg, is available in India as TT with low-dose diphtheria and pertussis (Tdap) vaccine (Boostrix by GlaxoSmithKline). In a fully vaccinated child, Tdap is administered in a single-dose intramuscular over the deltoid region at the age of 10 to 12 years. In children who have missed primary immunization with DTwP or DTaP and are older than 7 years of age, one dose of Tdap and two doses of Td are given at 0, 1, and 6 months. Common side effects include pain, swelling and redness at the site of injection in 70% of vaccinees.

Human Papillomavirus Vaccine (HPV)

Cervical cancer is the second most common cancer and is caused by oncogenic strains of human papillomavirus. Almost 100 serotypes of human papillomavirus have been identified, of which 15 to 20 are oncogenic. Types 16 and 18 account for 70% of the cases of invasive cervical cancer and the rest by serotypes 31 and 45. In addition, non-oncogenic human papillomavirus infection usually occurs because of direct skin-to-skin genital contact or through sexual activity; hence, vaccination should ideally be given before marriage or sexual activity.

Gardasil is a mixture of L1 proteins of human papillomavirus serotypes 16, 18, 6 and 11 with aluminum-containing adjuvant. The vaccine is recommended in women between 12 and 46 years of age and given 0.5 mL intramuscularly in three doses at 0, 2 and 6 months. It also provides protection against genital warts.

Cervarix is a mixture of L1 proteins of human papillomavirus serotypes 16 and 18 with AS04, which is a novel adjuvant system (aluminium hydroxide with monophosphoryl lipid A). Cervarix provides cross-protection against human papillomavirus 31 and 45. It is recommended in women between 10 and 45 years of age; a 0.5 mL dose is given intramuscularly at 0, 1, and 6 months. Recently, it is recommended that during 9–14 years, two doses of cervarix or gardasil administered at an interval of 6 months are sufficient.

Both vaccines are safe and common side effects include fever, local pain, redness, and swelling at the site of injection. Adolescent children, in general, are vulnerable to develop syncope following any vaccine shot. They should be given emotional support and counseling before vaccination. The vaccine should be given over the deltoid region while the child is sitting or lying down and the child should be observed for 15 minutes after the vaccination.

New Generation Vaccines

The currently available BCG against tuberculosis has poor protective efficacy and it merely prevents development of disseminated tuberculosis. The trials are underway to develop more effective subunit vaccines, DNA vaccine, and attenuated mycobacterial vaccine.

A highly attenuated NYVAC vaccinia virus strain has been utilized to develop a multiantigen-multistage vaccine candidate against malaria (NYVAC-Pf7). A recombinant *Plasmodium vivax* vaccine and a combination of malarial antigens with immune-boosting adjuvants and hepatitis B surface antigen are under development against all the four serotypes of malarial parasites.

A tetravalent live-attenuated vaccine against dengue fever has been developed in primary dog, kidney cells and is undergoing phase 3 trials in Thailand. A chimeric vaccine is under development by using attenuated YF virus vector (YF 17 D) in combination with all the donor genes from four serotypes of DEN 1 to 4. The chimeriVax system has been used to replace E gene of the 17 D YF vaccine with the analogous gene of the vaccine-targeted flavivirus (YF-DEN vaccine).

Other important candidates for vaccine development include human immunodeficiency virus (HIV),

21

respiratory syncytial virus (RSV), shigella, Group A and Group B streptococci (to prevent rheumatic fever) and hepatitis E and C, cytomegalovirus, Lyme disease, enterotoxigenic *Escherichia coli*, Epstein-Barr virus, schistosomiasis, bird flu, and *Helicobacter pylori*. The World Health Organisation has launched an initiative to produce vaccines against biological weapons, for example, anthrax, smallpox, plague, and hemorrhagic viral fevers, but their acceptance and commercial viability are doubtful.

Varicella Vaccine

Varicella or chickenpox may cause serious disease in adolescents and herpes zoster (shingles) during adult life. It is a live attenuated vaccine developed from Oka strain. Vaccine protects against development of severe chickenpox and shingles. The vaccine is administered in two doses, first dose alongwith MMR or between 15 to 18 months of age, followed by a booster at 4–6 years of age. The catch-up vaccine can be administered at any age (if an individual has not suffered from chickenpox) in two doses at least 3 months apart. A combined MMR-varicella (Priorix-Tetra) vaccine has been introduced recently to reduce the number of vaccine shots. It provides effective immunity but is slightly more reactogenic than isolated MMR or varicella vaccines.

Hepatitis A Vaccine

Most of the currently available hepatitis A vaccines are available from HM 175/GBM strains and grown on human diploid cell lines. The virus is formalin inactivated and adjuvanted with aluminium hydroxide. The vaccine is administered in two doses, first dose at 12 months, followed by a booster dose after 6–12 months. Live vaccine derived from H2 strain of the virus, attenuated by serial passages in human diploid cells (KMB 17 cell line) is also available. The live vaccine can be given in a single dose at the age of 12 months or preferably in two doses, the second dose is administered after 6–12 months of the first shot.

Typhoid Vaccines

The whole cell inactivated phenol-preserved vaccine has been replaced by new generation vi-capsular polysaccharide (Vi-PS) and Vi-polysaccharide conjugate vaccine. The vaccines contain highly purified antigenic fraction of Vi-capsular polysaccharide antigen of *S. typhi*, which determines virulence of the bacteria. Vi-polysaccharide vaccine is recommended after 2 years of age in a dose of 0.5 mL SC or IM. Revaccination is recommended every 3 years to maintain the immunity. In view of increasing incidence of typhoid fever below

2 years of age, Vi-capsular polysaccharide conjugate vaccines are preferred. Vi-PS is conjugated with tetanus toxoid (Typbar TCV®, Pedatyph®), can be administered below 2 years and produces both humoral and cellular immunity. The first dose is given between 9 and 12 months, followed by a single booster after 6 months to one year. A child with history of suspected or confirmed typhoid fever, may be vaccinated 4 weeks after recovery (when risk of relapse of typhoid fever is ruled out) if the child was not vaccinated in the past. The vaccine is stored between 2°C–8°C and should not be frozen.

VACCINES FOR HIGH-RISK CHILDREN

Influenza Vaccines

The influenza virus, a single stranded RNA virus, is classified into three main types A, B and C. The available vaccines include inactivated trivalent vaccines containing two influenza A strains (H1N1 or swine flu and H3N2) and one influenza B strain. A live attenuated influenza vaccine is also available which is administered through nasal route. Depending upon the circulating strain of influenza virus in the northern and southern hemispheres, the antigenic composition of vaccine is revised twice in a year. The commonly available vaccines are inactivated trivalent vaccines containing two influenza strains (H1N1 and H3N2) and one influenza B strain.

The vaccine is recommended in children with chronic systemic disease (especially cardio-pulmonary), congenital or acquired (HIV) immunodeficiency state, children on long-term salicylate therapy, laboratory personnel and healthcare workers and elderly subjects. The vaccine is given after the age of 6 months, in a dose of 0.25 mL in children between 6–35 months and 0.5 mL in children aged 3 years and above. Two primary doses, 4 weeks apart, are given to children between 6 months–9 years and a single primary dose to children 9 years and above followed by boosters once every year. Every year newly released stock of vaccine should be used preferably before the onset of rainy season.

Japanese Encephalitis Vaccines

Japanese encephalitis, a mosquito borne flavivirus disease is endemic in several parts of India. It has a case fatality rate of 30% and high percentage of survivors are left with permanent neuropsychiatric sequelae. Three types of JE vaccines are marketed in India. One live attenuated cell culture-derived vaccine (IMOJEV by Sanofi Pasteur) and two inactivated vero cell culture-derived vaccines (JEEV by BE India,

JENVAC by Bharat Biotech). The vaccine is administered to susceptible children living in endemic areas or during disease outbreaks. Two doses of inactivated vaccine are administered 4 weeks apart to children above one year of age. The need for boosters is still undetermined.

Meningococcal Vaccines

There are 13 known serotypes of *Neisseria meningitides* but 90% of disease causing isolates belong to serogroups A, B, C, Y and W–135. Meningococcal polysaccharide vaccines are either bivalent (A + C) or quadrivalent (A, C, Y, W–135). Meningococcal conjugate vaccines are preferred and are available either as monovalent or quadrivalent (Menactra by Sanofi Pasteur). The vaccine is recommended to high risk children (chronic debilitating disease, immunodeficiency state, laboratory personnel, during outbreaks, international travellers, pilgrims to Haj or endemic African countries. A single dose of quadrivalent conjugate vaccine is given after the age of 6 months. A booster dose may be given after 5 years if there is a risk of reexposure.

Rabies Vaccines

Rabies is an invariably fatal disease transmitted mostly through the bites, scratches or licks of rabid dogs. A number of safe and effective cell culture vaccines are available which include purified chick embryo cell vaccine (PCECV), human diploid cell vaccine (HDCV) and purified vero cell vaccine (PVCV). Post-exposure prophylaxis is given by administration of 4 doses of 1.0 mL each IM or SC on day 0, 3, 7 and 14, optional dose on day 28 in an immunocompromised child. In case of a bite by a pet dog or when a biting animal can be watched, three doses are enough if animal is normal on day 10 of observation.

Pre-exposure prophylaxis is recommended in high-risk individuals like children with pets, hostelers, postmen, wild life workers, veterinary doctors and their assistants. Three primary doses of vaccine are given on 0, 7 and 21 or 28 days followed by a booster dose after one year. In a vaccinated individual, only two doses (day 0 and 3) of vaccine are given for post-exposure prophylaxis. In these cases no rabies immune globulins (RIG) is needed.

Cholera Vaccines

The predominant strains of *V. cholerae* O1 include classical and Eltor. The available whole cell killed cholera vaccines have poor efficacy which lasts for 3 months. There is a possibility to develop a killed whole cell oral cholera vaccine. Cholera vaccine is recommended only during risk of an out break or when travelling or attending massive congregations like *Kumbh mela* and Haj tours. The vaccine is administered above the age of one year. Two doses are given 2 weeks apart, protection is achieved after 2 weeks of receipt of the second dose.

Yellow Fever Vaccine

The vaccination against yellow fever is mandatory for visitors to sub-Saharan African and Central/South America. The available vaccine is a live attenuated vaccine derived from 17D strain of the virus grown in chick 140 embryo cells. A single dose of vaccine is given to children above 9 months. The certificate of vaccination is valid for 10 years, beginning 10 days after the date of vaccination. Yellow fever vaccine is contraindicated during pregnancy, congenital and acquired immune deficiency states, chemotherapy, recipients of immunosuppressive drugs and transplants.

THE COLD CHAIN

In order to ensure potency of vaccines, they must be kept in cold conditions during transport and at the immunization center. The vaccines should be stocked neatly in the refrigerator and no more than one month's stock should be kept. It is preferable to use a purpose-built refrigerator which is meant for storage of vaccines but a double-door domestic regrigerator can be used but it should be dedicated entirely for storing vaccines alone. The live vaccines (measles, MMR, BCG, OPV, rotavirus, yellow fever chickenpox) should be kept on the top shelf below the freezer. The toxoids and killed vaccines should be stored in the middle shelf. The diluents may be kept in the door of the refrigerator. *No vaccine should be stored in the door of refrigerator and no food or drinks should be kept in the refrigerator meant for storing vaccines.* The door of the refrigerator should be opened only for taking out vaccine and frig should be kept clean and defrosted periodically. The frozen ice packs should be kept in the door and lower shelf of the refrigerator to keep it cool during power failures. The temperature of the refrigerator should be checked twice a day with a dial thermometer and kept between +4°C and +8°C. The left over reconstituted BCG vaccine should be discarded and "expired" vaccines should not be kept in the refrigerator. Cold boxes and vaccine carriers are used for transporting vaccines for short distances. They are used for transport of vaccines to primary health centers and subcenters and from the vaccine supplier to the hospitals and practicing pediatricians. Frozen ice packs are placed at the bottom and side of the thermocol box. The vaccines should be kept in polythene bags and then placed inside the vaccine carrier. The liquid vaccines (except OPV) and diluents should not be kept in direct contact with the frozen ice pack. BCG (after reconstitution), varicella, measles, MMR, rotavirus and human papilloma virus vaccines should be protected from light.

Preparing the Child for the Shot

Children should not be given threats of injections and doctors for modification of their behavior. Different children have different thresholds for pain and anxiety. Nurse should give an honest and simple explanation to the child depending upon his age and level of understanding. The child should be told that the shot would hurt a little (like a thorn or insect bite or hard pinch) but it will protect him from sickness that would hurt him much more than the shot.

Nursing Alert

Never administer any vaccine into the gluteal region due to slow absorption because of pad of fat and risk of injury to the sciatic nerve.

Infants should be placed on the examination table. Mother should stand on the head end side for holding the arms and comforting the baby while father or an attendant should firmly hold and stabilize the leg to be injected. The shot is given over the anterolateral or lateral part of mid-thigh. A squeaky toy and soothing words of mother provide comfort to the child. After the shot, baby should be picked up, caressed, cuddled and comforted while keeping the injection site pressed for a minute or so. Preschool children are best injected while sitting in the mother's lap which provides security and comfort. After the age of 4–5 years, it is preferable to give the vaccine shot over the outer side of upper arm (deltoid region) instead of thigh. The vaccines should be given with single use disposable needles and syringes.

Contraindications to Vaccines

Most children can be given vaccines unless they are critically sick. Children with mild fever, cough and cold and diarrhea can be safely given any vaccine. It is futile to give oral polio or rotavirus vaccine to a child with vomiting and severe diarrhea because vaccine will not be retained. Children with repeated convulsions or evolving neurological disease should not be given triple antigen containing whole cell pertussis vaccine (DTwP). When a child develops shock or inconsolable crying or

Nursing Alert

No killed and aluminium adjuvanted liquid vaccine (DTwP, DTaP, TT, DT, Td, hepatitis B, HPV, PCV) should be frozen and thawed. If these vaccines get frozen, they should be discarded.

convulsions after first shot of DTwP, he should receive DTaP or DT subsequently. Children with malnutrition and allergic disorders should not be denied vaccinations, infact it is more desirable that they must receive them. Live vaccines like BCG and oral polio vaccine should not be given to immunocompromised children (primary immunodeficiency disorder, cancer or leukemia, AIDS, etc.). Instead of OPV, they can be safely given IPV.

Common Side Effects of Vaccines

By and large most vaccines are safe and they do not produce any serious side effects. The side effects seen with some of the common vaccines are listed in **Table 21.2**. The common side effects of fever, pain and discomfort at the site of vaccination can be effectively controlled by administration of paracetamol. Just as an unexpected adverse reaction may occur to certain drugs (including life-threatening anaphylaxis), similarly vaccines may also produce some unusual side effects. Measles, MMR (measles, mumps, and rubella vaccine) and flu vaccines are prepared from egg protein. Children who are highly allergic to eggs may show adverse reactions to these vaccines. Anaphylactic reaction is extremly rare and is characterised by flushing, facial edema, itching breathing difficulty, syncope and cardiovascular collapse. It is a life-threatening emergency and managed as per guidelines summarized in the **Box 21.1**. Whenever there is an adverse reaction to the administration of the first dose of a vaccine, this fact must be brought to the notice of the doctor before second dose of the vaccine is given.

The vaccines are highly cost-effective and baby-friendly and no child should be denied the benefits of available vaccines. *It must be remembered that exclusive breastfeeding during first 6 months of life and timely administration of all vaccines is crucial to protect children against a variety of life-threatening infectious diseases.*

Future Developments

Due to rapid development of newer vaccines, it is posing logistic difficulties for their administration. Most children are expected to take 10–15 immunization shots between birth and school entry. Vaccines are likely to be available for prevention of malaria, dengue fever and AIDS in the near future. Novel attempts are being

21

Table 21.2 Common side effects of vaccines

Vaccine	Side effects*
BCG	A nodule appears 3–4 weeks after BCG vaccination. It may soften or ulcerate during next 2–4 weeks. No local application or fomentation is necessary. It heals by formation of a thin scar, indicating good "take" for effective vaccination.
DTwP or DTaP	There may be fever with pain, redness and swelling at the site of injection. A small painless nodule may remain for a few days. No local application or fomentation is required. DTaP is safer and produces less side effects but is less immunogenic. Paracetamol is useful for relief of fever and pain.
Oral polio vaccine	No side effects**
Rotavirus vaccine	Safe vaccine except rare occurrence of intussusception if vaccine is delayed beyond 6 months of age.
Hib vaccine	Fever, local pain and redness
Measles/MMR	Some children may get fever and mild skin rash 7–10 days after the vaccination. A child with egg allergy may show an adverse reaction to measles, MMR and flu vaccine.
Hepatitis B vaccine	Pain and redness at the site of injection. Some children with yeast allergy may show adverse reaction.
Typhoid vaccine	Local pain, fever, malaise and headache may occur. Oral typhoid vaccine may cause vomiting, diarrhea and abdominal pain in some children.
Chickenpox vaccine	Fever and mild papulovesicular skin eruption may occur rarely.

*Before giving the next dose of vaccine, ask the mother if the child had any significant reaction to the last dose of vaccine.
** OPV-related paralytic poliomyelitis is being increasingly reported from developed countries. These countries have changed their strategy and are giving IPV (injectable or inactivated or killed polio vaccine).

Box 21.1 | **Management of anaphylaxis**

1. Place the child flat on the bed and elevate legs.
2. Maintain airway and administer oxygen.
3. Administer epinephrine or adrenaline (1: 1000 solution 0.01 mL/kg/dose (maximum 0.5 mL) intramuscularly. The dose can be repeated after 3–5 minutes if required.
4. If shock supervenes, administer normal saline 20 mL/kg rapidly over 5–10 minutes through IV access.
5. The role of oral or parenteral corticosteroids is controversial. Oral antihistamines may be given for treatment of skin rash and itching.

made to develop vaccines against non-infectious diseases like allergic disorders, type 2 diabetes mellitus, hypertension, cancer, autoimmune diseases, Alzheimer disease, multiple sclerosis, addictions and for contraception. Oral vaccines (polio, typhoid, rotavirus and cholera vaccines, etc.) and nasal vaccines (influenza, measles and RSV vaccine) are convenient to administer. Injectable vaccines are painful and do cause discomfort, anxiety and scare both to the child and parents. There is a potential risk of transmission of dangerous diseases like hepatitis B, HIV and development of local abscess at injection site due to use of recycled unsterile non-disposable needles and syringes. A number of combination vaccines (DTP with killed polio vaccine, DTP with Hib, DTP with Hib, IPV and HBV, combined hepatitis A and B vaccine, MMR-varicella vaccines, etc.) have been produced to reduce the number of vaccine shots.

A pen-shaped device, which uses supersonic waves, has been developed to deliver drugs and vaccines without any pain. The vaccine "guns" are available for painless administration of vaccines but they are expensive and useful in hospital setting or community programs when a large number of children need to be vaccinated. Efforts are being made to deliver antigens of vaccines through fruits and vegetables. Genes from bacteria or viruses can be inserted into the genetic make-up of a fruit or vegetable, which then develops a foreign antigen or protein against the new gene. Bananas, potatoes, tomatoes and cabbage are being used to produce edible vaccines which are not destroyed or inactivated when the vegetable is cooked or deep fried. There is an interesting possibility and hope that in the near future, the doctor may prescribe bananas, potato chips or pre-cooked cereal infant foods which they can purchase from the "medicated fruits and vegetable" section of the chemists shop to vaccinate their children against various diseases in the most "child-friendly" manner.

Some Frequently Asked Questions (FAQs) about Vaccinations

What is the best interval between primary doses of vaccines?

The recommended interval between two primary doses of vaccines is 4–8 weeks. The interval should not be less than 4 weeks. The protective efficacy of vaccine is better when interval between two doses is more than 4 weeks.

21

21

If a dose of vaccine is missed, what should be done?

It is desirable that the child is vaccinated as per the recommended schedule to ensure early and effective protection. Mother should record the date of next vaccination on the calender or mobile phone as a ready reminder. However, if a dose is missed, it should be taken at the earliest opportunity. There is no need to restart the vaccination schedule again. The vaccine doses already taken remain valid because the immunological system has a good memory and responds effectively to the next dose of vaccine even when it is delayed.

What should be the minimum interval between two doses of different vaccines?

Most vaccines, whether killed or live, can be administered when available in a combo formulation or simultaneously at two different sites without any interference in their immune response. A live vaccine can be administered after an inactivated vaccine (or *vice versa*) without any concern regarding the minimum interval between two vaccines. Two inactivated or killed vaccines and antigen-based vaccines may be administered simultaneously or at any interval between the two doses. *However, a minimum interval of 4 weeks is recommended between the administration of two live vaccines.*

What should be done if there is no local reaction to BCG vaccination?

If there is no local reaction at the site of BCG vaccination after 8 weeks, the vaccine may be repeated. If there is no reaction even following properly conducted revaccination, nothing needs to be done. It has been shown that effective protection against tuberculosis is achieved even when there is no local "take" response.

Should OPV be given to a child who has suffered from polio?

Yes, it is desirable because there are three strains of polio viruses. Poliomyelitis occurs with one strain of polio virus and child would develop protection against that virus only. OPV is a trivalent vaccine (contains all the 3 strains of polio viruses) and should be given to the polio patient after recovery so that he is protected against other two polio viruses. In India, we have now shifted to bivalent OPV containing 1 and 3 strains of polio virus.

What is pulse polio immunization (PPI) program?

This is a special program launched by government of India in 1995 to eradicate poliomyelitis. In this program, all children under the age of 5 years, are given additional doses (in addition to the 7 doses taken under national universal immunization program) of OPV every

fortnight on predisgnated sundays. When simultaneously all under-5 children are administered OPV on the same day, there is massive excretion of polio vaccine virus in the stools causing displacement of the wild polio virus from the community. Even if the under-5 child had received OPV dose a day earlier, he must be taken to the health post for administration of OPV under PPI. Parents must cooperate with the public health authorities in this program to ensure that our country remains free of paralytic poliomyelitis.

How to vaccinate immunocompromised children against polio?

Oral polio vaccine cannot be given to immuno-compromised children (primary immunodeficiency disorder, cancer, leukemia, AIDS, etc.) because of risk of development of vaccine-related paralytic poliomyelitis. In such a situation, OPV should not be given even to the healthy sibling because of chance of transmission of live polio virus to the immunocompromised child. They should be vaccinated with an injectable or killed (IPV) vaccine. Three doses of IPV are given at an interval of 8 weeks, followed by a booster dose after one year of last primary dose.

What are the indications to give tetanus toxoid (TT) vaccine?

Tetanus toxoid is a very effective, safe and cheap vaccine to prevent occurrence of tetanus which is a life-threatening disease. It is preferable that TT boosters should be taken every 10 years throughout life to cover the risk of tetanus due to injuries sustained during the day-to-day activities. It is a mandatory vaccine for all military personnel. It is essential that every pregnant woman must receive two doses of TT 4 weeks apart during pregnancy to prevent occurrence of tetanus in her newborn baby. The second dose of TT must be taken at least 4 weeks before the anticipated time of delivery. Instead of TT, Td in which diphtheria antigen is present in low dose (5Lf) can be safely given to adolescents and adults.

Should tetanus toxoid (TT) be given to the child after every injury?

No, in a fully vaccinated child there is no need to give a repeat dose of TT or Td following a mild or moderate injury. However, a repeat dose of TT is required if the last immunization shot against tetanus (DTP, Td or TT) was taken more than 10 years before the occurrence of injury. Irrespective of the previous immunization status, a booster dose of TT or Td along with tetanus-specific human immune globulin must be given in cases of major burns and life-threatening automobile accidents with multiple open wounds.

Which children are at a greater risk to develop hepatitis B?

Children born to HbsAg-positive mothers (especially if positive for e-antigen), those receiving multiple blood transfusions and blood or plasma products and household contacts of HbsAg-positive family members are more likely to develop hepatitis B. These children may be given a booster dose of HBV every 5 years.

What should be done for a baby born to HbsAg-positive mother?

If the mother is a known carrier for hepatitis B virus, the baby must be protected both with passive and active immunization. The infant should be given hepatitis B immunoglobulins (HBIG 0.5 mL IM) along with first dose of HBV (at two different sites) within 12 hours of birth.

Should adults also be given hepatitis B vaccine?

Everybody needs to be protected against hepatitis B but if a person is already a carrier of hepatitis B virus (HbsAg-positive) the vaccine would be of no benefit. Therefore, the antigen status should be checked if an adult is to be given hepatitis B vaccine.

Can a child develop jaundice even after receiving hepatitis A and B vaccines?

Yes, because jaundice can occur due to at least 6–7 hepatitis viruses (A-F). Hepatitis due to HAV and HEV are water-borne while HBV and HCV are blood-borne.

Which vaccines can be safely given to pregnant women?

Live vaccines (OPV, BCG, chickenpox, measles, MMR, yellow fever) should not be given during pregnancy due to risk of causing fetal infection or congenital malformations. Yellow fever vaccine may be given with caution if risk of exposure to yellow fever outweighs the risk of vaccine. Alternatively, the pregnant woman can be issued a certificate of waiver on medical grounds to fulfill health regulations. Tetanus toxoid is a mandatory vaccine during pregnancy and should be given in two doses atleast 4 weeks apart, taking care that second dose is given atleast 4 weeks before the expected date of delivery. If a pregnant woman is bitten by a dog, she must be given human diploid cell antirabies vaccine as per the recommended schedule irrespective of the duration of the pregnancy. Antirabies vaccine should not be denied because rabies is an invariably fatal disease.

Which vaccines are credited to provide "post- exposure" protection?

Most vaccines are given to healthy children to equip them with protective antibodies to fight against any future encounter against natural or wild infection. Post-exposure protection is generally provided by administration of preformed equine or human antibodies as mentioned *vide infra*. In certain infections, vaccines can provide post-exposure protection if the incubation period of the disease is very long as in the case of rabies. Early post-exposure administration of vaccines are useful for prevention of rabies and tetanus and for prevention of measles, chickenpox and hepatitis A among family contacts. Earlier the vaccine is administered, the better are the chances for protection.

In what situations are disease-specific immuno-globulins life saving?

Disease-specific immunoglobulins of human origin (previously they were prepared as antisera mostly in horses or were equine in origin) are available for prevention and treatment of several life-threatening diseases. They are in short supply and expensive but are more effective and safe to administer without any risk of allergic or anaphylactic reaction. These include human tetanus immunoglobulins, hepatitis B-specific immunoglobulins, varicella-zoster immunoglobulins, rabies-specific immunoglobulins, respiratory syncytial virus immunoglobulins and rhesus (Rh) D immuno-globulins for prevention Rh-hemolytic disease of the newborn.

What is the immunization schedule in preterm infants?

In general, all vaccines can be administered as per the immunization schedule according to the post-birth age of the child irrespective of birth weight or period of gestation. However, as long as the neonate is in the neonatal intensive care unit (NICU), there is no risk of infection by vaccine-preventable diseases. It is, therefore, logical and practical to administer the "zero day" vaccines (BCG, OPV, hepatitis B virus vaccine) at the time of discharge when the infant is likely to the more mature to mount a better immunologic response. The subsequent vaccine schedule is planned keeping in mind the day of discharge as "zero day" of life. However, if mother is HBsAg-postive, the baby can be given hepatitis-specific immunoglobulins and hepatitis B vaccine within 48 hours of birth.

What are the recommendations for administration of vaccines to HIV-positive children?

Asymptomatic HIV-positive children can be given all vaccines. In symptomatic HIV-positive (AIDS) children, BCG and OPV are contraindicated. Inactivated polio vaccine (IPV) can be given for protection against polio-myelitis but BCG is denied.

21

What precautions should be taken for administration of vaccines to children with a bleeding disorder?

The vaccine should be given subcutaneously (instead of intramuscularly) with a thin needle (>24 G). The attendent should be asked to apply a form and sustained pressure (without rubbing) at the vaccine site for atleast 5 minutes.

What polio vaccination strategies are being followed in India after eradication of poliomyelitis?

Following launch of global eradication of polio by introduction of pulse polio immunization program, polio has been eradicated worldwide except isolated cases in Afghanistan and Pakistan. India was declared polio free on January 13, 2014. Inorder to maintain effective protection against poliomyelitis and reduce the risk of vaccine associated paralytic poliomyelitis (VAPP), India introduced two strategies. In addition to oral polio vaccine, it is recommended to administer inactivated polio vaccine (IPV) which is credited to enhance immunity and reduce the risk of VAPP. The government of India introduced the policy of administration of a single dose of IPV throughout the country in a phased manner w.e.f. November 2015. The second strategy was introduction of bivalent oral polio vaccine (b OPV containing polio virus 1 and 3) on 24th April, 2016 instead of conventional trivalent OPV (tOPV) containing three viruses. The logic behind introduction of bOPV is twofold. Firstly type 2 wild polio has been eradicated worldwide as early as 1999 and there is no need to continue vaccination against it. Secondly, b OPV is more effective and as immunogenic as monovalent oral polio vaccines. Instead of using two OPVs, each containing type 1 and type 3 polio viruses, it is convenient, equally efficacious and more cost-effective to administer b OPV containing two viruses.

What is the schedule for pre-exposure rabies vaccination?

In certain high-risk individuals such as veterinary doctors, dog trainers, animal handlers, laboratory workers, postmen, wildlife employees, pre-exposure rabies vaccination is advised. The optional indication for administration of pre-exposure rabies vaccine include children belonging to families having pet animals and children living in a hostel. Three doses of tissue culture vaccine are given on days 0, 7 and 28 days followed by a booster after one year. For post-exposure protection in an immunized individual, two doses of tissue culture vaccine are given on day 0 and 3. In immunized subjects, there is no need to administer rabies immunoglobulins (RIG). However, in case of all animal bites, the wound must be washed thoroughly and effectively with soap and water.

What is the schedule for rabies vaccination when a child is bitten by a pet dog or a neighbor's dog which is available for observation?

In such cases, the initial approach is identical even when dog is fully immunized because there is potential risk of transmission of rabies even when dog has been immunized. The wound should be washed thoroughly with soap and water. If a child has not received pre-exposure immunization, rabies immunoglobulins (RIG) 20 iu/kg is infiltrated around the bite if there are bites at multiple sites, face, neck and hands. Three doses of tissue culture vaccine are given on day 0, 3 and 7. If dog is normal and alive on day 7, there is no need for further doses of vaccine. However, a fourth dose of vaccine on day 21 or 28 may be given to complete pre-exposure prophylaxis schedule.

Can influenza vaccine be given to children with egg allergy?

There is a concern regarding safety of administration of certain vaccines, which contain egg protein such as measles, MMR, influenza and yellow fever vaccines. When there is a history of severe IgE-mediated reaction following intake of egg such as vomiting, facial swelling, difficulty in swallowing, stridor, breathing difficulty, widespread hives or anaphylaxis, it is preferable to avoid flu or other vaccines containing egg protein. In a child with mild or non IgE-mediated delayed reaction to egg protein, such as mild GI disturbances, localized swelling around perioral or diaper area, vaccine can be administered with caution. After vaccination, the child should be observed in the clinic for 15 minutes. If any allergic symptoms develop, the child should be managed by administration of epinephrine and antihistaminic.

Should measles, mumps, and rubella vaccine be given to male children? If MMR vaccine is missed in infancy, can it be given later in life?

Yes, MMR vaccine must be given to children of both sexes. Rubella during early pregnancy can cause devastating effects on the fetus while mumps in adolescent boys may be complicated by orchitis and infertility. According to latest recommendation of Indian Academy of Pediatrics, first dose of MMR (instead of measles alone) is given at 9 months followed by a booster during 15 to 18 months. If it is missed in infancy, the vaccine can be given at any age in two doses 4–8 weeks apart. If MMR vaccine is taken by a woman of childbearing age, pregnancy should be avoided for the next 3 months to circumvent the potential risk of development of rubella syndrome in the fetus.

BIBLIOGRAPHY

Handbook for vaccine and cold chain handlers. Ministry of Health and Family Welfare, Govt. of India and UNICEF 2010. Available online http://www.unicef.org/india/cold_chain_ book_final_ pdf.

Indian Academy of Pediatrics Committee on Immunization (IAPCOI). Consensus recommendations on Immunizations 2010. *Indian Pediatr* 2012: 49(7): 549–564.

Kimmel SR, Wolfe RM. Communicating the benefits and risks of vaccines. *J family practice* 2005, 54:51–57.

Vashishtha VM, Choudhury P, Bansal CP, Yewale VN, Agarwal R. IAP Guidebook on Immunization 2013–14, IAP National Publication House, Gwalior, 2014.

Vashishtha VM, Kumar P. Fifty years of immunization in India: Progress and future. *Indian Pediatr* 2013, 50: 111–118.

WHO best practices for injections and related procedure tool kit. March 2010, WHO/EHT/10.02 accessed from http://whqlibdoc. who.int/publications/2010/9789241599252_eng.pdf.

21

Growth and Development

Growth and development or maturation are two most distinctive attributes of children which distinguish them from adults. Growth refers to increase in body weight and height. Development refers to functional maturation of various neuromotor skills so that from a state of total dependence, the child gradually becomes independent in his day-to-day activities. In normal children, growth and development go hand-in-hand. But at times physical growth may be normal while neuromotor development is retarded and vice versa. Growth and development depends upon an interaction between genetic endowment or constitution and adequacy of nutrition, availability of safe and stimulating environment, freedom from diseases and developmental defects and love and affection by well-adjusted parents. *The basic aim and goal of pediatrics is to ensure that every child is assisted to achieve his or her optimal genetic potential for physical growth and mental development.*

Growth of Various Body Systems and Organs

There is a unique pattern of anatomic growth of various body systems and organs in children (**Figure 22.1**). The physical or somatic growth follows an S-shaped curve with two peaks of growth velocity, one during infancy and toddler age period and the other during adolescence. Neural or brain growth is maximal during fetal life and is completed by the age of 5–6 years. At birth baby has a large head size because 70% of the brain growth is already complete and 15% of the brain growth occurs during first year of life and remaining 15% during preschool years. Therefore, nutritional deficiencies and metabolic defects have profound effects on the integrity of brain and neuromotor development during late fetal life, infancy and preschool years. There is an excessive lymphoid growth in children as a protective response to prevent entry of pathogens through the nose and throat and generate high levels of cell-mediated and humoral immune responses to fight microbial diseases. School going

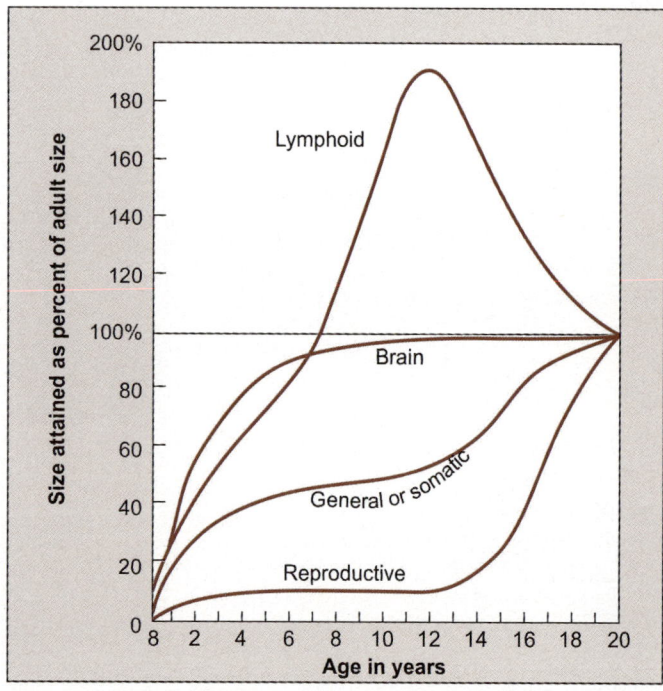

Figure 22.1 Different organs and tissues of the baby grow at different rates during childhood. See text for details

children do have large sized tonsils and adenoids as a protective mechanism to ward off droplet infections. Large tonsils or adenoids are an asset and not a liability or indicative of a disease in children. It is a common observation to find generalized lymph node enlargement in children as a normal physiologic response. The hyper-responsive lymphoid tissues tends to regress in size after the age of 12 years to achieve adult size when adolescence is completed. There is a minimal growth of genital organs during childhood. Adolescence is triggered by sudden release of gonadotropins from pituitary-hypothalamus axis around 10–12 years (10 years in girls and 12 years in boys) with appearance of secondary sex characters and sudden spurt in the growth of genitals which is completed by the age of 16 years in girls and 18 years in boys.

PHYSICAL GROWTH

Weight

The physical growth depends upon the genetic stock, adequacy of nutrition and freedom from illnesses. Growth is a steady continuous process but there are phases of very rapid growth. For example, maximum velocity of growth takes place during fetal life. Around 8 weeks of pregnancy, fetus weighs 1.0 gram while at birth (after 40 weeks) an average weight of baby is 3.0 kg (6½ lbs). Most babies double their birth weight by 4–5 months and triple it by one year (**Table 22.1**). Preterm and malnourished or asymmetric small-for-dates babies are likely to have relatively faster growth velocity. After birth, growth is extremely fast during first year of life and again during adolescence (phase of sexual maturation). Most infants are plump during early infancy but as their activity level increases they become lean and tall. Parents should not be unduly worried about the weight gain of their school going child because she is normally expected to gain around 2.5 kg weight in one year. Boys usually weigh more than girls except during 12–13 years of age when most girls weigh more than boys due to early onset of puberty in girls.

Road-to-Health card Isolated weight record does not provide any useful information regarding well being of a child but a serial or periodic weight record is more useful. Weight and height should be recorded on a Road-to-Health card during first 5 years of life (**Figure 22.2**). These measurements should be recorded every month (during visits for vaccinations) during first year, every 2 months during second year and every 3 months subsequently. Parents should understand the importance of growth charting and keep the Road-to-Health card in their safe custody. *The periodic and regular weight record provides valuable information regarding physical growth of the child as opposed to a single weight record*. The trend or slope of the weight curve is more important than its location on the chart. The growth curve of the healthy child should be directed upwards or it should run parallel to the 50th percentile line.

Corrected age About 10% of neonates are born prematurely without completing 40 weeks of gestation. For example, if a child is born on April 2, 1999 while his expected date of delivery was June 2, 1999, this means his gestational age at birth is 32 weeks. He will be zero day old on June 2, 1999. Therefore, the corrected postnatal age of this child on August 2, 1999 would be only 2 months (not 4 months). His physical growth and neuromotor development on August 2, 1999 would correspond to a normal 2 months old child. The concept of corrected age is used during first year of life.

Characteristics of a Healthy Child

Depending upon the genetic background and regional variations, healthy children vary a great deal in their weight and height at different ages. Some may be relatively taller than others, some may have narrower body frame with lighter bones while others may be broad-built depending upon the constitution and build of their parents. What is more important is the growth rate of the child and direction of his growth curve rather than any single weight record. Healthy child is likely to be active, energetic, happy and playful. There should be no cause for any concern when child is eating well, does not fall sick frequently, runs around and is busy with his naughty pranks. The overall vitality, exuberance and sense of well being are more important than actual weight of the child. Infact, active, wiry and restless babies expend so much energy in their day-to-day activity that they remain lean and never become chubby.

Body Mass Index

Inorder to provide optimal health care to children, we should try to ensure optimal nutrition by preventing under nutrition as well as over nutrition or obesity. Surveys have shown that in affluent families in India, around 20 to 25% of adolescent children attending public schools are overweight. These children are at an increased risk to develop obesity and its health consequences like metabolic syndrome X, type 2 diabetes mellitus, hypertension, coronary artery disease and osteoporosis in adult life. Body mass index (BMI)

Table 22.1 Average weight gain during childhood	
(A) Age	Weight gain
0–4 months	1.0 kg/month (30 g/day)
5–8 months	0.75 kg/month (20 g/day)
9–12 months	0.50 kg/month (15 g/day)
1–3 years	2.25 kg/year
4–9 years	2.75 kg/year
10–18 years	4.0–5.0 kg/year (upto 0.5 kg/month)
(B) Age	Weight gain
Weight at 4–5 months	2 × birth weight
Weight at 1 year	3 × birth weight
Weight at 2 years	4 × birth weight
Weight at 7 years	7 × birth weight
Weight in kg = (Age in years + 3) × 2	

Based on National Center for Health Statistics (NCHS) and WHO standards.

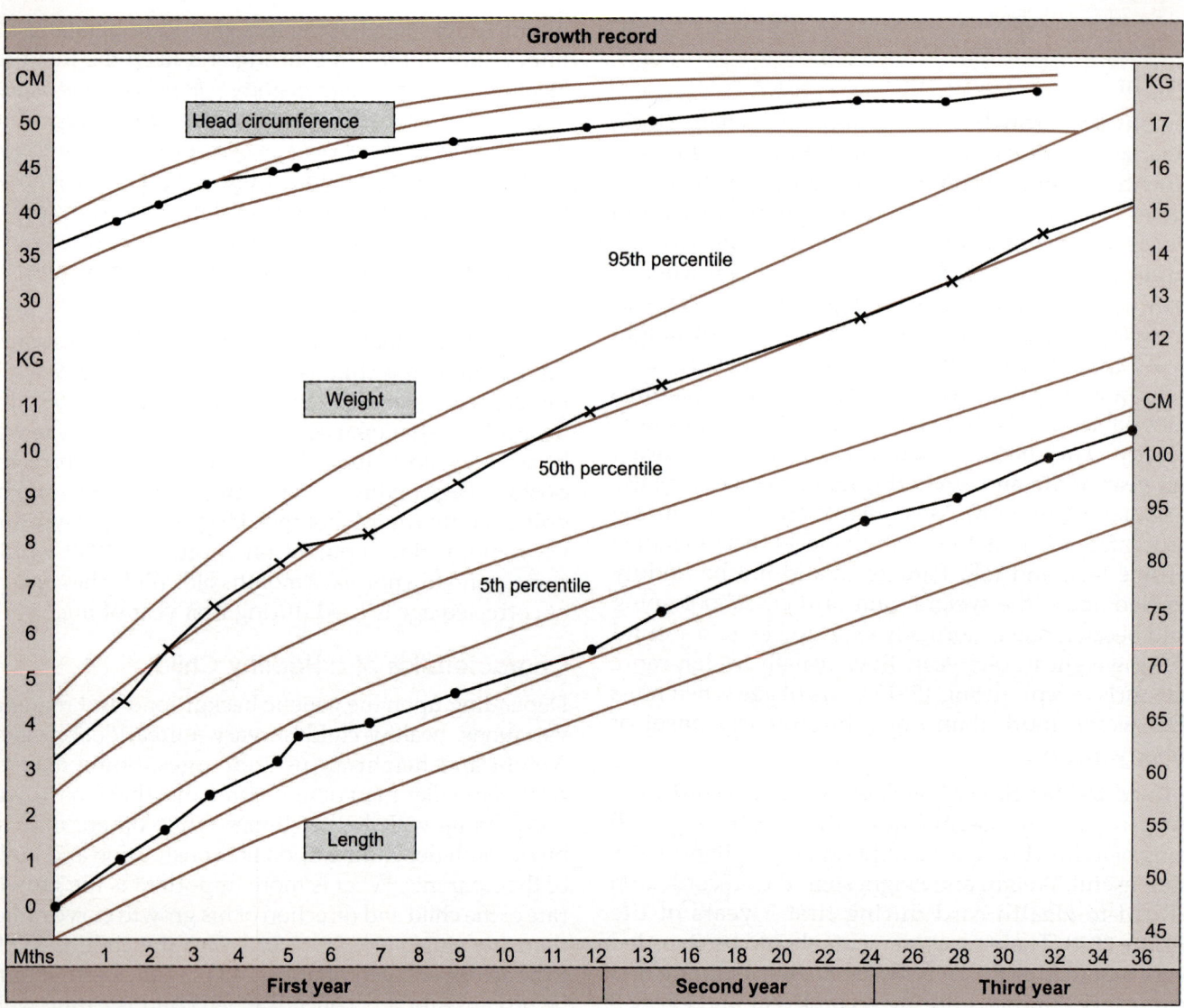

Note: Use corrected age during first year of life
Source: National Center for Health Statistics (NCHS)

Figure 22.2 Road-to-Health card for monitoring the growth of under-five children. The card also gives simple messages for immunizations, feeding and developmental milestones on the reverse. The mother should be explained the importance of growth monitoring and given the responsibility to keep the card in her safe custody. The periodic weight record provides valuable information regarding growth velocity of the child as opposed to a single weight on a particular occasion. The trend or slope of the weight curve is more important than its location on the chart. The satisfactory growth curve is directed upwards and lies parallel to the thick lines on the chart. If the growth curves is flat or directed downwards, the child needs urgent attention to identify the cause and reverse the trend. During early infancy, weight gain depends upon the gestational age, birth weight, health and well-being of the mother and adequacy of breastfeeding. By 1–2 years of age, most children would find their constitutional or genetic growth curve and maintain their growth velocity along their genetically appropriate growth curve. The growth chart serves as a useful tool to promote nutrition education and interaction between the health worker and mother

is calculated by the formula; weight in kg divided by height in meters^2. When BMI of a child is above 85th percentile of the median BMI-for-age of the reference population, the child is considered overweight, and when it is more than 95th percentile, the child is

diagnosed as obese. Body mass index takes into account body mass or weight in relation to stature or height but ignores the composition or distribution of body fat. It is likely to wrongly diagnose obesity in a body builder who has excessive muscle mass. Body volume index

(BVI) is now considered as a more reliable parameter of obesity, but it demands the availability of a special three dimensional full body scanner to accurately assess both the quantum as well as the distribution of fat provides computer-based data on BMI, waist circumference and waist-to-hip ratio.

Length or Height

Weight is more convenient and easier to record but length or linear growth is a more reliable parameter of physical growth. In infants below 2 years, length is measured by placing the child on an infantometer. When child can stand steady, his standing height can be measured which is more reliable than measurement of length. **Table 22.2** gives average height velocity of children during various age periods. When a child is otherwise healthy and free from any systemic disease, his ultimate height is dependent upon the height of his parents, constitutional factors and adequacy of nutrition. For example, children from Punjab and Haryana tend to be taller and heavier than those from the southern states of our country. *In a school going child when height velocity is less than 4 cm per year, it is a cause for concern.*

> ### Practical Tip
>
> *All attempts should be made to ensure optimal nutrition of pre-school children because height at 3 years is a reliable predictor of ultimate adult height. The short stature of adults in developing countries is largely due to poor physical growth during the first 3 years of life. According to National Family Health Survey 2005–2006 (NFHS–3), 38% of under-3 children are stunted in India.*

Prediction of adult height Every parent is keen to know how tall their child is likely to become when he or she becomes can adult. The ultimate adult height of a child depends on his or her constitution or genetic

endowment, adequacy of nutrition, freedom from chronic or recurrent diseases and developmental defects, stimulating environment with opportunities for physical and fun activities, and love and affection by well adjusted parents. Early growth pattern of the child and height of parents can be used to predict the ultimate adult height of the child. In a healthy child, who has no constraints (like congenital defects, systemic disease, dietary deficiency, emotional deprivation, etc.) his adult height can be calculated as follows:

Tanner's formula

1. Adult height = Height at 2 years × 2
2. Adult height = Height at 3 years × 1.37

Weech's formula

3. Adult height in inches:

   Boys = $0.545\,H_3 + 0.544\,P + 14.84$

   Girls = $0.545\,H_3 + 0.544\,P + 10.09$

   Wherein, H_3 is height of the child at 3 years and P refers to mean height of parents.

4. Adult height on the basis of mid-parental height:

   Boys = (Mother's height in cm + Father's height in cm)/2 + 6.5 cm

   Girls = (Father's height in cm + Mother's height in cm)/2 – 6.5 cm

   The calculated mid-parental height ±6 cm is considered as the predicted or target adult height of the child.

The Correlates of a Taller Child

Every mother wants her child to be tall like Amitabh Bachchan. The height of the child is dependent upon the genetic potential (Height of parents, grand parents, uncles, aunts, etc.) of the child, freedom from any developmental defect or systemic or endocrinal disease, adequacy of nutrition and health-friendly environment (love, emotional support, play activity, healthy environment, etc.). Parents cannot do anything to change the inherent genetic potential or genetic stock. But they must ensure that their child is able to achieve full genetic potential for height by providing her with a nutritious balanced diet with adequate calories, proteins and essential micronutrients. There are no "magic nutrient(s) and tonics" which are known to enhance the linear growth. The child should be provided with a healthy and clean environment, early and effective medical care, protection against vaccine-preventable diseases, recreational, sports and fun activities. Good balanced food, healthy and stimulating environment and freedom from illness are crucial to achieve full genetic potential for growth and

Table 22.2 Average rate of increase in height in children	
At birth	20 inches (50 cm)
Gain during 1st year	10 inches (25 cm)
Gain during 2nd year	5 inches (12.5 cm)
Gain during 3rd year	3.5 inches (7.5–10 cm)
Gain during 3–12 years	2–3 inches (5.0–7.5 cm/year)
Adolescence	
Girls	12–16 years: 8 cm/year
Boys	14–18 years: 10 cm/year

Based on National Center for Health Statistics (NCHS) 1987 and WHO 2006 Standards.

22

development. Unless there is a specific deficiency of a hormone there is no role of administration of hormones for increasing the height of the child. Indiscriminate use of anabolic hormones are harmful and should never be used for promotion of growth. Above all, parents should not have unnecessary concern for height, after all there are no virtues in being merely tall. What is more important for the parents is to mould the character and personality of their child in such a way that he has a pleasing outgoing manners, caring attitude, self confidence, poise, interest in arts (music, dance, painting, etc.) and qualities of a good human being.

Brain Growth

The birth weight of a newborn baby is 5% of the weight of an adult while weight of the brain at birth is 70% of an adult brain. Therefore, over two-thirds of the brain growth is completed during fetal life. Maternal health and nutrition during pregnancy have profound effect on the growth of the brain in utero. During first year of life, 15% of the brain growth occurs (importance of breastfeeding) while 10% of brain growth is achieved during 1–3 years of age (importance of balanced complementary feeds). By 5–6 years of age, almost total brain growth is completed. **Table 22.3** gives the growth velocity of the head during preschool years.

At birth, skull bones are separated by gaps or sutures and soft spots or fontanels to facilitate the growth of the brain. There are a total of six fontanels, an anterior, a posterior and four lateral, two on each side of the skull (anterolateral and posterolateral). The lateral fontanels are usually closed at birth while posterior fontanel usually closes by 3 months of age. Anterior fontanel is clinically important. It is located over the top of the skull, at the junction of frontal and parietal bones and is quadrangular in shape. It is normally flat and usually pulsatile due to transmitted pulsations of the cranial arteries. Anterior fontanel may be depressed by dehydration and it starts bulging (and pulsations may disappear) when intracranial pressure is increased. Anterior fontanel usually closes by the age of 12 to 18 months but may be large in size or remain open for a

longer period in children with rickets, hydrocephalus, cretinism, Down syndrome, thalassemia major, pituitary dwarf and certain developmental disorders.

The Process of Development

Unlike a calf or a colt who are up on their legs soon after birth and can search for their food, human baby is dependent and at the mercy of his parents and care takers for at least 4–5 years. The slow process of neuromotor development in human babies is the price we pay for highly evolved and complex brain that we are endowed with. Human brain is more sophisticated and versatile than any advanced computer. It is a most fascinating experience to watch children grow as they learn new skills and pranks every other week or month. The dependent baby gradually becomes more independent and interactive to explore the world around him. Development is a continuous process from conception to maturity and is intimately related to maturity of the central nervous system (CNS).

The sequence of development is identical in all children but rate of development varies from one child to the other. The child must hold his head and sit before he can stand and walk. The rate of development depends upon interaction between genetic potential and his environment. In certain families children learn to walk or speak earlier compared to others but normal children must be able to learn various skills within a normal range of development. The environmental factors which facilitate the process of development include stimulating home environment, emotional security, love and attention, optimal nutrition, ethnic and cultural factors. The stimulatory messages to the brain are received through special senses namely hearing (voices of parents and siblings, music, nursery rhymes, lullabies, etc.), sight (objects, pictures, flowers, lights, colors, etc.) and touch (caressing, cuddling, kissing, massage). The sensory inputs stimulate maturation of various areas of CNS. Children in orphanages tend to have slower rate of neuromotor development due to lack of environmental stimulation. In general, development is advanced in girls (especially development of language) compared to boys. Whenever there is a damage or disorder of the CNS before, during or after birth, it can adversely affect neuromotor development and intelligence.

Table 22.3 Head circumference in under-5 children (10th–90th percentile)

Age	Head circumference (cm)	Growth velocity
Birth	32.0–35.5	—
3 months	38.0–41.5	2 cm/month
1 year	43.5–46.5	2 cm/3 months
3 years	46.8–50.3	1 cm/6 months
5 years	48.1–51.5	1 cm/year
Adult	55.0–56.0	—

Practical Tip

Unlike other mammals, human baby has a relatively slow process of neuromotor development because she is endowed with a highly evolved and complex brain. Human baby is thus dependent and at the mercy of her parents and caretakers for at least 4 to 5 years of age.

Principles of Development

1. It is the most distinctive attribute of childhood and is a continuous process from conception to maturity.
2. Development is intimately related to the maturation of central nervous system.
3. The sequence of development is identical in all children but the rate of development varies from child to child.
4. The generalized mass activity of early infancy is replaced by specific and subtle individual responses. It is a common observation that when shown a bright object, an infant shows wild excitement by moving trunk, arms, legs and babbling while an older child merely smiles and reaches for the object.
5. The development proceeds in a cephalocaudal direction. The infant initially develops head control followed by ability to roll over, grasp, sitting, crawling, standing, and walking.
6. Certain primitive reflexes like grasp reflex and walking reflex must be lost before corresponding voluntary movements are acquired.
7. The development of language is early and advanced in girls as compared to boys.
8. Timing of dentition is unreliable for assessment of neuromotor development.
9. The child with odd-looking face does not necessarily have associated mental subnormality.
10. The attributes like creativity, future potentiality, IQ and mental superiority cannot be predicted in an individual child by developmental assessment.

The Sequence of Development

The development process proceeds from head downwards to the toes. Head control is achieved before a baby is able to use his hands, sit, stand and walk. The skills are not learnt overnight, the process is gradual and slow, gross incoordinated efforts are followed by attainment of perfection in due course of time.

The neonate is totally dependent on his mother for satisfaction of all his needs. Cry is the only signal to draw attention of the mother to his needs of hunger, discomfort and pain. He may momentarily look towards the mother or father but cannot fix his gaze. He is fascinated by flickering lights, bright objects and soothing music. He is comforted by cuddling, caressing and skin-to-skin contact. He is suddenly dazzled by a bright light and startled by a loud sound. He lives in his own world and seems to smile as if in a dream or while passing wind.

Social smile By about 4–6 weeks, the baby tries to fix his gaze and look into your eyes **(Figure 22.3)**. When you talk to him or tickle his chin, he responds by smiling. He cannot differentiate between you and a stranger and obliges everyone with an interactive smile. After a couple of weeks his smile becomes a broad grin and he expresses his pleasure by kicking wildly with his arms and legs and by cooing, babbling and gurgling sounds.

Head control When you pick up a newborn baby or young infant, you need to support his head with your hand or elbow while carrying him. By about 3–4 months, most babies achieve a satisfactory head control and you need not support their head while holding them **(Figure 22.4)**. At this stage when baby is lying on his abdomen, he can lift his head and shoulders off the cot and turn his head from side to side **(Figure 22.5)**.

Rolling over Most babies are able to roll over in bed once the head control is achieved. In India, since most babies are made to sleep on their back, they learn to roll over first from back to stomach and subsequently

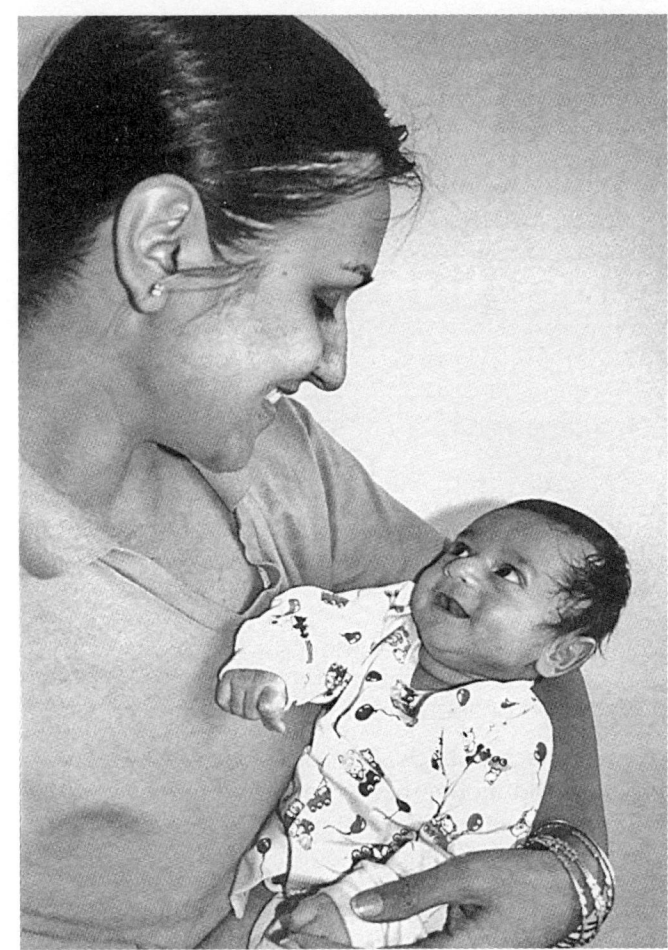

Figure 22.3 Baby is giving an interactive social smile at 6 weeks of age

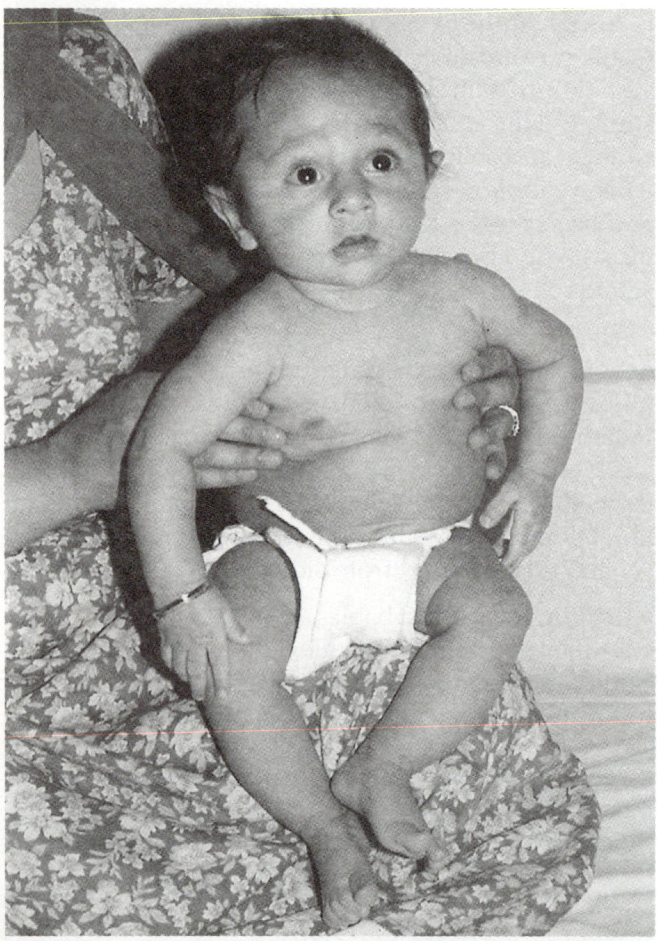

22

Figure 22.4 Baby is having steady head control at 4 months

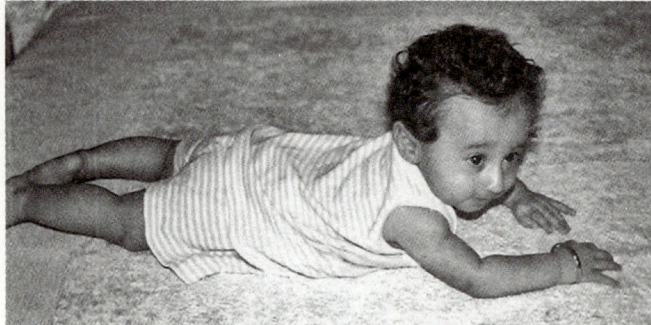

Figure 22.5 When placed on the tummy, head is lifted and chest is maintained off the bed and body weight is supported on the arms during 4–5 months of age

from stomach to back. The baby is achieving gradual mobility and mother has to be careful that he may not fall from the cot and hurt himself. The cot should have a side railing or pillows should be placed around the baby to protect him against the fall.

Sitting By about 5 months or so most babies can sit up with props of pillows or cushions. Mother can help the child to sit but she cannot hasten the process of

development because a new skill is achieved only when the specific part of the brain responsible for that skill matures. Initially baby is wobbly and takes the support of his arms to sit **(Figure 22.6)**. Subsequently he can sit by taking the support of one hand while playing with a rattle in the other. By 6–8 months, most children can sit independently without any support with their back straight and upright **(Figure 22.7)**. At this stage, child

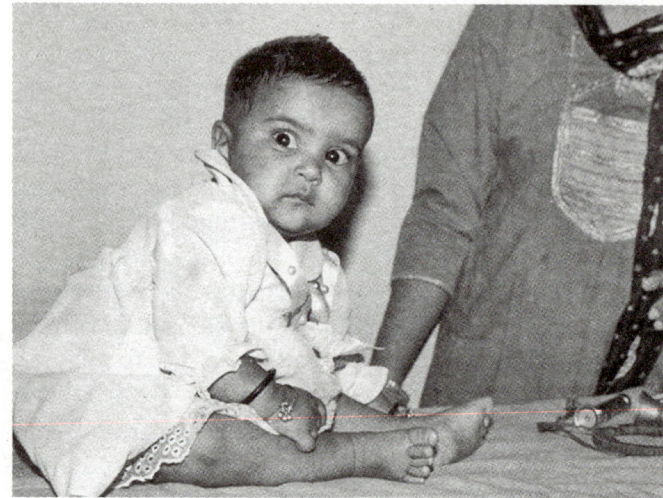

Figure 22.6 Sitting with the support of arms at 5 months of age

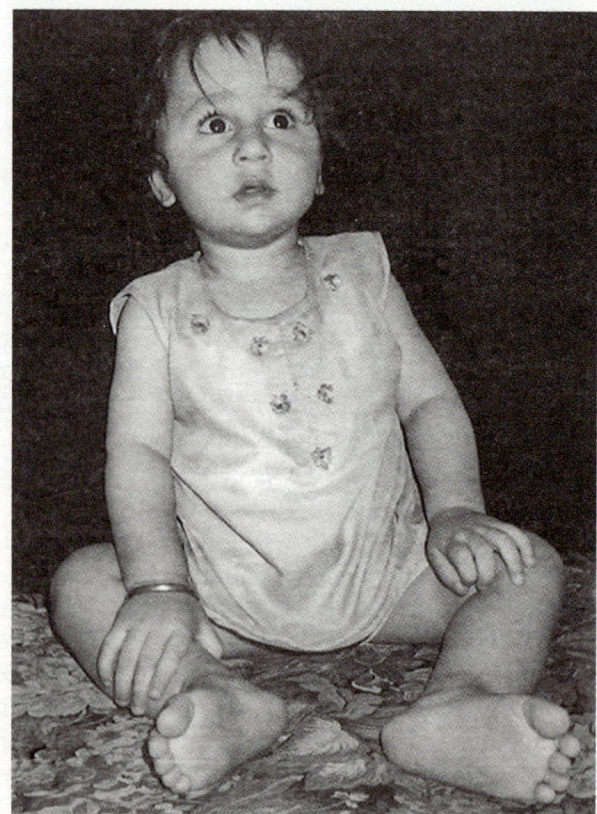

Figure 22.7 Sitting stable and independently with a straight back at 6 months

can pivot around on his bottom without losing his balance.

Crawling By 8–9 months, most babies develop control over their legs and trunk and begin to creep or crawl (**Figure 22.8**). Some babies learn to crawl on their buttocks giving themselves a push with their legs. Others crawl more gracefully on all the four limbs and he can reach virtually every corner of the house. The child is now ready to explore his environment by poking his fingers into every hole and "mouthing" every object that he can lay his hands on. The child now needs constant supervision and vigilance round-the-clock so that he is protected against various hazards during the process of exploration and learning. His hands, knees and leggings would remain dirty and soggy all the time. During this phase, make sure that he has no access to electrical wires, knives, blades, beads, pot of tea or pail of hot water, etc. You must keep dangerous and breakable things out of his way and reach.

Standing and walking By 9 months or so, most babies can hold on to furniture and stand with support (**Figure 22.9**). They can walk a few steps or cruise by holding your hand or furniture. By first birthday, most babies are able to take a few steps independently without any support. This is a moment of great pride for parents. Between 12 and 18 months, babies are able to walk fairly well though they are prone to frequent falls with minor bumps. Most parents buy a "walker" when baby is able to crawl so that he can move around on the props of the walker. But walkers are fraught with dangers of accidents and injuries and should preferably be avoided. Moreover, walkers eliminate the motivation and desire to walk independently because child can move around in the walker with a minimal effort.

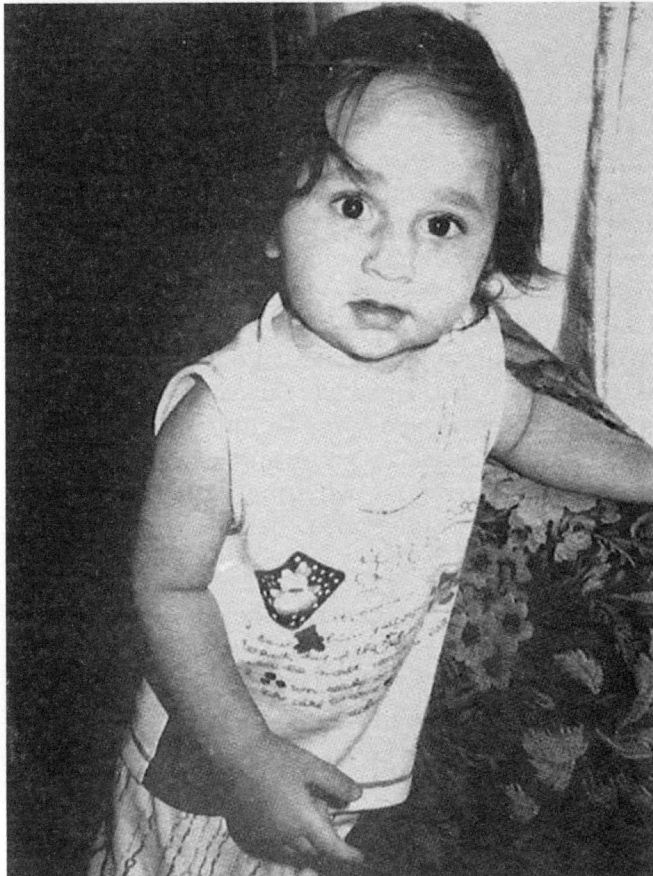

Figure 22.9 Standing with support at the age of 9 months

Holding Objects

Newborn babies have a grasp reflex. When a finger is placed in their palm, they automatically and involuntarily grasp it firmly but do not know how to release it. By the age of 3–4 months, a baby can deliberately hold an object like a rattle with his palm and fingers (like a monkey). The initial hold is crude and he cannot transfer the object from one hand to the other. Around 6 months, the baby wants to hold the spoon and tries to take it to his mouth. At this stage his coordination is poor and he succeeds in taking food to his nose or ears. But soon his coordination improves and he is able to do a better job. He can hold two objects in one hand and can transfer objects from one hand to the other. By the age of 9–10 months, he develops a finer grasp and can hold a button or a bead between his thumb and index finger (princer grasp). He can now pick up small objects from the floor and can indulge in all types of mischiefs unless he is closely supervised. By his first birthday, his grasp is mature, coordination is better and he can transfer objects from one hand to the other, can throw a ball, enjoys dropping and picking objects from the floor.

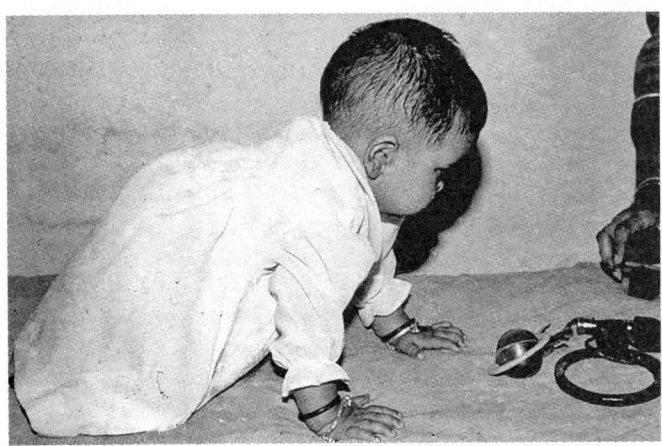

Figure 22.8 Infant is able to crawl and explore at 9 months

Milestones of Development

Every baby is unique and develops at his own pace but within the broad range of normality. Every normal baby will eventually smile, lift his head, babble, hold things, sit, crawl, stand, cruise and walk at his own pace. But children do need encouragement, cuddling, stimulation, interaction and confidence from parents and other people around them to achieve their full genetic potential. The process of development is continuous and child learns new skills as he grows. The child learns so many new skills and attributes at different ages that it is impossible to list all of them. Development is assessed in multiple spheres like gross motor, fine motor, social and adaptive, language, vision and hearing. There is a wide range of ages for acquiring various milestones which have been summarized below.

1–1½ months*

- Sleeps most of the time, cries when hungry, wet or uncomfortable.
- Fists are always kept closed or clenched.
- Blinks to strong light, startles, stretches or cries on loud sound.
- Stops whimpering on being picked up or by listening to a soothing sound.
- Turns towards the source of light and tries to fix his gaze and looks into mother's eyes.
- Gives a social smile (when talked to or tickled on the chin) and makes gurgling or babbling sounds.

3–4 months*

- Recognizes mother and he becomes more responsive and lively to mother's overtures.
- Starts to look at his hands which are mostly open and there is no grasp reflex.
- He can support his head when held in the lap or over the shoulder.
- When placed on the tummy, he raises his chest and head off the cot and turns the head to one side.
- He laughs aloud and shows his pleasure by gurgling sounds, vigorous movements of arms and legs.
- The anticipation of bath and feeds evoke coos, smiles, excited gestures and movements of limbs. Enjoys being bathed and gurgles happily when picked up or tickled.
- He can briefly hold a toy with his clumsy monkey-like grasp.
- Turns head towards sound of a bell or rattle.
- He can roll over from back-to-stomach and subsequently from tummy-to-back.

- He puts his fingers into his mouth especially when hungry or bored.

5–6 months*

- Can sit with support with prop of the arms for support.
- Supports all the weight of the body on the legs when made to stand.
- Can handle objects better and puts everything into his mouth.
- When offered a second toy, he drops the first.
- Squeals and chuckles when excited and during play activity and screams if annoyed.
- Smiles at his mirror image (**Figure 22.10**).
- May make sing-song noises and two syllable sounds like ma-ma, ba-ba.
- May show fear of strangers.
- Grabs toes and puts them in his mouth.

7–9 months*

- Can creep and crawl poking his fingers every where. He needs constant supervision and vigile against accidents and hazards of choking.
- Can pull himself up to stand by holding on to a piece of furniture.
- Can hold small objects like buttons, coins, peas, beads, etc. between his thumb and index finger.
- Pats his image in the mirror.
- Can hold a cup in both hands and hold finger foods like a piece of bread, biscuit or cake and take a bite.
- Makes constant non-sensible babbling and says repetitively ma-ma and da-da.
- Plays simple games like peek-a-boo, hide-and-seek and can clap his hands.

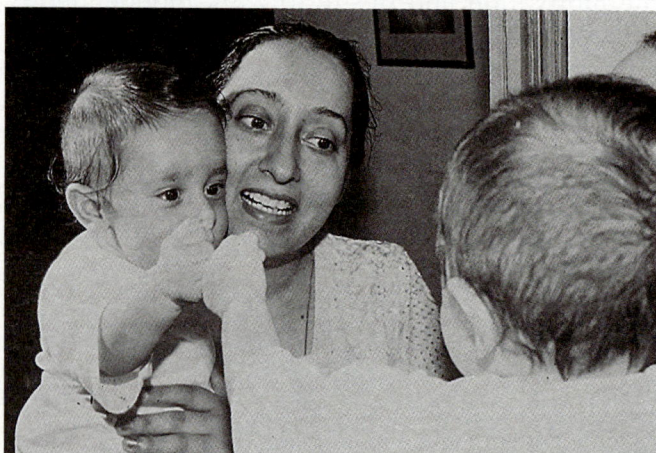

Figure 22.10 Baby enjoys and laughs on seeing his mirror image after 6 months of age

---

*In prematurely born babies corrected age should be used for evaluation of milestones of development. Refer to page 172 for understanding the concept of corrected age.

10–12 months*

- Can stand without support and walk or cruise with support, may take few steps independently.
- Can use a cup and small glass or feeder independently to drink water or milk.
- Holds a spoon but cannot use it effectively due to lack of coordination.
- Gives back the toy when asked.
- Enjoys finger foods.
- Uses gestures and shakes his head for "No" and understands the meaning of "No".
- Responds when called by his name.
- May kiss on request.
- Enjoys deliberately throwing toys and watching them fall.
- Uses a jargon speech.
- Enjoys playing hide-and-seek or peek-a-boo.
- Can say "bye-bye" and "ta-ta".

13–18 months

- Runs around and can crawl up and down the stairs without help.
- Enjoys picking up small objects from nooks and corners.
- Can drink with a cup and use spoon to eat but with spillage.
- Enjoys looking at picture books by turning 2 to 3 pages at a time.
- Plays with pushing and pulling toys.
- Makes tower of 3–4 cubes.
- Copies various household chores like sweeping, dusting and mopping.
- He develops awareness of bowels, may fidget or make gestures and sounds to express his toilet needs.
- Says 15–20 words and tries to recite nursery rhymes.
- Points to his own body parts like eyes, nose, ears, lips, etc. when asked.

19–24 months

- Obeys simple commands.
- Loves to run and like to be chased.
- Walks up and down stairs with two feet on each step.
- Usually possessive of his toys and shows jealousy when mother takes interest in another child.
- Enjoys dismantling toys and trying to mend them.
- Makes tower of 6–7 cubes.
- Can hold pencil between two fingers and thumb and scribble horizontal and vertical lines.
- Washes and dries hands.

- Fair control over the bowels and bladder.
- Tries to take off socks, shoes and pants.
- Uses own name to refer himself, loves songs and nursery rhymes and has a fairly large vocabulary.

24–36 months

- Goes upstairs by placing one foot on each stair, but comes down by placing both the feet on each stair.
- Can hop, skip and jump.
- Can pedal a tricycle (**Figure 22.11**).
- Can draw a circle.
- Enjoys saying "No" to everything.
- Can dress and undress himself (except buttons).
- Can kick a ball (**Figure 22.12**).
- Fully toilet trained.
- He becomes chatter box asking all sorts of questions all the time.
- May count up to 10 and recite nursery rhymes.
- Turns pages of a book one at a time.
- Knows his own sex.

Based on the achievement of various milestones, the developmental quotient (DQ) of the child can be calculated as follows:

$$DQ = \frac{\text{Developmental age of the child}}{\text{Chronological or corrected age of the child}} \times 100$$

A DQ of less than 70% demands detailed assessment of the child by a specially trained clinical psychologist. A number of developmental screening tools like Brazelton Neonatal Behavioral Assessment Scale, Gessel Development Scale, Bayley Scale of Infant Development (BSID), Denver Developmental Screening Test (DDST), Baroda Development Screening Test (BDST), Trivandrum Development Screening Chart (TDSC) and Goodenough-Harris Drawing Test can be used for assessment of development.

HEARING

Adequate hearing is essential for development of normal speech. Parents should carefully watch their child for his responses to various sounds. In young infants, a sudden loud sound may produce a startle response, blinking of eyes or change in his activity. At 4 months or so, the child would turn towards the sound of a rattle or temple bell or beating of a metallic plate with a spoon (**Figure 22.13**). As the child grows he will respond to the banging of the door, sound of music (by making dancing movements or gestures), and noise of

22

22

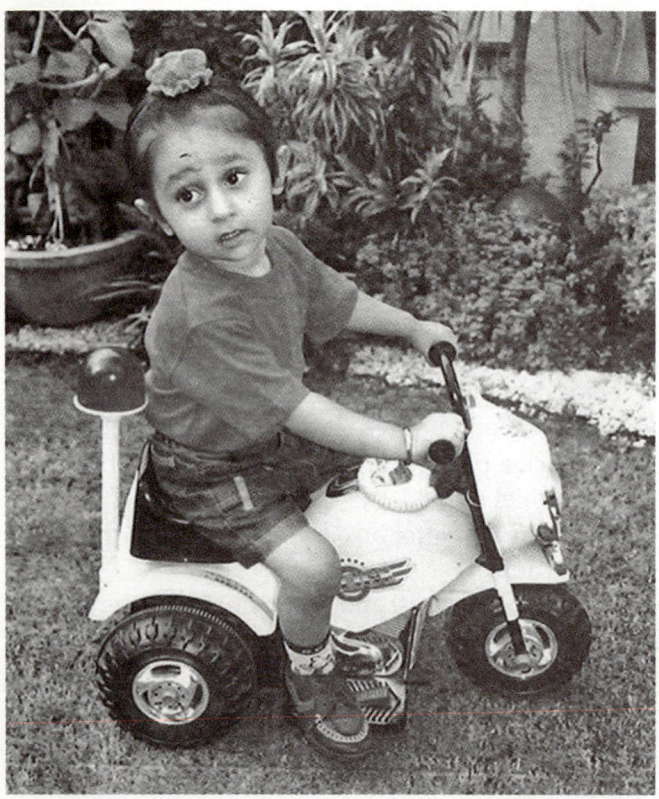

Figure 22.11 Rides tricycle at 2½ years age

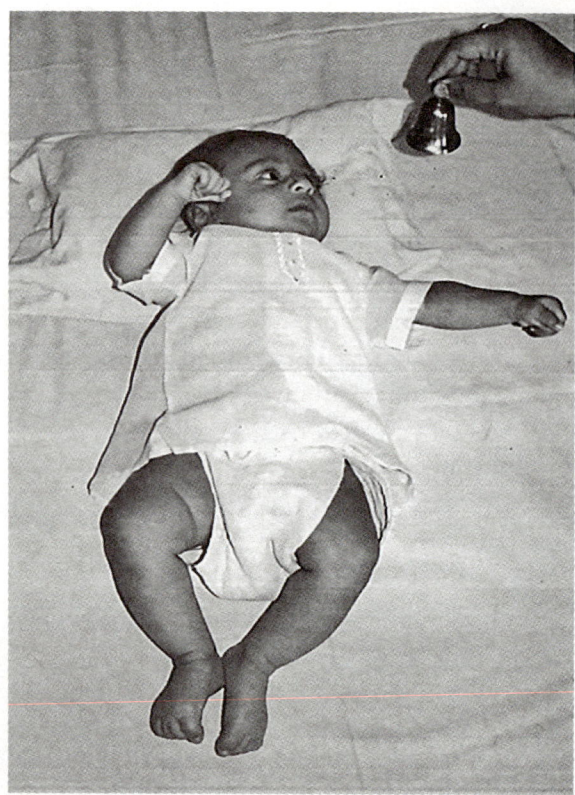

Figure 22.13 Baby turns towards the sound of a rattle or bell at 4 months of age

aeroplane. After one year, he will respond to his name when called from a different room. Whenever there is a doubt about the hearing capability of the child, he must be assessed by a pediatrician. A number of hearing tests viz. brainstem evoked response audiometry (BERA), otoacoustic emission (OAE) and behavioural audiometry are available to assess the hearing of the child. The infant must be screened for hearing at 3 months of age and when required, the hearing aid must be provided by the age of 6 months.

VISION

Newborn babies respond to bright light by blinking and turning their head towards diffuse light or a beam of torch light. The neonate can see clearly up to a distance of 12 inches and can appreciate different colors but red and black are perceived best **(Figure 22.14)**. Around 4–6 weeks, the child is able to fix his gaze and look into your eyes and give a social smile when talked to. He follows and looks towards a dangling red ring **(Figure 22.15)**. During first 6 months, infants love to look at stripes, checkerboards, bull's eyes and squares. By 3 months of age, he can see objects up to a distance of 10 feet. The acuity of vision gradually improves as child grows and reaches the adult level by the age of 6 years. When a baby is unable to see, he will not blink in

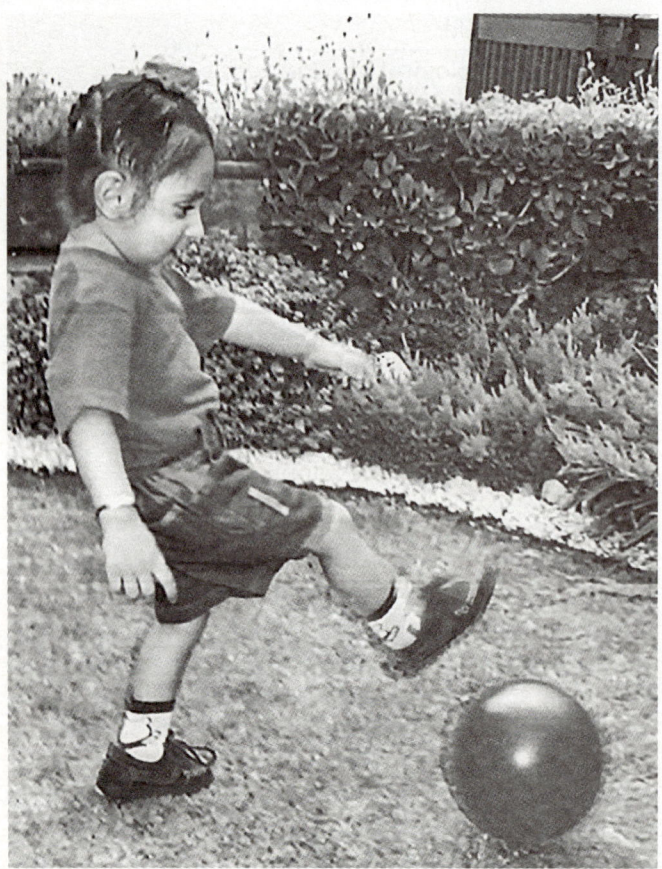

Figure 22.12 Able to kick a ball at 3 years of age

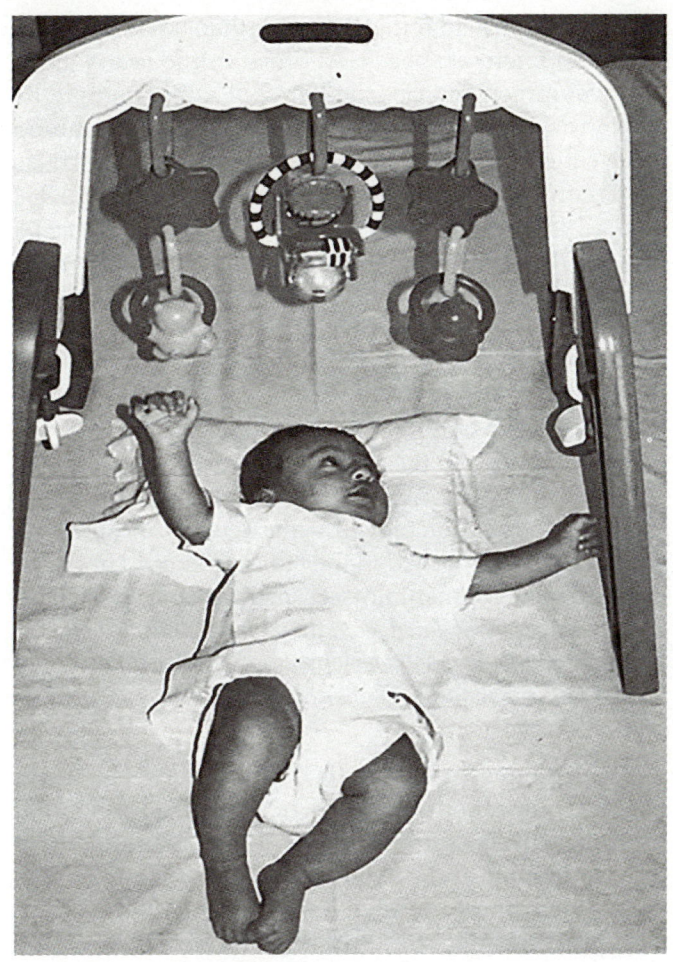

Figure 22.14 A neonate is attracted by bright colored toys dangling from a distance of about 12 inches

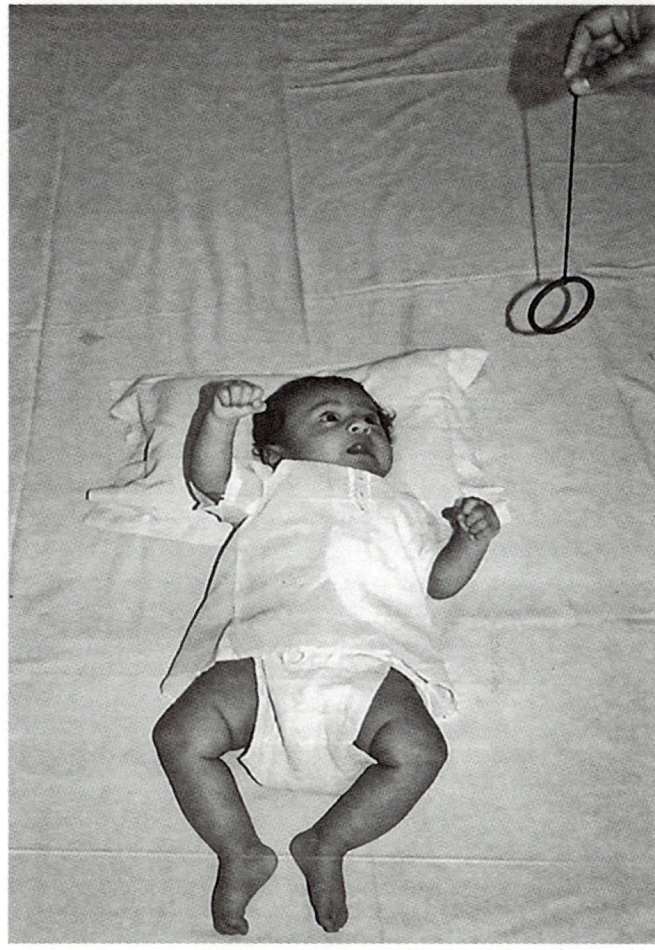

Figure 22.15 Follows a dangling red ring at 6 weeks of age

response to bright light, may have purposeless roving eye movements and persistence of squint or crossed eyes beyond 6 months. He may not give any blink response when you suddenly bring your finger towards his eyes. A blind infant is extrasensitive to noise and gets easily startled by sudden noise. Whenever there is doubt about the vision of the child, a consultation must be sought with an ophthalmologist for visual evaluation by a variety of modern tests like opticokinetic nystagmus, and visual evoked responses (VER).

SPEECH

Crying is the sole mode of communication during early childhood. Babies are able to signal all their biological needs and physical discomforts through cries and gestures. The earliest speech of a baby is cooing and gurgling sounds which are produced around 3 months of age. During next couple of months, he makes all sorts of sounds and noises which mean nothing to the caretakers (he may have his own meaning and purpose

attached to these meaningless sounds). By 6 months, a baby is constantly babbling and you may be able to discern words like "na-na, ma-ma, pa-pa, da-da", etc. Between 9 months and 1 year, the jargon vocabulary increases and the baby may use one sound for water, another for milk and yet another for mother and so on. The first word with meaning is usually spoken anytime between 9 and 15 months. During 1–2 years of age, vocabulary gradually increases and many children are able to express themselves and talk meaningfully. By second birthday most children are able to use pronouns like "I", "me", "you", etc. Some children may continue to indulge in "baby talk" much longer than others and it should be considered as normal. Most children are able to develop reasonable speech and vocabulary by 3 years of age.

Delayed speech Like other milestones of development, there is a wide age-range when normal children learn to speak. *Girls speak earlier than boys and this capability stands them in good stead throughout life!* Many parents get worried if their child is not speaking

22

by one and a half years because many of his age-mates have started speaking. If the child has achieved other milestones of development like sitting, crawling, standing, walking, etc. at the right time, there is no need to worry. He may outdo others later on and may indeed be a chatterbox in due course of time. It is not unusual to find a late talker, suddenly one day starts talking with meaningful words and sentences to the great surprise and pride of everyone. The development of speech depends upon both normal intelligence and normal hearing. Parents should make sure that their child hears normally. Ask the child to bring his favourite toy, shoes or potty from the next room. Call him when he is playing in the next room and watch whether he dances or responds to the tune of music. He should respond to every unusual sound and to the roar of an aeroplane.

High frequency deafness is an important cause of delayed speech. The child may respond to the whispers, clicks and clapping of the hands but is unable to understand human speech. He may be able to listen to a passing car, a banging of the door and door bell, so that parents can never believe that he is indeed deaf to certain high frequencies of sound. *Delayed speech or at times regression of speech after having achieved it, is an important feature of autism. Autistic children lack social interactions and live in a world of their own.*

It is important to remember that children can comprehend and follow commands and instructions much better before they have the capacity to speak. It is important that the mother should talk to her child while she feeds, bathes and plays with him. The baby will understand the rhythm and feelings of parental words long before he learns what the words actually mean. Early motor indicators of delayed speech include inability to lick lips with his tongue, poor swallowing or trying to push the food with his finger, drooling, inability to blow out the candles. Delay in the onset of speech most commonly occurs due to genetic or constitutional reasons. In certain families children learn to speak rather late. *Tongue-tie should never be considered as a cause for delayed speech.* Tongue-tie, malocclusion of teeth and cleft palate, etc. however, may affect the clarity of speech. Most normal children develop meaningful speech by the age of 3 years. It is believed that Albert Einstein caused good bit of anxiety to his parents as he spoke at the age of 4 years!

Developmental Delay

In normal children, developmental milestones are achieved within a wide range of ages. Children in certain families achieve some neuromotor skills earlier

and girls in particular mature faster than boys especially in development of speech. At times a child is advanced in development in a particular skill while he may be slow in achieving another. For example, it is a common observation that a child may start walking as early as 9–10 months but his speech may be delayed up to 3–4 years. *When there is retardation in all the developmental spheres, it is suggestive of mental retardation. However, isolated delay in walking may occur due to congenital dislocation of hips and isolated delay in speech may be because of deafness.* It is not possible to predict intelligence quotient (IQ) and personality or creativity of a child on the basis of developmental assessment.

Table 22.4 gives the upper age limits or target ages for achievement of major milestones of development. If a child has not achieved a particular milestone by the age limit mentioned in the table, he should undergo detailed developmental assessment. *The recommended corrected ages (calculated from the expected date of delivery) for undertaking detailed developmental assessment of a child are 4 months, 8 months, 12 months and then every 6 months till 3 years of age.*

Intelligence quotient (IQ) Intelligence includes child's comprehension, analytical ability, reasoning, memory and attention span. It is influenced by environmental and psychosocial factors and child's ability to properly receive and interpret stimuli from the environment. Several intelligence tests (like Stanfort-Binet and Wechsler) have been devised to measure a wide range of abilities including language development, drawing capability, spatial concepts, numbers, verbal and non-verbal reasoning, memory, and fine motor skills. In India, culture-specific tests for intelligence have been devised by the Central Institute of Education and the National Council of Education, Research and Training (NCERT). On the basis of results of the standardized intelligence test, the examiner can

Table 22.4 Target ages for achievement of major milestones	
Milestones	*Upper age limit**
▪ Social smile	2 months
▪ Stable head control	4 months
▪ Ability to recognize mother	6 months
▪ Ability to sit independently	8 months
▪ Crawling	9 months
▪ Standing without support	1 year
▪ Walking without support	1½ year
▪ Thumb-forefinger grasp	1 year
▪ Disyllabic babbling (ma-ma, da-da)	1 year
▪ Meaningful speech with sentences	4 years

* In prematurely born babies corrected age should be used.

calculate the mental age of the child. The mental age of the child, when compared with his chronological age (actual age in years) and expressed as a percentage gives his intelligence quotient (IQ).

$$IQ = \frac{\text{Mental age}}{\text{Chronological age or corrected age}} \times 100$$

There are some fallacies in interpretation of these tests. The child may not cooperate or he may not perform well due to tension and use of testing material with which he is not familiar. When a child is not doing well at school, these tests may be conducted to assess the IQ of the child. The child with an average ability has an IQ between 85 and 115. Children with an IQ of above 150 are exceptional or gifted children while an IQ of less than 50 is suggestive of severe mental retardation. There is an increasing evidence to suggest that IQ alone does not determine one's success in life. It is equally important to have good and balanced out going personality, confidence, self-esteem, determination, will power, easy adaptability, etc. which is expressed in terms of social, emotional and confidence quotients (SQ, EQ and CQ). It is hoped that in the near future people would look for spiritual quotient by assessing qualities like mental peace, poise, balance of mind, compassion and human qualities of heart (rather than head alone) as a barometer of real success in life.

How to have a Smarter Child?

Human brain is a most complex organ and superior to the most advanced computer. It is believed that if one were to create a computer to match the capabilities of an average human brain, it would have to be at least the size of England! Most of the brain growth takes place during fetal life and by one year of age 85% of brain development is completed. Brain contains high levels of phospholipids, long chain essential fatty acids (omega-3 fatty acids, docosahexaenoic acid and arachidonic acid), amino acids and antioxidants. It is true we are all a product of our heredity and environment. We are born with some in-built charateristics which are inherited from our parents and grandparents. According to psychologists, less than 10% of our characters are handed down to us in our genes while the rest of our thinking and behaviour patterns are learnt and most of the learning takes place in childhood. Our brain is divided into two equal halves or hemispheres. The left hemisphere is mainly responsible for logic, science, reasoning, cognition or analytical skills like language and mathematics. The cortex of the right hemisphere is responsible for development of artistic and aesthetic characteristics like music, dance, painting, platonic emotions, romance, extrasensory perception, intuitive thoughts, mythology, imagination and spirituality. Any activity that stimulates both hemispheres simultaneously promotes development of intelligence. In general, most women are predominently rooted in the right brain while men mostly exploit their left hemispheres. *Nutrition and stimulation during fetal life and preschool years are most crucial for enhanced growth and maturation of the brain.*

Nutrition

Mother's health, diet and emotions profoundly affect the growth and development of her fetus. She must take balanced nutritious food with high quantity of proteins, fresh green leafy vegetables, fruits and dairy products. Mother should take 2.6 g/day omega-3 fatty acids and 300 mg/day docosahexaenoic acid (DHA) during pregnancy and lactation. She must avoid smoking and taking alcohol during pregnancy which may adversely affect the fetal brain growth. After birth, the baby must receive breast feeding as long as feasible but at least for a minimum period of one year. Arachidonic acid and docosahaexenoic acid, two key fatty acids, choline, zinc, iodine and lactose are needed for the growth of brain. These essential brain nutrients are present in plenty in human milk. It has been shown that breast-fed babies have 8 IQ points higher cognition compared to bottle fed babies.

Stimulation

Babies have a biological and physiological need to learn. Any stimulation through his special senses (hearing, sight, taste, smell and touch) provided during fetal life and during first 12 months has more impact on the growth and maturation of brain than at any other time period in life. It has been shown that stimulation program can promote faster growth, improve neuromotor coordination, increase concentration span and improve baby's IQ by as much as 15 points.

Fetal life It is well known that fetuses respond to their mothers, heart beats and voice while still in the womb. We have several examples of learning in the womb in Indian mythology. Abhimanyu learnt in his mother's womb, how to enter *Chakarvyuh* when Arjun explained the principles and technique of the entry procedure to his pregnant wife Subadhara. It is believed that if mother recites *"Hanuman chalisa"* and *"Kirtan sohla"* every night throughout pregnancy, her baby is likely to be brave and fearless. After 5 months of pregnancy, mother can rock gently and slowly in a

> *"Apart from physical connection, there is a spiritual bond between the mother and her baby in the womb. Every emotion experienced by the mother is transmitted as vibrations and vibes to her baby. Mother's thoughts and perceptions have a profound effect on her unborn baby— She should be meditative and have positive and vibrant thoughts of love, peace and hope to touch the soul of her baby."*
>
> **— Meharban Singh**

rocking chair at the rate of 20 rocks per minute. It enhances neuromuscular development and coordination ability of the fetus. She can give positive suggestions to her baby whenever she is in a relaxed mood or before going to sleep. The fetus is most alert during the evening and night between 8 o'clock until about mid night. It seems when tired mother lies down for rest, her baby wakes up and kicks around. The in-utero behavior may continue even after birth, so that babies are usually more active, awake and cranky at night for several weeks after birth. Mother can call her baby by his pet name and say for example, "this is your mummy, I love you Karan, I adore you, you are going to be such a happy baby. You are going to be such a smart baby. You are going to be kind, generous and compassionate human being". She can repeat the suggestions 3–4 times every night. She can hum a soothing song, recite a nursery rhyme or sing a lullaby.

Infancy and childhood The best way for the baby to learn is when mother holds him and plays with him. The child should not be left alone in his crib or with his toys. Stimulate him when he is alert and attentive and not when exhausted, sleepy or hungry. We learn through exploitation of our special senses. Children should be taught the effective use and development of their senses i.e. how to keenly hear (listen), observe, touch, smell and taste. We perceive and appreciate the bounties and beauties of nature through our special senses which must be effectively harnessed. Music has tempo, rhythm, melody and harmony and it stimulates the brain in many ways. Babies love to listen to classical music. Young children are crazy to dance to the tune of Daler Mehndi. Extra stroking, touching, caressing, cuddling, skin-to-skin contact and massage are very stimulating. During first six months, infants love to look at black-and-white stripes, checker boards, bull's eyes and squares. Let the child focus and fix on these and other objects of different colors. Children are attracted by different colors though red color is appreciated most. Make sure that the child has at least 15 minutes of "tummy time" play every day. Babies learn through repetition and parents should repeat a stimulus till

habituation occurs and baby is no longer interested or he is bored. It is a great fun to actively interact and stimulate the baby and watch him learn and achieve perfection in newer skills. Children are more susceptible to a suggestion while going to sleep because their subconscious mind is more receptive. The messages of valour, courage, confidence, compassion, hard work, honesty, truthfulness given during the twilight state, are imbibed and acted upon during the waking hours.

The Gifted Child (Child prodigies)

Even before entry to school, children who demonstrate unusual curiosity, early language development and keen interest in books and magazines are likely to have advanced intellectual maturation. The exceptional capabilities of gifted child may be in the field of intellection or cognition (computer wizard or math genius), communication and fine arts like music, dance, acting and painting, and sports activities. The parents should be perceptive to appreciate and assess the unusual capabilities and qualities of their child so that they are effectively nurtured and harnessed. The child who is smarter than most of his classmates may get bored because the class work may appear too easy, repetitive and mundane to him. There is no real need to have special classes for gifted children or advance them to a higher class. A well-trained teacher can enrich the daily work of the extra-bright students so that they are adequately stimulated but they continue to interact socially with their age-mates.

The parents should spend more time with their gifted child to satisfy his curiosity and hunger for learning. They should be provided with greater exposure to the bounties of nature by traveling, trekking, visiting zoos, museums and so on. The capabilities of the gifted child can be further honed and harnessed by a specialized tutor to unravel his or her full inherent potential. Nevertheless, the parents should not be over ambitious and such children should be encouraged to develop a well-rounded balanced personality with emotional stability because arrogance may seriously compromise their contributions to the society. The world love child prodigies, the well known examples include Mozart, Beethoven, Ramanujan, Lata Mangeshkar, Zakir Hussain, Nadia Comaneci, mathematical genius Shakuntala Devi, and Budhia Singh (who ran marathon from Puri to Bhubaneswar at the age of 5 years). They certainly need special attention, encouragement, better opportunities and facilities for flowering of their full potential but they must be protected against exploitation by their parents, trainers and teachers.

22

The Left Handed Child (Southpaw)

The handedness is established by the age of 3 years. Most individuals are right handed (dominant brain on the left side) but about 10% people are left handed. Exact cause of left handedness is not known but there is some genetic predisposition. When one parent is left handed, there is 17% chance of a child being left handed, and when both parents are left handed, the probability increases to 50%. It is more common in boys than girls. Most left handers are intellectually bright (with greater mathematical capabilities) though the incidence of stuttering and learning difficulties is higher. Majority of left handed children are also able to use the right hand with fair dexterity (mixed handers or ambidexterous). Handedness is usually established by the age of 4 years. No coercive or punitive methods should be used to force the child to use right hand if biologically he is destined to be left handed. The manipulative tactics would never succeed but may lead to emotional disturbances. Allow the child to evolve and express himself the way nature has designed.

Some eminent scientists, artists and statesmen of the world including Albert Einstein, Alexander the Great, Napolean Bonaparte, Leonardo de Vinci, Hellen Keller, Beethoven, President Bill Clinton of America and Amitabh Bachchan have been lefties! But the world caters to the needs of the majority, i.e. right handers, while the left handers are allowed to fend for themselves by adapting and adjusting for the day-to-day goodies that are created for the convenience of right handers. A store in London has taken up the cause for lefties and sells a variety of articles to serve the special needs of southpaws.

BIBLIOGRAPHY

Khadilkar VV, Khadilkar AV, Choudhury P, Agarwal KN, Ugra D, Shah NK. IAP growth monitoring guidelines for children from birth to 18 years. *Indian Pediatr* 2007, 44(3): 187–197.

Rutter M. Nature, nurture and development: From evangelism through science toward policy and practice. *Child Develop* 2002, 73(1): 1–21.

Singh M. Growth and development. In: The Art and Science of Baby and Child Care. *New Delhi, CBS Publishers and Distributors Pvt. Ltd.*, 4th Edition, 2015, p135 to 153.

Singh M. Nutrition, brain and environment. How to have smarter babies? *Indian Pediatr* 2003, 40: 213–220.

Singh M. Nutrition, immunity and infections in children. *Sri Lanka J Child Health* 2003, 32: 35–39.

The World Health Organization website: http://www.who.int/childgrowth/standards/en/. Accessed on April 2nd, 2016.

22

23

Health Problems during Adolescence

Adolescence is associated with rapid physical growth, sexual maturation and emotional development. The physical changes and sexual maturation during adolescence are triggered by hormonal changes. Girls mature sexually and emotionally earlier than boys by about two years. That indeed is the basis for seeking a girl younger in age than the boy during an arranged matrimonial alliance.

There is a wide age ranges at which puberty begins. It is influenced by heredity, nutrition and general health. In girls pubertal changes take place between 10 and 16 years. A large majority of girls begin their sexual development at the age of 10 years and have their first menstrual period around 12 years of age. The average boy starts puberty two years later and achieves sexual maturity during 12–18 years. When pubertal changes start before 8 years of age in girls and prior to 10 years of age in boys, it is called precocious or early puberty and needs investigations. Puberty is considered to be delayed if no secondary sex characters are seen by 13 years in girls (lack of enlargement of breasts or thelarche) and 15 years in boys (lack of moustache). A nurse has an important role in interacting with adolescents and providing them emotional support, nutritional guidance, health services and counseling.

Physical Growth

Adolescence is associated with a sudden spurt of increase in height and weight. During this period the child will grow more quickly than at any other time period except the first year of life. The plump looking pre-adolescent child starts looking more muscular and lean due to increase in linear growth. During adolescence most girls gain 5–6 cm in height per year. The average duration of peak growth spurt in girls is 2½ to 3 years. After menarche (onset of menstruation) the girl would gain on an average of 2–3 cm per year for next 2 years or so. After this there is no further increase in height. Most boys gain 6–7 cm in height during adolescence every year which slows down to 4–5 cm per year between the ages of 16 and 18 years. There is no further linear growth in boys after the age of 18 years when complete pubertal maturation has taken place, with fusion of epiphyses with metaphyses of long bones.

During adolescence, girls on an average gain 3–4 kg body weight per year while boys gain at an average velocity of 6–7 kg per year. Physical growth is rapid during first 2–3 years of adolescence and then gradually slows down. During adolescence, boys gain on an average 20 kg (45 lbs) and girls around 10–12 kg (25 lbs) body weight. *Almost 50% of adult bone mass is achieved during the adolescent period.* During this period, appetite increases and teenagers must take adequate amount of balanced nutritious food to sustain their physical growth. Most boys look awkward and lanky with a "cracking" voice. It is a bit confusing for most boys at this stage because, they are no longer a child and neither a man as yet. Moreover, girls of the same age are at least two years ahead of boys in their physical, sexual and emotional maturation.

Diet during Adolescence

Adolescence is a vulnerable period to develop nutritional disorders, infective diseases and psychological problems. There is a rapid increase in weight and height and appearance of distinctive secondary sex characteristics of men and women during this period. The teenagers should ensure intake of energy-dense (boys 2,800–3,000 calories/day, girls 2,400–2600 calories/day) high protein nutritious balanced diet to support their physical growth and sexual maturation. The child should be encouraged to take plenty of pulses, legumes, soybeans, fresh green leafy vegetables, seasonal fruits, milk and milk products. Non-vegetarians may take poultry products (eggs, chicken), mutton, fish, etc. There is an increasing evidence, however, that vegetarian diet is more health-friendly and optimal nutrition can be maintained by taking vegetarian diet. Non-vegetarian diet due to its high salt, fat and cholesterol content is associated with increased risk of development of high blood pressure, coronary artery disease, heart attacks and carcinoma of colon. During adolescence, the child must be provided with extra supplements of calcium, iron and micronutrients especially iodine, vitamin A, vitamin C and zinc in their diet or through commercially available nutritional supplements. Zinc is essential for normal development of gonads.

Sexual Maturation

The sequence of sexual development is identical in all children but the rate of maturation may differ due to familial background, nutrition and general health status of the child. It is a unique process which is triggered by hormonal changes in the body. During adolescence there is elaboration of gonadotropin-releasing hormone (GnRH) from the medial-basal region of hypothalamus. The release of GnRH is pulsatile, being high at night and low during the day. This is followed by pulsatile release of luteinizing hormone (LH) and follicle-stimulating hormone (FSH) and secretion of testosterone which also shows a pulsatile rhythm.

When peak levels of sex hormones are achieved, there is a negative feed back between further rise in sex hormones and production of GnRH, FSH and LH. *The first sign of sexual maturation is enlargement of breasts in girls and increase in the size of testes in boys.* During 4–6 years, the boy becomes a man and the girl attains the status of woman. In most teenagers, this transition occurs smoothly and they establish their identity and individuality without any struggles with their parents or society. The stages of sexual maturation are quite distinctive and are different in boys and girls **(Table 23.1)**.

Girl becomes a woman Around the age of 10 years, breasts begin to develop as hard lumps under the nipples. They look conical initially and then become round and smooth. There may be itching, discomfort or mild pain in some girls. After breast development, pubic hair starts to grow followed by hair in the armpits or axillae. Around the age of 12 years, most girls would have their first menstrual period (menarche). The periods are infrequent during the first year or so. Pain and discomfort is also common during initial menstrual

Table 23.1 Stages of sexual development

Girls

Age (yr)	SMR* stage	Pubic hair	Breasts
<10	1	Preadolescent	Preadolescent
10–12	2	Sparse, lightly pigmented over medial border of labia.	Breast and papilla elevated to form mound, areolar diameter is increased.
12–13	3	Darker and coarse, beginning to curl.	Breast and areola enlarged, no contour separation.
13–14	4	Coarse, curly, abundant.	Areola and papilla elevated beyond the contour of breast to form secondary mound.
14–16	5	Adult feminine triangle, spread to thighs.	Nipple projects, areola part of general breast contour.

Boys

Age (yr)	SMR* stage	Pubic hair	Scrotum and testes	Penis
<10	1	None	Preadolescent (<4 mL)	Preadolescent
10.5–15	2	Scanty light colored over base of penis	Enlarged pink scrotum, texture is altered. Testes size 4–10 mL	Slight increase in size
12–15.5	3	Darker beginning to to curl	Larger scrotum, testes size 10–15 mL	Longer
13.5–16	4	Adult type but less in quantity	Larger with dark scrotum, testes 15–20 mL	Larger with increase in the size of glans and width of penis
16–18	5	Spread to medial sides of thighs	Adult size of scrotum and testes (20–25 mL) or maximal diameter of 4.0–4.5 cm	Adult size with average flaccid length of 9.16 cm and circumference of 9.31 cm

*Sexual maturity rating
Note: Axillary hair appear after 2 years of onset of pubic hair and coincides with development of facial hair in boys.
Testicular volume is measured with an orchidometer.

periods. At this stage, her body shape assumes a "feminine figure" with a full grown bust, narrow waist and wide hips. When there is no budding of breasts by 14 years or menstruation is delayed beyond 15 years, it is a cause for concern and consultation should be sought with an obstetrician.

Boy becomes a man Pubertal changes in boys begin around an average age of 12 years (two years later than girls). Initial change is increase in the size of testes and the scrotal sac. Throughout childhood, there is hardly any growth in the size of penis which rapidly increase in length and girth during adolescence. Pubic hair start growing followed by hair in the armpits and over the face. The voice cracks and deepens in boys at this stage. Unlike girls, where changes of sexual maturation are obvious to others by virtue of early breast development, the sexual development becomes obvious to others much later in boys when moustache and beard appear or voice starts cracking. In contrast to the girls, where onset of menstruation herald sexual maturity, there is no such obvious marker in case of boys. When there is no testicular enlargement by 16 years of age, it is a cause for concern.

Emotional and Psychological Changes

Teenagers go through a phase of tremendous emotional and psychological turmoil to establish their identity during this crucial phase of development. They want to be independent but are extremely anxious and insecure, and seek reassurance and support of parents. They need to be handled with care and understanding and should be provided with basics of family life and reproductive health education both at home and school. Firstly they have to come in terms with their new physical identity. They will develop their own distinct male or female emotional identity which is different from their peers. They start thinking about their role in society and what needs to be pursued in life to achieve financial self-sufficiency. They want independence to meet and mix with their friends of opposite sex to explore and develop their moral convictions and values in life. They start taking risks in life to enhance their self-esteem. The parental role is to help adolescents to safely take these risks by providing and setting some limits to their activities. Instead of preaching, the parents should try to understand the difficulties and problems of their teenager and be a friend and guide to them. They should be helped without hurting their ego. Adolescence is extremely vulnerable period for smoking, drinking, drug abuse, violence, suicide, sexual experimentation and pregnancy. The teenagers must have full confidence in their capabilities and they

should be assertive (not aggressive) to say "No" against unhealthy peer pressures (like smoking, drinking, drug abuse, and gambling) and should be able to take independent decisions depending upon personal perceptions and moral values in life. Parents should be vigilant regarding the type of friends their teenagers have and the nature of outdoor activities they are indulging without being too nosy or interfering with their freedom. They should be observant and keep a vigil but they should not spy on the child by reading his diary, searching his room, drawers or pockets.

Due to rapid physical and emotional changes, most adolescents are self-conscious about their body. They are worried about their pimples on the face, body ador and "cracking" of voice. They are confused with their identity, at one moment they feel like grown-ups and want to be treated as such, next moment they feel like children again and want to be cared like children. In trying to find their own identity, they often turn away from their parents and feel intense sense of loneliness. In order to relieve boredom and loneliness, they try to establish intimate ties with friends of the same age. Initially they establish their ties with friends of same sex to share their ever changing secrets and subsequently they try to establish emotional links with friends of the opposite sex.

Adolescents develop curiosity about sexual matters and they have sexual fantasies about their girl friends and classmates. Boys may experience night emissions or "wet dreams" in their fantasies. Masturbation is common at this stage to achieve sexual gratification. It is normal and without any adverse effects as long as it does not arouse any guilt feelings or sense of shame. Nevertheless, adolescent children should be encouraged to take part in outdoor activities instead of brooding or fantasizing all the time. Teenagers should be helped and guided to widen the scope of their interests by developing hobbies and activities to enhance their creativity and skills. They should be encouraged to spend their leisure time in body building, sports, reading, music, dancing, painting, and social welfare activities so that they have no time for being idle and aimless.

During this stage, most adolescents are extremely conscious of their appearance, hairdos, living style and dresses. They want to look modern and different from the conventional style of their parents. Sometimes their revealing dress styles may irritate and shock their parents. Most adolescents feel rebellious of constraints of society and strict discipline or rules imposed by their parents. Nevertheless, it is true that most of them need guidance and they want that there should be consistent rules or code of conduct which they can follow. The rules, however, should not be arbitrary, inconsistent or overbearing.

It is but natural for parents to know where the teenager is going for a party, who are the other mates, where he can be contacted in case of an emergency and when is he expected to come back home. Whenever there is a delay or change in plan, the teenager must call home well in time to inform and explain the reasons for delay. It is equally important that parents should also tell their children where they are going, how to reach them in case of an emergency and when they are expected to be back home. There must be a healthy and mutually respectful adult-to-adult relationship between parents and their teenagers. Teenagers should not be bullied or ordered by parents and parents should not be taken for granted by their children. Most parents do expect that their adolescent children must behave with due politeness and courtesy towards them and other family friends, teachers and relatives. And they should understand their obligations to assist their parents in the family chores and should have a sense of dignity and responsibility to feel as integral part of the family to share both happiness and hurdles.

Common Health Problems

Most adolescents have a *profuse strong-smelling perspiration* in their armpits, which may cause unpopularity with their school mates. They should maintain a good standard of personal hygiene and take a daily bath with soap and use body deodorants regularly. *Acne or pimples* on the face due to excessive secretion of sebum may cause embarrassment and disfigurement especially if they are squeezed. Girls may have painful and irregular menses (*dysmenorrhea*) especially during first 1–2 years of their onset of periods. Use of analgesic-cum-antispasmodic medication helps to relieve the pain and discomfort due to cramps.

Dysfunctional uterine bleeding is diagnosed when there is excessive, prolonged and painless menstrual bleeding. The common causes include pelvic inflammatory disease, fibroids, endocrinopathy, bleeding disorder or polycystic ovarian disease.

There is an increased incidence of tuberculosis during adolescence. They are prone to develop *infectious mononucleosis* because of EB virus infection and atypical pneumonia due to *Mycoplasma pneumoniae*. Unless sexual hygiene is maintained, adolescents are prone to develop vulvovaginitis, pelvic inflammatory disease (PID) and infertility later in life. During menses, the use of tampon (intravaginal pad) should be avoided because of potential risk of causing *toxic shock syndrome* (TSS) because of staphylococcal infection. *Headaches* are common because of anxiety, stress and migraines. *Thyroid disorders* (both hypo- and hyperthyroidism) may occur during adolescence. Mild enlargement of thyroid gland (goiter) is common during adolescence as a consequence of relative deficiency of iodine because of increased demands. *Mitral valve prolapse* ("floppy valve syndrome") is common among adolescent girls. *Musculoskeletal problems* such as scoliosis, kyphosis, slipped capital femoral epiphyses are common among adolescents. Adolescents are extremely vulnerable to *automobile accidents* while trying to establish their macho image. The *addictive behaviour* like smoking, drinking alcohol and substance abuse usually has its onset during adolescence (**Box 23.1**).

Unless properly cautioned and guided, teenagers are at an increased an risk to develop *sexually transmitted diseases* (STDs) and unwanted pregnancy by indulging in unsafe and unprotected sexual activities. There is high incidence of *depression and suicides* during this crucial phase of life. *Anorexia nervosa* (intense fear of becoming obese with extreme reluctance to eat) usually affects adolescent girls and is extremely difficult to manage. Hirsutism due to hormonal imbalance and polycystic ovarian disease (PCOD) may occur in adolescent girls. It is characterized by obesity, menstrual irregularities, acne and *metabolic derangements* like insulin resistance and type 2 diabetes mellitus. Nutritional requirements are markedly increased during adolescence due to rapid physical growth spurt. Teenagers are prone to develop *nutritional deficiencies* if they are not provided with adequate amounts of balanced diet. Iron deficiency anemia is extremely common especially among adolescent girls. They should be given supplements of iron and folic acid. Due to excessive intake of junk food and unhealthy sedentary lifestyle, *obesity* is emerging as an important public health problem in adolescents.

23

Box 23.1 **Common markers of substance abuse**

- Spending time alone with lack of communication with family members.
- A change in the choice of friends and way of dressing.
- Deterioration in school grades.
- Lack of energy, irregular eating habits and poor sleep.
- Blood-shot eyes and frequent "colds" or nose bleeds.
- Unexplained mood changes like irritability, hyperactivity and depression.
- Running away from home or attempting suicide.

Vaccinations

Most adolescents should have received uptodate vaccinations because of statutory requirement for admission to a regular school. A booster dose of MMR should be given during 5–10 years to enhance protection against rubella and mumps. A combined MMR-varilrix (Priorix Tetra) vaccine is available and a booster dose can be given during 5 to 10 years of age. A booster dose of Tdap (Boostrix) is given at the age of 10 years. Tetanus toxoid or Td boosters need to be taken every 10 years throughout life. A booster dose of hepatitis B vaccine is recommended by some health authorities at this age. Boosters of polysaccharide typhoid vaccine are required every 3 years. A purified vi-capsular polysaccharide *S. typhi* Ty_2 conjugated to tetanus toxoid (Typbar TCV) is available which provides lifelong protection after two doses. If natural chickenpox infection has not occurred and child has not been vaccinated against it, he should be protected because chickenpox is a serious disease during adolescence. Up to the age of 12 years, chickenpox vaccine can be given as a single dose, while older children are administered two doses at an interval of 6–8 weeks. In girls, two doses (0 and 6 months) of human papilloma virus vaccine can be given during 9–13 years and three doses (0, 1 and 6 months) after age of 14 years to prevent carcinoma cervix and genital warts.

School Health Program

Schools provide a captive population of children and account for 25% of the population of India. They are ideal places for purposes of health surveillance, provision of family life education, early identification and prevention of handicap or disability and promotion of health through inculcation of healthy life style. School health program is aimed to help children attain their optimal potential for physical growth, mental, emotional, sexual and educational development. The main objectives and components of school health program are listed in **Box 23.2**. School health services are delivered with the help and active involvement of a school pediatrician, nurse and teachers.

Role of a School Nurse

She should maintain the health, anthropometry and immunization records of school children. The school nurse provides the basic preventive, promotive and curative health care to children. Nurse should supervise the provision of healthy school environment like environmental sanitation, safe drinking water,

---

Box 23.2   **Services provided by school health program**

1. *First-aid care* for common health problems like fever, vomiting, pain abdomen, diarrhea, cough and cold, accidents, etc.

2. *Anthropometry*. Periodic record of weight, height, vision, hearing, blood pressure and nutritional status. Abnormalities if any, should be brought to the attention of parents.

3. *Family life education*. To provide regular nutrition, disease prevention, health promotion and sex education as a part of school curriculum.

4. *Healthy nutrition*. Improve nutrition of children with supplementary nutrition and mid-day meal program, providing healthy milk-based drinks or fruit-based drinks (avoiding unhealthy cola drinks) and nutritious snacks.

5. *Promotion of immunizations*. To ensure that all children admitted to the school are effectively immunized against all vaccine-preventable diseases and they are provided breakthrough immunizations in response to any epidemics like meningococcal meningitis, typhoid fever and chickenpox, etc. A booster dose of Tdap (Boostrix) is given at the age of 10 years.

6. Provision of *first aid and emergency care* for common diseases and accidents.

7. Early identification and referral of children with *learning disability* due to impairment of cognition, neuromotor incoordination, visual defect, deafness, specific learning disorders like dyslexia, attention deficit hyperactivity disorder (ADHD), dysgraphia, dyscalculia, emotional and conduct disorder, etc.

8. To increase *awareness of school* children regarding importance of personal hygiene, environmental sanitation, healthy food habits, safe drinking water, physical activity, sports, yoga, and meditation. The school authorities should ensure that the school premises provide high standard of these attributes for emulation by the students.

9. Promotion of *dental and eye health*.

10. To prevent spread of *communicable diseases* among children through epidemiologic surveillance, preventive inoculations, chemoprophylaxis (for meningitis), safe food and potable water supply, good sanitation and open spaces and healthy school environment.

11. *Teachers and ancillary school staff* should be free from communicable diseases because they come in close contact with children.

12. High-risk, sick or disabled children should be intimated to the parents and referred to appropriate health specialists for evaluation and management.

---

satisfactory toilets for boys and girls, adequate physical facilities (ventilation, proper lighting, comfortable furniture), safety and quality of food provided by the canteen. The nurse should assist the school authorities to provide healthy environment to ensure optimal physical, mental, social, emotional and spiritual well being of children. She should maintain the inventory of essential drugs in the school dispensary like paracetamol, betadine, antispasmodic syrup, sedative, antiseptic solutions (isopropyle alcohol, mercurochrome, betadine, antibacterial cream), antihistaminic, epinephrine, antiemetic, ice packs and sprays for sports injuries, dressing material like cotton and crepe bandages and occlusive tapes, etc.

BIBLIOGRAPHY

Dias PJ. Adolescent substance abuse. Assessment in the office. *Pediatr Clin North Am* 2002, 49(2): 269–300.

Greydanus DE, Rimsza ME, Newhouse PA. Adolescent sexuality and disability. *Adolesc Med* 2002, 13(2): 233–247.

Patton GC, Viner K. Pubertal transition in health. *Lancet* 2007, 369(9567): 1130–1139.

Venkaiah K, Damayanti K, Nayak MV, Vijayaraghavan K. Diet and nutritional status of rural adolescents in India. *Eur J Clin Nutr* 2002, 56(11): 1119–1125.

World Health Organization. Adolescent Health and Development, India. *Adolescent Health Document,* 2011.

23

24

Development of
Behavior and Personality

Children are innocents and carefree without any ill will, jealousy or malice towards anyone. They are full of life and energy and are constantly on the move. They are confident, fearless and friendly towards everyone. They are indeed spiritual in their characteristics and have all the attributes that saints and holy people endeavor to acquire. They have no desires or ambitions and they are fully absorbed in the "moment" with innocense and pure love. Early childhood is usually blissful with no responsibilities but all the fun and frolics. Parents should allow them to develop, flower and express their full innate potential without too much external control and regimentation. They should be reared with care, compassion, guidance and understanding to enable them to explore their environment and evolve as useful and responsible members of society. Every ugly thing told to the child, every shame, every fright or disdain given to him will remain like splinters in the flesh or subconscious mind to torture him throughout his life. As they grow, they learn various behavior characteristics from their parents, siblings, teachers and friends who serve as role models to them (see the quote). Therefore, if parents want their child to be honest, peaceful and happy, they should themselves attain that state of mind in the first place. Children gradually develop negative traits of anger and temper tantrums, fear, jealousy, greed, and possessiveness to control their small world to their advantage. They often blackmail their parents to get their demands fulfilled. They develop methods and techniques of their own to make the whole family revolve around them. They gradually develop control over themselves by developing their ego and try to control others as much as they can.

"The seeds of integrity, character and discipline are sown in childhood. They are planted by parents and tilled by the teachers."

— Meharban Singh

Children learn what they live with!

If a child lives with criticism,
he learns to condemn.

If a child lives with hostility,
he learns to fight.

If a child lives with ridicule,
he learns to be shy.

If a child lives with shame,
he learns to feel guilty.

If a child lives with tolerance,
he learns to be patient.

If a child lives with encouragement,
he learns confidence.

If a child lives with praise,
he learns to appreciate.

If a child lives with fairness,
he learns justice.

If a child lives with security,
he learns to have faith.

If a child lives with approval,
he learns to like himself.

If a child lives with acceptance and
friendship, he learns to find love
in the world.

If a child lives with serenity,
he learns to have peace of mind.

— Dorothy L. Nolte

The Role of Parents

Most parents are confused and have no goals or are uncertain about their hopes and aspirations regarding their children. Due to overwhelming pace of social change, parents are uncertain and worried as to what kind of a world awaits their children when they will grow to become adults. Is academic excellence in school

230

> *"If you want to give your child only one gift; let it be enthusiasm."*
>
> — **Bruce Barton**

the most important aim because it provides a lucrative job career? Do parents want their child to be individualistic or egoistic with a competitive edge in the highly commercialized society? Or do they want their child to learn to cooperate and at times renounce his own desires to give comfort and solace to others? Should children develop the ability and art of cooperation with others to sustain intimate human relationships in life? Do they want their child to evolve as a good human being with a wholesome and balanced personality with concern and compassion towards one and all? Is spiritual enlightenment the ultimate or supreme goal of every human being? Parents can mould their children depending upon their own perceptions and values in life. Parents must have a vision and a dream as to what they want their children to evolve as they grow up to become responsible adults in the society, which is full of virtues and vices. They can evolve as diamonds in this societal slush or get lost like millions of us in a seemingly purposeless rat race!

Producing children does not need any skills and is achieved as a natural biological instinct. But upbringing of children is an art which demands active efforts, concern, sensitivity and skills of parents. There is no doubt that children are born with different temperaments and developmental time tables. But how a child is raised has a lot to do with the kind of adult he becomes. The childhood is the most vulnerable and formative years of one's life. Children are truly at the mercy of their care takers to look after their physical, mental and emotional needs. Parents, teachers, siblings and friends have a profound effect to influence and mould the personality of children. *The seeds of personality and emotional disorders are sown in childhood. The successful adults do have pleasant memories of happy childhood while maladjusted adults are constantly haunted by the emotional scars of early life.* Children must be nurtured under close supervision, guidance, protection and discipline in the right proportion avoiding both excessive indulgence as well as the neglect. The parents must understand the basic or constitutional personality make up and aptitude of their children and provide them with the right stimulation, supervision and support to bring out the best in them (**Box 24.1**).

> *"Life without love is like a tree without blossoms or fruit."*
>
> — **Kahlil Gibran**

Box 24.1 Role of parents to mould their children

- Children need role models more than critics.
- Parents must set a good example for their children to emulate.
- Parents should say "No" when it is appropriate. Children do respect a firm denial.
- Give protection and security but do give your child freedom to explore the world. Never possess him.
- Children need your presence more than your presents.
- Treat and respect the child as you do to a grown up and never humiliate him.
- Assign household chores and responsibilities to your children.
- Children do as their parents do, and not what their parents say or want them to do.
- Be cautious and considerate what you say to your children. They do remember your bad and rude words when they grow up.

Love and security Love is a basic or fundamental emotional need which must be fulfilled. We all need and crave for love and affection from different people throughout our life from cradle to grave. Parents should love but never possess their child. The child should be treated as an independent being, a person in his own right and not a valuable asset or a possession of his parents. Child must be given comfort and security whenever he is distressed or in discomfort. Toys are a poor substitute for love; money can't buy love. It is wrong to believe that love consists of giving the child everything that he wants and buying for him expensive presents. Love causes no harm and no child can be spoilt by love! Children are spoilt by over-protection, over-indulgence and due to lack of consistent discipline.

> *"The tragedy is that most parents do love their children, but somehow don't know how to express it in ways that help the child feeling valued, respected and loved."*
>
> — **Rex Johnson**

24

Children who are reared with love and affection, are likely to have self-confidence, poise, grace and concern for others. They develop empathy and warmth towards other human beings. They would not have any complexes and conflicts in their personality. It is a tragedy that most parents do love their children, but somehow they don't know how to express it so that the child feels valued, wanted and respected. Children need love and appreciation from both parents. A father's love (or lack of it) is equally important for development of child's personality and good behavior. Lack of love or lack of acceptance either by mother or father is an important cause of lack of confidence, self-esteem, emotional instability, withdrawal, depression and anxiety. Many studies have shown that lack of father's love has a greater bearing on occurrence of disorders of personality, antisocial behavior and substance abuse in children.

> "There is more hunger for love and appreciation in this world than for bread."
> — **Mother Teresa**

Over-protection and over-indulgence Most educated parents now have only one or two children and they have very little time to look after them because of professional competition and career development. This situation often leads to over-protection, over-indulgence and constant fear and anxiety regarding the safety and well being of their children. They are mostly kept at home and not allowed to mix with other children and never left alone. The mother continues to feed him, dress him and attend to his toilet needs for too long when a child should be doing these activities independently by himself. The child may continue to sleep with his parents up to 10 years or even longer. The parents try to yield to all his wishes and demands whether reasonable or unreasonable. The situation becomes worse when grandparents are living with the family. They are likely to be more over-protective and indulgent and it is difficult for them to enforce discipline.

There are serious emotional consequences of over-protection and parental anxiety. The overprotected children are likely to become shy, introvert, and timid. They remain dependent, insecure and are unable to take decisions or face realities of life. These children are unable to cultivate friends and they lack the spirit of cooperation. They are more likely to have problems of food fussiness, temper tantrums, breath holding spells and conduct disorders. They may seek advice of their mothers throughout life in all matters leading to problems of adjustment in married life. Boys are likely to show greater fixation with their mothers (Oedipal complex) and girls with their fathers (Electra complex).

Favoritism and rejection Among all the parental attitudes, favoritism and rejection are most harmful. A son born after several girls or a good looking child or a bright and exceptional child is likely to be the favorite of his parents. The favorite child is not reprimanded, he is likely to receive more gifts and when he is in trouble with one parent, the other parent provides him protection and security. The favored child will show all the attributes of over-indulged child while the unfavored child would show signs of insecurity, lack of self-esteem and jealousy. The disfavored child will feel resentful against his parents.

Parental rejection occurs when child is unwanted (failure of contraception) or born with an unfavored sex. Rejection also occurs when child is not good looking or is clumsy and dull. At times the child is merely neglected without being rejected. The child may be constantly nagged, scolded and reprimanded. His shortcomings are exaggerated and he is shamed and belittled in the presence of others. Due to constant nagging and neglect, the child becomes insecure, shy and timid. He may develop excessive fears and night terrors. He would be jealous of favored sibling and other friends. He may develop antisocial behavior like aggressiveness, destructiveness, truancy and disobedience.

Parental example Children learn what they watch, not only at home but in school and society at large. Children are great imitators and it is essential that parents must set a good example. If parents are courteous and considerate and have the pleasant manners to say "please", "thank you" – the child is likely to copy them. Parents must demonstrate good habits of truthfulness, honesty, courage and morality in their day-to-day life for children to emulate.

> "Certainly, I do shout, fight, damage public property to serve the country as a politician. But, you are kids and must behave properly and play quietly."
> — **RK Laxman**

Hypocrisy, smoking, drinking, etc. are likely to breed similar traits in the child. Parents must try to inculcate good manners, good habits and virtues of human kindness by setting a good personal example. Do not order your child, always request the child what you want him to do. There is no harm in being polite to your child. If you are polite he will reciprocate and will be polite to others. If parents show bad temper, use abrasive or abusive language, are unloving, dishonest and selfish, there is no wonder their children would also develop all these traits. If there are constant fights among parents and violence at home, children are likely to become short tempered and aggressive. Children learn lot of aggressive traits from television and movies these days. Even cartoon films show lot of violence and many heroic stunts. If father is an alcoholic, the child is likely to be upset by his irrational, unpredictable and aggressive behavior.

> "Children have more need of role models than of critics."
> — **Joseph Jonbert**

The maladjusted parents The best safeguard to ensure hormonious development of personality and character of the child is to have well adjusted, happy, contented and mature parents. Children need both mother and father for their optimal care, development and emotional support. The parents must know the basic or constitutional personality make-up and aptitude of their children and provide them with the right kind of stimulation, supervision and support to bring out the best in them. *Happy and well-adjusted parents produce happy children while maladjusted parents produce maladjusted children who grow to become maladjusted adults.* When there are constant bickerings

> *"The child is the barometer of the family's emotional climate. Behavior and psychological problems in children are a reflection of interparental marital conflicts...."*
> — **John Apley**

and fights among parents, the child is scared, depressed and confused. The child loses interest in play activity and his school. He loses the zeal and enthusiasm in life. If a child sees the constant use of abusive language and violence at home, he is likely to become aggressive and antisocial in his behavior. The children of separated parents or single parent go through tremendous turmoil in their lives. When father is an alcoholic, children and their mother may become victims of his physical abuse. When a child is manifesting a serious behavior problem, it gives a signal that something is wrong in the family. The corrective measures and guidance is not required by the child but by his parents.

Attitude during adolescence Adolescence is a critical phase of child's development when he goes through tremendous physical, sexual and emotional changes. During this period, considerable tact is needed to handle children. Parents must show understanding and should avoid rudeness and threats during this vulnerable phase of life. They should establish a good channel of communication and rapport with their adolescent child and explain significance of body changes for a smooth transition from childhood to adulthood. Drug abuse is catching on in our society and parents should closely watch the activities and company of their children to curb this dreadful habit. Adolescents must receive formal family life and reproductive health education and importance of safe sex at this stage, so that they can make considered choices and decisions in life.

Discipline and punishment In our society, obedience seems to be the main criterion of discipline which is wrong. The child must have his own

individuality and should ask probing questions. A regular lifestyle with pleasant manners and clean habits are important aspects of self discipline. The efforts should be made to inculcate good habits early in life. *It is easier to form good habits in the first place but extremely difficult to break the bad habits.* The child should get up early in the morning, go to toilet, brush his teeth, take a bath, dress himself, take breakfast, go to school, do his homework regularly, play outdoors in the evening, etc. are essential components of disciplined life. There are some basic don'ts during early childhood that he should follow. He should be told not to scribble on the books or walls, not to jump off the sofas or climb on beds with shoes on. He should have regard for property of others and he should not hit, hurt or bite anybody without provocation. He should be agreeable and cooperative with his parents, friends and strangers.

Discipline must be taught with love, appreciation and tolerance instead of constant criticism and corporal punishment. The behavior of the child must be viewed in relation to his age and developmental status. Discipline must be consistent by all the care takers to avoid any confusion in the child's mind. Parents should not be unduly concerned about various emotional developmental phases of children like putting everything in the mouth, eating mud, thumb sucking, and fiddling with genitals, etc. They are transitory pheno-mena and disappear in due course of time. The child must learn to accept "No" and he must realize that he cannot have his own way in everything. He must learn to respect and prevent damage to the property of others.

Parents must differentiate between unintentional accidents and wrong doings because they need different ways of handling. Children should be allowed to make some mistakes and learn from them. Children do understand when you guide and explain to them. But they have short memories, you have to tell and train them again and again to ingrain the healthy family life concepts in their minds. Anger should not lead to anger and parents should not yell unnecessarily but be polite, understanding and sympathetic. They should have the patience and forebearance to explain to their child that what he did or demanded was unreasonable. And parents must love their child unconditionally irrespective of the nature of his behavior.

24

> *"Avoid extremes in life, follow the middle path."*
> — **Gautama Buddha**

Excessive discipline and no discipline are equally bad and parents must follow the "middle path" with some humour and common sense. Authority should be firm and consistent but parents should always remain kind and reasonable to give the sense of security to their child, which is essential for his emotional development. The child is confused if one parent condones while the other forbids or if grandparents allow him to do certain things which his parents do not allow him to do. Try to avoid corporal punishment as far as possible. Most of the times mere tone of mother's voice is more important to show displeasure rather than any punishment. The child can be denied a privilege (like not buying a toy or ice cream or keeping him indoor when he wants to play outside) as a form of punishment. The less you punish the child, the easier it becomes to discipline him. If parents resort to threats of punishment, very often the child will become used to it. Never use empty threats. Parents can show their displeasure by not speaking to him. But the anger should be short lived and a friendly atmosphere should be restored as soon as possible. It is important to remember that whatever may be the method of discipline, the child should continue to have the feeling that you still love and accept him. When a child does not take any notice of your "No-Nos" and continues to repeat the forbidden prank, never laugh over it. Babies enjoy the "no game" and if you constantly say "No" to whatever the child does, he enjoys doing it again and again.

> *"We constantly discipline our children throughout the day with negative commands—'don't do this', 'don't do that', 'don't jump', 'don't make noise'—without any positive commands as to "what actually they should do". No wonder their subconscious or core is corroded with negative vibes."*
>
> — **Meharban Singh**

Generally when father says something to the child, he is more likely to be listened to because mother keeps disciplining him the whole day by constantly telling him "do this", "do not do that", and child becomes used to her and starts ignoring her advice and threats. Father also wields the image of a boss in the family. Many mothers understand that coporal punishment is bad but they do not realize that constant scoldings, shaming, ridicules and sarcasms are worse and counter productive. Never embarrass or scold the child in front of strangers. It can harm the dignity and self-confidence of the child. Parents can criticize and mend the "unacceptable" actions of their child but they should not criticize the child. Parents must understand the genesis of the antisocial or bad behavior of the child and try to eliminate the root cause. They must remember that punishment is irrational because children (like animals) learn far better by rewards,

praise and encouragement than by blame and reprimands. It is a pity that on an average, parents say at least ten negative things to their children for one positive word of encouragement. It is a well known fact that children (like adults) are inspired and motivated by a pat on their back and are discouraged and humiliated by a kick at their bottom. Positive reinforcements, encouragement and rewarding good behavior works much better to build confidence and self-esteem.

Television and Behavior

It is an unfortunate fact that television (TV) remote and computer mouse are gradually replacing the toys and play activities of children. Television and cable have virtually revolutionized the lifestyle of people and have made outstanding impact on children. It is not uncommon to see a one and half year old infant playing with remote to change TV channels to the great amusement and annoyance of their parents and grandparents. Some parents use TV as a "baby sitter" for their toddler. By the age of 3 years, most children are already hooked to television and they have a list of their favorite programs.

It is true that selected TV programs like children's program, discovery channel, quiz program and cartoon films can be a great fun and learning experience for children. However, these programs cannot serve as a substitute for group activities, playing and reading. But watching violence, aggression and dangerous stunts in movies, WWF, AXN channel, cartoons and even commercials can have adverse effects on the mind and psyche of children. The children often get a message that violence is an acceptable way to deal with problems and it does not cause any real harm. Soap operas, prime time TV and many other popular programs may expose children to sexuality, smoking, drugs and alcohol abuse at a time when they are too young to understand their implications.

Some children may sit infront of "idiot box" drinking coke/pepsi and munching potato chips or crisps up to 4 hours in a day. The fast food and soft drinks commercials may have undesirable impact on the eating habits of the child. Children often get a distorted view as to what they should be eating and often get hooked to junk food. The TV crazy children often tend to become over weight, which adversely affects their physical activity in school with a vicious cycle of over eating, obesity and inactivity. They tend to become lazy, withdrawn and may avoid friendship with their classmates. Not only their social interactions are reduced but they may actually develop antisocial behavior exhibiting *dada giri*, violence and aggression in their day-to-day life. Moreover, watching television is a passive habit and it does not help the child to acquire the most important skills such as communication, fantasy, cooperation and leadership. It has been shown that kids who grow up watching TV rather than playing with toys and outdoor games are more likely to commit crimes later in life (Box 24.2).

At times, the girls of adolescent age group are concerned about their weight and many of them wish to look like the models they see on TV. They may resort to measures like drastic dieting or fasting without proper medical guidance resulting in subtle or overt nutritional deficiencies and increased vulnerability to develop infections and psychological fear of food (anorexia nervosa).

Parents should monitor TV viewing Television viewing is habit forming and may isolate the child from his classmates, teachers and even parents. Parents should encourage and enthuse their child to join enjoyable and constructive activities like sports, swimming, dancing, music, group activities like picnics, and trekking, etc. They should restrict their own TV viewing and child should be encouraged to watch appropriate child-friendly TV programs for a maximum of one hour in a day. Like other daily timetable of activities, child should have a time slot for watching TV so that you know in advance what options he has to watch. Whenever feasible parents should watch television with their child to make him become a critical and discriminating viewer. Parents should make him understand that the violence he sees on TV is make believe and just "made-up" and not real. They should criticize the characters that are dishonest, drink alcohol, smoke or use drugs or indulge in wreckless car driving. The child should be made to realize that most commercials are misleading and are merely advertisement stunts to promote their sales and the child must

---

Box 24.2 Hazards of excessive TV viewing

- Violent, aggressive and bullying behavior.
- Sleep deficit, poor attention span, decreased intellectual ability and falling grades in school.
- Reduced physical activity, greater munching of snacks and taking fizzy drinks or juices may lead to obesity.
- Eye strain, myopia and headaches.
- Early exposure to sex, violence, antisocial behavior and substance abuse.
- Increased incidence of sleep difficulties, night mares and perhaps enuresis.
- Risk of injury by imitating "stunts" shown on TV.
- Reduced communication, socialization, lack of cooperation and inability to make friendships.

Box 24.3 Guidelines for TV viewing by children

- Do not keep a TV set and iPad or Tablet or Mobile in the children's bedroom.
- TV viewing should be a family activity.
- Set time limits and monitor the programs being watched by your child.
- Explain that watching television is not the best way to spend leisure time and emphasize the need for various sports, social and fun activities.
- Encourage watching of sports, animal planet, children's quiz program, interactive TV programs, programs with pro-social and non-violent themes, etc.
- Explain that the programs are creations of fiction and they do not necessarily depict real life situation/s.
- Children should be made to understand that advertisements and associated stunts are commercial gimmicks and do not reflect the true virtues of the products being promoted.
- Parents should serve as role models to their children for censored and sensible viewing of TV.

---

appreciate the difference between "healthy" and "unhealthy" or undesirable foods and toys (Box 24.3). According to American Academy of Pediatrics, the "screen time" which include TV, internet, computer, videogames and cell phone usage should be restricted to 2 hours per day. Children below 2 years should have zero "screen time". Parents should spend a quality time with their children involving active interaction, play and fun activity. Reading a book to a child or telling a story of valour, courage or compassion is far more useful to stimulate mental faculties and develop humanistic qualities in children.

BIBLIOGRAPHY

Abubakar A, Van de Vijver FRJ, Suryani AO, Handayani P, Pandia WS. Perceptions of parenting styles and their associations with mental health and life satisfaction among Urban Indonesian adolescents. *J Child Fam Studies* 2015, 24(9): 2680–2692.

Aunola K, Stattin H, Nurmi J–E. Parenting styles and adolescent's achievement strategies. *J Adolesc* 2000, 23(2): 205–222.

Huver RM, Otten R, de Vries, Engels RC. Personality and parenting style in parents of adolescents. *J Adolesc* 2010, 33(3): 395–402.

Jeronimus BF, Ormel J, Aleman A, Penninx BWJH, Riese H. Negative and positive life events are associated with small but lasting change in neuroticism. *Psychol Med* 2013, 43(11): 2403–2415.

Roberts BW, Wood D, Smith JL. Evaluating five factor theory and social investment perspectives on personality trait development. *J Res Personality* 2005, 39: 166–184.

Rothbart MK, Ahadi SA, Evans DE. Temperament and personality: Origins and outcomes. *J Personality Soc Psychol* 2000, 78: 122–135.

24

25

Behavior and Habit Disorders

The factors governing the development of behavior and personality are discussed in **Chapter 24**. Every child needs tender loving care and a sense of protection by parents who are well adjusted and leading a happy married life. Children should have opportunities for development of independence, trust, confidence and self-esteem. Behavior and habit disorders may occur due to overprotection or rejection, pampering or over discipline and disturbed parent–child interaction because of broken family dynamics (single parent, divorce). Habit is a learned pattern of behavior that is repeated so often that it becomes automatic. There is a trigger or stimulus that initiates a response which becomes automatic in due course of time. Behavior problems in children are a reflection of interparental conflicts. Parents should follow a "middle path" in providing guidance and emotional support to their children. Extremes of manipulations and unrealistic discipline modalities are likely to cause behavior disorders. There may be adverse influence on children by mass media like television, radio and social networking sites on internet. Children with a chronic disease and disability may manifest with anxiety, stress and irritability. Social unrest, violence in society leads to changes in value system and economic insecurity which may have adverse effects on adolescent children. Nurses play an important role for prevention, early diagnosis and management of common behavior disorders in children.

Finger and Thumb Sucking

Some newborn babies put their fingers in the mouth as a signal of hunger. They drop the habit but around 3 months of age they again start putting their fingers in the mouth. When child has learnt grasping the objects at 5–6 months, he tries to take every object to his mouth. The habit becomes more persistent and pronounced because of irritation of gums due to teething. Finger sucking is often a symptom of hunger, boredom, shyness, teething, fatigue and sleep. Finger sucking

usually reaches its peak at 18–24 months and gradually disappears by the age of 3 years. During this stage, finger and thumb sucking is usually associated with sleep.

Finger and thumb sucking is a normal developmental feature but may become a habit in some children **(Figure 25.1)**. Persistent and compulsive sucking of thumb in older children is sign of insecurity, dependence, boredom and sleep ritual. Some people believe that thumb sucking is indulged by some children to satisfy their sucking needs if they were denied adequate sucking experience on breast or bottle. Bottle fed babies are more likely to suck their thumb because they are able to finish their feed quickly from a bottle and they resort to thumb sucking to fully satisfy their sucking urge. Thumb sucking has been blamed for a variety of ailments without any basis. It may produce soreness or callus formation over the thumb and occasionally malocclusion of teeth if habit persists beyond 5 years.

Treatment

The condition should be handled with care and compassion rather than aggression and disdain. The application of bitter substances over the thumb and use of restraining devices have limited utility. They cause psychological disturbances and may do more harm. Nothing needs to be done in young infants who put their fingers or thumb in their mouth while sleeping. Most children will grow out of the habit in due course of time. When thumb sucking is excessive and occurs both during the day and night in children over the age of two years, one should look for the cause. The common causes are insecurity, boredom and jealousy. The child should be distracted and provided greater opportunities for interaction and play activity. Children have lot of energy. We can give them paper, pencil, blunt scissors, clay or mud for modelling, building blocks, etc. to keep them occupied **(Figure 25.2)**. Constant nagging and reprimands cause unhappiness, resentfulness and more insecurity. The child should not

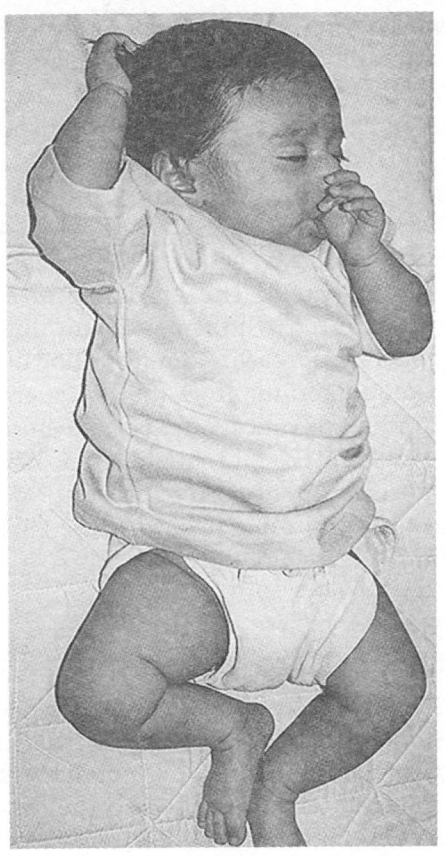

Figure 25.1 Thumb sucking at the age of 2 months. It is a temporary phenomenon and habit is dropped as the child grows

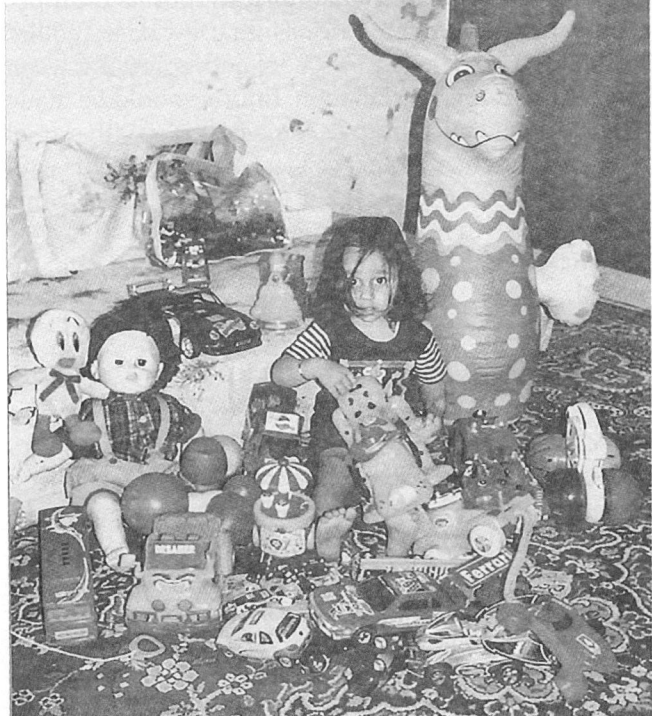

Figure 25.2 The child should be kept busy with toys and fun activities to distract him from thumb sucking

be ridiculed, teased, shamed or given threats. When parents make lot of fuss about his thumb sucking, he may deliberately continue to suck the thumb as an attention-seeking device. In an older child, a direct appeal can be made to him on the ground that its an infantile habit and that he is now a big boy/girl. The danger of thumb sucking lies not in the act of thumb sucking but in how you view and tackle it. Thumb sucking does not cause any harm to the permanent teeth because most children leave the habit by the age of 5 years.

Nail Biting (Onychophagia)

Nail biting usually begins around 8–10 years though occasionally it may start earlier. Toe-nail biting may be seen in some girls. The habit may continue into adult life or appear for the first time during adulthood. The common predisposing factors include insecurity, anxiety, jealousy and stress. Nail biting is socially unacceptable and is associated with increased risk of worm infestation. Inculcate the habit of keeping nails trimmed from early life. You can appeal to the sense of pride of the child because ridicule, teasing and scolding can do more harm. Anxiety and stress should be relieved by active participation in sports, dancing, music, yoga and meditation.

Pica (Mud eating, Geophagia)

During 1–2 years when children are passing through the "oral phase" of development or "mouthing", they try to put their fingers and every object into their mouth. The child may pluck his hair and swallow them or eat paper, chalk or crayons. Some children start eating mud or scrapings of plaster from the wall. There is a potential risk of development of diarrhea or worm infestation due to this perverted appetite. It was originally believed that pica may be a manifestation of calcium deficiency but there is no scientific basis for this. The condition is best managed by distraction, providing more play opportunities and by reducing the chances to pick up clay and mud. The child should not be left alone in the garden where he would have ample opportunities to eat mud. Scolding and frightening the child does not serve any purpose. Administration of iron supplement is associated with faster recovery because pica is now believed to be a symptom of iron deficiency anemia. In due course of time most children abandon the habit as their "mouthing" tendency gradually decreases.

Trichotillomania

There is repeated compulsive plucking of hair leading to significant hair loss. The peak age of onset is between 9–13 years. The disorder is more common in girls. It most commonly involves scalp hair leading to baldness.

25

Rare sites of hair plucking include eye lashes, eye brows, nose and pubic hair. The habit is triggered by local itching or because of stress, anxiety and depression. It may start as an attention seeking behavior. Some children may eat the plucked hair (trichophagia), which over a period of time may from a ball of hair (trichobezoar) in the stomach producing symptoms of anorexia, abdominal pain and non-bilious vomiting. It is often considered as an obsessive compulsive disorder (OCD). The child likely to have low self-esteem and shun socializing or making friends.

Treatment When hair pulling has not been observed by parents, other causes of hair loss such as alopecia areata, tinea capitis, malnutrition, traction alopecia and hypothyroidism should be excluded. Trichotillomania having onset before the age of 5 years, is usually self-limiting and resolves without any treatment. The condition is managed depending upon the underlying psychological disorder. Habit reversal training (HRT) and behavior modification strategies under the guidance of a child psychologist is recommended. Biofeedback, cognitive-behavior methods and hypnosis have been used with variable success. There is no specific pharmacological therapy but administration of tricyclic antidepressants like clomipramine and fluoxetine are credited to provide some benefit.

Obsessive–Compulsive Disorder (OCD)

Obsessive–compulsive disorder is a chronic distressing condition that can lead to severe impairments in social, academic and family functioning. Children with OCD are constantly anxious and worried to perform a task over and over again which adversely interferes with their everyday life. The exact cause of disorder is unknown. There is some evidence that OCD may occur when neurotransmitter serotonin is blocked which gives a "false alarm" resulting in unrealistic doubts and fears. The condition runs in families and seems to have a genetic basis.

The common *obsessions* include fear of dirt, contaminants and germs, need for symmetry and precision, preoccupation with body wastes, lucky and unlucky numbers, fear of illness, sexual thoughts, intrusive sounds, etc. The common *compulsions* and rituals include handwashing, teeth brushing, writing and erasing, collecting and hoarding, checking door locks, repetitive cleaning, going in and out of doors, etc. A number of other psychiatric conditions that are associated with OCD include anxiety disorder, depression, disruptive behavior disorder, attention deficit hyperactivity disorder (ADHD), learning disorders, and trichotillomania.

Treatment The condition is treated with behavioral therapy and medications. Cognitive-behavioral psychotherapy (CBT) involves gradually exposing the child to recognize his fears and reinforce their thoughts that they will not perform any ritual to resolve the fear. For example, a child who is afraid of dirt, may be exposed to something dirty, starting with something mildly bothersome and ending with something that may be grossly dirty. The guidance of a trained therapist is required who is consistent, logical and supportive in his approach. Administration of selective serotonin reuptake inhibitors (SSRIs) is credited to reduce the thought process, associated impulse and subsequent ritual. The child should be encouraged and inspired by constant support, praise and reward. It is important to keep in mind that it's the OCD that is causing the problem, not the child.

School Phobia

Most children are happy to go to school but some may have persistent and abnormal fear of going to school. It is an emotional disorder wherein child develops separation anxiety and cries while going to school and continues to cry when dropped to the school. The predisposing factors include over indulgent, overprotective and pampering behavior of the parents. The child is dependent and lacks self-confidence and becomes afraid in an unfamiliar environment. The condition is handled by emotional support and proper explanation to the child. During initial few days, mother can stay with the child in school and gradually wean him off by proper explanation. Efforts should be made to encourage the child to become friendly with school mates and teacher. Mother can leave some presents with the teachers who can give it to the child to gain his confidence so that in due course of time, the child gets adjusted and does not create any fuss while going to school.

Tics (Habit spasms)

Tics are stereotyped, awkward and repetitive movements of a particular part of the body. Most tics are acquired by imitation of a school mate, teacher or a member of the family. They may start as a symptom of a physical ailment and continue thereafter. Tics can occur any time after 3 years but are most common between 8 and 10 years of age. The common examples of tics are shrugging of shoulders, blinking of eyes, twisting of neck or dry coughing. Sometimes one tic disappears, only to be replaced by another. They are common in a child who is tense and whose parents are very strict and demand high standard of performance

25

and discipline. When a child gets attention due to tics their frequency increases.

Treatment Most tics are benign and usually disappear in a few days or weeks. The child should not be given undue attention or scolded because tics are beyond his control. Parents should try to identify any factors, which may be causing anxiety. Teasing and nagging should be avoided because they will aggravate the tics. The child should be made to relax at home and school and kept engaged in physical activities such as outdoor games and competitive sports. Participation in various group activities like music, dance, yoga and meditation is useful. At times tics-like movements may be early signs of a serious psychological or mental disorder. When tics are marked and persistent or associated with additional physical symptoms, a psychologist must be consulted.

Anorexia Nervosa

It is a rare disorder and usually occurs among teenage girls. There is intense morbid fear of becoming obese even though child is under weight. There is disturbed body image and lack of acceptance that the current body weight of the child is normal or below normal. There is extreme weight loss, cachexia and amenorrhea. The condition is usually associated with depression, anxiety, suicidal tendencies and obsessive–compulsive disorder.

The condition is difficult to manage and need compassionate handling. Psychotherapy is required to restore normal perception of hunger and satiety. Antidepressant and antipsychotic drugs are prescribed as indicated. Severely undernourished and cachectic patients require nasogastric feeding or parenteral nutrition.

Bulimia

It is characterized by episodes of binge eating with inappropriate compensatory behavior to prevent weight gain by self-induced vomiting, misuse of laxatives, diuretics and enemas to prevent excessive weight gain. The disorder is usually seen in adolescent girls and is commonly associated with depression and other psychoses. The condition is treated with a combination of psychotherapy (behavior modification) and use of antidepressants like fluoxetine. The child should be provided with emotional support to ensure motivation and adherence to psychotherapy.

Food Fussiness

The condition is common in preschool children belonging to affluent families. It is common in families with a single child or only male child who is pampered and given over attention. There is excessive concern on the part of mother (and other family members) to make the child eat the food of their liking. Mealtimes become minifights between the child and other family members. The child literally blackmails the parents who try all types of manipulations and pranks without any success. The condition is discussed in detail in **Chapter 15**.

Juvenile Delinquency

There is oppositional defiant behavior or conduct disorder as an expression of disobedience and disruptive behavior. It occurs because of lack of faith and communication betwen the parents and adolescent children. The child may join defiant group of peers who may indulge in *dadagiri* and may become victims of substance abuse. They may exhibit violent and destructive behavior and take part in dare devil macho acts and may come in conflict with juvenile justice system. The child may commit a criminal offence or display a variety of negative behaviors which are not allowed under the law, such as truancy from school, fights, damage to property, smoking, use of alcohol or illicit drugs.

Parents should be vigilant about the nature of the friends and extracurricular activities of their child. When there is excessive absenteeism from school or fall in academic grades, the parents should assess the situation and take corrective action. The child needs compassionate handling and taught about strategies for anger management, peer coping and problem-solving skills to tackle interpersonal conflicts. The child should be trained in the art of cooperation, mutual respect and ability to view the intent of others in a true perspective by avoiding any hostility and malice against others. Active participation in competitive individual and group sports (tennis, football, cricket, athletics) is useful to release anger, tension and stress. It diverts the attention of the child from hostile, violent and unproductive activities. The severely affected children may need de-addiction and care in a foster home.

25

BIBLIOGRAPHY

American Psychiatric Association. Diagnostic and Statistical Manual of Mental Disorders. Arlington VA (Ed). *American Psychiatric Association*, 5th edition, 2013.

Foster LG. Nervous habits and stereotyped behaviors in preschool children. *J Am Acad Child Adolesc Psychiatry* 1998, 37(7): 711–717.

Giannakopoulos G, Mihas C, Dimitrakaki C, et al. Parental separation and children's behavior/emotional problems: The impact of parental representations and family conflict *Acta Paediatr* 2009, 98(8): 1319–1323.

Graybiel AM. Habits, rituals and the evaluative brain. *Annu Rev Neurosci* 2008, 31: 359–387.

Hanna GL. Demographic and clinical features of obsessive-compulsive disorder in children and adolescents. *J Aus Acad Child Adolesc Psychiatry* 1995, 34(1): 19–27.

Huynh M, Gavino AC, Magid M. Trichotillomania. *Semin Cutan Med Surg* 2013, 32(2): 88–94.

Miller JM, Singer HS, Bridges DD, Waranch HR. Behavioral therapy for treatment of stereotypic movements in non autistic children. *J Child Neurol* 2006, 21(2): 119–125.

Rose EA, Porcerelli JH, Neale AV. Pica: Common but commonly missed. *J Aus Board Fam Pract* 2000, 13(5): 353–358.

Scahill L, Chappell PB; King RA, Leckman JF. Pharmacologic treatment of tic disorders. *Child Adolesc Psychiatr Clin North Am* 2000, 9(1): 99–117.

Singer HS. Motor stereotypies. *Semin Pediatr Neurol* 2009, 16(2): 77–81.

Common Developmental Disorders

Temper Tantrums

Sudden outbursts of anger in young children (usually 1–3 years) are called temper tantrums. The usual expression of anger is that the child drops on the floor and starts yelling and pounding with his hands and feet and even banging his head. He is not yet big enough to abuse or attack the parents. Children who are stubborn are likely to have more frequent and violent tantrums. The child with a chronic medical problem is also likely to become more temperamental, fussy and irritable with outbursts of temper tantrums. It helps the child to "let off his steam" to relieve his anger, frustration and helplessness. The tantrum may be sparked off when some demand of the child is unfulfilled, he is being forced to eat or his clothes are being changed or he is being given a bath, or merely for seeking attention. He is in a sullen mood and demonstrates development of his ego and individuality and is trying to send a message that "he cannot be taken for granted".

Treatment The best way to handle a temper tantrum is to show "intelligent neglect" when a child throws a tantrum. Mother should get away from the scene without showing any concern and reaction. The child often cools off quickly and meekly if mother goes about her own business in a matter-of-fact manner. It is unwise on the part of mother to counteract his tantrum by showing her own temper. Mother should not shout but be firm and considerate. Never scold the child or argue with him but handle the situation with common sense and patience. Every wish of the child should not be fulfilled and he must learn to handle frustration from time to time. The child should be helped to feel angry about fewer things and he should be encouraged to communicate his anger without throwing a tantrum. Many young children do understand when you try to explain to them the futility of their prank. Parents should remember that a young child understands a lot more language than he can express. The mother should

not feel helpless and at the mercy of the child otherwise he will "black mail" and make it a habit to get what he wants. If parents try to honor and fulfill every demand and wish of their child, then there is no end to it. Hunger, fatigue and boredom are common causes of outbursts of temper tantrums. Be sure that the child is getting enough sleep, having his meals on time and is occupied playing with his friends and with toys. After the age of 4 years, children learn and demonstrate other ways and means to express their anger and frustration.

Breath Holding Spells

In some children temper tantrum may be followed by a breath holding attack. The child gets angry (due to unfulfilled demand or frustration) or gets hurt, cries loudly (by putting his heart and soul into it) and after a long uninterrupted cry, holds his breath and becomes blue. Rarely, the attack may lead to a fit or convulsion. When enough carbon dioxide accumulates in the body by holding the breath, it provides the necessary trigger to the breathing center in the brain and child starts breathing again. After the spell the child may continue to cry and whimper and start asking for the same demand which triggered the attack. The spells usually occur in children between 6 months and 3 years of age but in some babies they may start as early as newborn period. There is a strong familial predisposition and affected children may have an underlying autonomic dysregulation. These spells occur in over sensitive and over demanding babies of anxious, concerned and apprehensive parents and grandparents. It would appear that breath holding spells are a sort of "black mailing" tactics on the part of the child to get his demand fulfilled. The episode is so frightening to the family that many a times the parents give-in to the demands of the child. The reaping of the reward after the spell sets a vicious cycle wherein the child repeats the spells as and when an opportunity arises to get a wish or demand fulfilled. The child learns to use these spells as a tool to get what he wants and makes parents feel helpless and at his mercy. These children are very demanding and lack patience or coping skills to manage their frustration, disappointment and anger.

Treatment The breath holding spells are harmless and do not pose any danger to the life or brain of the child. The frequency of spells increases if parents or grandparents show extreme anxiety and panic during the attack and when the child is pampered and rewarded after the spell. There is no need to panic or sprinkle cold water on the face of the child. Parents should accept the spell coolly and with confidence that no harm will come to the child by holding his breath. If mother starts shouting or create undue panic and alarm, the child is likely to hold his breath more often and for a longer period. Parents should try to reduce episodes of frustration by meeting some of his genuine or minor demands. At times, when it appears that the child is going to hold his breath, he can be pinched when he will start breathing again. Parents should be advised to follow a sensible middle-of-the-road approach and should not succumb to all the pranks and demands of their child. Administration of iron supplements may reduce the frequency and severity of breath holding spells if child has iron deficiency anemia. The spells usually disappear by the age of 3 years when child learns other ways and means to express his anger and frustration.

Tribulations with Toilet Training

Toilet training should neither be aggressive nor left to the whims or fancies of the child but a common sense approach should be followed. The mother should not be over anxious or rigid in her approach. There are no rigid rules and mother should follow a flexible approach depending upon the development of the child.

Bladder Control

Newborns pass urine almost after every feed with a frequency of 8–10 times in a day. As the child grows, the capacity of bladder increases, the child is able to hold urine for a longer period of time. Mother should be observant and identify the time when child is most likely to void. Most babies are likely to pass urine on waking up. The child may indicate urinary urgency by touching or holding his genitals and becoming restless and uncomfortable. If his subtle gestures are ignored, the child is likely to void and wet his nappies or create a mess by splashing his hands in the pool of urine. The observant mother can hold the baby over the wash basin or make him sit on a potty, when he shows subtle signs to void. If child is unwilling to void, he should not be

forced and mother should handle the situation in a relaxed manner. Avoid using unnecessary force and coercion which may lead to rebellious attitude. After the age of 2 years, the child can be taken to the bathroom to void. When given proper toilet training, most children become dry during the day by the age of 2–3 years. Occasional accidents may occur when child is engrossed in play, is unhappy, tired or unwell and when he is in an unfamiliar environment.

Bowel Control

During early life, passage of urine and stools are involuntary activities without any control to initiate the process, delay it or stop it at will. When rectum is full of feces, further pressure following a feed leads to opening up of the anal canal and evacuation of stools. There may be some straining efforts or facial grimaces before and during the process. The child may become still, stop playing, strain a little or look intently into mother's eyes. The mother must be observant to identify the "signals" and "best time" for placing the child on the potty. When potty training routine is established on a regular basis for a couple of days, the mother would know when to place the baby on the potty. During potty session, the child can be kept busy with toys or a picture book. When efforts at potty are rewarded, the child should be appreciated to strengthen the process of conditioning. When child is unwilling to sit on the potty, he should not be forced or cajoled, instead he should be left alone for a couple of days before trying again.

Aggressive potty training is counter productive and is likely to make the child rebellious. Around the age of 2 years some children may develop a possessive attitude and they "do not let go" or relax to evacuate. At times, the passage of hard stools lead to formation of a crack or fissure in the anus with coating of stools with streaks of blood. The process of evacuation becomes a painful procedure and child becomes reluctant to sit on the potty leading to development of intractable constipation (obstipation). Many a times, the child may go to a corner and may evacuate stools while standing. The condition should be handled by proper dietary advice, use of stool softeners and proper psychological guidance to the parents.

When adequately trained, most children become independent and can look after their toilet needs by 3 years (entry to play school) of age. At this stage the child can wash his bottom when water is poured by the mother or school attendant. Girls should be taught about the importance of washing bottom from "front-backwards" to avoid the potential risk of soiling vulva with feces as a safeguard against ascending urinary tract infection. After washing the bottom, the child should be trained to wash his hands with soap and water and explained about the importance of personal hygiene.

Speech Problems

Baby talk In some children initial speech is like a "baby talk" with lisping while others develop a clear and distinct speech. Children have their own vocabulary for common objects; *mum* for water, *toti* for *roti*, *buboo* for *milk*, *bum-bum* for car, *tha* for gun, etc. Children start making cute little sentences like *toti nahin thani* (I don't want to eat), *mein maloon ga* (I will beat), *ta ta mujeh kahani sunao* (cha-cha tell me a story), *meirey ko nahi dana* (I don't want to go), *aap dao* (you go), etc. The family should take it in a matter of fact manner as a part of growing. Parents should never imitate the child by repeating the words in the same manner. They should not make him self conscious and uneasy by drawing his attention to mispronunciation. The child is not yet mature enough to pronounce better and more clearly at this stage. By your corrective methods he will feel more confused and helpless and may develop hesitancy in his speech. It is best to leave him alone and make no attempts to correct him. When grown ups also start imitating his "baby talk" and start appreciating that how "cute" he talks, he will continue with his habit much longer for seeking attention. At times, a child who has been talking normally, may regress back to "baby talk" when he is upset or on arrival of a new sibling. When parents talk to him like a grown up person, he will gradually get over the baby talk in due course of time.

Stammering (Stuttering) Some children between the ages of two and three years may get stuck, stumble or repeat certain words and lose the rhythm and flow while speaking. Disorder may run in families and is more common in boys than girls. About 5% of preschool children stutter at some point and most children grow out of it without any special help. Only when the speech difficulty persists beyond 2–3 months and it interferes with communication, it is labelled as stuttering. Some children may have normal speech for some time and then suddenly develop stuttering without any obvious cause or due to an emotional upset. The stuttering becomes worse when child is anxious, tired, ill or excited and the situation becomes worse when mother herself is tense. The child is frustrated when he feels that mother is not paying any attention to what he is saying. Stutterers often speak normally when alone and when singing, talking to animals or reciting nursery rhymes.

Treatment Stuttering is usually a temporary speech defect and can be resolved by proper handling. Parents must pay full attention and listen patiently to what the child has to say. He should not be hurried but encouraged to speak slowly and loudly. The child should feel that you are interested in what he is saying, and not in how he is saying it. He can be asked to sing a song or recite nursery rhymes alone infront of a mirror. Parents should try to build his self-esteem by praising him for all the activities he is doing correctly without drawing any attention to his speech difficulties. Mother should set aside some relaxed time each day to play and talk with him slowly and clearly in a simple language. The child should never be chided or shamed by making fun of him or imitating him. The family should seek the help of a speech therapist if stuttering persists beyond the age of 4 years. It is desirable that the child should have normal speech by the time he starts going to school otherwise he may feel embarrassed or humiliated by other children.

Sleep Problems

Children differ widely regarding their physiological need for sleep. The duration of child's sleep depends upon his age, personality, intelligence and constitution (genetic factors). Some children take a lot of time to go to sleep, some have a deep sleep while others have a light sleep and keep turning and tossing the whole night. The newborn baby sleeps most of the time. At 3 months most babies are likely to have three or four sleep periods and at one year they are likely to have two or three sleeping sessions. Many children discard their afternoon nap by about 3 years (entry to play school). The active, energetic and brighter children tend to sleep less while placid, slow and relatively inactive children are likely to sleep more.

The bedroom The newborn baby often sleeps with mother in her bed or in a baby cot placed next to her bed. The baby needs constant care, feeding and change of nappies. After 6–9 months, his cot can be moved to a corner in the same room. In our country due to shortage of space and cultural habits, children continue to sleep in the same bed with parents or in a separate cot in the same room till the age of 7–8 years or even longer.

Disturbed night sleep The depth and soundness of sleep decreases as child grows. Newborn babies sleep soundly but are awakened by hunger as they need to be fed at night during first 8–10 weeks. Sleep may be disturbed by wet nappy, insects and mosquito bites. Hot weather, over clothing and exposure to cold are common causes of sleep disturbances. Sleep may be disturbed by anal itching due to pinworms. Children

26

are known to awaken up with a sudden scream due to a nightmare or at times by entry of pinworms in the vagina. Sleep may be disturbed due to a blocked nose because of cough and cold or use of a heater or hot air blower. After 2–3 years, the child may cry because he wants to pass urine. A common cause of sleep disturbance is the presence of parents in the same room. The child is likely to be disturbed by their talking, coughing, snoring, late night TV watching or other noises. Mother has to get up early in the morning to send the children to school or prepare food, whereas the father is in no hurry and would prefer to sleep a little longer. Whenever feasible, it is desirable that when a child is older than 3 years he should sleep in a separate room.

Sleep-time rituals Most babies are fussy and fretful while falling asleep. The fussiness becomes worse if they are unwell, tired or hungry. Some children are more active, wiry and alert and they take a long time for "winding down" at the end of the day. The child may be desperately sleepy but he wants to remain active and enjoy the overtures of doling parents and grandparents. Some children put their fingers into their mouth, bang or roll their head at bed time while falling asleep. Many children like to be gently rocked on the mother's lap, patted on the back or want to be taken for a ride in the car to fall asleep. Around 18 months, the child may like to hug a favourite teddy bear or a doll while falling asleep **(Figure 26.1)**. The list of sleep-time rituals and demands may go on increasing during this phase, e.g. child may ask for a drink, may want to keep the door open or light on, like to have light music or want the TV on, etc. Most children discard these rituals after the age of 3 years.

Handling sleep problems It is important both for the child and parents to have a good night's sleep to wake up fresh, charged and energetic to enjoy another day. When falling asleep becomes a perpetual daily ordeal or child is having disturbed sleep, it is most tiring and challenging for parents and an important cause of bad temper and marital disharmony. It is wrong to let the child have prolonged spells of crying every night or smack him or put him to sleep with drugs. A child who has had an enjoyable day time activities, without undue frustration and had a "healthy fatigue" (not overtired or overstimulated) is likely to have less difficulty in falling asleep. The child should not be hungry and preferably given a cereal feed last thing at night to prolong his night's sleep. *Drugs should never be used to break a bad habit or for putting a healthy child to sleep.* Many children fall asleep while listening to a story or a lullaby. Mother should

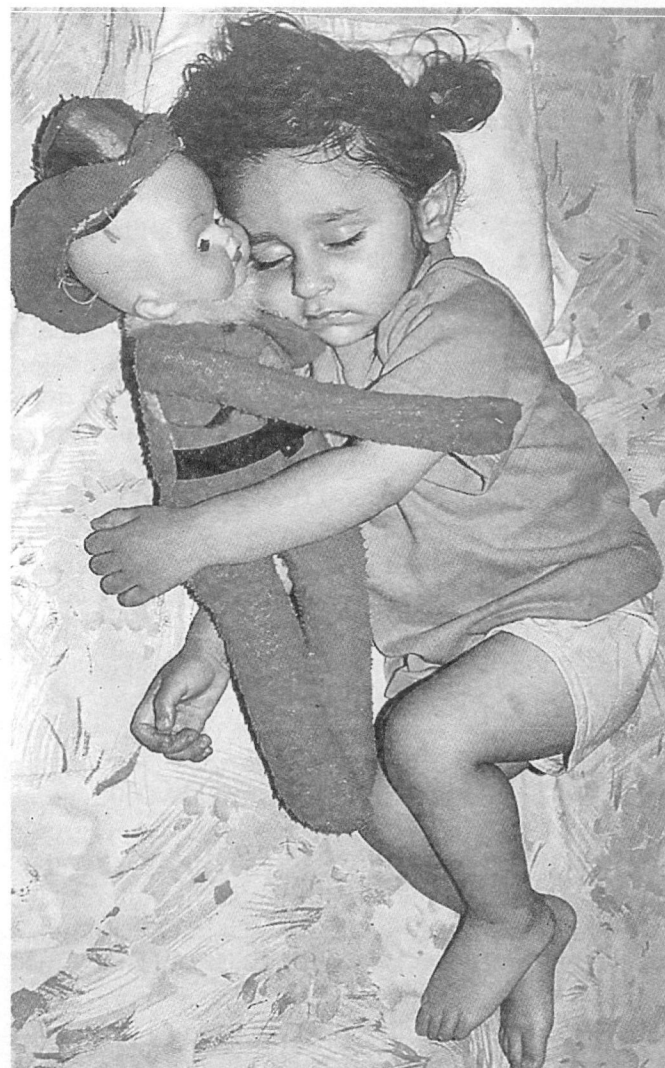

Figure 26.1 The toddler is sleeping by hugging his favorite doll

identify the time when her child falls asleep with least fuss. The best time, place and "harmless sleep-time rituals" should be exploited to facilitate the process from wakefulness to sleep. Avoid playing exciting games just before bed time. Mother must stick to his child's established sleeping routine otherwise he will become cranky and irritable. Do not offer any bribes or rewards for going to sleep. The child should have a comfortable and loose night dress. The room should be cool, comfortable and well ventilated. The child should be adequately covered and nicely tucked by avoiding both over clothing and exposure. It is unwise to leave a crying child in his bed room to teach a lesson or to break a habit. Some fathers come home so late that either the children have gone to sleep or they are getting ready for it. The child wants to spend some time with the father whereas the mother is anxious that he should go to bed. Many a times mother becomes helpless and she is at her wits end and needs all the understanding and sympathy of her husband to tide over this difficult period. The parents should handle the crisis together with common sense, patience, good humor and matter of fact manner.

Nightmares and Night Terrors

Children start having bad dreams between the ages of 3–5 years. The exact cause is not known but they may occur because of stress and frustration during the day time. Due to a bad dream the child wakes up crying and screaming. Mother should comfort and cuddle him saying everything is alright and he was just having a bad dream and dreams are not real. After he is comforted, you can ask him about the details to identify the issue bothering him. Give him the assurance and comfort that he should not worry and you are always close to him to protect him. Mother should stay with him until he falls back to sleep. At times young girls may scream at night when pinworms may wriggle into their vagina.

Night terrors are much less frequent and occur due to temporary disturbance in the brain. Night terrors tend to run in families. They are more common in boys and usually occur during the age of 5–7 years. During night terror, child starts screaming loudly but his eyes are wide open with a blank stare. The child looks frightened, has a rapid breathing and marked sweating. The child does not respond to mother's shouting or vigorous shaking as if he is in a trance. It is difficult to wake him up. *When the night terror goes off, the child has no scare or memory of the event because it is not dependent on a dream.* About one-third of children with night terrors also experience sleep walking. Mother should hold and comfort the child during the episode of night terror till he goes back to sleep again. When child is having frequent night terrors, parents should consult a neurologist or child psychologist.

Sleep Walking (Somnambulism)

Sleep walking runs in certain families and is usually a self-limited condition. During sleep, the child stands up with glassy stary eyes and starts walking. He may have mumbling speech and some semi-purposive activity like urinating or opening a cupboard. The child will go back to his bed of his own and sleep again. He will have no memory of the event next day. Some children may wander out-of-door and at times may hurt themselves. Most sleep walkers give up the habit in a couple of months. When sleep walking is frequent, child can be given diazepam at bedtime under supervision of a child psychologist.

Teeth Grinding (Bruxism)

It is generally believed that teeth grinding during sleep is a sign of worm infestation though there is no scientific basis for it. Even children from developed countries, where there is hardly any incidence of worm infestation, grind their teeth in sleep. The exact cause of teeth grinding is unknown but it may be a symptom of tension due to unexpressed anger and resentment during the day. In some children, teeth grinding may be accompanied by talking during sleep. The child should be encouraged to participate in the play activities and should learn to express his anger and resentment without any undue restraint. Bedtime should be made enjoyable and relaxed by narrating a story or talking with the child regarding various pleasant and unpleasant experiences of the day. It is important to remember that praise and encourage-ment boost the confidence of the child and reduce tension.

Rocking and Head-banging

Some infants may start rocking their body or banging their head soon after they start sitting or crawling. Some children may just roll their head on the cot side-to-side leading to loss of hair. Head-banging is more frightening to parents as they are worried about the injury to the head and are concerned whether the child has low intelligence or autism. It may be due to headache, discomfort of teething or irritation in the ears or a symptom of hearing or visual loss. Rocking may be a feature of self-stimulation like thumb sucking or a sign of boredom, anxiety and stress. Many a times it is difficult to identify the underlying cause of body rocking and head banging and both may coexist in a child. A soft rug may be placed under the cot to reduce the pleasing vibrations during rocking.

Bedwetting (Nocturnal enuresis)

Voiding of urine during sleep is called bedwetting or nocturnal enuresis. Depending upon the family background and neuronal maturation, many children are dry at night after their first birthday but some may continue to wet their bed at night upto the age of 3 years. This is in accordance with other developmental milestones which have a wide range of achievement among normal children. Most children should become dry at night by the time they start going to a regular school. About 5 percent children do not achieve bladder control at night by the age of 5 years and are labeled to have nocturnal enuresis. The condition is more common in boys than girls. Enuresis may be primary, i.e. the child never achieved bladder control or after having

26

achieved the bladder control at night for a period of 6 months or more, the child starts wetting the bed again (secondary enuresis).

Causes

The exact cause of bed wetting is not known. It seems children with enuresis have a small capacity of bladder and they are blessed with a deep or sound sleep. The sensation of full bladder does not wake them up and they void during sleep. Children with secondary enuresis may have underlying stress or emotional disturbance. The common causes of stress are arrival of a new baby, a move to a new home, a transfer to a new school or exposure to scary movies or videos. There is increased familial tendency of bed wetting in certain families indicating hereditary or genetic basis. Most children with bed wetting do not have any urinary symptoms during day time. When there are associated symptoms related to micturition during the day like frequency of passing urine, difficulty in voiding or passage of excessive quantities of urine, underlying kidney disorder should be ruled out by proper laboratory investigations. Bed wetting may undermine the self-esteem of some children and interfere with their social development and peer relationships. School-age children who continue to wet at night are reluctant to accept invitation from their friends to sleepover and avoid joining overnight education and recreational tours.

Treatment

The condition is best handled with sensitivity, understanding and compassion. Most children would respond to general measures without any medications. The child should be asked to restrict his fluid intake to at least 3 hours prior to bed time. He should be advised to take early dinner and avoid taking rice and milk at night. He should be asked to empty the bladder before going to sleep and repeat several times that "I will not wet my bed today". These positive thoughts get lodged in the subconscious mind to strengthen his will power to achieve bladder control. He should be asked to maintain a calender of dry and wet nights. The child should be encouraged and rewarded for dry nights by words of praise, pat on the back, golden stars or gifts. He should be constantly encouraged and supported by positive thoughts to control the habit. Punitive action and reprimands are counter productive and should be avoided. Parents should avoid nagging, scolding or belittling the child when he fails in his attempts to achieve a dry night. Instead he should be encouraged and reassured that "you have the ability and will power to control it." During the daytime, the child should be encouraged to drink plenty of liquids and asked to hold the urine as long as possible till the urge to pass urine cannot be further controlled. This procedure enhances the capacity of the bladder.

Specific therapy

Most children are able to achieve bladder control at night by following the above mentioned general measures. The use of "moisture alarm" or "potty pager" and drugs have a limited role due to high risk of relapse. The "moisture alarm" consists of a small sponge pad that is worn within the *pajamas*. There is an electrical sensor in the pad which is attached to an alarm box. The alarm serves as a conditioning device. When sponge pad becomes wet, the alarm is triggered thus waking up the child. After several nights of alarm use, the child may get conditioned to prevent the ringing of alarm by waking up before voiding. Some "deep sleepers" may not wake up to the noise of alarm, wherein a parent should take the responsibility of awaking the child when alarm goes off. If a "moisure alarm" device is not available, even an ordinary alarm clock can be tried. Over a couple of days, identify the exact time when the child wets his bed which is usually fixed and constant. The child can be conditioned to wake up before the accident by setting the alarm 15–30 minutes before the anticipated time of wetting the bed. The use of medications should be delayed till the age of 8 years and they should be taken strictly under the guidance and supervision of a physician. The commonly used drugs include antidepressant namely imipramine (25–50 mg at bedtime for 3–6 months) or oral desmopressin or nasal sprays (DDAVP 10–40 mg at night), which are continued until child remains dry at night for atleast 28 days. The drug therapy is associated with several side effects and there is high risk of relapse on cessation of treatment.

Fiddling with Genitals

It is natural that when a child learns to grasp objects around 5–6 months, he touches his own body organs including genitals. There is nothing wrong or bad about it and if it is ignored the child will stop it soon. He may touch the genitals as a signal to pass urine. Many mothers feel that it is dreadful for the child to touch his genitals and they use aggressive tactics to stop it. Some children may rub their thighs together or make rhythmic rocking movements of the pelvis. The child may appear to be lost in his own world and his face may be flushed. This may occur due to local irritation because of nappy rash or anal itching due to pinworms. No fuss or scene should be created when child manipulates his genitals. He should be distracted and if there is any local cause of itching it should be priately treated. It must be understood that touching the genitals is a phase of normal development to explore body organs and should not be viewed as an evidence of sexual perversion. It is important to realize that aggressive parental attitudes and actions are more harmful than the transitory phase of genital stimulation. The correct matter-of-fact attitude on the part of parents is very important. The boredom of the child should be relieved by providing more interaction and play opportunities.

Masturbation (with ejaculation in boys and orgasm in girls) is extremely common among adolescents. Contrary to the common belief, it does not give rise to weakness, impotency, blindness, insanity or pimples. The physical act itself is not harmful but the associated guilt feelings may lead to depression and emotional disturbances. The child should be encouraged to channelize his energy to outdoor activities by cultivating friendships and participating in sports, dance, yoga and meditation.

BIBLIOGRAPHY

Cheifetz AT, Osganian SK, Allfred EN, et al. Prevalence of bruxism and associated correlates in children as reported by parents. *J Dent Child* 2005, 72: 67–73.

DiMario FJ Jr. Prospective study of children with cyanotic and pallid breath holding spells. *Pediatrics* 2001, 107: 265–269.

Glazener CM, Evans JH, Peto RE. Alarm intervention of nocturnal enuresis in children. *Cochrane Database Syst Rev* 2005, (2): CD002911.

26

Fluids and Electrolyte Disturbances

Next to oxygen, water is the most essential element for life. The integrity of human life depends upon the stability of internal environment which is constituted by water, electrolytes and acid-base components. Water constitutes the largest component of our body. In a term newborn baby, total body water constitutes 75–80 percent of body weight which gradually declines to 60 percent by one year of age **(Figure 27.1)**. Water is distributed inside the cells (intracellular fluid or ICF) and outside or around the cells. The extracellular fluid (ECF) is distributed in-between the cells (interstitial fluid, inside the blood vessels like plasma) and transcellular spaces (like CSF, intestinal juices, pleural and peritoneal cavities, synovial fluid, etc.). The distribution of water in the body compartments is shown in **Table 27.1**.

Table 27.1 Distribution of total body water as percent of body weight

Fluid compartments	Infants	Older children
Intracellular fluid (ICF)	40%	35–40%
Extracellular	35–40%	20–25%
Interstitial	–	15%
Intravascular (plasma)	–	5%
Transcellular (CSF, serosal cavities, synovial fluid, etc.)	–	1–3%
Total body water	75–80%	55–65%

Electrolyte Composition of Body Fluids

Body fluids contain electrolytes which are electrically charged either positively (cations) or negatively (anions). Sodium (140 mEq/L), chloride (103 mEq/L) and bicarbonate (25 mEq/L) are the principal electrolytes in the extracellular fluid (plasma) while potassium (158 mEq/L) and phosphates (95 mEq/L) are principal electrolytes inside the body cells **(Table 27.2)**. The internal homeostasis of the body is maintained by a complex regulatory mechanism by virtue of thirst, renal

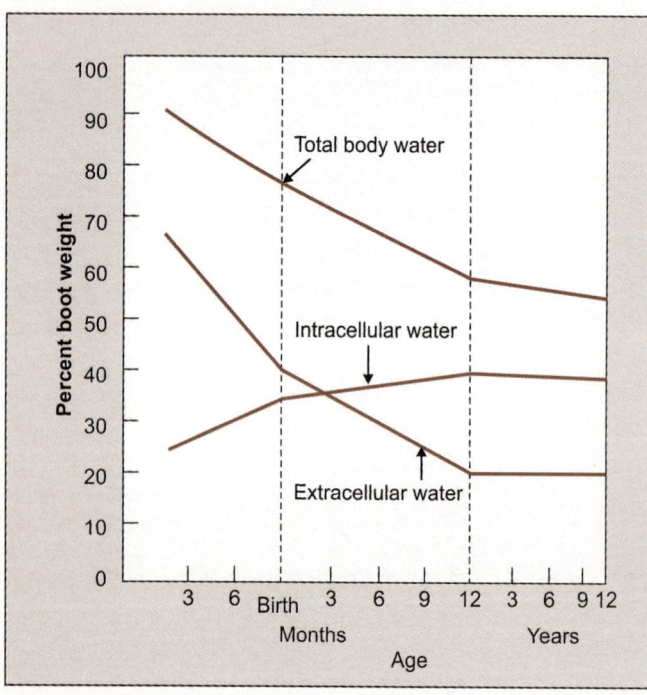

Figure 27.1 Physiological changes in total body water and ratio of intracellular to extracellular water from fetal life to maturity. Refer to text for details

Table 27.2 Electrolyte composition of body fluids

Electrolytes	Intracellular fluids	Extracellular fluids	Interstitial fluids
Cations (mEq/L)			
Na^+	9.0	140	147
K^+	158	4.5	4.0
Ca^{++}	3.0	5.0	2.5
Mg^{++}	30	2.0	1.0
Anions (mEq/L)			
Cl^-	4.0	103	114
HCO_3^-	10.0	25	30
Phosphates	95	2.0	2.0
Proteins	65	15	—
Organic acids	4.0	6.0	7.5
Sulfates	22	—	1.0

mechanism, hormones (ADH, cortisone, aldosterone) and Na^+-K^+ – adenosine triphosphate-dependent pump at the cellular level. These homeostatic regulatory mechanisms are immature or unsatisfactory in children and they are completely dependent and at the mercy of care takers to look after their needs for fluids and electrolytes.

MAINTENANCE FLUID REQUIREMENTS

The requirement for fluids and electrolytes depends upon the metabolic rate of the body. For every 100 kcal metabolized, a child needs 125 mL water, 3 mEq of sodium and 2.5 mEq of potassium. Because 10–15 mL water is produced in the body during the oxidation processes involved in metabolism of food, therefore, it works out that the child needs 100 mL of water for every 100 kcal consumed. The body loses fluids and electrolytes through urine, stools, skin (sweating and insensible water loss) and lungs (water vapors) which must be replenished every day to maintain internal homeostasis. Daily maintenance requirement of fluids and electrolytes of children is usually calculated on the basis of body weight **(Table 27.3)**.

Newborn babies The daily maintenance fluid requirements are higher in newborn babies specially those born preterm. Preterm and LBW babies have additional insensible fluid losses due to use of radiant heater, phototherapy, low humidity in the nursery or incubator, greater surface area and increased metabolic rate. The maintenance fluid requirement depends upon their birth weight. The fluid requirements are low during initial few days when they are unwell and unstable and gradually increase as the caloric intake increases **(Table 27.4)**.

Maintenance fluids are administered as N/5 solution prepared by taking 800 mL of 5% dextrose (10% dextrose in newborn babies), 200 mL of physiological or normal saline, 10 mL potassium chloride 15% (only

Table 27.4 Daily maintenance fluid requirements in neonates (mL/kg)

Birth weight (g)	Days 1–2	Days 3–14	Days 15–30
Term infant	70	80	90–100
1751–2000	80	110	130
1501–1750	80	110	130
1251–1500	90	120	130
1001–1250	100	130	140
751–1000	105	140	150

when child has passed urine) and 20 mL sodium bicarbonate 7.5% solution. Alternatively ready-made maintenance fluids like isolyte-P can be given.

Children are more Prone to Develop Disorders of Fluids and Electrolytes

Dehydration and electrolyte imbalance is more common in children (especially infants) as compared to adults due to following reasons:

1. They have a large body surface area leading to excessive insensible water losses.
2. They have poor capability to concentrate urine leading to excessive urinary losses of water.
3. Infants have higher metabolic rate and greater caloric needs per kg (120 kcal/kg in infants compared to 40 kcal/kg in adults).
4. There is rapid turnover of water in infants because their daily maintenance requirements are around 15% of the total body water (as opposed to 5% in adults).
5. Children are more prone to develop frequent episodes of diarrhea and vomiting.
6. Children are at the mercy of parents and care takers to satisfy their thirst and fluid needs.

Dehydration

Dehydration occurs due to net loss of body water. The most common cause of dehydration in children is acute gastroenteritis. Inadequate intake of water, vomiting,

Table 27.3 Daily maintenance requirements of fluids and electrolytes

Component	By body weight*	By caloric intake**
Water		
Up to 10 kg	100 mL/kg	100 mL/100 kcal
11–20 kg	1000 mL + 50 mL/kg for extra weight above 10 kg	
>20 kg	1500 mL + 20 mL/kg for extra weight above 20 kg	
Sodium	3–4 mEq/kg	3.0 mEq/100 kcal
Potassium	2–3 mEq/kg	2.5 mEq/100 kcal
Chloride	3–4 mEq/kg	3.0 mEq/100 kcal

*Calculated on the basis of actual body weight of the child (not the expected or optimal body weight)
**One year old infant needs 1000 kcal/day (100 kcal/kg/day) plus additional 100 kcal (or 100 mL fluids) per day for each year of age

27

excessive urinary losses of water (diabetes mellitus, diabetes inspidus, diuresis) may lead to dehydration. **Table 27.5** outlines common clinical features of dehydration and its classification. When pre-illness weight of the child is known, sudden weight loss is a reliable criterion to assess the presence or severity of dehydration. Skin turgor is assessed by pinching the skin over the abdomen and chest and observing its recoil back to normal shape. When skin tugor is lost, the skin recoils back slowly or remains pinched for a long time **(Figure 27.2)**. It is difficult to assess dehydration in a malnourished or marasmic child because loss of skin turgor and sunken eye balls are seen because of loss of subcutaneous fat.

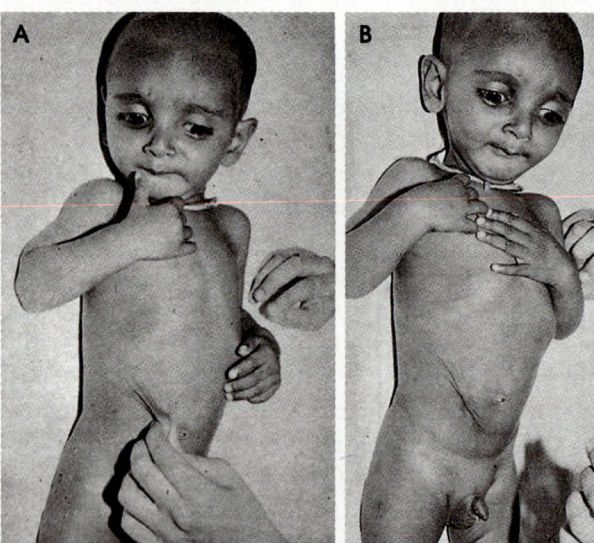

Figure 27.2 Method for elicitation of skin turgor. The abdominal skin is pinched, lifted and released (A). When skin turgor is lost due to dehydration (or marasmus) it takes several seconds before the pinched skin assumes its unwrinkled appearance (B). Note the sunken eyes of the child

On the other hand, in chubby children, the diagnosis of dehydration may be delayed because skin turgor may be preserved even when they develop some dehydration. In these children, excessive thirst, dry mucosa, reduced urine flow, metabolic acidosis or shock are more reliable indicators of dehydration.

Most cases of dehydration are isotonic (no change in serum sodium level) because of proportionate loss of water and sodium from plasma. In hypertonic dehydration (serum sodium >145 mEq/L) skin turgor, blood pressure and urine output are relatively well maintained while in hypotonic dehydration (serum sodium <130 mEq/L) there is excessive loss of skin turgor and early onset of hypotension and shock.

Serum electrolytes (sodium and potassium), blood urea, serum creatinine and acid-base status should be checked. Blood urea may be elevated due to hemoconcentration and renal hypoperfusion but serum creatinine of more than 2 mg/dL in a dehydrated child suggests coexisting renal dysfunction.

Oral Rehydration Therapy

In children with acute gastroenteritis, oral rehydration therapy (ORT) should be started to prevent dehydration. When some dehydration has occurred, and there is no persistent vomiting or abdominal, distension and child is accepting oral feeds, he can be rehydrated with ORT. WHO oral rehydration solution (ORS) is used for prevention and treatment of dehydration **(Table 27.6)**.

ORS and plain water should be given ad libitum depending upon the thirst. When some dehydration is present, provide ORS at a rate of 50–80 mL/kg over 4–6 hours and reassess again. The ongoing losses in the diarrheal stools should be replenished at a rate of 50–100 mL per stool in infants below 2 years and 200 mL per stool in older children. The infant with diarrhea should be encouraged to take breast feeds and other milk feeds without any dilution. Children on complementary

Table 27.5 Assessment of hydration status			
Signs	*No dehydration*	*Some dehydration*	*Severe dehydration*
Thirst	Not thirsty	Thirsty and drinks eagerly	Drinks poorly or not able to drink
Condition	Well, alert	Restless, irritable	Lethargic or unconscious
Eyes	Normal	Sunken	Very sunken and dry
Tears	Present	Absent	Absent
Mouth and tongue	Normal	May be dry	Very dry
Skin turgor	Normal	May be reduced	Grossly reduced
Urine output	Normal	Oliguria	Severe oliguria or anuria
Shock	Nil	Nil	May be present
Acidosis	Nil	Nil	May be present
Weight loss (% of body weight)	Nil	Between 5–10%	More than 10%

27

Table 27.6 New low-osmolality WHO ORS formulation

Ingredients	g/L		mOsm/L
Sodium chloride	2.6	Sodium	75
		Chloride	65
Potassium chloride	1.5	Potassium	20
Trisodium citrate	2.9	Citrate	10
Glucose, anhydrous	13.5		75
Water (mL)	1000	Total osmolality	245

Abbreviation: WHO-ORS, World Health Organization's oral rehydration solution.

feeds should be advised to take *khichadi*, curd, banana and half-boiled egg. Fruit juices and fizzy drinks should be avoided.

Intravenous Rehydration Therapy

Indications

1. Severe dehydration with acidosis and/or shock.
2. Persistent vomiting.
3. Abdominal distension due to paralytic ileus.
4. Nonpassage of urine for more than 6 hours in an infant and more than 12 hours in an older child.
5. Inability to take oral fluids when child is too sick or comatosed.

Fluid requirements The child needs daily maintenance fluid requirements, correction of deficit (depending upon severity of dehydration) and replacement of concurrent fluid losses (due to vomitings and loose motions). **Table 27.7** provides the calculation of IV fluid requirements in a moderately dehydrated infant and rate of infusion during first 24 hours of intravenous rehydration.

After correction of dehydration and when child is able to drink and there is no vomiting or abdominal distension, ORS can be started along with IV fluids for next 4–6 hours. When ORS is being tolerated and child is stable, IV fluids are stopped.

Rate of infusion In young infants and newborn babies, it is preferable to use syringe-based infusion pump to ensure accuracy of fluid administration. In children, a micro-drip burette set can be used to give IV fluids. When infusion is given at a rate of 20 drops/min, it delivers 15 mL of fluids in one hour (microdrip provides 80 drops per mL while ordinary drip set provides 20 drops per mL).

Monitoring The following clinical and laboratory parameters should be monitored by the nurse when IV fluid therapy is given for dehydration:

1. Vital signs every 1 hourly.
2. Check infusion rate every one hourly.
3. Intake and output chart. Concurrent fluid losses through stools, vomitings or NG aspiration should be recorded and replenished. Urine should be collected by attaching a test tube or a condom in a male baby and a urine collection bag in a girl. Record the time when urine is first passed after starting IV infusion.
4. Signs of dehydration.
5. Signs of overhydration like puffiness, enlarging liver size and rales at the bases of lungs.
6. Check for extravasation of fluids, redness and thrombophlebitis at IV site.
7. Abdominal distension or paralytic ileus.
8. Weight record every 12 hourly.

Table 27.7 Calculation of IV fluid requirements in a moderately dehydrated (7% body weight loss) 10 kg infant

Requirements	Type of fluids	Volume
Maintenance	N/5 saline in 5% dextrose	100 mL/kg=1000 mL
Deficit	N/2 saline in 5% dextrose	70 × 10=700 mL
Concurrent losses	N/2 saline in 5% dextrose	For 3 stools*=300 mL
Total		2000 mL
Rate of Infusion		
0–1 hour	20 mL/kg	200 mL normal saline or Ringer's lactate
1–8 hours	½ Deficit + 1/3 Maintenance	350 mL N/2 in 5% dextrose + 350 mL N/5 in 5% dextrose + 7 mL KCl (15%)**
9–24 hours	½ Deficit + 2/3 Maintenance + Ongoing losses (say 3 stools)	350 mL N/2 in 5% dextrose + 750 mL N/5 in 5% dextrose + 300 mL N/2 in 5% dextrose + 14 mL KCl (15%)**

*100 mL for each stool in infants

**Potassium is added once child has passed urine. Add potassium chloride (15%) 1 mL to every 100 mL of fluids as soon as urine flow is established. Never inject potassium chloride as a bolus

Abbreviations: KCl, potassium chloride; N/2, half-normal saline; N/5, one-fifth normal saline.

27

ELECTROLYTE DISTURBANCES

Hyponatremia

It is defined as serum sodium level of less than 130 mEq/L. Hyponatremia occurs due to water retention (congestive heart failure, nephrotic syndrome, renal shut down, hepatic failure, hyperglycemia, sepsis), sodium loss (diarrhea, sweating) or by both mechanisms. Syndrome of inappropriate secretion of ADH or anti-diuretic hormone (SIADH) is an important cause of water retention (due to lack of urination or anti-diuresis) in critically sick children with multi-organ failure or pneumonia and meningitis.

Clinical features The diagnosis is usually made on estimation of serum electrolytes because symptoms appear when serum sodium falls below 120 mEq/L. The child may have circulatory collapse, drowsiness, seizures and coma.

Treatment Asymptomatic hyponatremia is treated by restriction of fluids. Symptomatic hyponatremia is treated by IV infusion of 3% saline, 10 mL/kg at a rate of 1.0 mL/min to correct sodium deficit by 5 mEq/L. This should be followed by administration of normal saline or N/2 saline slowly to achieve serum sodium level around 135 mEq/L. The total deficit of sodium in a case of hyponatremia is calculated as follows:

Sodium deficit = 0.6 × body weight (kg) × (135 − observed serum sodium)

The rate of correction should not exceed 10 mEq/L in 24 hours and total correction is usually achieved in 48 hours.

Hypernatremia

Hypernatremia is defined as serum sodium concentration of more than 150 mEq/L. The common causes include net water loss (diarrhea, vomiting, diuresis, burns, rapid breathing) or excessive intake of sodium (ORS with high salt content or administration of ORS in the absence of diarrhea).

Clinical features Skin turgor and blood pressure are maintained better in hypernatremic dehydration. Skin of abdomen gives a doughy feel (like kneaded wheat flour). The child has marked thirst, CNS irritability with high-pitched cry, seizures and pronounced metabolic acidosis.

Treatment If the child is in shock or severely dehydrated, rapid infusion of Ringer's lactate or physiological saline in 5% dextrose is given to correct hypovolemia (20–30 mL per kg per hour). When child is not in shock, it is preferable to correct hypernatremia through oral route or by a feeding tube. The correction should be done slowly to achieve a fall in serum sodium level by 0.5 mEq/L per hour (about 10 mEq/L during 24 hours) by feeding N/2 glucose saline solution. When hypernatremia is rapidly corrected, child may develop convulsions because of water intoxication. Administer 3–5 mL/kg of 3% saline or 20% mannitol IV to reduce cerebral edema. Hypocalcemia occurs during treatment of hypernatremia and should be corrected by adding calcium gluconate to the infusate.

Hypokalemia

Hypokalemia is defined as a serum potassium concentration of less than 4.0 mEq/L. The common causes include G1 losses (vomiting, diarrhea, gastric aspiration), urinary losses (prolonged use of diuretics, renal tubular acidosis, steroid therapy) and during shift of potassium from plasma into the cells (alkalosis, insulin therapy during diabetic ketoacidosis). Children with protein-energy malnutrition have low body potassium due to poor muscle mass and are very vulnerable to develop hypokalemia.

Clinical features There is muscular weakness, hypotonia and abdominal distension due to paralytic ileus. ECG changes (prolongation of QTc, inversion or flattening of T wave and depression of ST segment) and cardiac arrhythmias are common.

Treatment Potassium deficit should be corrected slowly over 24–48 hours. Potassium is administered at a rate of 40 mEq/L (KCl 15% solution provides 2 mEq potassium per mL) when urine flow is established. In severe life-threatening hypokalemia with ECG abnormalities, rapid correction of serum potassium using a concentrated solution (200 mEq/L or 20 mEq in 100 mL saline) is recommended. The infusion is given with an infusion pump at a rate of 0.30–0.35 mEq/kg/ hour till ECG changes revert back to normal. This modality of therapy is particularly useful in those situations where administration of large volumes of fluids can be dangerous such as acute renal failure, hemolytic uremic syndrome and protein-energy malnutrition.

Hyperkalemia

Hyperkalemia is defined as a serum potassium level of more than 5.5 mEq/L. The common causes include renal dysfunction (oliguria, acute or chronic renal failure, adrenal insufficiency) and shift of potassium from cells to extracellular fluid compartment during acidosis, sepsis, acute hemolysis and tissue necrosis due to a variety of causes including severe hypoxia.

Clinical picture Muscular weakness, cardiac arrhythmias and bradycardia are common. First degree heart block, ventricular fibrillation and cardiac arrest

27

may occur. ECG shows prolonged PR, tall T waves, shortened QT interval and wide QRS complexes.

Treatment Intake of potassium is completely stopped. Calcium gluconate (10%) 0.5–1.0 mL/kg over 5 minutes should be given intravenously as a life-saving measure to reverse electrophysiological abnormalities. Sodium bicarbonate (7.5%) 1–2 mL/kg IV bolus or infusion over 20 minutes moves potassium into the cells. Glucose (10–20% solution) 0.5–1.0 mL/kg along with insulin 0.1–0.2 units/kg (or 1.0 unit for every 5 g of glucose) infusion is started. In children with hyperkalemia due to chronic renal failure, sodium polystyrene sulfonate 1.0 g/kg in 10% dextrose (1.0 g in 4 mL) oral or per rectum is given every 4–6 hourly to enhance excretion of potassium from the gut. Peritoneal dialysis is indicated if serum potassium exceeds 6.5 mEq/L or there is cardiac arrhythmia.

Hypocalcemia

Hypocalcemia is diagnosed when serum total calcium level is less than 8.0 mg/dL or ionized calcium is less than 4.0 mg/dL or <0.8 mmol/L. Calcium is essential for myocardial contractility and is involved in the control of vascular tone and action of several drugs and hormones. In sick children, hypocalcemia is commonly seen during sepsis, exchange blood transfusion and following correction of metabolic acidosis. Other causes of hypocalcemia include vitamin D deficiency, increased urinary losses, hypoparathyroidism and excessive intake of phosphates.

Clinical features Hypocalcemia is usually asymptomatic and picked up either on ECG or estimation of serum calcium level. The common symptoms include increased neuromuscular irritability, muscle spasms or tetany, laryngospasm (stridor), positive Chvostek and Trousseau signs, cardiac arrhythmia and cardiac failure. Electrocardiogram may show 2 : 1 atrioventricular block, low voltage, and prolonged QoTc (>0.2 sec).

Treatment Symptomatic hypocalcemia is treated by slow intravenous administration of 2 mL/kg (up to maximum of 10 mL) of 10% calcium gluconate (0.45 mEq or 9 mg/mL) under cardiac monitoring. Intravenous calcium boluses can be given every 6 hours for 3 days followed by oral supplements of elemental calcium 40 – 80 mg/kg per day. When hypocalcemia is unresponsive to calcium administration, magnesium sulfate 0.2 mL/kg of 50% solution is given intramuscularly in two doses 12 hours apart.

Metabolic Acidosis

Metabolic acidosis occurs either due to excessive production of or decreased excretion of H^+ ions, or excessive loss of bicarbonates from the body. The common causes of metabolic acidosis include severe diarrhea (bicarbonate loss in stools), diabetic ketoacidosis, hypoxia, shock, salicylate poisoning and acute renal failure.

Clinical features Metabolic acidosis becomes symptomatic when pH falls below 7.2 and base excess is more than –10 mmol/L. The most important compensatory mechanism is hyperventilation to get rid of CO_2 (to reduce carbonic acid) and excretion of H^+ ions in urine leading to fall in $paCO_2$ and passage of acidic urine respectively. There is rapid and deep breathing (Kussmaul breathing) with signs of peripheral vasodilatation. Severe acidosis leads to myocardial depression, increased pulmonary vascular resistance, depressed cellular and cerebral metabolism due to hyperkalemia.

Treatment Prompt treatment of underlying condition (acute diarrhea, hypoxia and shock) is associated with correction of metabolic acidosis. Sodium bicarbonate is the drug of choice for treatment of severe metabolic acidosis (pH <7.2, base excess > –10 mmol/L) and its dose is calculated by the following formula: *mEq of bicarbonate = Body weight (kg) × base deficit (desired – actual bicarbonate) × 0.3.* One-half of the calculated bicarbonate is given immediately and the remaining over 12–24 hours. Sodium bicarbonate (7.5 % solution provides 0.9 mEq bicarbonate/L) is diluted with equal volume of distilled water or double volume of 5% dextrose before administration. Concurrent administration of potassium is recommended to safeguard against development of hypokalemia due to shift of K^+ from ECF into the cells. Following correction of acidosis, hypocalcemic tetany may occur due to fall in ionized calcium level. Calcium gluconate 10% (0.5–1.0 mL/kg) is administered slowly intravenously to correct hypocalcemia. *Calcium gluconate should not be added to the infusate containing sodium bicarbonate due to risk of precipitation.* Sodium overload should be kept in mind while correcting acidosis with sodium bicarbonate.

Acute Renal Failure

Intake of fluids whether oral or IV should be restricted to 300–400 mL/m² (15–20 mL/kg or 30–40 mL/100 kcal) per day. Urine output should be recorded by an indwelling urinary catheter and replaced every 4–6 hours. Non-urinary fluid losses are replaced by 10% dextrose without any electrolytes. Hyperkalemia or hypokalemia should be treated as discussed *vide supra.* Patients with volume overload, critical hyperkalemia and worsening consciousness are treated with

27

peritoneal dialysis. Body weight should be monitored every 12 hours and efforts should be made to ensure fall in body weight by 0.5–1.0 percent everyday.

Burns

The fluid deficit in burns is calculated by Parkland formula, i.e. 4 mL/kg per percent of burn area. The deficit amount along with maintenance fluid needs are administered during 24 hours. One-half of the total amount is given in 8 hours and the remainder during the next 16 hours. The fluids should contain 120 mEq/L of sodium, 20 mEq/L of bicarbonate and made isotonic with chloride and dextrose. Ringer lactate is most suitable during first 24 hours. Potassium is added after 24 hours when urine flow is established. Colloids (plasma and albumin) are usually started after 24 hours because when administered early, they may leak through the damaged capillaries.

Mannitol (0.5 g/kg) may be administered after 4–6 hours to promote diuresis and prevent hemoglobinuria.

Fluid requirements from second day onwards are usually three-fourth of the first day requirements. The patient should be closely watched to ensure urine output of 1–2 mL/kg per hour and care should be taken to prevent development of overhydration and pulmonary edema.

BIBLIOGRAPHY

Decaux G, Soupart A. Treatment of symptomatic hyponatremia. *Am J Med Sci* 2003, 326(1): 25–30.

Greenberg A. Hyperkalemia: treatment options. *Semin Nephrol* 1998, 18(1): 46–57.

Moritz ML, Ayus JC. Intravenous fluid management for the acutely ill child. *Curr Opin Pediatr* 2011, 23(2): 186–193.

Singhi S. Hyponatremia in hospitalized critically ill children: Current concepts. *Indian J Pediatr* 2004, 71(9): 803–807.

Singhi S, Sasidaran K. Fluids, electrolytes and acid-base disorders. In: Medical Emergencies in children. Singh M (Ed). *New Delhi, CBS Publishers and Distributors, Pvt Ltd*. Revised 5th Edition 2016, p 65–89.

Traditional Healthcare Practices in Children

The traditional or cultural practices are time honored rituals and beliefs which are prevalent in a community and they may pertain to a wide range of activities. Every community has its own way of rearing children, which is ingrained in the society through traditions established over centuries. The customs and cultural practices pertaining to mothercraft and child care are passed from one generation to another, from grandmother to mother and to their daughters and grand children. The ancestral or conventional child care practices are by and large based on core knowledge and wisdom although some of them may have emerged purely from intuition and superstition. The traditional practices are influenced by the education level, socio-economic status and value system of the family and community.

It is neither possible nor feasible to provide modern medical care to all the people of a developing country, which is bogged by numbers, illiteracy and economic poverty. There is no doubt that a combination of modern and traditional healing is appropriate to serve the health needs. However, the rapidly changing life style and introduction of modern medicine has caused confusion in the minds of tradition-bound people and their promotors in the Indian system of medicine. There is evidence to suggest that traditional health care practices have a definite link with the science of Ayurveda.

Utility of Traditional Healthcare Practices

The conventional or traditional health care practices have become part and parcel of our life style. They are available at the door-step of the people and are readily acceptable to the society. Above all, they are cheap and can be utilized by a large segment of our community. The traditional practices and home remedies are promoted by village healers, midwives, physicians practising Indian system of medicine (Ayurveda, Siddha, Unani), charltans, quacks and of course wise old people of the community. The traditional practices are so ingrained in the minds of people that it is difficult to change them even when they are identified to be useless or harmful.

TYPES OF TRADITIONAL HEALTHCARE PRACTICES

Traditional healthcare practices can be categorised into four main sub-groups: useful, harmful, inoccuous and of uncertain utility. Nurse must be conversant with common customs and beliefs pertaining to health care of children in the area or community in which she works.

1. **Useful traditional practices** A number of traditional health practices for the care of newborn babies are useful and based on sound scientific basis and logic (Box 28.1). They must be promoted and actively encouraged in the society. These practices are appropriate to serve our health needs as they are based on simple technology. A large number of diseases are minor and self-limited and it is desirable to treat them with safe and cheap home remedies.

Box 28.1 List of useful traditional healthcare practices

1. Delivery at mother's place.
2. Isolation of the mother-child dyad for 40 days.
3. Oil massage.
4. Universal and prolonged breastfeeding and wet nursing.
5. Instillation of colostrum in the eyes to prevent conjunctivitis.
6. Use of a cup and spoon or "*paladay*" for top feeding.
7. Baby sleeping on mother's bed and latter avoiding to turn her back towards the baby.
8. Use of honey, basil (*tulsi*) and ginger tea for common cold.
9. Washing hands before taking meals.
10. Rinsing mouth after taking a meal.

2. **Harmful traditional practices** A large number of customs and cultural practices prevalent in our country for mothercraft and child rearing are positively harmful **(Box 28.2)**. Many traditional practices have undergone lot of changes and developed certain aberrations over the years and they have become unacceptable in the context of current scientific understanding. These practices are dangerous and should not be followed. Nurse should educate parents against the hazards of these cultural practices. It is essential that community must be educated so that harmful rituals pertaining to child care are stopped.

3. **Innocuous or inconsequential practices** A large number of traditional practices are apparently harmless or innocuous but are widely practised **(Box 28.3)**. Though most of these practices are harmless but their utility is doubtful and they may lead to delay in seeking medical aid with resultant deterioration of the child.

4. **Traditional healthcare practices of doubtful or uncertain utility** A number of popular child rearing practices are of uncertain or doubtful utility **(Box 28.4)**. There is a need to systematically study the utility, futility and possible dangers of these traditional

---

> **Box 28.2** **List of harmful traditional healthcare practices**

1. Eating less and restricting certain foods during pregnancy.
2. Conducting delivery in a dark and ill ventilated room.
3. Use of rags/dirty clothes during delivery conducted at home.
4. Using ineffective and harmful resuscitation procedures like splashing water on face, squeezing onion in front of nose, vigorous and prolonged slapping, making loud noises, roasting placenta, etc.
5. Use of unsterile knife or blade for cutting the cord.
6. Application of ash, cow dung, catechu, turmeric, etc. on the umbilical stump.
7. Bathing the baby at birth.
8. Discarding colostrum and delaying breastfeeding.
9. Giving water to breastfed babies.
10. Avoiding certain foods during lactation such as pulses, legumes, vegetables, some fruits, etc.
11. Discrimination against girl child.
12. Opium for diarrhea/crying child.
13. Use of *kajal* in the eyes.
14. Use of pacifiers or dummy nipples.
15. Dilution of milk for bottle-fed babies.
16. Castor oil for constipation and diarrhea.
17. Delayed weaning and giving inappropriate weaning foods.
18. Branding the baby with religious symbols to expel evil spirits.
19. Instillation of oil and urine in the ear for ear ache.
20. Exanthematous diseases viewed as personification and wrath of goddesses (*mata*).
21. Starving a child with fever and diarrhea.
22. Delaying introduction of complementary feeds.
23. Wrapping the baby with fever in a blanket.
24. Blaming teething for a variety of diseases.
25. Blind faith and demand for injections.

> **Box 28.3** **List of innocuous or inconsequential traditional healthcare practices**

1. Giving prelacteal feeds: glucose water, honey, jaggery water, tea, donkey's milk, *ghutti*, etc.
2. Nose and ear piercing, talisman, amulets, removing "*Nazar*" by burning lahi, chillies and alum.
3. Circumcision as a religious ritual.
4. Tying neem leaves on the door of the house to prevent infections.
5. Massage of anterior fontanel.
6. Keeping knife under the pillow to protect the infant against harmful spirits.

28

Traditional healthcare practices of uncertain or doubtful utility

1. *Janam ghutti*.
2. Gripe water.
3. Boiled water containing anisi, cummin seeds, ilaichi for the mother after delivery.
4. Use of a variety of traditional galactagogues: garlic, ginger, coconut, jaggery, *bajra*, *ghee*, fenugreek, *panjeeri*, *sonth*, *khaskhas*, *sathavari*, pepper, neem, margosa, *jeevanthi*, etc.
5. Brandy for cough and cold, and pneumonia.
6. "Hot" and "Cold" foods.
7. Avoiding exposure of pregnant women to eclipse.
8. Use of copper, steel and magnetic bracelets.

practices. The blind faith in the traditional health care practices of doubtful utility may lead to nonacceptance of modern system of medicine.

Under the garb of tradition, many substandard and undesirable commercial preparations like gripe water and *janam ghutti* are being promoted and sold over the counter. Gripe water may have alcohol content while *janam ghutti* is credited to provide relief both for constipation as well as diarrhea. Nevertheless, there is a need to preserve the good and useful traditional practices for the care of children and weed out the harmful cultural beliefs and practices by health education. There is a need to launch a compaign through media against balatant advertisements by manufacturers of various formulations of doubtful utility and safety.

BIBLIOGRAPHY

Bolukbasi N, Erbil N, Altunbas H, Arslam Z. Traditional practices about child care of the mothers who own 0–12 month baby. *Int J Hum Sci* 2009, 6: 166–176.

Mattock ES. Traditional medicine is being practiced successfully. *Brit Med J* 2003, 327: 989–9810.

Roy LC, Torrez D, Dale JC. Ethnicity, traditional health beliefs and health-seeking behavior. *J Pediatr Hlth Care* 2004, 18(1): 22–29.

Singh M. The challenge of child health in the villages. *Swasth Hind* 1991, 35: 59–61.

28

29

Birth Defects

During first 3 months of pregnancy (phase of embryogenesis), various organs of the baby are being formed. His eyes, ears and nose are taking shape and various organs like brain, heart, lungs and kidneys, etc. are being formed. During this critical phase of development of the fetus in the womb, if anything goes wrong in his environment, baby can develop structural defects. Occurrence of viral fever (especially rubella or German measles) and intake of certain medicines during this crucial phase may be lead to development of structural defects or congenital malformations. There is an increased risk of development of birth defect if fetus is exposed to X-rays during the period of embryogenesis. Nutritional deficiencies (especially folic acid) may be associated with increased risk of defective development of brain and spinal cord (neural tube defects) and cleft lip.

The overall incidence of major *congenital malformations*, causing a functional disability or cosmetic handicap, is around 2 percent in general population. Birth defects, especially those due to chromosomal abnormalities, are more common if mother is elderly (above 35 years of age). When there is missed abortion (spotting of blood during early pregnancy) or failed abortion following intake of certain drugs (taken to abort a fetus of unwanted sex), there is a greater likelihood of having a baby with birth defects. Genetic defects (inborn errors of metabolism) are more common among couples who are close blood relatives. Birth defects are more common is preterm and low birth weight babies. But in a large majority of birth defects (over 90%), no obvious cause is identified, it is merely a quirk of nature and viewed as will of God.

Birth defects may be limited to a single organ of the baby or there may be multiple defects affecting several organs causing a life-threatening emergency with high chances of producing a serious physical and neuromotor disability. Infants with birth defects may need multiple surgical procedures and prolonged rehabilitation and follow-up by a large number of specialists. Some infants with serious birth defects may die in the womb. Every parent is thus gravely concerned and worried to have a healthy baby. Most parents heave a sigh of relief when they are told that their newly born baby is normal and without any significant or serious birth defects.

COMMON BIRTH DEFECTS

Birth defects may involve any organ of the baby but they most commonly involve skin, muscles, bones and central nervous system. Baby with serious birth defects are often born prematurely or they fail to have satisfactory growth in the womb resulting in the birth of a low birth weight baby (<2500 g), which is small-for-dates and has intrauterine growth retardation (IUGR).

Birth Marks (Nevi)

Vascular nevi They may be flat or raised above the surface. They may be present at birth or appear subsequently during early childhood.

Salmon patch (stork bite) They present as dull pink areas of skin over the nape of the neck, forehead and upper eyelids (angel's kiss) in over 40 percent of newborn babies. They usually fade away during infancy but pink areas over the upper part of the neck may persist.

Portwine stain (nevus flammeus) They present as deep red or purple-red patches on one side of the face, neck or limb. They may be associated with vascular malformation of the brain (with intracranial calcification) and seizures (Sturge-Weber syndrome). Skin defect can be minimized by use of cosmetics or treated by laser therapy.

Strawberry mark (cavernous hemangioma) They appear as dark-red or pinkish skin patches raised above the skin surface like a strawberry. They are compressible on pressure. During first 5–6 months of life, they grow in size along with growth of the baby. They spontaneously disappear over the next 2–3 years leaving behind pale and slightly raised skin. When large in size they can be treated by local application of a cream containing corticosteroids, and oral intake or topical application of beta blockers.

Pigmented or pale nevi A large number of birth marks with different colors (brown, coffee with milk, blue, black, etc.) may be seen at birth or appear subsequently during early childhood **(Figure 29.1)**. They may be flat or raised above the surface of skin. Similarly pale or white (decreased or absent skin pigmentation) birth marks of different sizes and shapes may be present on the skin. There is no specific treatment and they are managed by application of cosmetics or laser therapy.

Musculoskeletal Defects

Extra or fused fingers and toes (polydactyly and syndactyly) There may be extra finger or toe on the thumb (big toe) or little finger (little toe) side in the hands and feet. The extra finger or toe may be normally attached or attached with a thin tag of skin. At times some of the fingers and toes may be fused (syndactyly) with each other with inability to make fine manipulations of hand. The anomalies of fingers and toes may be isolated or associated with other abnormalities in various systems of the baby. The anomalies of fingers and toes are minor but they cause lot of embarrassment to the child. The extra and fused finger or toe can be surgically excised and repaired by a plastic surgeon at an early age. When extra digit is attached merely by a thin tag of skin, it can be tied with a nylon thread and it would drop off within a day or so. This should, however, be done under medical supervision.

Bowed legs (genu varum) Most normal babies have curved legs at birth. When a baby lies flat on the bed with feet touching each other, there may be a gap of up to 5 cm between the knees **(Figure 29.2)**. When child learns to walk, the bowing or curvature becomes less and child often develops knock-knees. In some families, there is greater tendency to have bowed legs but it should not be a cause for concern. When bowing is marked or limited to one side, rickets and developmental bone defect should be excluded.

Knock-knees (genu valgum) Most preschool children have knock-knees and it is not of any significance. When child stands erect with both knees touching each other, a gap of upto 5 cm between the

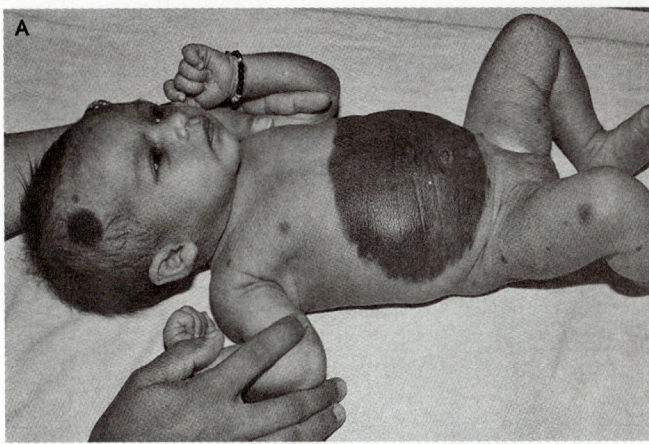
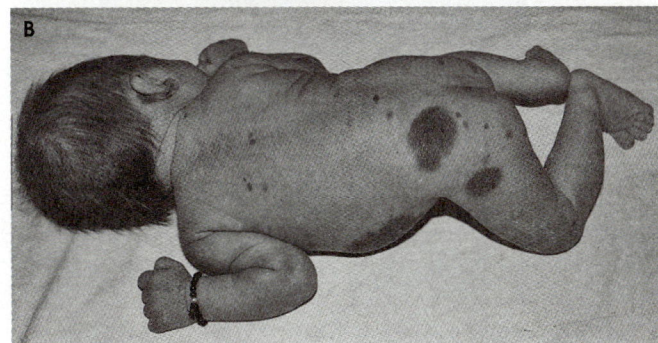

Figure 29.1 Giant pigmented nevus over the abdomen (A) with smaller pigmented nevi over the face, back and buttocks (B)

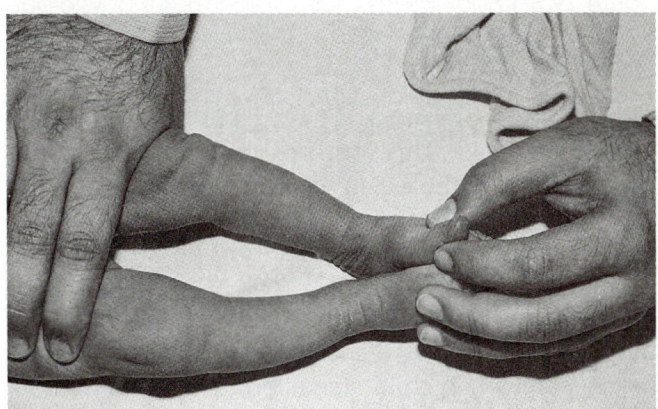

Figure 29.2 Bowed legs (genu varus). It is common and physiological during first 2 years of life. The distance between the knees is usually less than 5 cm when both ankles are closely opposed

feet is normal **(Figure 29.3)**. The knees may rub against each other while walking. Overweight children may have greater degree of knock-knees. Knock-knees may occur due to rickets (vitamin D deficiency) and developmental defect. The knock-knees usually disappear by the age of 7 years. When deformity is persistent or more marked, orthopedic surgeon should be consulted.

29

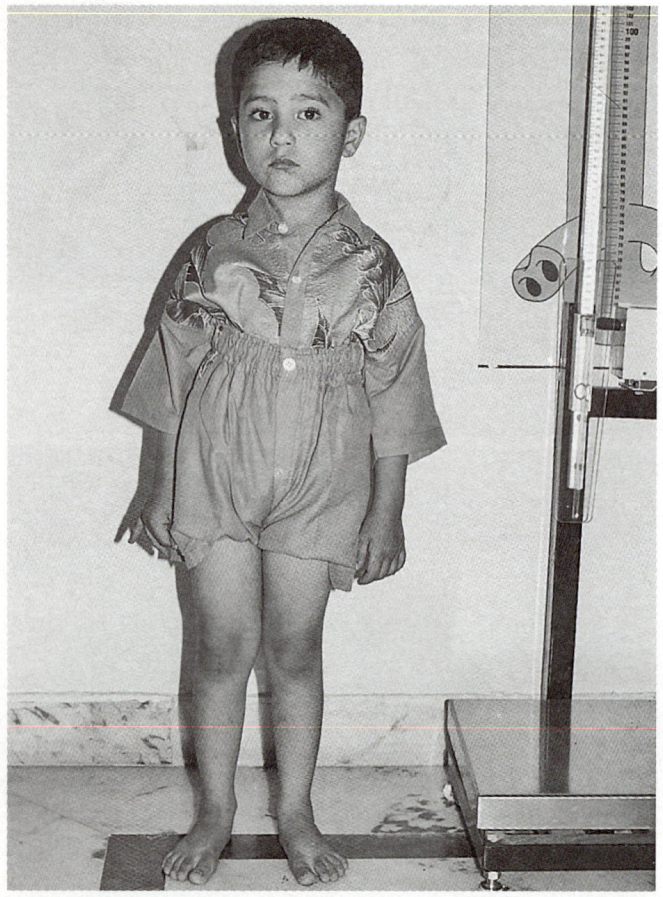

Figure 29.3 Knock knees (genu valgum). It is physiological during 2–5 years of age

Flat feet (pes planus) In infants, flat feet are normal because bones are soft and the arch of the feet is filled with a fatty pad. This obscures the normal curve on the inner side of the feet giving a flat appearance to the feet. When infant walks with wet feet, it leaves behind complete impression of the feet on the ground. The normal appearance of flat feet disappears by the age of 2 years. After this age, flat feet is diagnosed when the inner side of the heel of shoes wear off and arch of the feet is poor when child stands on his toes. When the child stands, the whole foot touches the ground instead of the inner side being raised a little bit off the ground. There may be pain in the feet and difficulty in running. Physiotherapy and special shoes with insoles and inserts (orthoses) are recommended for treatment. Ask the child to walk or run on toes and try to spread out the toes as widely as possible. Child can be asked to pick and hold pebbles or marbles between the toes and sole. Stretching excercises of tendo-Achilles by forcibly trying to touch the dorsum of the foot with shin are useful when there is shortening of Achilles tendon.

Club foot (talipes equinovarus) The defect may be on one side or both sides and occurs due to crooked position of the baby in the womb because of less quantity of amniotic fluid. The foot is stretched downwards (plantar flexed) and turned inwards (adducted) **(Figure 29.4)**. The upper surface of the foot cannot be made to touch the front of the leg (shin) by dorsiflexion. It may be associated with a spinal deformity (spina bifida, meningocele) in some babies. Early physiotherapy (foot is pulled outwards and then dorsiflexed to touch the shin) and application of plaster of paris cast can correct the deformity. The cast has to be changed frequently and treatment is carried out for several months. The foot would become entirely normal and child would be able to walk normally if early and effective treatment is instituted.

In-toeing (pigeon-toed) The child walks or runs with forefeet turned inwards (like a pigeon) instead of pointing straight forward. The child may stumble or trip by striking the toe of one foot against the heel of the other. The condition affects both limbs but one side is affected more than the other. The condition usually runs in families and has hereditary basis. The deformity occurs because of rotational problems of the bones of lower extremities. The forefoot is adducted at the tarsal-metatarsal joint (metatarsus adductus). In about 10–15% cases, dysplasia of the hip may be associated.

Most cases of in-toeing resolve spontaneously as the child grows. There is no role of exercises, special shoes and braces. When there is severe bending of toes inwards due to metatarsus adductus (like club feet), physiotherapy, special shoes and casts may help. When deformity is rigid, the condition is treated with a cast extended above the knee which is kept flexed 20–25 degrees to facilitate walking. The cast is changed biweekly and correction is achieved after 3 to 4 cast

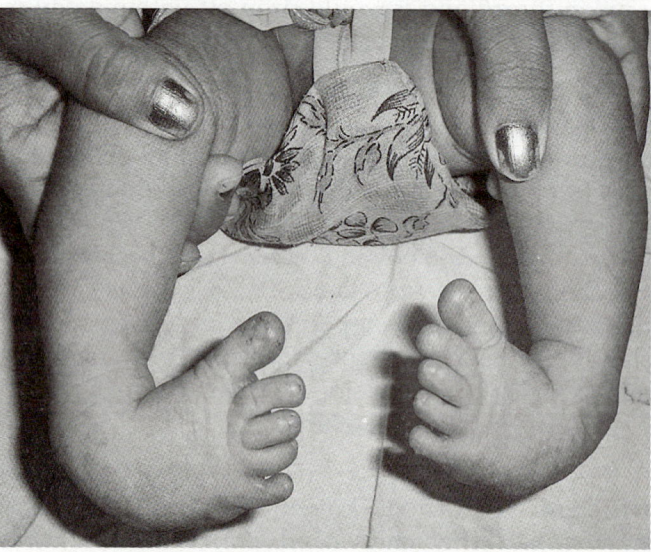

Figure 29.4 Bilateral club feet

changes. When in-toeing due to twisting of the thigh and leg bones is severe and persists beyond the age of 10 years and is causing difficulty in walking, surgical correction by an experienced orthopedic surgeon may be considered.

Out-toeing (Duck feet)

Out-toeing of forefeet is less common and may occur due to flat feet, external tibial torsion and in-utero positioning of feet. It is more common during late childhood or adolescence, and is usually unilateral. It is more common in obese children with retroversion of femur. The condition may be associated with patellofemoral pain. In most cases, no treatment is required because change in shoe wear, bracing, physical therapy and chiropractic manipulations do no help. In a severe care, osteotomy may be done to correct the deformity.

Toe-walking

The child walks on toes without putting any pressure on the heels or any other part of the foot. Toe-walking is common in toddlers when they start walking. They usually adopt normal walking pattern as they grow older. If a child continues to walk on the toes beyond the age of 3 years, he should be evaluated by the pediatrician. The common causes of toe-walking include spastic child (cerebral palsy) with shortening of tendo-Achilles, Duchenne muscular dystrophy, foot drop (peripheral neuropathy) and autism spectrum disorder.

The majority of cases of toe-walking are habitual and they usually resolve without any treatment. When tendo-Achilles (tendon behind the ankle) is shortened or taut, stretching exercises are advised by forcibly dorsiflexing the foot (tryng to touch dorsum of the foot with the shin) to stretch the tendo-Achilles. When toe walking is marked and unrelieved by stretching exercises, a brace or splint can be worn to keep the Achilles tendon stretched. In severe cases when physical measures fail to relieve the condition, surgical procedure can be done by an orthopedic surgeon to lengthen the Achilles tendon.

Calcaneovalgus Deformity

The deformity of foot is like a mirror image of club foot and occurs due to in-utero cramped up position. The ankle is dorsiflexed and foot is abducted, everted or pronated. The dorsum of the foot is maintained close to the shin. Most cases can be managed by physiotherapy by passive plantar flexion and inversion of foot. When foot cannot be plantar flexed to neutral position and there is fixed or rigid calcaneovalgus

deformity, the condition is managed by graded application of plaster casts over 6–8 weeks as in the case of club feet.

Genu Recurvatum

It is a benign disorder characterized by hyperextension of the knees due to laxity of ligaments or abnormal in-utero positioning. The condition is usually bilateral. Skiagram of the knees should be taken to exclude subluxation. In dislocation of knees, the tibia is shifted anteriorly and laterally in relation to the femur. Congenital fibrosis of the quadriceps is frequently associated with the subluxation and dislocation of knees. Genu recurvatum is treated by passive streching exercises and repeated cast changes to provide stability to the knee joints. The subluxated and dislocated knee is best managed by open reduction because stretching exercises and cast changes may result in damage to the epiphyseal plate.

Cleft Lip (Hare lip)

The baby is born with a cleft in the upper lip. There may be two clefts one on either side, with the central part of the lip jutting or protruding out **(Figure 29.5)**. The nose appears flat and asymmetrical. These infants have difficulty in sucking from breast or bottle. They are best fed expressed breast milk (EBM) with a spoon or *paladay* or rubber-tipped medicine dropper. Infant should be fed slowly by keeping the head in the upright

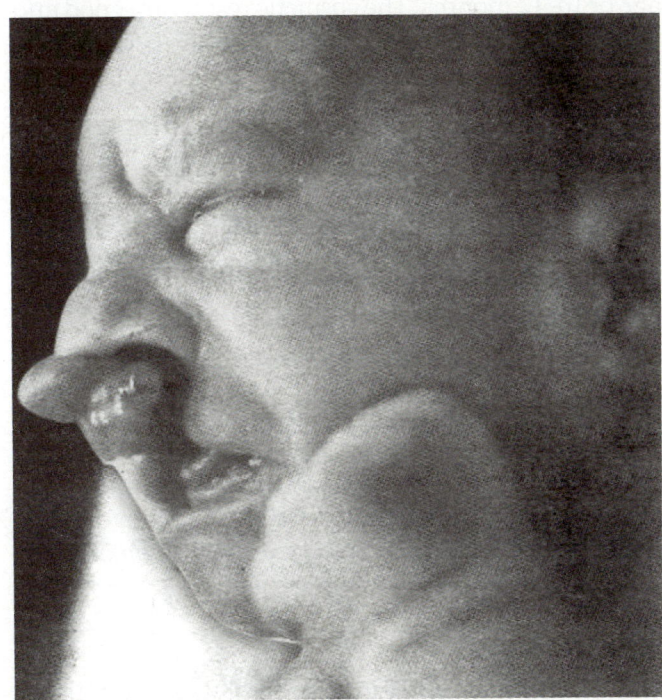

Figure 29.5 Bilateral cleft of the primary and secondary palute

position to avoid choking. Nasal blockage and congestion may interfere with feeding and breathing. In some cases of bilateral cleft lip, gavage feeding is preferred during the first few days. It is desirable to get the lip repaired before the baby leaves the hospital or the repair can be done within the first few weeks of life. Early surgical repair within 1–2 months is associated with better cosmetic results. After surgery wound is kept aligned with a Logan Bow and hands of the baby are restrained by affixing them to the sides of the diaper.

Cleft Palate

Cleft in the palate (roof of oral cavity) is usually associated with cleft lip but may occur as an isolated anomaly **(Figure 29.6)**. Isolated cleft palate may be assoicated with ventricular septal defect. Although cosmetically less frightening, it seriously interferes with feeding in early life and causes difficulties in speech (nasal twang and indistinct speech) later in life. The baby is unable to suck at the breast or bottle and feeding is associated with risk of regurgitation through the nose and aspiration into the lungs. The baby should be fed sitting in an upright position with a wide flat teat which can close the gap in the palate. Most mothers find it easier to feed EBM with a spoon or *paladay*. You can get a device or a prosthesis made by the dentist to temporarily close the gap in the palate for feeding purposes. The surgical repair is recommended at the age of 10–12 months. The cosmetic results are good and quality of speech is normal when repair is done by a plastic surgeon.

Umbilical Hernia

Herniation of intestines through the umbilicus is a common disorder. It is more common in preterm babies and infants with reduced muscle tone (rickets, cretinism, Down syndrome). Straining (due to constipation and crying) may aggravate the hernia while swelling may become less or disappear during sleep **(Figure 29.7)**. The herniated intestines can be easily pushed back into the abdomen by gentle pressure. There is no risk of strangulation in umbilical hernia and swelling disappears spontaneously between 6 months to 2 years of age. There is no need to put a coin over the umbilicus and strap it. This may further weaken the overlying skin and delay the recovery.

Inguinal Hernia

Herniation of intestines into the scrotal sac through the inguinal canal in the groin is called inguinal hernia. There is a soft boggy swelling which appears on

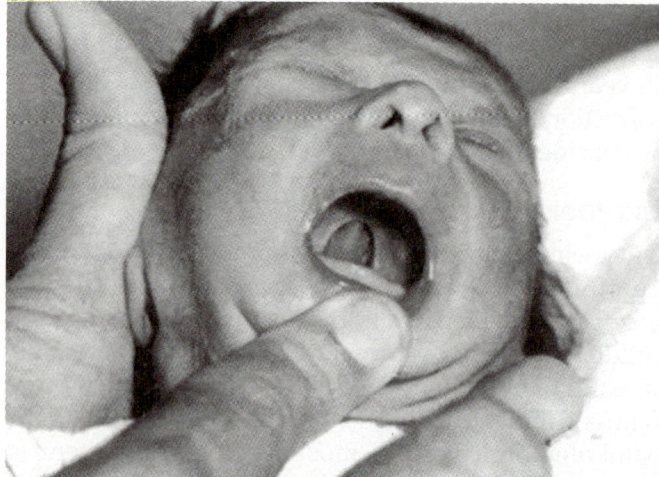

Figure 29.6 Isolated cleft palate. The infant also had ventricular septal defect

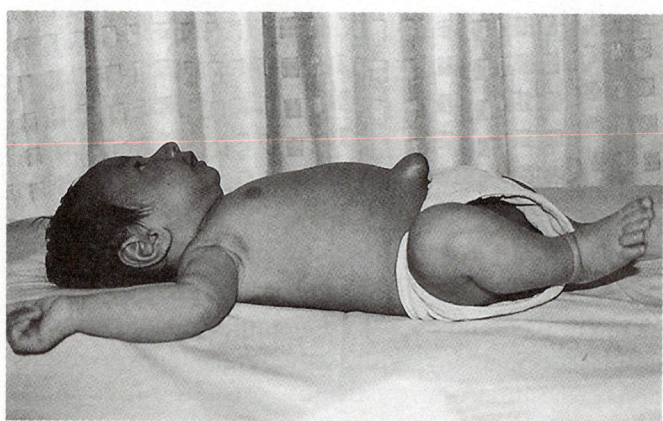

Figure 29.7 Umbilical hernia. No bandage should be applied as hernia spontaneously disappears after a few months

straining or crying and disappears on lying down and during sleep. The intestines can be pushed back into abdomen by gentle pressure. The hernia may be on one side or both sides. It may be associated with undescended testis. The swelling will not be transilluminant due to presence of loops of intestine. Inguinal hernia is associated with a serious risk of strangulation and should be operated by a pediatric surgeon as early as possible. The wait and watch policy should not be followed in case of inguinal hernia.

Hydrocele

The collection of fluid around one or both the testicles is called hydrocele. The testes may not palpable on the affected side due to watery, boggy swelling of the scrotal sac. The swelling is transilluminant and not reducible by rest or pressure. Hydrocele is common in healthy newborn babies and usually disappears spontaneously by 3 months of age.

Spina Bifida

There is a gap in the spinal cord through which coverings of the spinal cord (meningocele) or part of the nervous tissue of the cord (myelomeningocele) may protrude out **(Figure 29.8)**. There is evidence to suggest that neural tube defects may occur due to deficiency of folic acid during conception and embroyogenesis. The defect may occur at any site but is most common over the lower back (lumbosacral area). There is a soft round swelling in the midline over the lower back which may be covered by skin or it may be covered by the meninges or there is no covering of the spinal cord with oozing of cerebrospinal fluid (CSF). The lower limbs may appear wasted and paralyzed. The baby may not have any spontaneous movements of legs and may not withdraw the leg on pinprick. At times there may be constant dribbling of urine or incontinence of stools. Hydrocephalus may be present at birth or appear later in life after repair of spinal defect.

In some cases of spina bifida, there is no protrusion of meninges or spinal cord and condition is called as spine bifida occulta. The gap or defect in the spine can be detected on clinical examination and confirmed by taking a skiagram of spine.

Nursing care The baby should be placed on his tummy. When swelling is covered with skin it can be operated electively after a few days. The open or uncovered swelling should be protected against

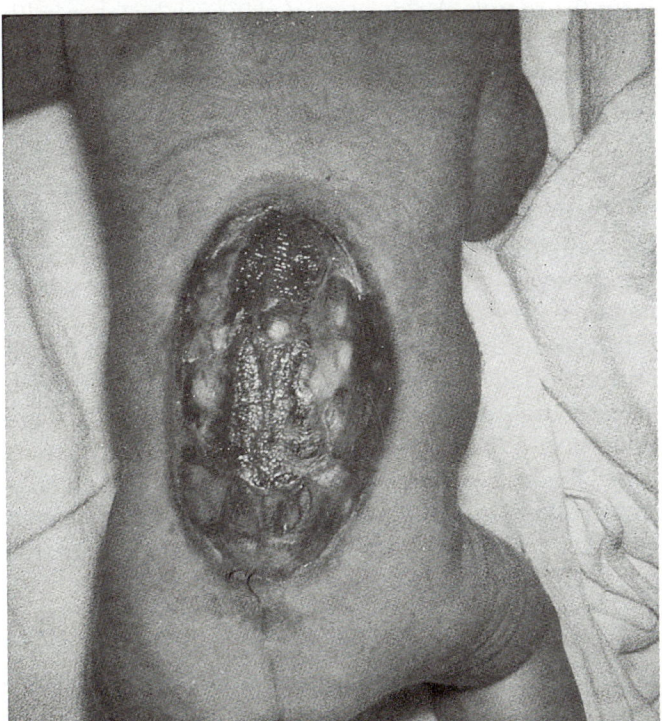

Figure 29.8 Open meningomyelocele

development of superadded infection. It is recommended to apply an antiseptic lotion like betadine or mercurochrome. The perineal area should be kept scrupulously clean and effectively covered with a plastic sheet to minimise the chances of contamination. Surgical repair should be done as early as possible before it gets infected. It is futile to get it operated if defect is associated with severe paralysis of lower limbs, marked deformity of the spine and severe hydrocephalus. When urinary retention is present, the nurse or mother should empty the bladder by gentle manual compression every two hours. Care should be taken to prevent development of bed sores. The occurrence of a similar defect (neural tube defect) in the next pregnancy can be prevented by administration of folic acid during periconceptional period (before missing the period and first 8 weeks of pregnancy).

Hydrocephalus

Hydrocephalus may occur in association with neural tube defect or Arnold-Chiari malformation. There may be obstruction to the flow of CSF due to congenital malformation or increased production and decreased resorption of CSF because of intrauterine or postnatal meningitis. Hydrocephalus may be present at birth or develop subsequently.

The head is large in size with skull bones widely separated. The anterior fontanel is large in size and bulging. There is excessive production or poor drainage of CSF. Veins may be prominent over the forehead and face. The eyes are often rolled downwards so that white part of the eyes (sclera) is visible below the upper eye lid (sun-setting appearance) **(Figure 29.9)**. It may be associated with irritability, vomiting and slow neuromotor development. Ultrasonography of the brain through anterior fontanel is helpful in screening newborn babies. In older children CT scan or MRI of brain with or without contrast is useful to assess the degree of ventriculomegaly and its possible etiology. Acetzolamide 50–100 mg/kg/day in 3 divided doses may be given to reduce CSF production. Nurse should provide emotional support and guidance to the family for long term follow-up.

Hydrocephalus may get spontaneously arrested or it may be progressive. Regular monitoring of head circumference once a month is important to assess the velocity of increase in head size for diagnosis of arrested or progressive hydrocephalus. Several surgical procedures are available to "shunt off" extra CSF into the abdominal cavity or superior vena cava. Ventriculo-peritoneal (VP) shunt is the most popular procedure. Early operation gives good results and should be done if brain is not damaged.

29

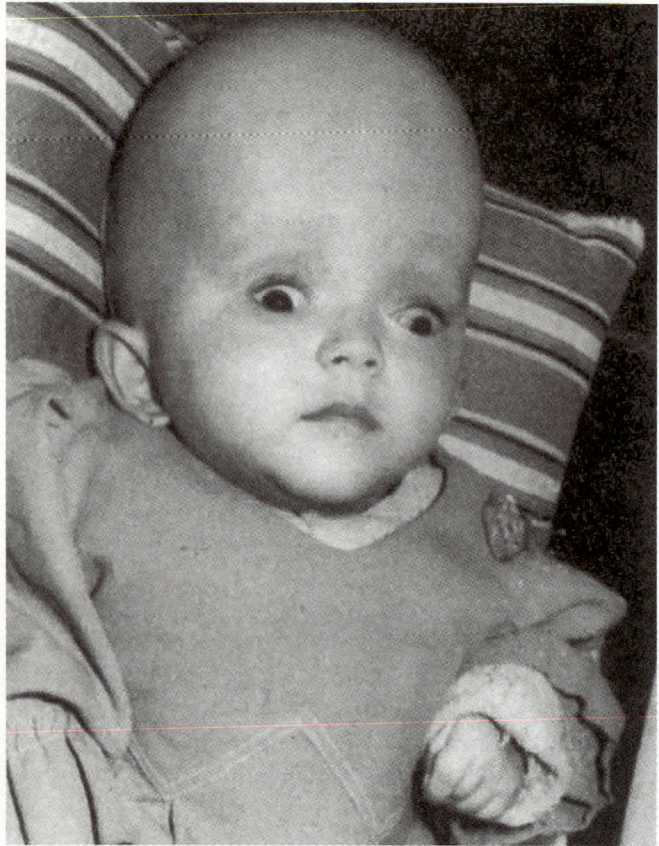

Figure 29.9 Hydrocephalus in an infant who was operated for meningocele during neonatal period

Microcephaly

In this condition, head is smaller in size than normal. The head may be small in size due to poor growth of the brain. Microcephaly may occur due to brain damage from a variety of causes including intrauterine infection and infection by recently recognized zika virus. These children may have mental retardation and other CNS abnormalities. Unfortunately, nothing can be done to treat this condition because we do not have any satisfactory brain tonics. At times, the head size may remain small because of early fusion of one or more of the sutures between the skull bones (craniosynostosis) which does not allow the brain to grow in size. This condition can be treated by an early surgical procedure to break the fusion between the skull bones so that the brain can grow in size.

Esophageal Atresia

There are atleast six types of esophageal atresias with or without tracheoesophageal fistula (TOF). In over 85 percent of cases, esophagus ends in a blind pouch about 4–6 cm from pharynx. The lower end of esophagus communicates with trachea through TOF. Saliva and oral secretions will pool in the upper pouch of the esophagus while gastric contents may regurgitate through the TOF and cause aspiration pneumonia involving upper lobe of right lung.

Clinical Features

Early diagnosis is important to prevent complications and improve the outcome. The presence of maternal polyhydramnios and single umbilical artery in a preterm or LBW baby should alert the nurse to look for atresia of the esophagus. The newborn baby has excessive drooling of frothy saliva and there is choking and cyanosis when baby is given the first feed. Aspiration of gastric contents may lead to development of pneumonitis in the upper zone of right lung. About one-third of infants with esophageal atresia have other associated anomalies of heart, gastrointestinal tract and genitourinary system.

> **Practical Tip**
>
> *Choking and coughing with first feed and drooling and frothing of saliva from mouth in a neonate are highly suggestive of esophageal atresia. Presence of air bubble in the stomach or aspiration pneumonia in the upper zone of right lung are suggestive of tracheoesophageal fistula.*

Diagnosis

A stiff rubber catheter cannot be passed into the stomach and it goes only up to a distance of 8–10 cm from the mouth. A skiagram of chest can be taken with catheter in-situ but without using any contrast. The presence of air bubble in the stomach indicates the presence of TOF.

Nursing Care

The baby should be nursed in a supine position with head slightly raised. The esophageal pouch should be sucked every 5 minutes or continuously with a gentle negative pressure of about 50 cm H_2O. Antibiotics and intravenous fluids are administered. Ligation of fistula and esophageal anastamosis is performed through extrapleural route as early as possible as a single stage operation. When atretic segment of the esophagus is long, feeding gastrostomy and ligation of fistula is undertaken initially followed by plastic repair of esophagus after 6–8 weeks. These infants need intensive supportive and nursing care.

Imperforate Anus

The child is born without any anal opening and he cannot pass the stools. The condition can be easily diagnosed at birth by looking at the bottom and not finding the anal hole. Nurse can easily identify the anomaly while trying to take the rectal temperature of the baby. In some female babies, there may be an abnormal channel between the rectum and vagina (rectovaginal fistula) so that stools are passed through the vagina. "High" anomaly is more common in boys and is usually associated with a fistula with urinary bladder or urethra with passage of meconium in urine. The baby must be seen by a pediatric surgeon immediately. A skiagram of abdomen is taken 6–8 hours after birth in a lateral position with the infant held upside down after placing an opaque object (coin) over the anal dimple. When distance between the coin and air in the rectum is more than 2 cm it indicates a high defect. More commonly lateral invertogram or cross table X-ray of the infant with elevated buttocks (knee-chest position) is more useful to find whether anomaly is high or low. When obstruction is low down, it can be managed by simple modified cut-back procedure. In case of a high obstruction, the surgical repair is undertaken in two stages. When a colostomy has been performed, the skin around the wound should be kept clean and covered with a protective barrier cream. The condition needs prolonged nursing care, medical management and emotional support.

Down Syndrome (Mongol baby)

It is the commonest chromosomal defect (1:800 live births) wherein there is an extra chromosome 21 (Trisomy 21). The defect is more common among babies of elderly mothers (>35 years). The child has soft rounded features with a flat nasal bridge and a small and flat head with a large anterior fontanel. The eyes are placed wide apart and are slanted upwards and outwards (Figure 29.10). The mouth is small and usually open with protrusion of tongue. Ears are small and located at a lower level. Instead of two horizontal creases in the palm (head and heart lines), there may be a single palmar crease (simian crease) and little finger is usually small and incurved (Figure 29.11). The hands are small. There is increased space between 1st and 2nd toes with a deep furrow (sandle toe). The muscles are flabby and child's limbs can be placed in any position. The developmental milestones are delayed and child has mental subnormality of varying grade. There may be other associated defects like deafness, visual defects (cataract, squint, nystagmus), structural defects of the heart (ventricular septal defect or endocardial cushion defect) and intestines (duodenal atresia and Hirschsprung's disease). The diagnosis can be easily made by looking at the baby and can be confirmed by analysis of chromosomes (karyotyping).

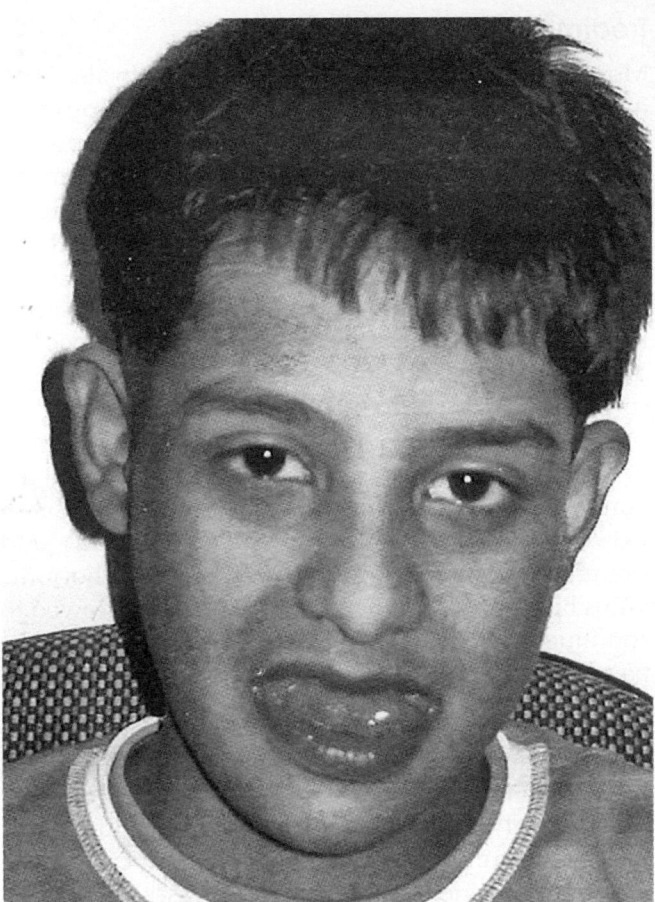

Figure 29.10 Typical facial features with protrusion of tongue in a 12-year-old child with Down syndrome

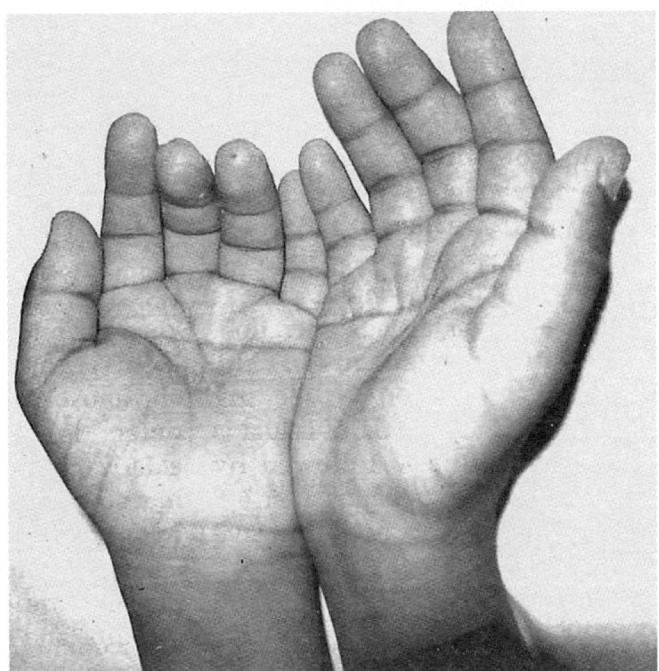

Figure 29.11 Small hands with a single horizontal palmar crease (simian crease) and incurved little finger in a child with Down syndrome

29

Treatment

Mongol babies are pleasant, lovable and docile. They have great love for music and dance. They are prone to develop frequent chest infections and should be protected against exposure. There is no specific treatment. Rarely hypothyroidism may be associated which is treated with eltroxin. The child should not be sent to a regular school. The parents should join and interact with the members of the Down syndrome Association for emotional support and guidance. The associated defects in the heart and intestines may need surgical correction. Parents should seek genetic counselling for prospects of having a normal child. It is extremely rare to have two children with Down syndrome in the family. It is possible to make antenatal diagnosis of Down syndrome during early pregnancy by ultrasound examination and chromosomal studies on chorionic villus biopsy. The normal pregnancy can be allowed to continue, while medical termination of pregnancy can be advised when mother is carrying a baby with Down syndrome.

PREVENTION OF BIRTH DEFECTS

Pre-marital genetic counselling and avoidance of marriages among close relatives can reduce the incidence of genetic or hereditary diseases. Girls must be protected against development of German measles by timely administration of MMR vaccine. It should be remembered that the safest age for reproduction in women, is between 20 and 30 years. During pregnancy, self-medications should be strictly avoided (especially during first 3 months) and drugs should be taken only on the advice of an obstetrician. Among married women, X-ray examination (and even medications!) should be limited during 2 weeks after menstruation (when it is sure that woman is not pregnant) to avoid inadvertant exposure of the embryo (young fetus) to the harmful effects of X-rays. When couple is planning to have a baby, mother should take a balanced and nutritious diet (including supplements of folic acid) and she should avoid smoking and drinking alcohol. No attempt should ever be made to abort the fetus of unwanted sex by taking any medicines.

BIBLIOGRAPHY

Agarwala S, Mitra DK. Timing of surgery for common pediatric surgical conditions. *Indian J Pediatr* 1996, 63: 769–774.

Robb J. In-toeing and out-toeing gait. In: Pediatric Orthopedic Diagnosis. *Springer India*, 2015, pp 207–220.

Stahli LT. Lower limb. In: Fundamentals of Pediatric Orthopedics. *Philadelphia, Lippincott Williams and Wilkins*, 4th edition, 2008, p135.

The Child with a Handicap

The child is considered to have a handicap if a disability in his body or mind interferes with his ability to lead a normal independent life in society. The challenged or disadvantaged children need supervised care with utmost consideration and compassion. According to some surveys conducted in India, about 8–10% of individuals suffer from some form of disability.

TYPES OF HANDICAPS

The child may have one or more of the following handicaps:

1. Blindness
2. Deafness
3. Leprosy
4. Bone, joint or muscle disorders: Congenital malformations, joint and bone infections, muscular dystrophy, and fractures, etc.
5. Central nervous system disorders: Mental retardation, cerebral palsy, paralytic poliomyelitis, and congenital malformations, etc.
6. Congenital malformations and chronic diseases of heart, lungs, kidneys, liver and other body organs.
7. Chromosomal disorders like Down syndrome.
8. Socially handicapped children due to interparental conflicts, broken family, loss of parent(s), poverty, lack of educational opportunities, lack of emotional support and tender loving care. These adverse social factors are important correlates of orphan child, abused child, addicted child, street children, child labor, destitute child, exploited or victimized and delinquent children.

Prevention of Handicaps

Premarital health check and counselling of would-be-couples is important. There is a greater risk to give birth to children with genetic or hereditary defects if parents are blood relatives (like first cousins). Reproduction should be limited between 20 and 35 years of age because an elderly mother has a greater risk to give birth to a child with a chromosomal disorder especially Down syndrome. Mother should avoid cigarette smoking and drinking alcohol during pregnancy. No attempts should be made to identify the sex of the fetus with the intention of aborting the girl fetus. During first 3 months of pregnancy mother should avoid taking any medicines and exposure to X-rays unless advised by the doctor. Intake of supplements of folic acid before and during early conception has been shown to reduce the incidence of neural tube defects and cleft lip.

Regular medical check-ups and proper care during pregnancy under the guidance of an obstetrician is most desirable. The delivery must take place in a center having adequate facilities both for the care of mothers and newborn babies. Pediatrician and a specially trained nurse must be present at the time of delivery to provide immediate basic care including resuscitation to the newborn baby. Perinatal distress factors, such as hypoxia, hypothermia, acidosis, hypoglycemia and hyperbilirubinemia, should be prevented, identified early and managed promptly to prevent brain damage. Routine screening of all newborns for cretinism, G6PD deficiency and phenylketonuria is advocated for early diagnosis and prompt management. The child must receive all the immunizations as per the recommended schedule. Hearing loss may occur due to loud noise and intake of ototoxic drugs such as aminoglycosides and furosemide. Sound is measured in decibels (dB) and 60 dB is intensity of normal speech. Noise louder than 85 dB including sound produced by hair dryers, squeaky toys, loud music, and fire crackers, etc. can cause irreversible damage to ears. Screening for deafness should be done around 3 months of age and whenever indicated hearing aid should be provided before the age of 6 months. Early detection of the handicap, proper management and rehabilitation are essential to reduce the severity of disability.

30

The Parental Attitude

Parents should not have the guilt feelings that child's handicap is somehow due to their fault. They should not blame each other or family doctor and the hospital to relieve the feelings of guilt. The child should be accepted as the ordain of nature or will of God. The child should be looked after with due care, understanding and compassion. *Parents should not harbour any feelings of guilt, self-pity, anger and shame. They should have the courage and confidence to accept that God has chosen them to look after the special child because they have the patience and compassion to provide him necessary care and protection.*

It is important that family should have a positive and optimistic approach in handling the child. Parents must accept the child in a matter-of-fact manner and should not feel embarrassed in public in the company of their challenged child. The child should be encouraged to maintain his self-esteem and face the disability with confidence and courage. He should be provided opportunities for regular interactions with relatives, family friends and other children. While it is essential for parents to provide tender loving care and greater attention to their disabled child, but it is equally important that other normal children should not be neglected. When parents do not have any normal child, they should seek genetic counseling regarding the risk of handicap or a similar problem in future babies. When there is no increased risk or risk is minimal (worth taking), parents should be advised to plan for another pregnancy when the disadvantaged child has reached the age of 3 years. Both the parents should discuss this issue with the family physician in a dispassionate and relaxed manner.

Indian Disability Act

The government of India has enacted Indian Disability Act in 1995 with the objective of providing equal opportunities to persons with disability to protect their fundamental rights and to enable them to have full participation in public life. Seven categories of disabilities have been included under the purview of the Act, i.e. blindness, visually impaired, hearing impaired, leprosy, locomotor disability, mental retardation and mental illness. According to the Act, a number of concessions and facilities are provided to disabled persons and Institutions dealing with various types of disabilities. Disabled persons are entitled to 75% concession by rail travel (along with one attendant) in any class and 50% concession by air travel (without any attendant). The disabled persons or their wards are allowed a deduction of INR 40,000.00 from their total income for income tax purposes.

Treatment and Rehabilitation

The care of a handicapped child is a challenge and it imposes a great physical and mental strain to the parents and may cause disharmony in the family. Whenever possible, the family should get some help for housework so that mother does not get exhausted. The mother needs some relaxation and time for looking after herself and other kids.

During the last decade, many more facilities for management of disabled children have become available but these are still very inadequate in our country. The parents often ask, "Doctor, will my child be alright when he grows up"? It must be remembered that the handicap is unlikely to disappear as the child grows but child may learn new skills and adapt with age. However, with gentle and patient handling, love and understanding, the problem can be tackled under the supervision of several experts. Depending upon the nature and severity of disability, the child with a handicap may require different kinds of treatments and rehabilitation measures. The family may need to seek the expert guidance of an ENT surgeon, eye specialist, orthopedic surgeon or pediatric surgeon for evaluation and definitive management of disability. Nurse will need to work closely with a physiotherapist, occupational therapist, speech therapist, psychologist, medical geneticist and a medical social worker.

The aim of the rehabilitation program is to help the handicapped child to achieve his optimal potential as far as physical, mental, educational, emotional, vocational and social capabilities are concerned within the constraints of his disability. Whenever feasible these children should be provided education and learning opportunities in the mainstream or regular schools. They should not be admitted in any boarding school because the normal environment of the home is very helpful for their growth and development. This also helps the normal siblings to understand the nature of handicap and provide support to the family. Special efforts should be made to provide them with vocational training and guidance so that they can live a near normal independent life.

Besides the government and non-government organizations, parents of affected children (like mental retardation, Down syndrome and thalassemia, etc.) have formed support groups to provide information and help to the families of affected children. Parents can share their worries and anxieties with other parents and it provides them a consolation that they are not the only one faced with such a problem. These parents' groups provide first-hand information to deal with day-to-day problems encountered during the long-term care of handicapped children including procurement of special medicines, equipment and other specialized facilities, which are extremely useful. Above all, such groups provide invaluable moral and emotional support to parents. Some children with severe mental or physical disabilities like mental retardation, learning disorders, blindness and deafness require education in special schools.

Efforts should be made to train the child in day-to-day activities so that he can independently look after himself. He should be provided vocational guidance as he grows to undertake simple tasks and jobs to achieve social independence. The associated medical problems like seizures, hearing and visual difficulties should be managed by drugs, hearing aids and speech therapy. Parents should be realistic in their expectations while rearing and caring for the child with mental retardation. The child is likely to learn more skills as he grows but he is unlikely to have normal intelligence.

It is important to remember that some individuals with handicaps may have specialized capabilities in certain specific fields. These capabilities should be harnessed by proper guidance and encouragement to the child. It is well known that Milton's visual impairment and Beethoven's hearing handicap did not deter them to make outstanding contributions in the fields of poetry and music. It is amazing that the physically disabled living legend Stephen Hawking, the propounder of unification of quantum physics and theory of relativity, has made contributions akin to the caliber of Albert Einstein.

CEREBRAL PALSY (Spastic Child)

Cerebral palsy is defined as non-progressive neuromotor disorder of cerebral origin due to abnormal brain development or brain damage in fetal life, during delivery, at birth and early infancy. The exact incidence depends upon several epidemiological factors and varies between 2 and 5 per 1000 live births. The child may have convulsions, visual and hearing defects and mental subnormality. There is stiffness or spasticity of limbs (more in the lower limbs which may cross each other like a scissor) with inability to sit, stand, walk and difficulty in holding objects at the expected ages of their achievement. There may be irregular move-ments or tremors of the limbs and sometimes of the body. The degree of mental retardation is variable and may be absent in some patients. The speech is often delayed and lack clarity. There is generally no hereditary predisposition to have another child with cerebral palsy. The most common causes of cerebral palsy include extremely premature babies, lack of

oxygen to the brain at birth (birth asphyxia), severe jaundice during first week of life, metabolic disorders (low blood glucose), infection of the brain and intracranial hemorrhage.

Early markers of cerebral palsy It is possible to make an early diagnosis of CP by 4 months of age by looking for following clinical markers:

1. Episodes of inconsolable and unexplained crying, feeding difficulties, lip smacking or chewing movements, excessive sensitivity to light and sound producing startle response.
2. Persistent neck tonic or asymmetric posture beyond 4 weeks of age.
3. Absence of social or interactive smile by 6 weeks.
4. Clenched fists with thumbs adducted and flexed across the palms (cortical thumbs) beyond 8 weeks.
5. Paucity or absence of cycling or fidgety limb movements during first 6–12 weeks of life.
6. Persistence of automatic reflexes (Moro, grasp, asymmetric neck tonic) beyond 4 months.
7. Lack of stable head control or rolling over by 4 months.
8. Slow head growth.

Management The family should be given social and emotional support to handle the child with sensitivity, courage and fortitude. A great deal can be done with the help of appropriate physiotherapy by ensuring proper movements and exercises of different groups of muscles. *Massage should not be done as it may further increase muscle tone and spasticity.* The child should be made self-reliant to feed, bathe and dress himself even when he takes a long time and does it awkwardly. Some children with cerebral palsy have unique or specialized capabilities like interest in painting and instrumental music. Parents and health care professionals must identify these and other special attributes and harness them effectively by guiding and inspiring the child. After getting hands-on instructions from a physiotherapist, family should continue the exercises and manipulations at home. There are special institutions for spastic children in several big cities and their expertise can be effectively utilized. Drugs and surgical procedures are available to reduce spasticity. These children must be provided with routine immunizations as per the recommended schedule. The

Nursing Alert

Massage is contraindicated in children with spastic diplegia because it is likely to further increase the muscle tone.

30

family should be discouraged to use any "brain tonics", which are promoted in various systems of medicine. Due to swallowing difficulties, they may have to be fed with a liquid or a semi-liquid homogenized diet. Prokinetics (domperidone) and ranitidine are given for treatment of feeding difficulties and gastroesophageal reflux. Avoid over feeding because they have a tendency to become obese due to lack of physical activity.

MENTAL RETARDATION (Mental Subnormality)

Children with mental retardation have an impairment in their intelligence and they have limited ability to adapt and deal with day-to-day activities and environmental situations. Mental retardation may occur due to a variety of causes. The child's brain may suffer damage due to various factors, while in the mother's womb (genetic, chromosomal disorders like Down syndrome, fragile-X-syndrome and Klinefelter syndrome, developmental defects, intrauterine infections, thyroid deficiency), during labor and delivery (birth asphyxia, birth injury), at birth or subsequently (metabolic disorder, meningitis, encephalitis and head injury). In over 50% cases of mental retardation, no cause is found.

Clinical features There is global retardation of all the developmental milestones. There may be evidence of facial dysmorphism and congenital malformations suggestive of a chromosomal disorder. There may be microcephaly (brain damage, craniosynostosis) or macrocephaly (hydrocephalus, porencephaly). Early diagnosis of cretinism (congenital hypothyroidism) should be made by newborn screening and identification of early clinical markers such as prolonged physiological jaundice, lethargy, hypotonia, umbilical hernia, intolerance to cold, constipation and lack of social smile by 6 weeks of age. There may be associated neuromotor disability, spasticity and seizures. Feeding difficulties and regurgitation may lead to failure to thrive and frequent infections. Eyes should be examined for squint, nystagmus, cataract, visual acuity and abnormalities in the retina. Speech and hearing should be assessed.

Diagnosis Children with mental subnormality are late in achieving all the milestones of development. They are late in acquiring muscle control and movements, recognition, speech, language and learning skills. Some children with mental retardation may have additional problems like convulsions, spasticity of muscles, visual difficulties, deafness and behavior problems. Their head size may be small (microcephaly) due to poor growth of the brain. Some may have a large

head size due to hydrocephalus. On the basis of intelligence quotient (IQ) and severity of disability, mental retardation is classified into five grades:

1. *Borderline* (IQ 71–90) Dull normal and educable in a regular school.
2. *Mild* (IQ 51–70) Educable with special efforts.
3. *Moderate* (IQ 36–50) Trainable but not educable.
4. *Severe* (IQ 21–35) Not trainable and cannot look after toilet needs.
5. *Profound* (IQ <20) They need custodial care.

> **Practical Tip**
>
> *Children with mental retardation have global retardation in all the developmental parameters, i.e. gross motor, fine motor, social, adaptive, and speech. Isolated deafness may be associated with delayed speech or deaf mutism while isolated delay in walking may be due to congenital dislocation of hip/s.*

Laboratory investigations Intelligence quotient $\left(\dfrac{\text{mental age}}{\text{chronological age}} \times 100 \right)$ should be assessed to grade the severity of mental retardation. Urine should be screened for common inborn errors of metabolism. Cretinism should be ruled out by estimation of triiodothyronine, thyroxin and thyroid stimulating hormone (TSH). Karyotyping is done if there is facial dysmorphism or clinical suspicion of Down syndrome, fragile-X syndrome and Klinefelter syndrome. Routine CT scan or MRI studies of brain are not advised.

Management The child with mental retardation must be identified early so that he is provided stimulation through his special senses (music, lullabies, bright objects, colors, lights, touch, caressing, smell, taste, etc.). Detailed assessment and investigations may be undertaken to identify the cause. Certain genetic or metabolic defects and deficiency of thyroid hormone (cretinism) can be managed by administration of specific medicines. Their specific capabilities, if any, should be identified and effectively harnessed. Some children love to enjoy music and dance. *It must be recognized that there are no specific drugs or tonics to enhance intelligence and money and resources should not be wasted to buy them.*

CHILD WITH A LEARNING DISABILITY

In this competitive world, academic performance is the key to success in professional life along with additional attributes like good personality, communication and social skills, confidence, courage and enthusiasm.

About 20% children face various types of learning disabilities with suboptimal academic performance. They are physically or apparently normal children without any obvious disability.

Causes Scholastic backwardness has a multifactorial etiology and following conditions should be excluded:

1. Specific learning disability (SpLD) because of inability to read (dyslexia), write (dysgraphia) or perform mathematical calculations (dyscalculia).
2. Disorders of hearing, vision and speech.
3. Mental subnormality.
4. Attention deficit hyperactivity disorder (ADHD).
5. Autism spectrum disorder (ASD).
6. Emotional and conduct disorder.
7. Environmental and social factors.
8. Medical disorders due to chronic diseases like bronchial asthma, type 1 diabetes mellitus and collagen vascular and autoimmune disorders.

Assessment Children with learning disability should be assessed by a team of specialists namely pediatrician, clinical psychologist, audiologist, speech therapist, special educator and a counselor. Specialized tests are available for evaluation of intelligence quotient and assessment of academic skills. Specialized questionnaires are available for making the diagnosis of dyslexia, attention deficit hyperactivity disorder (ADHD) and autism spectrum disorder (ASD).

DYSLEXIA

Dyslexia is the commonest cause of learning disability and is characterized by difficulties in reading, spelling or writing. Around 10–15 percent children are affected who may have either normal or above normal intelligence. Boys and girls are equally affected. The exact cause of dyslexia is not known and it appears that there is defective neurological wiring because of genetic or acquired factors.

Clinical features Early recognition of dyslexia is important because slow learning may adversely affect the confidence and self-esteem of the child. These children may be taunted by classmates and ignored by teachers, leading to isolation, anxiety and depression. The child may be labelled as lazy, careless, stupid, indisciplined or mentally subnormal. In desperation the child starts missing school and he may even drop out of school. The following difficulties in learning and other associated problems should alert you to the possibility that the child may be dyslexic.

1. The child is slow in learning skills of reading and spelling though he is competent in other skills like oral class work, art and craft, puzzles and games. The child tends to write slowly and hesitatingly wriggling as he writes, at times contorting the face and protruding his tongue. Hand writing and drawing skills are poor.
2. He is confused over right and left direction of alphabets which appears as mirror image of each other like "b", "d", "p", "q". The child may read "was" as "saw", "pit" as "tip", "pan" as "nap", "car park" as "par cark", etc.
3. He is unable to follow and perform actions in a sequential order such as describing the days of the week or months of the year. He has difficulty in reciting nursery rhymes or remembering the exact sequence of a story.
4. The child may be clumsy and may have difficulty in dressing, buttoning, tying shoe laces and often get confused between right and left.

Management Early recognition of the problem is important so that confidence and self-esteem of the child are not adversely affected. The child should be assessed by an educational psychologist for diagnosis and management of the condition. The child should be examined for any visual or hearing defect. The commonest cause of difficulty in reading is low level of intelligence which should be excluded by assessing IQ. The dyslexic child should remain in the mainstream school and encouraged to pursue other activities and hobbies of his interest. They should be given coaching in phonetics by special educators. They can be provided help by computer based reading programs. Among the good ones that promote phonemic fluency include Read, Write and Type, Learning System, and Read Naturally and Readit. The mother should educate herself in the concept of phonemes (breaking every word or sound into several parts) and phonetics to provide training to her child at home.

To encourage these children to study in a regular mainstream school, the school authorities are authorized to give certain concessions to these children during block assessments and terminal examinations. These provisions include (i) giving extra time and overlooking spelling mistakes, (ii) exemption of second language such as Sanskrit and substituting it with art and craft, (iii) providing a writer to a child with dysgraphia and (iv) giving exemption to algebra and geometry and substituting it with lower grade of mathematics.

ATTENTION DEFICIT HYPERACTIVITY DISORDER (ADHD)

This descriptive name is more appropriate than the old nomenclature of "minimal brain dysfunction". The disorder affects 1.5 percent children, boys are affected

30

5 times more often than girls. Its prevalence is relatively less in India than in the West. The exact cause of disorder is unknown but there is a familial tendency and some derrangement of chemical neurotransmitters in the brain. There is controversial link between diet and hyperactivity in children. There is no evidence whatsoever that excessive intake of sugar is associated with hyperactivity. However, food additives, dyes, preservatives, caffein and vitamin C-rich foods may trigger hyperactivity in some children. There is some correlation between ADHD and low intake of omega-3 fatty acids and docosahexaenoic acid (DHA).

Clinical features The developmental milestones are usually normal and some children may have above normal intelligence. Learning disabilities and school problems due to hyperactivity and poor attention span are seen in 10–30 percent children. The affected children are restless, hyperactive, inattentive, impulsive, unable to sit still and are perpetually "on the go" as if "driven by a motor". They are constantly on the move, fidget, squirm, aimlessly touch and poke their fingers into everything. They are unable to sit through a TV program or listen to a story due to short attention span. They have an impulsive behavior, blurting out answers before completion of questions and have trouble waiting for their turn or standing in a queue. Their behavior becomes worse in crowded places and infront of guests. They are aggressive in their behavior and uncooperative with their classmates and have difficulty in cultivating friendship. They may have antisocial behavior like disobediency, defiance, lack of discipline, destructiveness, fire setting, and inflicting harm to others. They have associated language and learning disability due to easy distractibility and short attention span.

Differential diagnosis The condition should not be over diagnosed and diagnosis should be delayed till child goes to a regular school when concept of rules and discipline is more likely to be followed by children. Temper tantrums and "spoilt" child due to overattention and overindulgence should be excluded. Normally outgoing, ebullient, wiry and energetic children should not be wrongly labelled as ADHD. Hyperactivity and inattention are also recognized features of low intelligence, epilepsy, poor vision, hearing disability and intake of certain medications which should be ruled out. It is important to remember that a highly intelligent child may become hyperactive or inattentive because he is bored with the teacher or mother. The child should be evaluated by a psychiatrist and clinical psychologist for making a definitive diagnosis.

Management In India, there are lack of facilities and expertise to treat children with ADHD and counsel their parents and teachers. They should be handled with due care and compassion. They should not be spanked or penalized for their "naughty" behavior. They should be given supervised tasks to improve their attention span. It must be realized that child's behavior is not intentional, it is involuntary or spontaneous. The child should be encouraged to take part in physical activities, sports, yoga and meditation. Paradoxically drugs which are known to cause hyperactivity and restlessness provide relief to these children. These drugs include methyl phenidate, pemoline and dextroamphetamine and are given after the age of 6 years. They should be used under the close supervision of a doctor due to potential risk of serious side effects.

AUTISM SPECTRUM DISORDERS (ASD)

Autism is a pervasive developmental disorder that affects a child's communication, social skills and behavior. The main defect in children with autism is their lack of development of "theory of mind" i.e. realization that other people exist around them who have their own thoughts and desires which are different from theirs. The condition is believed to affect 2 per 1000 individuals in the West. The disorder is 4 times more common in boys than girls. Autistic children are difficult to diagnose and they are often confused with mental retardation. There is a wide spectrum of disorders due to autism and condition is better called as autism spectrum disorder. The condition may be likened to a major psychiatric disorder like infantile "schizophrenia" and its exact cause is unknown. There is a familial tendency with an abnormality in the neurotransmitters or brain chemicals. Recent studies have shown reduced activity in the prefrontal and parietal cortex with reduced number of Purkinjee cells in the cerebellum and a less number of tightly packed neurons in the limbic area. Lack of emotional support and interaction by one or both the parents is a recognized predisposing or precipitating factor. There is no evidence that thiomersol contained in MMR vaccine has any role in the causation of autism.

Clinical features These children may have normal development upto certain age and then regress in their social interactions and communication skills. The manifestations are usually evident by the age of 2 years. The autistic children live in their own world and do not like to be held or cuddled and they have no or only brief eye contact. They lack emotional warmth and social interaction. They may have strange compulsive and repetitive movements or stereotypic behavior like rocking, bouncing, head banging, swinging, spinning objects and flapping or twisting their hands. The child may be fascinated by visual stimuli like flickering or moving lights and fans. They have other abnormal behavior like toe-walking, sniffing, licking or smelling objects. Speech may be absent or they may have gibberish and repetitive (echolalia) language of their own. They may have immense liking towards some inanimate object (like teddy bear) and react violently to any change in their environment and daily set routines. There may be diminished response to pain and lack of startle response to a sudden loud noise. Some children may have severe sleep problems. They may have associated mental subnormality and epilepsy (Box 30.1).

Treatment The child and family dynamics should be evaluated by a psychiatrist and an experienced child psychologist for making a correct diagnosis and excluding other conditions especially mental retardation. These children should be handled with utmost care, emotional support and compassion under the guidance of a specially trained psychologist. Intensive and early speech therapy, behavior modification, play activities and social skill therapy are most useful. They need structured and supportive environment with plenty of individual attention. The role of drugs is limited. A variety of alternative treatments like dietary restrictions (exclusion of gluten and dairy products), dance, yoga, reiki and foot reflexology have been tried with variable results. Other dietary restrictions that have been found to be useful include avoidance of caffeine containing aerated drinks, canned juices and processed foods. Drug therapy is

---

Box 30.1 Salient features of autism

- No babbling by 12 months, no single words by 16 months, no two words phrases by 24 months.
- Any loss or regression of language or social skills at any age.
- No gestures or saying bye-bye by one year.
- No pretend playing.
- Short attention span.
- No eye contact.
- Lack of response when his name is called from behind at one year of age.
- Mostly self-occupied with no interest to make friends.
- Repetitive behavior like throwing of toys, rocking, hand flapping, head banging, etc.
- Resistance to change an established routine or ritual.
- Limited or lack of facial expression.
- Limited gestures or non-verbal communication.

---

indicated for children with aggressive or abusive behavior, severe hyperactivity and mood disorder. As these children grow older, they tend to become more aggressive and often display self-injurious behavior. Prognosis for recovery is poor.

NURSING MANAGEMENT

Public health nurses play a crucial role to assist the family to cope with a child having disability. The nature of precise disability of the child should be identified and quantified by clinical assessment and necessary laboratory support. The family should be explained about the nature of disability and special capabilities and potentialities of the challenged child which can be harnessed to improve the confidence of the child and provide emotional courage to the family. Nurse should plan various components of care of the handicapped children in health care institutions and community with effective participation and involvement of parents. She should assist the family to make the child independent in his day-to-day activities with minimal need for help and support. The family should be assisted to strengthen effective relationship and bondage so that children with handicaps are not socially isolated. The nurses should create awareness in the society for prevention, early identification and effective management of children with handicaps. The nursing management of children with disabilities is handled with following protocol.

Nursing Assessment

A complete history is taken to identify the predisposing conditions, socioeconomic and education status, number of children, parent-child interactions and social support system of the family. A thorough physical and neurological examination is conducted to identify the nature and severity of disability. A complete assessment is undertaken with the help of a number of specialists and relevant laboratory investigations with special focus on functioning of various special senses like cognition, hearing, speech and vision.

Nursing Diagnosis

A complete list of nursing diagnoses should be screened to identify various disabilities and handicaps of the children.

1. Anxiety and stress levels of parents and family members.
2. Gender of affected child or children and number of normal children.
3. Ability of the family of cope with the challenged child.

4. Growth and development status of the child.

5. Is disability limited to one functional area of the body or there is widespread involvement of several components of functioning?

6. Is disability hereditary in nature and need for genetic counseling?

7. Ability of the child to look after day-to-day activities. (independently or with some help) like, physical mobility, toilet care, bathing, dressing, self feeding and hygienic care.

8. Communication and social interactions.

9. Status of special senses like hearing, vision, touch, taste and smell.

10. Physical mobility.

11. The need for pharmacotherapy: Seizures, hyperactivity, mood alterations, swallowing difficulties and gastroesophageal reflux, constipation and spasticity/rigidity, etc.

12. Sleep pattern and behavior alterations.

13. Nutritional status and concerns. Avoidance of both under nutrition as well as obesity.

14. Susceptibility to infections and status of immunizations.

15. Involvement of the family with normal children, if any.

16. Level of awareness, knowledge, commitment and continued care of the family towards disabled child.

17. Special assets, capabilities and interests of the affected child should be identified.

Planning Care

A complete plan should be formulated to provide immediate care and long term emotional, financial and social support and follow-up. The various experts which are likely to be involved in the care and rehabilitation of the child should be identified and informed. Their specific roles and goals should be recorded and intimated to the family. Depending upon the nature of disability, a large number of specialists are likely to provide care and support to the child. The list includes clinical psychologist, child developmental psychologist, neurologist, ophthalmologist, pediatric surgeon, orthopedic surgeon, audiologist, physiotherapist, occupational therapist, behavior therapist, speech therapist and so on. The time schedule of management with each specialist should be formulated and family provided support and encouragement for regular follow-up. The family should be guided to contact various non-government organizations (NGOs) and Associations of Parents who provide care and guidance to families with specific disabilities. It is a great relief and support to the family to know that they are not alone in handling their "special child" and they can share their concerns and difficulties with parents of similarly affected children.

Nursing Interventions

Nurses are most important or key members of health care team to provide assistance, guidance and emotional support to the families with handicapped children. The interventions are planned depending on the nature and severity of the problem keeping in mind the immediate or short-term and long-term goals. The care can be provided at home, ambulatory clinic, health care facility and day care boarding facility and vocational training centers. The goal of management is to ensure that the disabled child is able to exploit all his capabilities to become independent to look after his day-to-day needs and is able to integrate with family and society as a useful member of the community.

BIBLIOGRAPHY

Alexander AW, Slinger-Constant AM. Current status of treatments for dyslexia: Critical review. *J Child Neurol* 2004, 19(10): 744–758.

Biederman J, Faraone SV. Attention-deficit hyperactivity disorder. *Lancet* 2005, 366 (9481): 237–248.

Karande S, Gogtay NJ. Specific learning disability and the right to education 2009 Act: Call for action. *J Postgrad Med* 2010, 56(3): 171–172.

Sukumaran TU. Poor scholastic performance in children and adolescents. *Indian Pediatr* 2011, 48(8): 597–598.

Common Symptoms in Children

FEVER

Fever is the commonest signal or symptom of disease in children. It provides a warning that some thing is wrong with the child. Like all mammals, human beings are homeothermic and they maintain their normal body

> "Humanity has but three great enemies; fever, famine and war. Of these by far the greatest, by far the most terrible, is fever."
> — **Sir William Osler**

temperature between a narrow range of 36.8°C ±0.4°C (98.2°F ±0.7°F). There are diurnal variations in body temperature with lowest in the morning (maximum oral temperature of 37.2°C or 98.9°F) and highest in the evening (maximum oral temperature of 37.7°C or 99.9°F). *The body temperature is more unstable in children and diurnal variations are more marked especially during summer months.* In summer, oral temperature of up to 37.7°C or 99.9°F in the evening is normal and should not be labeled as low-grade fever. The normal body temperature is maintained by a thermostat located in the brain behind the third eye (anterior hypothalamus). The thermostat tries to maintain normal body temperature by ensuring a balance between heat production (metabolic activity, muscular activity, shivering) and heat conservation (flexed posture, wearing warm clothes) on one hand and heat loss mechanisms (heat loss from body by conduction, convection, radiation, evaporation, dilatation of blood vessels, sweating, wearing light or no clothes) on the other hand. The body temperature may rise due to various bodily activities such as physical (exercise), physiological (heavy meal), mental (studies, stress), and emotional excitement (joy, anger) because of surge of catecholamines. Fever occurs when heat production exceeds heat loss and is diagnosed when oral temperature goes above 100°F or 37.8°C.

Recording Body Temperature

A clinical glass thermometer (35°C–42°C and 95°F–108°F) is used to record the body temperature. Unlike an ordinary room thermometer, the clinical thermometer is provided with a constriction at the bottom end of the mercury column. Due to constriction, the mercury column does not fall after recording the body temperature. Thermometer must be vigorously shaken to let the mercury column drop below 37°C or 98°F before recording the next temperature. Hold the thermometer by its upper end (the end opposite the bulb) between your thumb and finger. Shake the thermometer with a sharp, snappy or jerky motion to drive the mercury down. Skin temperature in infants and preschool children is quite reliable. Axilla (armpit) or groin should be dried with a cloth and bulb of thermometer is placed snugly by tightly holding the arm against chest or flexing the thigh over abdomen. Thermometer should be left in place for at least 2 minutes before reading the temperature. If a thermometer is placed in a wet axilla or groin, it will give erroneously low temperature. In school going children, oral temperature is recorded by placing the thermometer under the tongue and asking the child to breathe through the nose. Digital thermometer is safer than mercury thermometer for taking oral temperature in children. Oral temperature should not be taken immediately after intake of a hot or cold drink. In critically sick children and infants, rectal or core body temperature is recorded. Infant is placed in a supine position and nurse holds both feet with one hand and inserts the thermometer with the other hand. It is wise to keep the penis covered in a boy because insertion of a rectal thermometer may cause urination. Older

---

Practical Point

In peak summer, oral temperature up to 99.9°F in the afternoon is normal and should not be labeled as low grade fever.

31

children are placed in a lateral or side-lying position, taking care that they do not roll over while thermometer is in the rectum. The rectal thermometer has a small rounded mercury bulb. After lubrication with vaseline, it is inserted upwards and backwards for 2–3 cm and baby is held tightly to prevent any movements of legs. It needs some practice to read a conventional glass thermometer. Roll the thermometer gently in your fingers till you see the mercury column.

Digital thermometers are easy to read and they give an audible signal when temperature has been recorded. Thermocrystal strips are available to record temperature of the forehead. They are convenient to use at home but are unreliable. Eardrum temperature can be recorded with a thermoscan which works on the principle of infrared technology. It is a useful device in a busy clinic of the doctor because temperature read-out is obtained within one second. Thermoscan probe is inserted into the ear canal after holding the pinna. In order to get a clear view of the eardrum, pinna is pulled straight backwards in infants and upwards and backwards in older children. While tugging the ear, thermoscan probe is snugly inserted into the ear canal and activation button is pressed till a beep is heard **(Figure 31.1)**. The digital read out of the temperature appears on the monitor. **Table 31.1** gives normal ranges

Nursing Tip
In most healthy children, forehead is warm to touch because of excessive flow of blood to the brain. It should not be considered as a sign of fever. When trunk is warm while extremities are cold to touch, it is suggestive of fever.

of body temperatures at different sites. By practice and experience, one can reliably assess (accuracy ±0.5°C or 1.0°F) the temperature of the child with one's hands by touching the forehead and chest or abdomen. Most normal children have relatively warm forehead because of high flow of blood to the brain. Some children have warm hands while others may be endowed with less warm or cold hands. It should be remembered that skin temperature is 0.4°C (0.75°F) lower than oral temperature while rectal or eardrum temperature is 0.4°C (0.75°F) higher than oral temperature.

Physiologic Basis of Fever

Fever occurs through a series of metabolic steps that are mediated and triggered by infectious agents or their toxins (endotoxins and exotoxins). They initiate an inflammatory response by production of pyrogenic cytokines such as interleukins, tumor necrosis factor and interferons in an attempt to eliminate the infectious

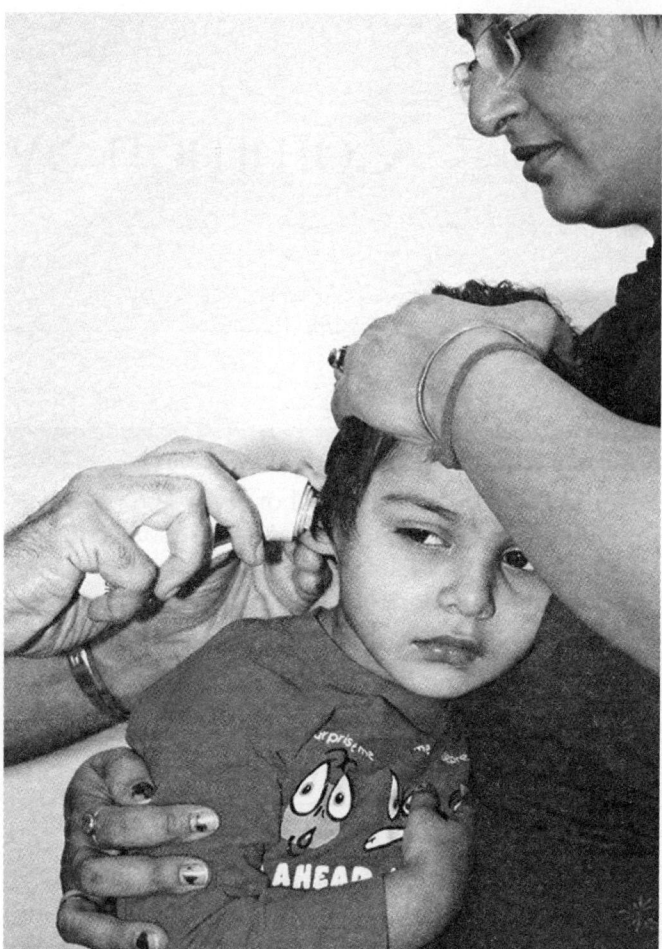

Figure 31.1 Method for recording eardrum temperature. The child is restrained by the mother or a nurse and thermoscan probe is inserted into the ear canal while tugging the earlobe upwards and backwards. When activation button is pressed, a beep is heard and digital read out of the temperature appears on the monitor within one second. It is a useful device for use in a busy ambulatory clinic but its reliability depends upon the expertise and skill of the user

Table 31.1 Normal body temperatures at different sites		
Site	*Temperatures*	
Axillary	34.7–37.3°C	94.5–99.1°F
Oral	35.5–37.5°C	95.9–99.55°F
Rectal	36.6–38.0°C	97.9–100.4°F
Thermoscan	35.8–38.0°C	96.4–100.4°F

agent or neutralize their toxins. The inflammatory agents induce the production of cyclo-oxyenase-2 (Cox-2) enzyme in the brain which catalyzes the production of prostaglandins (PGE_2) from arachidonic acid. The PGE_2 reduce the activity of cyclic adenosine monophosphate and raise the thermoregulatory set point in the hypothalamus at a high level, i.e. above the normal or mandatory set point of 37°C or 98.4°F **(Figure 31.2)**. Thermostat sends regulatory messages to the sympathetic blood vessels and prefrontal cortex to cause vasoconstriction, cold extremities, feeling of chills, rigors or shivering, assuming a flexed posture, taking a blanket, etc. in an attempt to raise the temperature of blood perfusing or surrounding the thermostat to match with the higher set temperature. *It is a common observation that extremities become cold before the body temperature shoots up.*

Mode of Action of Antipyretics

The antipyretic agents block Cox-2 enzyme, and thus prevent conversion of arachidonic acid to PGE_2. The conventional nonsteroidal anti-inflammatory drugs (NSAIDs) like ibuprofen block not only Cox-2 in the brain but also Cox-1 in the stomach and kidneys thus causing adverse effects like dyspepsia, gastrointestinal bleeding, reduced renal perfusion and risk of bleeding by interfering with the integrity and aggregation of platelets. The exact mode of action of paracetamol is not known, but it possibly blocks Cox-2 and Cox-3 in the central nervous system without having any effect

Nursing Tip

In a febrile illness, core body temperature is elevated but extremities are cold, while in heat stroke both trunk and extremities are warm to touch.

on Cox-1. That is why paracetamol is safer and gentle on the stomach with minimal gastrointestinal and renal side effects. Newer antipyretics (like aceclofenac, diclofenac) are also safer because they are specific inhibitor of Cox-2 and have no adverse effect on Cox-1 in the stomach and kidneys.

Types of Fever

Due to wide-spread use of antipyretics, the character or pattern of fever is often altered.

- *Continuous.* Fever is continuous as body temperature never touches normal and daily fluctuations are less than 1°F. Examples: Localized viral and bacterial infections.
- *Remittent or hectic.* Fever is continuous with wide (>2°F) variations in daily body temperatures. Examples: Viremia, septicemia, abscess.
- *Step-ladder type.* Fever is mild to moderate in severity at onset and gradually increase in severity reaching a peak level after 5–6 days. Example: Typhoid fever.
- *Intermittent.* Body temperature touches normal daily (quotidian) or fever occurs on alternate days (tertian) or after every 2 days (quartan). Examples: Malaria, tuberculosis **(Figure 31.3)**.
- *Pel-Ebstein.* Fever lasts for 3–10 days followed by afebrile period of several days. Examples: Hodgkin disease, lymphoreticular malignancy.

Associated Symptoms

The site of infection or cause of fever is suspected on the basis of associated or localizing symptoms:

- *Nil:* Viremia or septicemia
- *Sore throat:* Tonsillitis, pharyngitis, herpangina
- *Cough and coryza* (running nose): Common cold, influenza
- *Pain ear:* Acute otitis media
- *Pain chest, cough, rapid or difficult breathing:* Bronchopneumonia
- *Vomiting and diarrhea:* Acute gastroenteritis
- *Dysuria or frequency of micturition:* Urinary tract infection

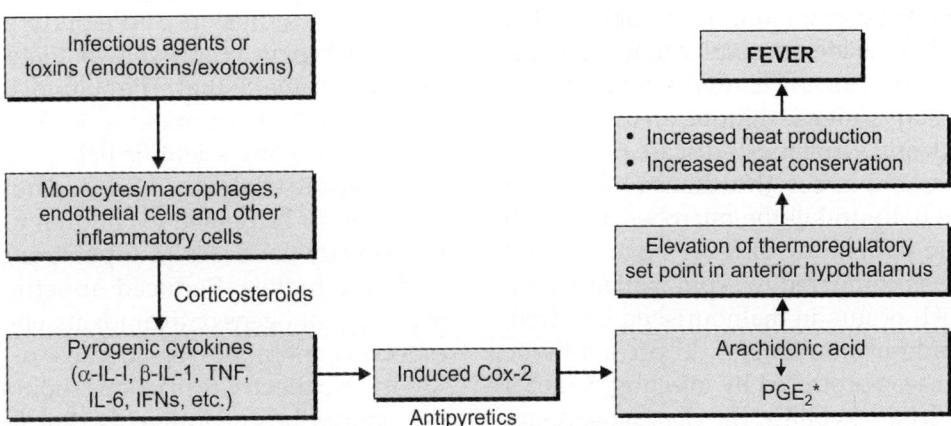

Figure 31.2 Pathogenesis of fever

Cox-2, cyclo-oxygenase-2; IFNs, interferons; II, interleukins; PGE_2, prostaglandin-E_2; TNF, tumor necrosis factor
*PGE_2 in circulation produce body aches and arthralgias

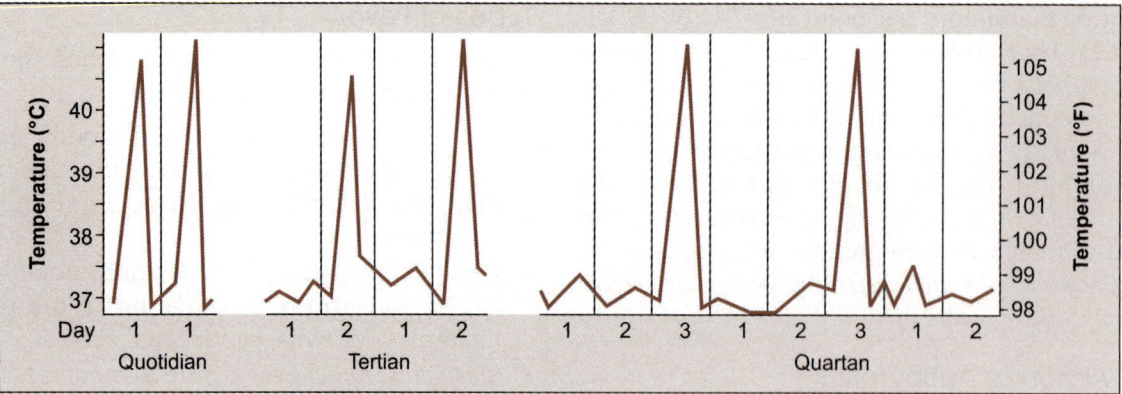

Figure 31.3 Types of intermittent fever

- *Headache, vomiting, photophobia, neck stiffness, alteration in consciousness*: Encephalitis, meningitis
- *Vomiting, anorexia and jaundice:* Viral hepatitis
- *Pain and swelling of joints:*
  - Single joint: Pyogenic or tubercular arthritis
  - Multiple joints: Rheumatic fever or rheumatoid arthritis

Common Causes of Fever

Fever occurs due to a variety of causes but the commonest cause of fever in children is acute viral infection like common cold. Sore throat due to tonsillitis is common in school going children. Other common causes of fever include malaria, typhoid fever, tuberculosis and urinary tract infection. These conditions should be excluded whenever fever persists beyond one week. Fever may occur following administration of some vaccines in children. Hyperthermia can occur due to exposure to high environmental temperature during hot summer months.

Fever is a friend not a foe Nature is supreme and has a profound biological wisdom. Fever heralds the onset of disease and provides a useful signal that some thing is wrong. Fever is not an "illness" but a response on the part of the body that it is fighting an infection. It inhibits the growth and virulence of disease producing pathogens. Fever enhances the disease fighting capabilities of the body to kill the microbes. It is well known that septic patients with fever have a better chance to survive as compared to septic patients with hypothermia which occurs in malnourished children, cancer patients and newborn babies. In pre-antibiotic era, artificial fever was produced by injecting malarial parasites to treat tertiary syphilis. *Therefore, unnecessary reduction of mild to moderate fever (<37.8°C or <100°F) may be likened to "disarming the body which is trying to fight an enemy".*

Hazards and Adverse Effects of Fever

Young children, specially between the ages of 6 months and 3 years, have a tendency to suddenly shoot up their body temperature and they are vulnerable to develop febrile convulsions due to immaturity of the brain. Fever makes the child uncomfortable and increases his needs for fluids and cause tachycardia and rapid breathing. Fever leads to increased metabolic rate with greater consumption of oxygen and increased production of carbon dioxide with dangerous consequences in children with pneumonia and cardiac disease. There is excessive thirst, hot dry skin, passage of scanty high-colored urine. Fever often leads to nausea, loss of appetite, negative nitrogen balance and weight loss. Most viral fevers are associated with flushed face, discomfort, body aches and headache. High grade fever may lead to delirium and confusion.

Nursing and Supportive Care of a Child with Fever

Most viral fevers are self-limiting and child needs good supportive and symptomatic care. When fever is due to a contagious disease, the child should be kept away from other youngsters and elderly people. The child should be kept in a cool, well-ventilated room with light and comfortable clothes. The cultural belief that keeping the child with fever under a fan leads to pneumonia does not have any scientific basis. The child should be encouraged to take extra fluids and nutritious diet. Food should never be denied to children with fever because they already have loss of appetite and their metabolic needs are higher. Reduced appetite is often due to invading pathogens or their toxins, effect of medications (especially antibiotics) and because of reduced physical activity. No dietary restrictions should be imposed and they should be encouraged to eat food and fruits of their liking and choice. The cultural practice of denying certain foods to children with fever does not have any scientific basis in the modern system of medicine.

> *"Fever is a friend, not a foe—never try to give it a knocking blow!"*
>
> — **Meharban Singh**

Antipyretics should be given to children with previous history of convulsions due to fever, high grade fever (oral temperature of >38.5°C or >101°F), children with breathing difficulty and when there is discomfort and body aches. Unnecessary use of antipyretics for treatment of mild fever should be avoided. Paracetamol or acetaminophen is a safe and an effective antipyretic with minimal side effects **(Table 31.2)**. It can be safely used in children with bronchial asthma as it does not enhance bronchial reactivity. It should be used in a correct dose (15 mg/kg/dose every 4–6 hours). The drug should be administered in a precise dose with the help of a syringe or a graduated plastic measure provided by the manufacturer. The use of a teaspoon should be avoided because they are variable and not of a standard size. When fever goes beyond 42°C (>104°F) despite adequate antipyretic therapy, effective sponging of the body with tap water is recommended. Ice cold water should not be used for hydrotherapy because it is likely to cause shivering and discomfort with further rise in body temperature. The child should be placed under the fan to assist cooling by evaporation. When fever occurs due to heat stroke there is no role of antipyretics. These children should be managed by aggressive physical cooling methods like use of cooling blanket, iced water bath or total body sponging with cold water. The physical cooling methods should be

stopped as soon as body temperature drops to 38°C (100°F) to prevent the risk of over cooling. The site of infection and possible pathogens causing the disease should be ascertained or identified by detailed clinical assessment and laboratory investigations. "Shotgun" antibiotic therapy with multiple drugs should be avoided and a specific antibiotic should be used depending upon the diagnosis. Antibiotics should not be indiscriminately misused as antipyretics. *Efforts should be made to treat the child rather than the thermometer!*

Low Grade Fever

Many children are diagnosed to have low grade fever and subjected to unnecessary investigations. The usual story is that the child had an episode of high grade fever (viral fever or some other acute infection like typhoid fever) but parents continue to record the body temperature (either on their own or on the advice of a physician) even when initial disease has settled. They find that the child is running low grade fever (oral temperature 37.2–37.8°C or 99–100°F) especially in the afternoon and evening. A number of consultations are sought and investigations are done to identify the cause of fever without realizing that it is the normal diurnal pattern of body temperature of the child. The child is otherwise well, active and without any discomfort. He is playful and his appetite is good. Infact, there is nothing wrong with the child if his temperature is ignored. He wants to go to school but parents think he needs rest. All investigations including erythrocyte sedimentation rate (ESR) are normal. No further investigations should be done and parents need to be reassured that there is nothing wrong with the child. Further recording of body temperature should be stopped and child sent to school.

A number of diseases, however, are known to start with a low grade fever. They are often associated with other symptoms of an underlying disease process like loss of appetite, lack of vigor and enthusiasm, easy fatigability, inability to play, pallor (due to fall in hemoglobin), and poor weight gain or loss of body weight. Depending upon the site of the disease process, additional symptoms like cough, dysuria (discomfort while passing urine), bowel disturbances (constipation or diarrhea), body aches or bone pains, etc. may be noticed. ESR (which is a non-specific marker of a large number of diseases) is often elevated. These children do need expert medical advice and a battery of investigations are done to identify the cause of underlying disease process. A large number of diseases like tuberculosis, chronic infections, lymphoreticular malignancy and autoimmune diseases may have this symptom complex.

31

Table 31.2 Common side effects of antipyretic agents		
Adverse effects	*Paracetamol*	*NSAIDs**
Skin rash	+	++
GI side effects	±	++
Bronchial reactivity	±	+
Bleeding risk	–	+
Hepatotoxicity in therapeutic doses	±	(Idiosyncratic)
Nephrotoxicity**	+	++
Seizures	Nil	+ (Mefenamic acid)
Fluid retention	Nil	+
Hypothermia	Nil	+
Drug interactions	+	++
Infants <6 months of age	Licensed	Not licensed
Pregnancy	Licensed	Not licensed

GI, gastrointestinal; NSAIDs, nonsteroidal anti-inflammatory drugs.

*Except newer Cox-2 specific agents which are safer.

**According to National Kidney Foundation of United States of America, paracetamol is the antipyretic of choice in patients with renal disease.

31

VIRAL FEVER

There are over 200 viruses which are known to cause non-specific flu-like illnesses. Viral diseases can occur throughout the year but they are usually activated during change of weather, i.e. during a sudden transition from winter to summer and from summer to winter. It is true that viral infections are more common during winter but epidemics are known to occur during any abrupt change and extremes of weather or environmental temperatures due to air-conditioning. The viruses may lie dormant in the throat and get activated during sudden exposure to the cold environment or on drinking chilled water, soft drinks and taking ice-cream, etc.

These infections are highly contagious and spread both through direct contact and by dissemination of infected air droplets during conversation and bouts of coughing and sneezing. Children get the infection from household contact or through contact with other children in the creche, nursery or school. The disease is most infectious one day before the onset of symptoms and during the initial 2–3 days of illness. Due to existence of a large number of respiratory viruses and relatively short duration of immunity following an episode of infection, most children suffer from 4–6 episodes of viral infections every year. Viral infections are the leading cause of absenteeism from the schools.

Diagnosis

There is a sudden onset of fever with headache and body aches. Sore throat and irritation of nose with a watery discharge is common. At times there may be watering and redness of eyes. Dry hacking cough and sneezing are common. Nasal congestion leads to blockage of nose. In some viral infections, the symptoms of cough and cold may be absent. There is general malaise, feeling of being unwell, headache, body aches and loss of appetite. Most viral infections are self-limiting and resolve spontaneously within 4–5 days. Superadded bacterial infections may lead to spread of infection to the middle ear, sinuses and lungs.

Prevention

There are effective and safe vaccines for a large number of specific viral infections like poliomyelitis, measles, mumps, rubella, chickenpox, influenza, yellow fever, and Japanese encephalitis. But no vaccination is available for the prevention of non-specific flu-like viral infections, because a large number of viruses are known to produce these manifestations. The viral infections spread by direct contact through dissemination of infected air droplets which are thrown out during speaking, bouts of coughing and sneezing. The patient contaminates his hands by touching his mouth and nose and transmits infection through indirect routes by touching others by handshaking and through contaminated fomites (non-living objects like towels, handkerchief, crockery, furniture, etc.). The risk of spread of infection is reduced by adopting following measures.

- During an epidemic, avoid visiting crowded places like cinema halls, religious congregations, and using public transport system as far as possible.
- Sudden exposure to an extremely hot and chilled environment should be avoided.
- Avoid drinking extremely chilled water, soft drinks and ice-cream as far as possible.
- The mouth and nose should be covered with a handkerchief while coughing and sneezing.
- Patients and healthy individuals should frequently wash their hands with soap and water.
- Try to keep away from an infected person in school.
- Isolation at home is neither feasible nor practical and many household contacts who are susceptible would contract the disease.

Treatment

There are no antiviral drugs for the treatment of non-specific viral infections. The disease is self-limiting and spontaneous recovery occurs in 4–5 days. Simple home remedies like taking hot drinks, soups and tulsi tea or ginger tea and honey in hot water provide soothing relief to the throat. The inflamed throat should not be exposed to food items like condiments, lemon, chillies, fried foods, chilled drinks, ice-cream, etc. The child with fever should be kept in a cool well-ventilated room. The clothes should be light and made of cotton fabric. He should be encouraged to drink plenty of liquids and take a balanced nutritious diet comprising of fresh vegetables, fruits and milk products.

Fever and discomfort due to headache and body aches should be relieved by taking a safe antipyretic-analgesic drug like paracetamol. The cough mixture containing antihistamines are commonly prescribed but they have limited utility and may even worsen the nose block by drying the secretions. Infants are unable to blow their noses. Nasal secretions can be sucked with the help of catheter attached to a syringe or suction bulb after instillation of few drops of normal saline. Gargles with hot water containing table salt and steam inhalations provide more comfort and relief than medicines. Antibiotics are not only useless, but they

Box 31.1 **Some do's and don'ts for treatment of viral infections**

Do's

- Drink plenty of liquids and hot drinks.
- Cough and sneeze after covering your nose and mouth with a handkerchief.
- Frequent washing of hands with soap and water, blowing of the nose after rinsing with water and mouthwashes with a mild antiseptic liquid can ward off the infection.
- Take a nutritious and balanced diet with plenty of fresh green leafy vegetables and fruits.
- Steam inhalations and gargles with hot water containing common salt are more beneficial than medicines and cough mixtures. Paracetamol is safe and effective for relief of fever, headache and body aches.

Don'ts

- Avoid taking excessively chilled water and soft drinks.
- Avoid the habit of touching your face or scratching your nose.
- Avoid exposure to sudden changes in the environmental temperature. The room and car should be kept comfortably cool and not excessively chilled.
- Avoid visiting congested public places as far as possible.
- Avoid consumption of chillies, fried foods and condiments. Avoid junk foods.
- Avoid use of medicated nose drops. Saline water (0.6% solution of sodium chloride) is an effective and safe nasal decongestant without any side effects.
- Avoid taking self-medications including unnecessary antibiotics and antihistamines.

may actually be harmful both to the patient and society by emergence of antibiotic-resistant microorganisms. They are indicated when there is a superadded bacterial infection. **Box 31.1** highlights some do's and don'ts for the treatment of viral infections.

FEVER DUE TO HYPERTHERMIA

Heat Exhaustion

Heat exhaustion occurs due to loss of water and salt because of excessive sweating in summer. During hot summer months, if a child trecks or plays out doors in the sun for a long time, he can develop heat exhaustion. The skin is cool and wet (due to marked sweating) with mild or no elevation of body temperature. The child complains of headache, weakness, fatigue and dizziness and may have nausea and vomiting.

The child should be made to rest in a cool place under the fan or infront of a desert cooler or an air-conditioner. He should be given plenty of fluids. A cool lemon drink with salt and sugar or ORS is most refreshing to replenish the loss of fluids and salt due to excessive sweating.

Heat Stroke (Heat Hyperpyrexia)

During hot summer months when a child is exposed to sun for a long period, his heat-regulatory mechanisms may fail leading to marked elevation of body temperature. The body temperature may suddenly rise to above 41°C (106°F) and child becomes drowsy and delirious. He may develop convulsions. Skin is hot and dry without any sweating. Most vital organs of the body may get damaged due to extremely high body temperature. Hepatic transaminases are markedly elevated.

Treatment The child should be immediately removed from hot environment. All clothes should be removed and child wrapped in a thin wet sheet. He should be placed in front of an air conditioner or under a fan. He can be given a bath with cold water. If conscious, child should be given plenty of fluids (water, *nimbu-pani, sherbat, ORS*) to drink. Every effort should be made to bring down the body temperature as far as possible. *There is no role of giving antipyretic drugs because thermostat is not set at a higher temperature in these children.* When a child had seizures or is drowsy he should be promptly shifted to a hospital in an air-conditioned vehicle. These children are managed by aggressive cooling methods like use of iced water bath, total body sponging with ice cold water and use of cooling blanket. Dehydration and electrolyte disturbances should be managed by intravenous administration of fluids and electrolytes.

Prevention Over-clothing should be avoided and children should not be allowed to play outdoors for long periods during hot summer months. The sports activities and physical training program should be restricted to early morning or late evening during summer. Light and loose cotton clothes are better than clothes made of synthetic material. Children should be encouraged to drink plenty of liquids with extra salt during hot and humid summer months. *Infants should never be left alone in a stationary or locked car during shopping sprees, because of potential risk of life-threatening hyperthermia.*

ACHES AND PAINS

Pain and discomfort are the most common signals of disease. Infact, disease (dis-ease) literally means lack of ease or comfort. Pain is a protective mechanism on the part of the body so that timely action is taken to seek medical help and prevent further damage to the tissues. Threshold for pain varies widely in different individuals depending upon the genetic or constitutional background. Some children are very brave, others are timid and easily frightened with

31

> | Box 31.2 | **The PQRST pain assessment** |
>
> **P** = Are you having **P**ain now?
> **Q** = **Q**uality of pain—sharp, burning, tingling, colicky, boring
> **R** = **R**adiation of pain
> **S** = **S**everity of pain as assessed to assign a score from 0 (no pain) to 10 (maximum pain)
> **T** = **T**iming or duration of pain

various grades in between. Pain is subjective and often associated with emotional components like anxiety, fear and terror. Children with recurrent aches and pains are more sensitive to pain, are easily scared in unfamiliar or stressful situations, cry more often during blood sampling or vaccinations and often avoid playing games due to fear of hurting themselves. Pain is usually associated with physiologic responses of stress (due to release of catecholamines, cortisol, endorphins) and vagal stimulation like rapid heart beats (palpitation), rapid breathing, rise in blood pressure, flushing, sweating, and dilatation of pupils. Endocrinal responses to pain include hyperglycemia because of release of cortisol and glucagon and suppression of insulin. Pain may adversely affect body defences and immune mechanisms thus slowing the healing capabilities of the patient. Medical science has not invented any device (algometer or dolometer) to objectively assess the severity of pain. In older children, the severity of pain can be graded as mild, moderate, severe and excruciating. Alternatively the child can be asked to grade the severity of pain on a scale of 0 (none) to 10 (worst pain). In infants and preschool children, the severity of pain can be gauged on the basis of facial expression rating scale based on drawings of faces. Pain can be assessed by the acronym PQRST **(Box 31.2)**.

Infants and preschool children are unable to provide any clues to the severity, site and type of pain and they merely cry. The common practice of frightening and "blackmailing" children with threats of doctors and injections is strongly condemned. Instead, efforts should be made to create a doctor-friendly and hospital-friendly perceptions among children by giving them age-appropriate explanation and information when they are being taken to a doctor or hospital.

BODY ACHES

At times, we may not be able to cure a disease but we must provide comfort and symptomatic relief from discomfort and pain. The common causes of pain and discomfort in children include pain because of vaccinations, everyday pains such as body ache, headache, growing pain, toothache, sprain, and minor

injury, and dysmenorrhea. Body aches and myalgias may occur during the course of viral infections, collagen vascular disorders, chronic fatigue syndrome, or fascial myositis, trauma and inflammation of subcutaneous tissues, joints and bones. Pain and anxiety may occur during various diagnostic and therapeutic procedures and should be managed by an appropriate sedative or analgesic agent.

Headache

Headache is a common complaint in school-going children. It may occur as a non-specific symptom in association with fever because of any cause (viral fever, malaria, typhoid, and so on). Frequent episodes of headache or severe headache may occur because of diseases of the organs of the head and face (i.e. brain, eyes, ears, nose, throat and teeth). When headache occurs at school, after completing homework or on watching television, it may be because of defective vision or fatigue of muscles of eyes because of their malalignment. Headache in association with frequent cough and colds with persistent purulent nasal discharge is usually because of sinusitis. Caries teeth may be diagnosed because of headache. Episodes of headache with vomiting are suggestive of a raised intracranial pressure due to any cause. Triad of fever, headache, and vomiting of acute onset is suggestive of meningitis. Migraine typically causes episodes of one-sided headache that runs in certain families. The attack may be precipitated by exposure to bright light, loud noise, excessive intake of salt, emotional stress; sleep deprivation or excessive sleep; and premenstrual tension. Intake of nuts, chocolates, cheese, tea, and coffee may trigger the attack. There may be initial symptoms (aura) of seeing stars or zigzag figures in the eyes. The child would prefer to lie down in a quiet, dark room. Headache may be pulsating in nature because of spasm and dilatation of the blood vessels of the scalp. Headache is usually localized to one side but may involve the whole head. Vomiting may occur in severe cases. The episodes of migraine may occur at intervals of 1 to 3 months. The disorder is more common in sensitive and bright children. Migraine is more common among adolescent girls. Hypertension is uncommon in children but should be ruled out by recording blood pressure.

Treatment

Most headaches in association with fever are self-limited and disappear when fever resolves. Paracetamol (15 mg/kg) or ibuprofen (7.5 to 10 mg/kg) is a safe and effective analgesic for providing symptomatic relief. Aches and pains at multiple body sites along with headache are usually because of psychological factors. Depending on the associated symptoms and clinical suspicion, a further consultation is often required with an ophthalmologist, otolaryngologist, dentist, and neurologist. Treatment of migraine needs administration of specific medicines such as sublingual ergotamine tartrate or sumatriptan succinate for aborting an attack. Administration of an over-the-counter formulation containing acetaminophen, aspirin and caffeine (Excedrin) provides dramatic relief. Application of cold pack and intake of coffee may provide dramatic relief. When attacks of migraine occur frequently, administration of flunarizine hydrochloride, propranolol, cyproheptadine, and topiramate is recommended to reduce the frequency of further attacks. Exercise of eye muscles is required for the relief of headache owing to imbalance of eye muscles. Biofeedback, self-hypnosis, yoga, or meditation can be tried as an alternative to pharmacological treatment.

Growing Pains

Children between 2 and 10 years of age often complain of pain in the legs (calf and thigh muscles), especially during the evening. The child is healthy, active, and playful. Pain is usually because of fatigue caused by excessive exertion and playful activity throughout the day. Because children are actively growing during this period, the condition is often labeled as "growing pains." Hot water bath and massage are useful to provide relief. When discomfort is marked, a safe analgesic such as paracetamol provides prompt relief. The presence of associated nutritional anemia should be treated with a hematinic. The disorder is self-limiting and spontaneously disappears in due course of time. When aches and pains are present at multiple body sites (e.g. legs, arms, chest, abdomen and head), it is usually suggestive of a psychological or an emotional disorder. When pain is localized to the joints or bones, it should be investigated to identify the cause.

Toothache

Toothache is very common and is one of the most severe forms of pain. Pain is usually deep seated, sharp and boring in character. It is aggravated by eating food and on taking hot and cold drink. Pain may be referred to the face and ear or there may be headache without any obvious pain over the tooth. It is usually caused by caries or cavities and infection of the gums and root of the tooth. Eating nuts or hard food and impaction of gritty food in between the teeth may produce sudden toothache. Eruption of wisdom tooth is often associated with pain.

Treatment Local application of clove oil and intake of a safe analgesic such as paracetamol usually provides prompt relief. Advice of a dentist must be taken for use of an appropriate antibiotic and definitive treatment. Regular and correct brushing of teeth, avoidance of sweets and candies, and rinsing of mouth with water after every meal are useful to prevent caries. Cleaning of teeth with hard brush, neem twig (*datun*), and gritty tooth powder (*manjan*) can rub off the protective enamel of teeth. These should be avoided. Regular preventive checkup by a dentist every 6 months is recommended for early recognition and treatment of any problems of the teeth and gums.

Dysmenorrhea

When menstrual periods are associated with marked discomfort and pain, it is called dysmenorrhea. Dysmenorrhea is common in teenage girls, especially during their initial menstrual periods. Pain and discomfort can be relieved by giving paracetamol. Local fomentation with a hot-water bottle kept over the suprapubic region and perineum provides relief. A combination of antispasmodic and an analgesic such as dicylomine hydrochloride and mefenamic acid is useful to relieve the painful contractions of the uterus. Dysmenorrhea may be associated with high levels of prostaglandins E_2 and F_2, which are likely to respond to the administration of prostaglandin synthetase inhibitor. Naproxen (500 mg at the onset of menses followed by 250 mg every 6 to 8 hours for 24 hours) has been found to be effective in most cases of primary dysmenorrhea. Most adolescent girls are anemic, and must be given a hematinic containing iron and folic acid.

PAIN MANAGEMENT

Pain and discomfort must be relieved to provide comfort and improve the quality of life. Relief of pain is associated with reduced morbidity and enhanced survival by reversing neuroendocrinal responses that are associated with pain. **Figure 31.4** summarizes the choice of analgesics and sedatives for various painful conditions and situations in children. The commonly used analgesics and sedatives with their doses are listed in **Table 31.3**.

Indications to Give Analgesics

Pain control is one of the most important components of palliative care to provide comfort to the patient. Analgesics and sedatives must be prescribed in children to relieve pain and anxiety. Emotional support, comfort of mother's lap, cuddling, and caressing are useful to

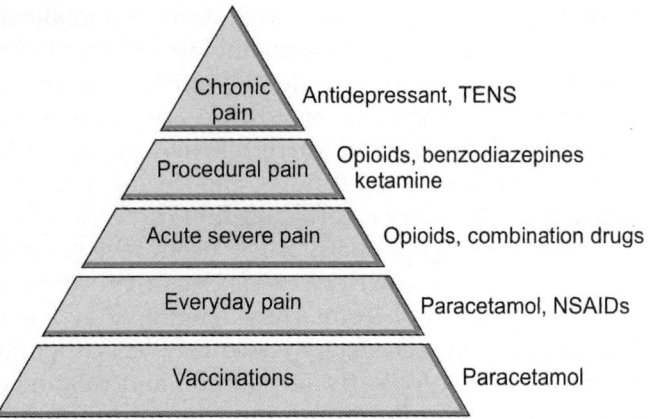

Figure 31.4 Pyramid of pain and indications for use of various analgesic agents

NSAIDs, nonsteroidal anti-inflammatory drugs; TENS, transcutaneous electrical nerve stimulation.

provide comfort and relieve fear and anxiety of painful procedures.

Newborns

Pain in newborns is often unrecognized and undertreated. There is no doubt that neonates do feel pain, and nalgesics should be routinely prescribed during their medical care. Sucrose (1 to 2 mL of 20% solution) or sucking at dummy nipple or breastfeeding provides comfort during minor procedures by virtue of distraction and possibly because of the pharmacological effect of sucrose. Surface anesthetic should be used before heel stick and venipuncture and the baby should be comforted by skin-to-skin contact, cuddling and caressing after the procedure.

Paracetamol is the drug of first choice for relief of pain because of traumatic and instrumental delivery,

Table 31.3 Doses of analgesics and sedatives used in children	
■ Analgesics	
□ Paracetamol or acetaminophen	15 mg/kg every 4–6 h up to a maximum of 60 mg/kg/d (10 mg/kg for infants younger than 6 mo)
■ NSAIDs	
□ Acetylsalicylic acid	15 mg/kg every 4–6 h
□ Ibuprofen	7.5–10 mg/kg every 8 h
□ Naproxen	5.0–7.5 mg/kg every 12 h
□ Indomethacin	1 mg/kg every 8–12 h
□ Diclofenac sodium	1.5 mg/kg every 8 h
■ Opioids	
□ Morphine	0.1–0.2 mg/kg IM or IV
□ Pethidine (meperidine)	1–2 mg/kg IM or IV
□ Codeine phosphate	0.5–1 mg/kg oral every 4–6 h
□ Fentanyl	1–5 µg/kg IV slowly
■ Sedatives and hypnotics	
□ Chloral hydrate	25–75 mg/kg oral
□ Triclofos sodium	10–20 mg/kg oral
□ Benzodiazepines	
• Diazepam	0.1–0.2 mg/kg IM or IV
• Midazolam	0.5–0.75 mg/kg oral or rectal
	0.25–0.5 mg/kg nasal or sublingual
	0.05–0.15 mg/kg IM or IV
□ Ketamine[a]	1–2 mg/kg IV slowly
	3–5 mg/kg per dose IM, oral, rectal
□ Propofol	1–2 mg/kg IV followed by 100–200 µg/kg/min as a constant infusion
□ Dexmedetomidine	1–2 mg/kg IV followed by 100–200 µg/kg/min as a constant infusion
■ Local anesthetics	
□ Regional or deep	Local nerve block, epidural, or spinal
□ Surface agents	Lidocaine or prilocaine-lidocaine mixture (Ametop, Emla, or Emlap cream)

Abbreviations: d, day(s); h, hour(s); NSAIDs, nonsteroidal anti-inflammatory drugs; IM, intramuscular; IV, intravenous; mo, month(s).
[a]Ketamine causes amnesia and it has synergistic effect with midazolam.

congenital fracture, cellulitis, abscess, osteomyelitis and arthritis. *Paracetamol is the only analgesic licensed for use below 6 month of age.* Nonsteroidal anti-inflammatory drugs (NSAIDs) are not recommended for use in newborns and infants as analgesics. Effective analgesia, preferably by use of opioids, should be provided for conducting procedures such as intubation, assisted ventilation, chest drainage, circumcision and laser/cryotherapy for retinopathy prematurity.

Children

Paracetamol is the drug of first choice for treating pain and discomfort associated with vaccinations, teething, viral infections, growing pains and non-inflammatory conditions such as headache, dysmenorrhea and sprains/sport injuries. NSAIDs are recommended when paracetamol fails to provide adequate relief and for the treatment of painful inflammatory conditions such as localized infections (cellulitis, abscess, fascial myositis, arthritis and osteomyelitis) and autoimmune or connective tissue disorders. In children with severe or intractable pain, opioids are most useful and may be combined with paracetamol to have a synergistic effect.

PAIN OF PROCEDURES

During various procedures, fear and anxiety are often out of proportion to the actual pain. Depending on the age, the child should be given relevant information regarding the procedure. The child must be given the comfort and confidence of parental presence. The infant should preferably be kept in the mother's lap, which provides security and confidence to the child. Parental humor, distraction, praise and reassurance provide comfort and emotional support to the child during the procedure. The procedure can be explained on a dummy animal to relieve the anxiety and fear of the child. A topical anesthetic or systemic analgesic-sedative must be used whenever feasible. Chloral hydrate, triclofos sodium, and promethazine are useful to sedate the child for radioimaging and neurophysiology studies. Tissue biopsies and diagnostic procedures such as gastrointestinal endoscopy are best performed after the administration of midazolam with or without ketamine. There is a synergistic effect when midazolam is coadministered with ketamine. Apart from relieving pain, ketamine has the added advantage to produce amnesia. Opioids are used for emergency room suturing and dressing, intubation and for relief of postoperative pain.

PAIN ABDOMEN

Abdominal pain is one of the most common symptoms in children. The pain may be acute and sudden in onset or child may complain of pain off and on over a period of time.

Acute Pain Abdomen

Pain abdomen due to sudden onset and short duration may occur due to infection or inflammation of any organ of abdomen or spasm of a hollow organ (intestinal colic, renal colic, biliary colic). The pain starts suddenly and may be associated with fever, vomiting, diarrhea or constipation, loss of appetite, inability to void urine or dysuria, jaundice, etc. During evaluation of acute abdominal pain, ask site or location of pain, severity and character, timing in relation to food, radiation of pain and associated symptoms like fever, vomiting, bowel disturbances, urinary symptoms, and jaundice. In acute appendicitis, pain usually starts at the epigastrium (above the naval) and then it moves to the right lower quadrant (iliac region) of the abdomen. Pain is usually associated with fever, loss of appetite and vomiting. The common causes of acute abdominal pain are listed in **Box 31.3**.

Recurrent Pain Abdomen

This is a common problem in school-going children. When episodes of abdominal pain occur frequently over a period of 3 months, they are called recurrent abdominal pains. The pain is vague, mild and is usually pointed vaguely to the mid-abdomen area (over the umbilicus) by the child. Pain lasts for a brief period, child is generally well, takes his food normally and plays around but every now and then complains of momentary episodes of abdominal pain. The pain may be due to a prank by the child to miss the school or avoid drinking milk. Some children may have genuine abdominal pain and flatulence after drinking milk due to deficiency of lactase (lactose intolerance). Children with psychogenic pain may have pain at multiple sites of body like headache, chest pain and pain in the limbs. Many children identify themselves with other family members (especially their mother) and start complaining of similar or identical symptoms. These children are otherwise healthy and active, feeding and playing normally. They do not have any other associated symptoms referable either to the bowels or urinary system. The above mentioned symptom complex is due to functional or psychological abdominal pain **(Box 31.4)**.

The common physical causes of recurrent abdominal pain in children include worm infestation, giardiasis,

31

> **Box 31.3** **Common causes of acute abdominal pain**

Gastrointestinal system
Gastroesophageal reflux disease (GERD), dyspepsia, peptic ulcer disease, enteritis, colitis, inflammatory bowel disease, irritable bowel syndrome, diverticulitis, appendicitis, necrotizing enterocolitis, helminthiasis or giardiasis, intestinal obstruction, constipation, food allergy, lactose intolerance, over eating and dietary indiscretion.

Hepatobiliary system
Hepatitis, liver abscess, congestive hepatomegaly, bile stone, choledochal cyst, cholecystitis.

Genitourinary system
Urinary tract infection, nephritis, hydronephrosis, calculus, dysmenorrhea, oophoritis or orchitis, ovarian or testicular torsion, ectopic pregnancy.

Pancreas
Acute pancreatitis, pancreatic stone.

Spleen
Splenitis, infarction (sickle cell disease), infective endocarditis, hydatid cyst, trauma.

Miscellaneous conditions
Mesenteric adenitis, Henoch-Schonlein disease, collagen vascular disorder, diabetic ketoacidosis, lead toxicity, acute intermittent porphyria, abdominal migraine, visceral epilepsy.

Referred pain
Spinal tumor, pleurisy and basal pneumonia.

Psychogenic or functional pain

> **Box 31.4** **Common features of psychological abdominal pain**

- Vague, mild and brief episodes of pain abdomen usually during the daytime.
- Pain mostly occurs at home but not in school or during playtime.
- Pain may occur in relation to meal times as a prank or attention seeking behavior.
- Child does not cry due to pain.
- Pain is pointed by the whole hand vaguely over mid-abdomen.
- There may be associated aches and pains over the head, chest, limbs, etc.
- Child is active, playful and has normal appetite.
- There are no other associated symptoms pertaining to bowels or urinary system.

urinary tract infection, gastroesophageal reflux, dyspepsia, peptic ulcer disease, etc. The pain may occur due to excessive food indulgence, food allergy or milk intolerance. There may be associated symptoms like nausea, vomiting, retrosternal burning sensation, loose

motions or frequency of micturition, and failure to thrive. The child may wake up at night due to pain and pain is usually severe enough to make the child uncomfortable or cry. The pain may be located at a site other than mid-abdomen and is generally pointed by the child with his finger tip rather than the whole hand. The characteristics of organic abdominal pain are listed in **Box 31.5**.

Treatment

In large majority of children, recurrent abdominal pain is due to functional or psychological reasons. It may be due to anxiety, an emotional upset or merely an attention or advantage seeking behavior. It may be a feigning behavior or prank by the child to miss school or avoid milk or skip early beakfast. The child may be sympathesizing or identifying himself with the mother or father who may have a similar problem. Parents should avoid talking about their own symptoms or illness in front of kids. Children are very sensitive and they can easily sense any tension among the parents

Practical Tip

When abdominal pain is momentary and vague, pointed with the whole hand placed over the navel, it is likely to be functional. When the site of pain is pointed with a finger and is further away from the umbilicus, it is more likely to have an organic cause.

and express it through their physical symptoms. Parents should try to identify any adverse psychological factors in the family dynamics or at school which may be the root cause of his abdominal pain. Avoid undertaking unnecessary investigations unless symptoms complex suggests the possibility of a physical or an organic cause.

A policy of "intelligent neglect", distraction, denial of any secondary gain or advantage (like missing the school or sleeping with parents), "suggestion" and use

> **Box 31.5** **Features suggestive of organic abdominal pain**

- Child winces or cries due to pain.
- Child may wake up at night due to abdominal pain.
- The episodes of pain may last for several minutes or hours.
- Associated symptoms like nausea, vomiting, loose motions, constipation, urinary symptoms, and loss of appetite, are common.
- The location of pain is usually at a site other than mid-abdomen and is pointed out by the child with his finger (rather than whole hand).
- There are no aches and pains in other parts of the body.

of inoccuous home remedies (like *pudin hara* or *ajwain*) or antispasmodic medicines are useful for management of recurrent abdominal pain due to psychological causes. Identification and modification of adverse underlying psychological dynamics would provide long-lasting relief. Although worm infestation is common in our country but it is unwise and unnecessary to deworm the child whenever he complains of abdominal pain.

APPENDICITIS

Appendicitis is caused by inflammation of appendix but predisposing factors are not well recognized. It may occur at any age but the condition is more common in adolescents and young adults. There may be hereditary predisposition in certain families.

Clinical Features

The classical features are abdominal pain, vomiting and fever of acute onset. The pain usually starts from upper abdomen (epigastric region) and then moves over to the McBurney's point in the right iliac fossa which is located at the junction of outer two-thirds with inner one-third of the line joining the iliac crest with umbilicus. Pain is associated with vomiting, anorexia and moderate fever. When a child with abdominal pain can jump down from the examination table, he is unlikely to have acute appendicitis.

The child looks sick and toxic with tenderness at the McBurney's point. When surgery is delayed, appendix may rupture and produce an appendicular lump and at times peritonitis. Laboratory support is provided by polymorphonuclear leukocytosis and ultrasound examination of abdomen.

Treatment

The child is kept nil orally and administered intravenous fluids and antibiotics while preparations are made for surgery. Appendicectomy is done by conventional method or with the help of a laparoscope. If appendix has ruptured and a lump has formed, the patient is treated conservatively by bed rest, Ryle's tube aspiration, intravenous fluids and antibiotics. After recovery, the child is taken for elective appendicectomy after 6 weeks of conservative treatment.

Nursing Care

1. Provide emotional support to the family and allay the fear and anxiety of the child regarding surgery.
2. The child should be kept nil orally and vital signs monitored. Any deterioration in the condition of the child, worsening of pain and abdominal distension should be reported to the surgeon.

3. After surgery, early ambulation is encouraged. Oral fluids are started on the next day followed by semisolids as the child feels comfortable, passes wind and there are audible peristaltic sounds in the abdomen.

INTUSSUSCEPTION

Intussusception, as the name signifies, is invagination or entry of a part of the proximal gut into the adjoining distal gut leading to acute intestinal obstruction. The most common site of intussusception is ileocolic but it may occur at any site. The exact cause is unknown but it may follow acute diarrhea or localized inflammation or lymphoid tissue enlargement in the gut. The first generation oral rotavirus vaccine was withdrawn due to occurrence of intussusception as an adverse effect.

Clinical Features

The disease is more common in first born male infant. The classical manifestations include onset of acute diarrhea followed by sudden cessation of diarrhea, episodes of inconsolable crying due to intestinal colic with passage of blood-stained currant-jelly stools. The right lower quadrant of abdomen may feel empty while a sausage-shaped mass may be felt in the right upper quadrant of epigastrium. In advanced cases, the invaginating gut (intussusceptum) may be felt on rectal examination. When diagnosis is delayed there is vomiting which becomes bile-stained with progressive distension of abdomen. Infant may look sick, toxic and dehydrated. In late stages, gangrene and perforation of gut may occur. Skiagram of abdomen in upright position shows air fluid levels. Ultrasound examination of abdomen is diagnostic.

Treatment

1. Nasogastric tube is inserted to decompress the abdomen and infant kept nil orally.
2. Intravenous fluids are administered to correct dehydration and electrolyte imbalance.
3. Vital signs, abdominal girth and urine output are monitored.
4. In an early case without any complications, medical management is attempted with a barium or saline enema under ultrasound guidance.
5. When medical treatment fails or infant has associated complications, laparotomy is done and intussusception is reduced. When gangerene has set in, excision of gut with end-to-end anastomosis is done.

31

31

PEPTIC ULCER

Peptic ulcer is uncommon in children but may occur in school-going children and adolescents. Ulcer develops in the second part of duodenum due to imbalance between pepsin, acid and enzymes of stomach. It is caused by an infection with bacteria called *Helicobacter pylori*. It is aggravated by intake of spicy, fried foods, pickles, chocolates, cola drinks, tea and coffee, etc. Stress, anxiety and worry are recognized aggravating factors. The common symptoms are dyspepsia, bloating, burning pain in the upper abdomen and behind the chest bone. The symptoms may occur during sleep due to gastroesophageal reflux and when stomach is empty.

Treatment

Dyspepsia and burning sensation are usually relieved by taking cold water, milk, yoghurt, bland food and antacids. Intake of spices, chillies, fried food, smoking, cola drinks, tea and coffee should be avoided. Avoid intake of aspirin, ibuprofen and other NSAIDs which are known to increase the severity of hyperacidity and may cause upper GI bleeding. Paracetamol is the drug of first choice for treatment of fever and pain in these children. Symptomatic relief is obtained by intake of antacids, sucralfate and ranitidine. *Helicobacter pylori* should be treated with specific drugs like amoxycillin, tinidazole and omeperazole.

EXCESSIVE CRYING

In young children, cry is the only signal or language to express their need and draw attention to their discomfort, hunger and painful or unpleasant conditions. Periodic crying in infants is most commonly due to hunger, thirst, uncomfortable environment, over or under clothing, wet nappies and boredom. An intelligent and perceptive mother and nurse can differentiate between the cry due to hunger and cry as a signal of discomfort. Most parents are quite used to episodic crying of their infants but persistent or protracted and inconsolable crying is frightening to parents and should be handled with urgency and sensitivity.

Causes

Excessive crying and restlessness most commonly occurs due to benign physiological conditions. Inconsolable crying may occur due to a painful condition originating from any of the body system (Box 31.6). Detailed history should be elicited to identify preceding events and associated symptoms. Presence of fever suggests underlying infective condition. The child should be carefully examined from "top-to-toes"

Box 31.6   **Causes of excessive crying in infants**

Central nervous system
Raised intracranial pressure due to meningitis/encephalitis, bleeding, space occupying lesion, brain-damaged infant.

Cardiovascular system
Arrhythmias, congestive heart failure, veno-occlusive disorder.

Respiratory system
Blocked nose, acute suppurative otitis media, pneumonia, bronchospasm.

Gastrointestinal system
Aphthous ulcers, herpangina, hand-foot-mouth disease, intestinal colic, mesenteric adenitis, gastroesophageal reflux disease, appendicitis, incarcerated hernia, intussusception, pinworms.

Genitourinary system
Urinary tract infection, renal colic, torsion of testis, orchitis and oophoritis

Musculoskeletal system
Unrecognized trauma, dislocation of elbow or shoulder, osteomyelitis or arthritis, scurvy.

Miscellaneous conditions
Temper tantrums, insect bites, open diaper pin, DTwP vaccine, foreign body in the eye or nose, poisoning, drugs.

---

after taking off all the clothes to exclude common conditions like intestinal colic, inflammatory condition, unrecognized trauma (nursemaid's elbow), diaper rash, incarcerated or obstructed hernia or torsion of testis. Most crying infants are quietened and consoled when picked up or gently rocked. When crying is precipitated or aggravated when baby is picked up, it is suggestive of a painful condition in the musculoskeletal system. Night crying is common in infants and is most disturbing and troublesome not only to tired parents but also to the neighbors. The common causes of night crying include "evening colic", nasal congestion, diaper rash, pinworms, insect bites, gastroesophageal reflux disease (GERD) and bronchospasm. In about two-thirds of cases, cause of excessive crying can be indentified by taking good history and conducting detailed physical examination.

Laboratory investigations are rarely required and should be planned depending upon the clues obtained on clinical assessment.

Management

Child should be provided comfort by holding, rocking and cuddling. Symptomatic relief should be provided when serious life-threatening conditions have been excluded. Analgesics like paracetamol and ibuprofen are useful for relief of pain due to inflammatory and traumatic conditions of musculoskeletal system. Application of asafetida (*hing*) around navel, decoction of carom seeds (*ajwain*) and anethi seeds (*sonf*); and antispasmodics are useful for relief of intestinal colic. Specific management depends upon the underlying cause of crying. Several severe or life-threatening disorders like intestinal obstruction, incarcerated hernia, torsion of testis, appendicitis and intussusception would need urgent surgical intervention.

BIBLIOGRAPHY

Cote CJ, Wilson S. American Academy of Pediatrics, Working Group on Sedation. Guidelines for monitoring and management of pediatric patients during and after sedation for diagnostic and therapeutic procedures: an update. *Pediatrics* 2006; 118(6): 2587–2602.

Devanarayana NM, Rajindrajith S, De Silva HJ. Recurrent abdominal pain in children. *Indian Pediatr* 2009; 46(5): 389–399.

Harnden A. Antipyretic treatment for feverish young children in primary care (Editorial). *Brit Med J* 2008; 337: 1409.

Singh M. Symptomatic management of fever in children: A rational approach. *Indian J Pract Pediatr* 1999; 1: 75–80.

Singh M. Pain in children: practical issues and concerns. *Indian J Pract Pediatr* 2001; 3: 146–149.

Sullivan JE, Farrar HC. Section on Clinical Pharmacology and Therapeutics Committee on Drugs. Fever and antipyretic use in children. *Pediatrics* 2011; 127(3): 580–587.

31

Common Disorders of Skin

Skin is the largest organ of the body and provides a protective covering. Skin manifestations may be localized (contact dermatitis, eczema, acne, insect bites, etc.) or generalized throughout the body (viral or bacterial infections, autoimmune disorders, drug allergy, urticaria, etc.). Insect bites and allergic reactions are characterized by itching. Inflammation and exudation are seen in association with eczema and infections. Skin lesions are classified into the following subtypes depending upon their clinical morphology.

Types of Skin Lesions

Macules It is circumscribed lesion of the skin, not raised above the surface. It may be an area of redness or erythema, depigmented (pale) or pigmented (dark brown or black) patch on the skin.

Mole A pigmentary nevus is called a mole.

Freckles They are small, less than 1.5 cm, discrete brown macules that appear on the sun-exposed areas of skin. The condition is inherited as an autosomal dominant trait in light-skinned red-haired individuals. They are commonly seen on the face, trunk, upper shoulders, sparing the mucous membranes.

Papules A circumscribed pinhead sized compact lesion raised above the surface of skin is called a papule. When it is large in size, it is called as a nodule or a tumor.

Vesicles A circumscribed skin lesion or a small blister containing clear fluid like a dew-drop is called a vesicle. Large vesicles are called blisters or bullae.

Cysts The circumscribed tumors containing semisolid or fluid contents are called cysts. The typical examples include epidermal cyst, dermoid cyst, sebaceous cyst and branchial cyst.

Pustules When a vesicle or blister is filled with pus, it is called a pustule. When pus collects in the subcutaneous tissues, it is called an abscess. Pyogenic bacteria produce an abscess with all signs of inflammation (redness, warmth and pain) while tubercular bacilli produce a cold abscess without any inflammatory signs.

Wheals It is characterized by a pale papule inside the dermis which is surrounded by irregular erythema or flare. The itching is marked and intense.

Petechiae Pin-head-sized macules due to extravasated blood are called petechiae. They cannot be blanched on pressure.

Purpura The large areas of extravasated blood under the skin are called purpura or ecchymoses. They are seen as reddish or blue patches which cannot be blanched by pressure with a finger or glass slide. They may be flat or slightly raised above the surface.

Cradle Cap

Some newborn babies develop a brown crust on the top of their scalp. This forms due to collection of natural secretions of hair follicles and skin (sebum) of the scalp. It is a form of dandruff. There is nothing special that needs to be done and it gradually disappears by daily shampooing and brushing the scalp. Do not try to forcibly remove it. Mother can apply some milk cream or coconut oil and shampoo the scalp every day with savlon after 15–20 minutes. The crusts will gradually come off with washing and gentle brushing but it may take several days or weeks to completely resolve. No oil should be applied on the scalp after shampooing the hair.

Dandruff (Seborrhea, *roosi*)

Dandruff is very common in children who have oily skin. The follicles of scalp hair secrete an excess of oily material (sebum) which dries up to form whitish flakes on the hair of scalp. At times, even eye brows and eye lashes may show white flakes of dandruff. There is itching over the scalp. The hair should be washed daily with a shampoo. Do not apply any oil over the scalp hair. The comb or brush should be washed frequently and should not be shared by anybody else. If dandruff persists, a medicated shampoo containing savlon and antifungal agents (2% ketoconazole) should be used.

Perianal Soreness

Perianal soreness or redness around anus is common in bottle fed babies especially following a bout of diarrhea. Anal soreness and itching at night may occur due to threadworms. Other causes of anal itching include constipation, anal fissure, rectal prolapse, fungal infection, amebiasis and insertion of foreign body. After the passage of stools, baby should be cleaned lightly and gently with wet cotton. Keeping the baby in a prone position and exposing the buttocks to the air (preferably sun light) in a warm room is followed by prompt recovery. Mother can apply a zinc oxide containing baby cream or a bland oil (coconut oil) which hastens recovery. Never apply mustard oil which can produce severe irritation in the perianal area.

Nappy Rash (Diaper rash)

The common form of rash at the bottom affects areas covered by the diaper but often spares the creases of the groins. The affected skin becomes red and thickened. The rash occurs due to maceration of the skin caused by a prolonged contact with a wet and

> ### Practical Tip
> *Soakable diaper should be worn only during social visits or when a baby has diarrhea. Routine use of diaper or plastic covered napkin at home is an important cause of nappy rash.*

soiled nappy. The use of a tight fitting rubber or plastic panties and soakable diapers is the main culprit. In boys, foreskin of penis may be severely affected causing difficulty in passing urine. When nappy rash persists for more than 3 to 4 days, superinfection with *Candida albicans* commonly occurs. Candidal infection is usually associated with erythema (redness) and pimples or vesicles over the margins of nappy rash.

> ### Practical Tip
> *Avoid excessive use of soap and water in washing the nappy area. Alcohol or antiseptic lotions should not be applied over the axillae, groins and genitalia due to smarting and risk of fungal infection.*

Treatment The soakable diaper or plastic panties should not be worn at home. The baby must be cleaned and dried immediately after passage of each urine and stool. The bottom should be kept dry as far as possible. Mother must have liberal supply of nappies so that she can change a wet nappy immediately after each voiding. The nappies should be thoroughly rinsed in water to get rid of all traces of detergent and soap. They should be sun dried and ironed to kill the germs. Keeping the baby naked and exposure of buttocks to air and sunlight is usually followed by prompt recovery. Local application of a bland oil or a soothing cream containing zinc oxide and calamine facilitates recovery. When candidal superinfection is suspected, local application of a cream containing nystatin or miconazole is followed by prompt resolution.

Eczema (Atopic dermatitis)

It is an allergic disorder of skin and can occur at any age. The exact cause is unknown but there is hereditary predisposition for skin allergy, allergic rhinits (hay fever) and bronchial asthma among family members (atopic family). It is a chronic (long lasting) condition with frequent remissions (spontaneous periods of recovery) and relapses (flare-ups). The flare-ups may occur due to exposure to various allergens like dust mites, mold, pollen of flowers, seafood, animal dander or intake of foods like milk, eggs, orange juice, nuts, soy and wheat products. Infections and skin irritants like use of soap, detergent, wool and nylon clothing may aggravate the skin condition. Emotional disturbances like anger, anxiety, frustration, and hostility are also known to trigger the condition. In infants, cheeks, wrists and extensor surfaces of arms and legs typically develop papulovesicular, often weeping or wet lesions. In older children, dry maculopapular lesions are mostly distributed over the flexor surfaces of extremities, neck, wrists and ankles. There is eosinophilia and elevation of serum IgE level. Eczema is not contagious to other siblings or family members. Breast feeding protects the child against development of eczema and disease is much less common in India than the western world.

Diagnosis In infants, skin lesions start from cheeks and forehead. There is marked redness with tiny vesicles (likes dew drops) which rupture to give wet appearance. The oozing of serum may dry up to form scabs over the surface of active skin lesions. The infant is irritable and uncomfortable due to marked itching. During recovery skin may become thick and dry because of marked scaling. Fever and pustules may appear because of superadded bacterial infection. The disease is chronic with frequent flare-ups and remissions. The skin lesions may progress to involve flexural (towards the side where joints bend) areas or

32

creases of neck, elbows, wrists, knees and ankles. The flexural areas have a greater tendency to sweating and irritation. Infants with cradle cap (seborrhea, dandruff) may develop skin manifestations which are similar to atopic dermatitis. These children do not have any allergic tendency or genetic predisposition and are likely to recover faster.

Treatment Parents should be vigilant to identify any trigger factors that aggravate the skin condition. The elimination of suspected or known trigger factors would lead to prompt recovery and complete cure. Bathe or shower the child daily with plain luke warm water. Do not apply any soap because they are known to irritate and dry the skin. After the bath, dab the child dry with a soft cotton towel without rubbing. Apply a moisturizer or emollient cream over the skin immediately after the bath and at night. Antihistaminics are useful for relief of itching and irritability and to provide restful sleep to the child. Antibiotics are useful when there is superadded bacterial infection. Topical corticosteroids may be used to promptly control the flare-ups. Corticosteroid cream or ointment should be applied on the affected areas once or twice daily. As soon as recovery starts, corticosteroid cream should be applied once daily (after a bath) or on alternate days for 3–4 weeks. Probiotics (lactobacilli) may be given to prevent the entry of allergens through gut. The child should wear non-irritating full-steeve dress made of pure cotton. The clothes should be thoroughly rinsed after washing to effectively remove all traces of detergent. The nails should be kept trimmed and clean to prevent skin abrasions due to itching.

Boils (Impetigo)

Children are very prone to develop superficial infection of the skin during summer and hot and humid rainy season. Boils or pyoderma occur due to excessive sweating and poor personal hygiene. They may be aggravated by eating too much sweets or mangoes. Initially red pimples develop which enlarge in size and get filled with pus. Later on, these get covered with scabs. Boils can occur at any site but are more common over skin creases (neck, armpits, groins), buttocks and legs. Fever and pain may occur when there are multiple large sized boils.

Treatment During hot and humid months child should be given a daily (preferably twice a day) bath with an antiseptic soap (dettol or savlon soap). The nails should be kept trimmed to prevent scratching of skin. The child should have a towel of his own which should not be shared by others. Local application of an antiseptic lotion (betadine, mercurochrome or gentian

violet) or an antibiotic skin cream is useful if there are few scattered skin lesions. Pain and fever can be relieved by giving paracetamol. When boils are large in size or increase in number, an appropriate antibiotic should be given. In children with recurrent episodes of pyoderma, nasal carrier of staphylococci should be eradicated by topical application of an ointment containing mupirocin or fucidin.

Prickly Heat (Miliaria rubra)

During hot and humid weather, prickly heat is common in children. The baby's skin is more delicate and skin rash appears due to retention of sweat in the sweat glands and its spillage into adjacent tissue. There is a fine maculopapular pinkish skin rash which starts from neck and front of chest and then spreads over the whole body. The child is uncomfortable due to itching.

Treatment Keep the child cool and comfortable by frequent bathing or sponging. After the bath, let the skin dry spontaneously under a fan without rubbing with a towel. The baby should be kept in a cool room with a minimum of soft cotton clothes. Local application of calamine lotion or a soothing talcum powder relieves itching.

Skin Rash

Tiny pink spots of diffuse skin rash over the trunk or whole body is common in children. A large number of viruses are known to produce skin rash or exanthemata. Certain specific viral infections like measles, German measles (Rubella) and chickenpox produce characteristic features which are described in **Chapter 18.** Skin rash especially with bleeding manifestations may occur due to life-threatening viral and bacterial infections. Transient rose spots may occur over the trunk in fair complexioned children with typhoid fever. Diffuse redness of skin (erysepalis) with a strawberry tongue and pharyngitis are characteristic features of scarlet fever. Skin rash may occur as an adverse or allergic reaction to a variety of drugs. Allergic reaction to insect bites may produced generalized skin rash (papular urticaria). Itching is common if skin rash is due to allergy. Waxing and waning type of skin rash may occur in certain auto-immune or rheumatic diseases.

Treatment When a child develops skin rash, all medications should be stopped. Viral rashes disappear spontaneously while allergic skin rash responds to oral administration of an antihistaminic. Measles, German measles and chickenpox can be prevented by timely administration of specific vaccines against them.

Urticaria (Hives, *chhapaki*)

It is an allergic manifestation of skin reaction. The child may be allergic to certain types of foods, drugs, insect bites and at times to certain infections. In many cases, no cause is found. There may be a family history of skin allergy. The child is predisposed to develop other allergic disorders like "allergic colds" (Hay fever), eczema and bronchial asthma. There is sudden development of blotchy red patches with pale papules in the centre (wheals) over the whole body. Itching is most intense making the child extremely uncomfortable. Rarely, it may be associated with swelling of larynx or wind box with breathing difficulty (stridor). The skin lesions may disappear on its own and recur on and off for several days.

Treatment If a child is taking any drug, it should be stopped immediately. There is no role of local medications. The itching and skin lesions respond to administration of antihistaminic drugs such as hydroxyzine hydrochloride, cetirizine dihydrochloride and loratadine which is a long acting selective peripheral H$_1$ antagonist. In severe cases, corticosteroids may be given for a short period. Avoid the intake of chillies and condiments. The antihistamines should be stopped gradually over a period of several days or weeks to prevent relapse.

Papular Urticaria

It is a common, intensely pruritic disorder caused by an allergic response to insect bites. The fresh lesions are papules with a punctum on an erythematous base mostly distributed over the extremities. Most cases occur in susceptible children during summer and after rainy season due to mosquito and flea bites. Excoriations and secondary infection may lead to hyperpigmentation in older lesions. Measures should be taken to prevent breeding and bites by mosquitoes. Administration of antihistamines and local application of calamine-based lotion provides relief from itching and facilitates resolution of skin lesions.

Scabies

Scabies occur due to infection by a tiny flea *Sarcoptes scabiei var hominis*. Infection occurs due to poor standards of personal hygiene. It is common to contract the infection when family visits a hill station and stays in a guest house or a substandard hotel. The child may get scabies from his classmate or during out of town school trips. When one member of the family gets scabies, it is common for others to get cross infection. The child develops small pin-sized pimples over the body especially areas with creases (neck, armpits, groin), genitalia, wrists and webs between fingers and toes. The classical lesion is a linear or S-shaped burrow, a grey thread like serpentine tunnel with a minute black dot at the end. The face is usually spared except in infants. There is marked itching which is worse at night. The disease is highly contagious and several family members are affected simultaneously.

Treatment Ensure good standard of personal hygiene to prevent scabies. Child should be given a bath every day and his underclothes changed daily. The bed sheets should be washed frequently and sun-dried. The bed may have to be placed in the scorching sun to get rid of fleas. The whole family should be treated at the same time to prevent cross infection. A number of lotions and creams containing 25% benzyl benzoate, gammabenzene hexachloride or crotamiton and permethrin 5% are available for local application. A single application at night followed by a repeat application after one week is enough. The antiscabies lotion or cream should not be applied on the face. Ivermectin 0.2 mg/kg single dose oral is a useful adjunct in children above 5 years of age. Itching may take a long time to resolve. The child may be given promethazine hydrochloride (Phenergan) or hydroxyzine hydrochloride (Atarax) for relief of itching. The nails should be kept trimmed and clean to prevent skin abrasions and superadded bacterial infection. Infected scabies is treated with a suitable antimicrobial agent followed by topical therapy. It is recommended that all household and close contacts should be treated with scabicide agent even if they do not have any overt skin lesions.

Warts

They are flat or dome shaped skin lesions with rough surface caused due to benign proliferation of the epithelium or epidermis of mucous membranes and skin by infection with human papillomavirus (HPV). Skin lesions may occur at any site but are most common at hands and feet. There is no itching.

Treatment Most warts regress spontaneously or by auto-suggestion. Local application of salicylic acid or trichloroacetic acid, electrodessication or cryosurgery is advocated for resistant cases.

Molluscum Contagiosum

It is characterized by discrete, pearly, skin-colored dome-shaped smooth papules varying in size from 2–5 mm. The center may be depressed or umbilicated. They are caused by a poxvirus and occur in clusters at any site in the body. Immunodeficient children are more vulnerable and may develop multiple or large lesions.

Treatment Molluscum contagiousm is a self-limited disease and most lesions disappear spontaneously or by auto suggestion. Topical application of liquid nitrogen or 0.9% cantharidin is useful for treatment of isolated lesions.

Lice and Nits

The presence of lice and nits in the scalp and hair is an index of the standard of personal hygiene of the child and family. These parasites are transmitted from one child to the other or from an adult infested with lice. They can also occur due to sharing of combs. Lice do not thrive on pets and do not infest furniture. There is marked itching over the scalp and you can see the nits (eggs of lice) as shining white particles on the hair. The lice may be seen sticking on the comb or they may fall on the ground during combing.

Treatment Shampoo and comb the hair daily and maintain a good standard of personal hygiene. Some lice and nits can be removed by combing with a fine-bristled comb. Many preparations with DDT and lorexane are available and they can be applied. Shampoos containing permethrin or pyrethrins (perlice lotion) are useful. After shampoo when hair are still wet, thoroughly apply perlice lotion. After half an hour, rinse the scalp with water and comb the hair with a fine-bristled comb. Care should be taken to prevent the entry of these medicines into the eyes. Ivermectin 0.2 mg/kg single dose oral is a useful adjunt, in children above 5 years of age.

Acne Vulgaris (Pimples, *keel muhanse*)

Acne vulgaris is a polymorphic eruption that occurs due to increased secretion of sex hormones during adolescence. It is a self-limited inflammatory disorder of pilosebaceous glands with excessive secretion of sebum. The common predisposing factors include genetic predisposition, level of androgens and emotional stress. Seborrhea of the scalp and face due to excessive secretion of sebum may coexist. It is slightly more common in boys than girls. The common aggravating factors include oily skin, eating imbalanced diet, having too much sugars and chocolates and humid weather. Intake of certain drugs like steroids, androgens, antitubercular agents and anticonvulsants may induce and aggravate acne. Pimples, black heads (comedones), nodules and pustules form on the fore-head and face. In severe cases lesions may occur over upper back and shoulders especially in boys.

Treatment Wash the face with soap and water several times in a day. Do not apply any cosmetics and moisturizer cream over the face. The skin lesions should not be touched or squeezed as it may lead to formation of unsightly pitted scars. Oral intake and topical application of erythromycin, tetracycline or clindamycin are recommended. Topical retinoids and 5% benzyl peroxide cream should be applied on the face at night. Patient should be advised to take a balanced diet with plenty of fresh green leafy vegetables and fruits.

Dermatophytoses or Ringworm

Dermatophytoses are superficial skin infections caused by fungi. Fungi thrive in the keratin layer of skin at sites which are moist and wet. The typical skin lesion is ring-shaped coin-sized red-colored plaque with pupules at the elevated border. The central area shows clearing with thin scabs. Itching is marked. Depending upon the site of lesion, ringworm is classified as tinea capitis (scalp), tinea corporis (body), tinea cruris (groins and upper thigh), tinea pedis (foot) and tinea unguium (nails).

Treatment Ensure strict personal hygiene and avoid sharing of towels, caps and scarves. Topical application of antifungal creams (clotrimazole 1% or miconazole 2% or ketoconazole) twice a day for 2–4 weeks is curative. Systemic therapy with griseofulvin or flucona-zole or ketoconazole or terbinafine is recommended for 8–12 weeks for treatment of fungal infection of scalp, feet and nails.

Pityriasis Versicolor

The condition is caused by a commensal yeast, *M. furfur*. It is characterized by perifollicular scaly (pityriasis refers to scales) macular skin lesions with variable pigmentation (hypopigmented, brownish or erythematous) in adolescent children. The fine branny scales are aggravated by gentle scratching with a glass slide. The lesions are typically distributed over the neck, front of chest and proximal parts of upper extremities. Topical therapy with ketoconazole or terbinafine or selenium sulfide lotion is curative.

Pityriasis Alba

There are ill-defined hypopigmented macules with fine scales on the face of preschool children. The lesions are asymptomatic and clear up spontaneously. Many parents wrongly believe them to be a marker of worm infestation or a deficiency disorder. The etiology is unknown but they are often ascribed to infection by *Staphylococcus albus*. Mother is asked to scrub the face with soap and water at least twice a day followed by application of an antibiotic cream and mild emollients. It may take one month for the lesions to resolve.

32

Acrodermatitis Enteropathica

It is a rare disorder of zinc transport due to defective gene located on chromosome 8q24.3. Breast milk contains compensatory zinc-binding ligand that facilitates absorption of zinc. The manifestations start after 1–2 weeks of weaning from breastfeeding. It is characterized by triad of acrodermatitis (peripheral or acral parts of the extremities) with special predilection of body orifices, diarrhea and alopecia.

It is characterized by eczematous scaly skin rash which becomes vesicular, bullous, pustular or desquamative, involving peripheral parts of extremities, perioral and anogenital areas. There may be superadded bacterial or fungal infection. Serum zinc level and alkaline phosphatase activity are low. The condition is managed by administration of optimal nutrition, control of superadded bacterial and fungal infections and supplements of zinc (1–2 mg/kg/d elemental zinc in two divided doses) for one month.

BIBLIOGRAPHY

George A, Rubin G. A systematic review and meta-analysis of treatments for impetigo. *Brit J Genl Pract* 2003, 53: 480–487.

Gibbs S, Harvey I, Sterling JC, Stark R. Local treatments for cutaneous warts: Systematic review. *Brit Med J* 2002, 325: 461.

Gibbs S, Harvey I, Sterling JC, Stark R. Local treatments for cutaneous warts. *Cochrane Database Syst Rev* 2003, (3): CDO01781.

Higgins EM, Fullar LC, Smith CH. Guidelines for the management of tinea capitis. *Brit J Dermatol* 2000, 143: 53–58.

Sladden MJ, Johnston GA. Common skin infections in children. *Brit Med J* 2004, 329(7457): 95–99.

32

Teething and Oral Health

Teething is a physiological process and is not expected to cause any significant problems in the child. Some babies are born with a tooth, which is considered as a bad omen without any basis. If a natal tooth is loose, it should be removed because of risk of aspiration. Milk teeth start erupting anytime during 6–9 months of age but in some babies they may be delayed upto first birth day or even later. The delayed teething in healthy babies is usually due to familial or hereditary reasons. When teething is delayed in a child, ask for family history of delayed eruption of teeth. Teething is not delayed either due to nutritional factors or developmental retardation. Teething should not be used as a milestone of neuromotor development. When eruption of teeth is delayed beyond the age of one year, rickets, cretinism and hypopituitarism should be ruled out. Non-eruption of any tooth (anodontia) is a classical feature of ectodermal dysplasia.

Common Symptoms due to Teething

Historically every ailment has been ascribed to teething. According to Indian folklore, teething has been blamed to cause fever, common cold, severe diarrhea, convulsions and even death! *The truth is that teething is a harmless physiological process and is not associated with any serious health consequences.* Teething may be associated with irritability, drooling of saliva and mouthing, i.e. child putting his fingers or every object in his mouth. Drooling may cause skin rash or dryness over the angles of the mouth and chin. These symptoms are due to irritation of the gums when tooth is erupting. The child may become irritable, cranky and refuse to take his food. Discomfort is worse when child is cutting his first tooth or molars (around 1 year). At times the toddler may touch or pull at his ear because pain of tooth eruption may be referred to the ear. Teething is never a cause of watery diarrhea or fever. However, in some infants, the stool frequency may increase (say from 1 to 2 stools/day, it may go up to 3–4 stools/day) and they may become green in color. The child may wake up more often at night due to discomfort. He needs to be comforted, cuddled and solaced. A large majority of children, however, do not manifest any "teething troubles" and teeth erupt as a matter of routine.

The eruption of milk teeth continues during the age of 6 months to 2½ years. During this period, the inquisitive and restless toddler is likely to put many dirty things in his mouth, i.e. soiled fingers, small objects, nibbled food particles, toys, etc. which may lead to development of watery diarrhea due to infection. This should never be ascribed to teething. Infact, whenever a child is genuinely sick, it should never be attributed to teething and child should be examined for an underlying disorder.

Nursing Care

There is no medicine which is known to promote or facilitate teething though practically every mother gives homeopathic medicine calcaria phos! The child should be given soft nutritious home-made weaning foods with sufficient intake of calcium (milk and milk products), vitamin D (fats, oils, exposure to sunlight) and vitamin A (green leafy vegetables and yellow colored fruits). A number of teething powders and syrups are advertised but they have no proven utility. Due to irritation of gums, the baby likes to chew on a rubber ring or plastic toys. Avoid giving toys having small, loose parts which can dislodge and cause aspiration. The toys should not be made of brittle plastic material which a child may chew into small bits and get choked. Alternatively, a big piece of hard biscuit, rusk, toast or a cold peeled carrot can be given to the child to chew. If a child is cranky and irritable, he can be given a safe analgesic like paracetamol and/or a sedative like phenergan. Mother can apply teething gel containing a mild local anesthetic over the swollen gums with her finger. Just rubbing or massaging the swollen gums with index finger (after washing hands with soap and water) may provide comfort and relief.

DENTITION

Teeth buds are formed as early as 6 weeks of intrauterine life. The human dentition, like most of the mammals, consists of two generations of teeth. The first generation is known as the deciduous or temporary dentition (milk teeth) and the second as the permanent dentition. The logic for two sets of dentition is based on the fact that the jaw of the infant is small and it can accommodate only a limited number of teeth. Since teeth once formed cannot increase in size, a second set of dentition consisting of larger-sized and greater number of teeth is required to fill the bigger jaw of the older child.

Milk teeth (primary or temporary or deciduous teeth) The time of eruption of milk teeth is in accordance with genetic clock. In some families, children erupt their teeth by 6 months of age while in others it may be delayed till the first birth day. Delayed or early dentition are not related to the nutritional or developmental status of the child. It is not unusual to see a healthy and chubby infant without any tooth by 9 months or 1 year of age because his parents cut their teeth late. In general, eruption of teeth in the lower jaw (mandible) usually precede the dentition in the upper jaw (maxilla). The teeth in both the jaws appear in pairs, one on either side. The lower central incisors are usually the first teeth to erupt around 6 months of age. Subsequently, the child on an average would gain one tooth every month (for example 1 year old child is likely to have 6 teeth, if first tooth erupted at 6 months) till the complete set of 20 milk teeth has erupted by the age of 2 to 2½ years **(Table 33.1)**. Milk teeth are white in color and have a smooth edge. They can be kept clean with a wet piece of gauze or damp cloth after feedings. If milk teeth are well looked after, it is more likely that the permanent teeth will grow in their correct position. Mother should avoid giving a bottle feed or fruit juice during sleep as it may facilitate the process of tooth decay. Occasionally milk teeth may erupt in a crooked fashion but generally it has no adverse implications for eruption of permanent teeth.

Permanent teeth In school-going children, milk teeth are shed followed by eruption of permanent teeth. The first molars of permanent teeth appear at the age of 6 years (without loss of any deciduous teeth) and are called as "6 years molars". There is no pain or discomfort when a tooth is shed. In order to console the child, as a ritual the shed tooth is often hidden under the pillow and replaced by a tiny toy as a gift by the fairy. Around 6 years of age central incisors and first molars are shed to make place for eruption of permanent teeth. During 9–13 years, due to eruption of permanent canines, the teeth in the centre of upper jaw become crowded giving an appearance of "ugly duckling". Mother should not be worried about this temporary physiological phenomenon because in due course of time the teeth become well aligned. By the age of 12–13 years, a set of 28 permanent teeth are usually well in place. Third molars or wisdom teeth do not erupt in all individuals but only in some by the age of 17–22 years. Eruption of wisdom teeth may be associated with discomfort and pain due to constraints of space in the jaw. In contrast to milk teeth, permanent teeth are ivory-white or off-white in color and have a finely serrated edge. Parents should inculcate good habits, early in life, to ensure that children maintain their teeth and gums in good condition **(Box 33.1)**.

Brownish Staining of Teeth

Pearly white well-aligned teeth are an asset and owner's pride. The foundation of teeth is laid in the mother's womb at 6 weeks of fetal life. Good health and nutrition of the mother during pregnancy lays a sound foundation for baby's teeth. Intake of tetracyclines during pregnancy should be avoided as it may get

33

	Milk teeth		Permanent teeth*	
Teeth	Lower jaw	Upper jaw	Lower jaw	Upper jaw
Central incisors	5–7 months	6–8 months	6–7 years	7–8 years
Lateral incisors	7–10 months	8–11 months	7–8 years	8–9 years
Canines	16–20 months	16–20 months	9–11 years	11–12 years
First premolars	—	—	10–12 years	10–11 years
Second premolars	—	—	11–13 years	10–12 years
First molars	10–16 months	10–16 months	6–7 years	6–7 years
Second molars	20–30 months	20–30 months	12–13 years	12–13 years
Third molars	—	—	17–22 years	17–22 years

Table 33.1 Eruption of teeth

* Before permanent teeth erupt, the milk teeth are shed

 **Tips to keep teeth healthy and sparkling**

- Establish the habit of regular brushing of teeth twice a day after the age of 2 years.
- Avoid bottle feeding while the toddler is asleep.
- Avoid giving tinned juices and fizzy drinks.
- Do not give chocolates and candies as rewards. Color-free and sugar-free chewing gum is teeth-friendly and acceptable alternative after 4–5 years.
- Encourage eating of a crunchy fruit (apple, guava, pear) after meals and after "sweet encounters".
- When a colored medicine (like iron) is given follow it with a bite of crunchy fruit or vegetable (apple, carrot, cucumber) or by few sips of water as a safeguard against discoloration of teeth.
- Caries of primary teeth should not be ignored and must be treated for the sake of health and alignment of permanent teeth.
- The age old Indian custom of rinsing the mouth after meals or snacks should be encouraged.
- Consult a dentist every 6 months!

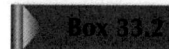 **Correct method of brushing the teeth***

- Hold the tooth brush just under the gum line at an angle of 45°. Gently jiggle the brush (short jerky up and down and to and fro motions) or move it in tiny circles over the teeth and gums. Brushing for 2 minutes is adequate.
- Use tip of the tooth brush to brush the insides of each tooth both in the upper and lower jaw with same jiggling movements.
- Use light back and forth motions to brush the chewing surfaces of upper and lower teeth.
- Gently brush the tongue. Avoid the use of a sharp metal tongue cleaner.
- Massage the gums with your fingers after brushing.
- School-going children should be taught flossing of teeth (cleaning the gaps in-between the teeth with a thread).

*Avoid the use of a hard brush. It is not so much the brand of tooth paste but the correct technique of brushing which is more important to have trouble-free teeth.

deposited in the tooth buds leading to premanent yellow staining of teeth. Children should not be given tetracyclines during first 8 years of life due to risk of yellow-staining of permanent teeth. Poor orodental hygiene and intake of colored medications (especially iron containing syrups) may cause brownish discoloration of teeth. When a child is given oral iron or any other colored medication, it should be followed by sips of water or intake of a crunchy fruit like an apple or pear. The enamel of teeth may become mottled and brown in color if the flouride content of water is high (>2 parts per million). Severe jaundice during newborn period may cause yellow staining of permanent teeth.

Care of Teeth and Gums

Children need healthy, well aligned, sparkling white teeth for chewing, clarity of speech and a charming smile. Teeth care should begin as soon as the milk teeth start erupting. Mother can clean the teeth of her baby with a gauze piece rolled around her index finger. After 2 years, baby tooth brush with extra soft bristles can be used (Box 33.2). A bright colored brush with favourite cartoon characters is more readily accepted by the child. During preschool years, mother should brush the teeth twice a day, morning and before going to bed. It is convenient for the mother to place the baby's head on her lap so that she can see his teeth better. She should use the correct circular movements so that healthy habit of brushing teeth is established. Use a tiny bit of

fluoride-free tooth paste so that there is no harm even if it is swallowed by the baby. There is no need to use a fluoride-rich tooth paste because in several parts in India, the fluoride content of water is high. Due to tropical climate, we also tend to drink lot of water. Moreover, tea and certain spices like cumin seeds (*jeera*), turmeric (*haldi*) and black pepper are rich in fluoride. Baking soda or common salt has no virtue to keep the teeth white and shining.

The correct technique of brushing teeth is more important than the use of any specific brand of tooth paste but it should have a pleasant acceptable taste. The child should not have any foul breath. Avoid use of battery-operated brushes. The child should not do any pranks or run around with a tooth brush dangling in his mouth, because it may cause serious injury to the oral cavity. Eating fruits with a hard pulp (apple, guava, pear, etc.) after a meal is useful to "floss out" food debris stuck inbetween the teeth. The age-old practice of rinsing the mouth after every meal must be promoted. It effectively removes food particles, starches and sugars which are known to cause proliferation of germs. When a child is given any sweet or a colored medicine like iron tonic, it should be followed by a sip of water as a safeguard against discoloration of teeth. Dental care and maintenance of good orodental hygiene are associated with several health benefits. There is evidence to suggest that chronic infection or inflammation of gums is a risk factor for adverse pregnancy outcomes (intrauterine growth restriction), coronary artery disease, respiratory infection, rheumatoid arthritis and type 2 diabetes mellitus.

Caries and Cavities

When teeth and gums are not kept properly cleaned, bacteria and food particles combine with saliva to form a sticky material called dental plaque that sticks to surfaces of teeth. Bacterial growth (*Streptococcus mutans*) is facilitated when oral cavity is loaded with starchy food and sugars (chocolates, sweets, soft drinks, fruit juices, etc.). Giving a bottle feed or fruit juice to the child during sleep is not advised due to potential risk of causing caries. If plaque is not removed and there is continued growth of bacteria and production of acid, it dissolves the mineral content of teeth (enamel and dentin) leading to development of caries and formation of cavities. There may be tooth ache with swelling and bleeding of gums. Caries teeth is an important cause of bad breath and bad taste in the mouth. It may lead to formation of tooth abscess, headache, and even sepsis. There is recent evidence to suggest that decay of teeth and diseases of gums are associated with increased risk of heart disease later in life. The help of a dentist must be sought for proper management of the affected teeth and prevention of its further spread to other teeth. In children, dental appointment should preferably be sought in the morning when child is fresh after a good night's sleep because he is likely to be tired and irritable in the evening.

It is often argued about the need for treating the carious milk teeth because they are going to eventually fall off and get replaced by the permanent teeth. But it is recommended that they must be treated for two reasons. Firstly they are used for biting and chewing food for 5–6 years and secondly early loss of milk teeth may deform the jaw with a possibility of malocclusion of permanent teeth.

Malocclusion of Teeth

Normally upper jaw teeth are located a little in front of lower jaw teeth. In certain families, this difference may be more pronounced and upper jaw may look over-hanging and prominent while chin looks a bit receding. At times chin may be prominent and just forwards while upper lip seems to recede. These are developmental or familial variations producing some cosmetic characteristics but without causing any difficulty in eating, chewing or biting. Rarely, prolonged thumb sucking may cause dental malocclusion. When teeth do not erupt in a symmetrical manner and they are too crowded and malaligned or they tend to protrude out, the help of a dental surgeon (orthodontist) must be sought for timely bracing and alignment. Orthodontic treatment is started after the age of 14 years when jaw is fully developed and 12-year molars have erupted. When management is delayed or ignored it may cause a lot of embarrassment to the child later in life.

Avulsion of Tooth

Tooth may get knocked out of the mouth by an injury or accident. Nothing needs to be done if it is a temporary tooth, because its place will be taken up by the permanent tooth in due course of time. When a permanent tooth is knocked out, it can be reimplanted if proper precautions are taken. Hold the tooth by its crown (the part which is visible in the mouth or used for chewing) under the running tap to wash the root. Do not scrub or rub the tooth to avoid damage to the attached tissue which is required for reattachment. Insert the tooth back into its socket, place a folded gauze piece or soft cloth over it and let the child bite it gently to keep it in place. If parents are scared to reimplant the tooth, it should be placed in a cup of cold milk (without sugar) or in saliva and child taken promptly to the nearest dentist. Reimplantation is usually successful if it is achieved within 30 minutes of avulsion. The child should avoid eating anything for next couple of hours followed by liquid and soft diet for the next 2 days or so.

Fluorosis

Fluorine deficiency is a recognized risk factor for development of caries but in areas where fluoride content of drinking water is in excess of 2 parts per million (>2 mg/L) the population is at risk to develop fluorosis. The enamel of the teeth gets mottled and becomes brown and hypoplastic. Fluorosis may produce crippling deformities of long bones, spine and joints. Radiological features include osteosclerosis (thickly dense bones) and at times osteoporosis and osteomalacia may occur due to secondary hyperparathyroidism because fluorine is known to interfere with calcium metabolism.

Teeth Grinding (Bruxism)

Refer to **Chapter 26** for details.

BIBLIOGRAPHY

Douglas JM, Douglas AB, Silk HJ. A practical guide to infant oral health. *Am Fam Phys* 2004, 70(11): 2113–2120.

Griffen AL. Pediatric oral health. *Pediatr Clin North Am* 2000, 47: 138–140.

Owais AI, Zawaideh F, Bataineh O. Challenging parent's myths regarding their children's teething. *Int J Dental Hygiene* 2010, 8(1): 28–34.

Selwitz RH, Ismail AI, Pitts NB. Dental caries. *Lancet* 2007, 369: 51–58.

Sonis A, Zaragoza S. Dental health for the pediatrician. *Curr Opin Pediatr* 2001, 13: 289–295.

Wake M, Hesketh K, Lucas J. Teething and tooth eruption in infants: A cohort study. *Pediatrics* 2000, 106(6): 1374–1379.

33

34

Diseases of Ear, Nose and Throat

Developmental Aspects

A number of ENT diseases are more common in children due to structural and physiological peculiarities. The lymphoid tissue is hyperreactive in children in an attempt to ward off day-to-day infections and entry of allergens in the body. Tonsils and adenoids are physiologically large in size to serve their protective mechanisms. Cervical lymph nodes readily enlarge in size in response to ENT infections and it should not cause undue anxiety and concern. Eustachian tubes (ducts connecting nasopharynx with middle ear) are short, soft and more horizontal in children thus predisposing the child to develop acute otitis media (AOM) especially when baby is bottle fed or feeding is done in a supine position. Associated developmental defects of lips and palate further predispose to the development of AOM.

Epistaxis is a common problem in children because septal blood vessels are superficial and lie in close proximity to the bone or cartilage under cover of thin mucous membrane (Little's area). Children are more prone to put their fingers or foreign bodies in the nose leading to epistaxis. Infants are more likely to develop stridor because of narrow air passages, relatively large tongue, hypertrophy of tonsils and adenoids, collapsibility of upper airway and floppy epiglottis due to lack of supporting cartilage. Children are more vulnerable to develop sudden choking due to inhalation of foreign bodies and are more likely to present with insertion of foreign bodies or entry of insects in the nose and ear canal.

COMMON COLD (Upper Respiratory Infection)

Common cold is the most common acute respiratory infection in children. Most children are likely to suffer, on an average, 4 to 6 episodes of common cold in a year. It is the commonest cause of absenteeism in schools. Common cold is caused by over 200 antigenically distinct viral agents. The infection occurs throughout the year but is more common during change of weather and in winter. It is a highly contagious disease with direct spread from an infected person by coughing and sneezing or through hands and by contact with infected clothes like, towel and handkerchief of the patient. The patient with common cold is most infectious a few hours before the onset of symptoms and 1 to 2 days after the illness has appeared. A patient with common cold in the family would transmit the infection to most of the family members. Children attending the nursery or play schools and day-care centers get frequent episodes of cold due to greater risk of exposure.

Clinical Features

It is characterized by fever, cough, sneezing, and running of the nose. There may be sore throat, headache and body aches. Nasal congestion leads to blockage of the nose. Infants become miserable due to blockage of nose because it interferes with their sleep and feeding behavior. There may be irritability and restlessness because of fever, body aches and nose block. There is general malaise and loss of appetite. The bout of cough may be followed by vomiting in infants. Some children with common cold may develop associated viral diarrhea.

Common Complications

Common cold is a self-limited disease and most cases resolve spontaneously within 3–5 days. "Common cold like" symptoms may herald the onset of several serious childhood disorders like measles, chickenpox, mumps, whooping cough, acute poliomyelitis, etc. Superadded bacterial infection and its spread may lead to development of acute sinusitis, acute otitis media and pneumonia. Sinusitis should be suspected by purulent nasal discharge, persistent headache and tenderness over the forehead and cheek bones. Acute otitis media is characterized by reappearance of fever, irritability due to ear ache and pus discharge from the ear. Rapid breathing, chest retractions and refusal of feeding are suggestive of development of pneumonia. In some children common cold constitutes an important trigger to increase bronchial reactivity in children who are predisposed to develop attacks of bronchial asthma.

Differential Diagnosis

Children with allergic rhinitis (hay fever) show persistent watery nasal discharge with frequent exacerbations. There is no fever, nasal discharge is watery and sneezing is marked. Cough is minimal or absent. There may be itching in the eyes and nose. Antihistamines are useful in these patients for prompt relief of nasal symptoms. These children are more vulnerable to develop features of bronchial allergy in the from of bronchial asthma.

Streptococcal pharyngitis must be differentiated from common cold because of its potential risk to cause serious complications like acute rheumatic fever and post-streptococcal acute glomerulonephritis. Early treatment of acute streptococcal pharyngitis with a specific antibiotic is mandatory for recovery and prevention of complications.

Treatment

There is no specific treatment for common cold which is a self-limiting condition. It is said that untreated common cold lasts for 7 days but when you treat, it disappears in one week! Symptomatic treatment is given to provide comfort and relief. Give paracetamol (15 mg/kg/dose) for relief of fever, headache and body aches. Aspirin should be avoided in children with viral respiratory infection because of potential risk of development of Reye syndrome. Home remedies like tulsi tea, ginger and honey in warm water, chest rub with a liniment containing eucalyptus and menthol, steam inhalation and gargles with warm water containing table salt are useful and effective to provide comfort. Cough mixtures containing nasal decongestants, antihistamines and cough suppressants are not necessarily superior to home remedies. Antihistamines may worsen the nose block by drying the secretions. In children predisposed to develop asthmatic bronchitis, antihistamines may worsen the chest symptoms due to drying of secretions which becomes viscid and thick.

Infants with common cold may feel miserable due to nose block. They cannot feed or breathe properly and become irritable. Avoid medicated nose drops because they are known to cause local irritation and may produce rebound blockage of nose when the effect of medicine wanes off. Saline (0.6% solution of sodium chloride in water) nose drops are effective and safe to relieve nasal congestion. Keep the nose clean with a cotton bud or suck out nasal secretions with a soft bulb suction device because young children cannot blow out their nasal secretions. The use of nose drops should be restricted to 4–5 days. Placing the infant on abdomen may assist in draining the nasal secretions. Steam inhalation and application of rub liniment (over the chest and neck) containing eucalyptus and menthol are useful to relieve nasal congestion. To avoid irritation of the delicate skin of an infant, dilute the rub ointment with an equal quantity of a cold cream before application. Keeping the head raised and warm with a woollen cap, especially in winter, is also useful to reduce nasal congestion.

Give plenty of warm liquids in the form of plain water, milk, tea, and soups, etc. They are soothing to the throat and keep the secretions thin and liquified. The child should be encouraged to take good nutritious diet without any unnecessary restrictions. The food items which are known to cause irritation in the throat (like fried items, condiments, ketchup, cold drinks, spices, lemon, synthetic colors, etc.) should be avoided.

There is no role of an antibiotic in an uncomplicated case of common cold. The antibiotic may be required if their is a superadded bacterial infection. Thick nasal secretions, pain in the ear (due to middle ear infection), severe headache (due to sinusitis), spread of infection to the lungs (development of pneumonia) and persistence of fever beyond 3 days or reappearance of fever should be treated with an appropriate antibiotic.

Prevention

There is no effective vaccine as yet against common cold because it is caused by a large number of viruses. Flu vaccine (Two primary doses 4 weeks apart followed by boosters every year) can be given to prevent occurrence of influenza and H1N1 (Swine flu). Good nutrition with adequate intake of micronutrients maintains adequate body defences to ward off infections. Breast feeding provides protection against a variety of infections including common cold because human milk is replete with a large number of protective factors. Avoidance of over crowding, reduced exposure to cold and environmental pollutants may reduce episodes of respiratory infections. The children should be properly clothed and effectively covered during winter. Isolation at home is virtually impossible. The patient should cover his mouth and nose while coughing and sneezing. Frequent hand washing and use of personal towel and handkerchief is recommended to reduce risk of transmission of infection.

34

ALLERGIC RHINITIS (Hay fever)

Allergic rhinitis is an IgE-mediated inflammation of the nasal mucosa in response to exposure to airborne allergens such as pollen, dust mites, animal dander and mold. The symptoms usually start in school-going children. There is sudden onset of nasal itching, sneezing and profuse watery nasal discharge (coryza or rhinorrhea). Unlike common cold, there is no fever. Nasal itching leads to grimacing, picking at the nose or upward rubbing of nose with an open palm. There may be itching and watering from eyes due to associated allergic conjunctivitis. Nasal congestion is more marked at night leading to mouth breathing and disturbed sleep. The symptoms of allergic rhinitis may be followed by wheezing due to allergic bronchitis or bronchial asthma. Allergic rhinitis can be easily differentiated from viral rhinopharyngitis (common cold) on the basis of clinical assessment **(Table 34.1)**.

Treatment

Avoidance of offending allergens is curative but difficult to achieve. Bedroom (bed sheets, mattresses, curtains, carpets) should be kept free of dust, dust mites and molds. Air conditioners should be provided with high-efficiency particulate air (HEPA) filters to reduce the risk of exposure to dust. If dander of the pet is the culprit, the family may have to send it to a friend's place. A combination of montelukast with cetirizine is useful to control the symptoms and can be given on a long term basis. Nasal congestion can be controlled by giving intranasal steroid sprays (mometasone furoate, fluticasone propionate) by giving 1–2 puffs in both nostrils at night and on waking up in the morning.

ACUTE TONSILLITIS (Streptococcal pharyngitis)

It is not uncommon that a child is brought for consultation with the complaint, doctor "my child has tonsils". True every child has tonsils but that does not mean they are causing trouble. Tonsils are two pads of lymphoid tissue, deep in the throat, one on either side. These can be seen as small rounded projections in the throat on asking the child to widely open the mouth. They serve as protective sentinels in the throat to attack the germs which enter through the mouth. *Tonsils are normally relatively large in size in children between 5–10 years of age to provide enhanced protection during this vulnerable period.* The mere size of the tonsils should not be a cause for concern. They shrink in size and assume adult proportions after 10–12 years or during adolescence.

Practical Point

ENT examination is mandatory in every child with an unexplained fever. Most errors in clinical practice are made by cursory or incomplete examination rather than due to lack of knowledge or skills.

Clinical Features

The infection of tonsils is most commonly caused by Group A *Streptococcus hemolyticus*. It is also called "strept" throat. The child develops high grade fever, pain in throat and headache without any watering from

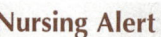

Nursing Alert

Nurse should guide the mother or provide assistance to restrain the child for examination of throat with a wooden spatula and eardrum with an otoscope. Most children cooperate when they are properly handled.

Table 34.1 Salient differences between allergic rhinitis and common cold		
Features	*Common cold*	*Allergic rhinitis*
Age	Common at all ages	Common after 4 years
Predisposing factors	Contact with a patient at home, creche or school	Family history or genetic susceptibility
Fever	Common	Absent
Nasal discharge	Watery at onset, gradually becomes thick and greenish	Watery and profuse with nasal itching
Sneezing	Occasional	Marked
Cough	Common	Absent or intractable if bronchial reactivity is triggered
Nasal congestion	Mild to moderate	Marked and may be associated with hypertrophy of a nasal polyp or adenoids
Progression to wheezing or reactive airway disease	May occur	More common

the nose. The tonsils become large, walnut sized, angry-red in color with whitish patches or pus points called follicles.

Treatment

Paracetamol (15 mg/kg/dose) or ibuprofen (10 mg/kg/dose) is given for symptomatic felief of fever, sore throat and headache. Gargles with warm saline water is useful to relieve sore throat. Avoid intake of chilled water and ice cream. The condition should be promptly treated with an antibiotic like penicillin, erythromycin or cephalosporin or amoxycillin. The antibiotic therapy must be given for atleast 10 days to prevent complications. When "strept" throat infection is inadequately treated there is a potential risk of development of rheumatic fever (and rheumatic heart disease) or acute glomerulonephritis during recovery.

Tonsils should not be removed just because they look large in size as they are known to perform important function of preventing the entry of pathogenic bacteria in the body. There is a wrong belief that removal of tonsils would improve the growth of the child. Now a days doctors are more considerate and conservative in removing the tonsils. An episode of tonsillitis can be easily treated with an appropriate antibiotic and unnecessary tonsillectomy should not be performed. If a child is having repeated episodes of tonsillitis he can be put on long-term penicillin therapy orally or through injections. In the present day era, there are limited indications or justifications for removal of tonsils except peritonsillar abscess.

Peritonsillar Abscess (Quinsy)

It is a rare complication of acute tonsillopharyngitis. The condition is suspected when there is high-grade fever, marked toxemia, dysphagia, drooling, harshness of voice and trismus (lock jaw). There is asymmetric tonsillar enlargement or bulge in the oropharynx.

Treatment The child should be admitted to the hospital under the care of an ENT specialist. The antibiotic of choice include amoxicillin with clavulanic acid (50–100 mg/kg/d of amoxicillin base every 6 to 8 hr) and metronidazole (7–5 mg/kg every 12 hr) through intravenous route. Alternatively, clindamycin hydrochloride 10 mg/kg can be given intravenously every 8 hours to provide coverage against methicillin-resistant *Staphylococcus aureus* (MRSA) and anerobic infections. Abscess should be drained by needle aspiration followed by tonsillectomy after control of infection. Some specialists recommend open surgical drainage with removal of tonsils during the acute stage.

STRIDOR

Refer to **Chapter 38** for details.

ADENOIDS (Pharyngeal Tonsils)

Adenoids comprise of lymphoid pads of tissue which are located deep down in the nasopharynx. Adenoids cannot be seen on opening the mouth but unfortunately they create more serious problems than tonsils. They try to tackle and ward off germs and allergens which enter the body through the nose. In some allergic children the adenoids become very large in size and they block the nasal passages in the back of nose or nasopharynx. The child is unable to breathe through his nose and keeps his mouth open, both during the day and while sleeping. There is constant trickling of phlegm over the back of throat causing irritating cough, persistent nasal discharge, foul breath, and nasal twang in the voice. There is excessive drooling of saliva and snoring. Enlarged adenoids may block the Eustachian tube (channel between the nasopharynx and middle ear) leading to repeated attacks of ear infection. Adenoids produce characteristic facies (rather "unintelligent looks") with an open mouth, drooping of jaw, drooling and expressionless face. If diagnosis is confirmed by an ENT specialist and when there is history of repeated attacks of acute otitis media, adenoids can be removed by a surgical procedure. The older practice of removing adenoids and tonsils en block is no longer recommended.

EARACHE

Earache is common in children and usually occurs due to middle ear infection (acute otitis media), herpes zoster oticus, otitis externa, insertion of foreign body, wax, and trapping of insect or fly in the ear canal **(Box 34.1)**. At times toothache is referred to the ear. Infant may cry and point to his affected ear. Some children pull at their ears or rub them when they are tired, sleepy, bored or hungry. Do not put any oil in the ear, it may clog the wax and lead to development of fungal infection. Infants with dandruff tends to have similar scales in the ear canal leading to constant itching. Wax is formed by normal secretions produced by the glands in the outer part of ear canal. It helps to trap dust and other small particles and provides protection to the ear drum. No attempt should be made to remove normal wax from the ears.

Treatment

Pain and discomfort can be relieved by administration of paracetamol or ibuprofen and a sedative like chloral hydrate or promethazine hydrochloride. Warm

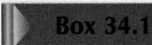

Box 34.1 **Common causes of earache in children**

Otogenic causes
- *External ear*
  - □ Wax
  - □ Trauma
  - □ Otitis externa
  - □ Herpes zoster
  - □ Foreign body or trapped insect
- *Middle ear*
  - □ Acute suppurative otitis media
  - □ Otitis media with effusion
  - □ Complicated chronic suppurative otitis media

Non-otogenic causes
- Caries teeth
- Stomatitis and gingivitis
- Pharyngitis and peritonsillar abscess
- Teething
- Cervical lymphadenitis
- Mumps
- Dysfunction of temporomandibular joint

34

fomentation over the ear provides comfort. Wax and foreign body visible at the opening of the ear canal may be removed with a small forceps. Never push a hair pin, match stick, tooth pick or cotton bud to remove the wax or insect. Focussing bright light into the ear canal may at times attract the mosquito to fly out. When a large plug of wax is formed, it may cause local irritation and hearing difficulty. When wax is solidified and impacted, local instillation of wax softener drops for a few days would facilitate removal of wax by aspiration. *Never pour any oil drops into the ears (and nose) of children.*

ACUTE-OTITIS MEDIA

Children commonly develop middle ear infection (otitis: ear infection, media: middle) following an attack of cough and cold, flu or upper respiratory tract infection. Most cases are viral but bacterial superinfection may occur because of *S. pneumoniae, S. aureus, H. influenzae type b* and *M. catarrhalis.* There is a channel or tube (Eustachian tube) which connects middle ear with posterior part of the nose or nasopharynx. When tube gets blocked due to

Nursing Alert

Ear canal can be moistened with a cotton bud soaked with coconut or olive oil but never pour any oil into the ears and nostrils of children!

inflammation, middle ear infection sets in. When children are fed in lying down position, they are more likely to develop middle ear infection by blockage of the tube by milk. Acute otitis media is more common in bottle fed babies and in children with cleft lip and/ or palate.

The condition should be suspected when a child with common cold develops fever and pain in the ear. Infant would have marked irritability, excessive crying and he may pull at his affected ear. Nose is usually blocked. When eardrum perforates, pus is discharged through the ear which is associated with relief of earache. It may lead to significant loss of hearing.

Treatment

Every child with cough and cold should be monitored for early diagnosis of acute otitis media before perforation of drum occurs. Paracetamol and a sedative should be given for relief of earache. Local fomentation with a hot pack provides symptomatic relief. There is no role of eardrops but saline water nose drops (or steam inhalation) are recommended to relieve nasal congestion and relieve blockage of Eustachian tube. Antibiotics like amoxicillin, amoxicillin-clavulanic acid, cefoprox, cefuroxime axetil for 10 days and a nasal decongestant are recommended. When ear drum is bulging, early tympanostomy (putting Grommet drainage tube through ear drum) is recommended to prevent perforation of drum. Whenever there is perforation of the eardrum, swimming should be avoided or done by wearing ear plugs.

SINUSITIS

The sinuses are air-filled spaces which are situated inside the facial bones behind the forehead (frontal), inside the cheek bones (maxillary) and around the eyes (ethmoid). These air-spaces normally serve the purpose of providing resonance to the voice. In children with persistent cough and cold, the sinuses may get infected because they are connected to the nose and the upper part of the throat. The "cold" symptoms becomes persistent with continuation of fever, persistence of cough, headache (and tenderness over forehead or cheek bones) and yellowish-green pus discharge from the nostrils. There may be soggyness and black circles under the eyes, blocked nose and nasal or non-resonant voice.

Treatment

Steam inhalation and instillation of saline water drops in the nose are useful to relieve nasal congestion and for drainage of pus from the sinuses. Paracetamol or ibuprofen is recommended for relief of headache. Appropriate antibiotic and docongestant are recommended for 10–14 days.

EPISTAXIS (Nose bleed)

Nose bleeding is common in children. It usually occurs without any obvious injury. It occurs during dry weather or due to use of hot air blower in winter resulting in formation of thick crusts in the nose. Nose picking often leads to bleeding. Bleeding may occur during "cough and cold" due to frequent blowing or cleaning of the nose. Rarely insertion of a sharp object or a large finger nail into the nose may lead to bleeding.

First-aid It is frightening to see a child bleeding from the nose but mother must remain calm. There is no need for any alarm or panic as bleeding stops spontaneously within a few minutes. Make the child sit up with head slightly bent forwards. He should be asked to pinch both the nostrils with a clean handkerchief or a paper napkin while breathing through the mouth **(Figure 34.1)**. Apply a cold pack on the nose if child is old enough to allow it. When bleeding is massive or persistent lasting for more than 5–10 minutes and when it is occurring

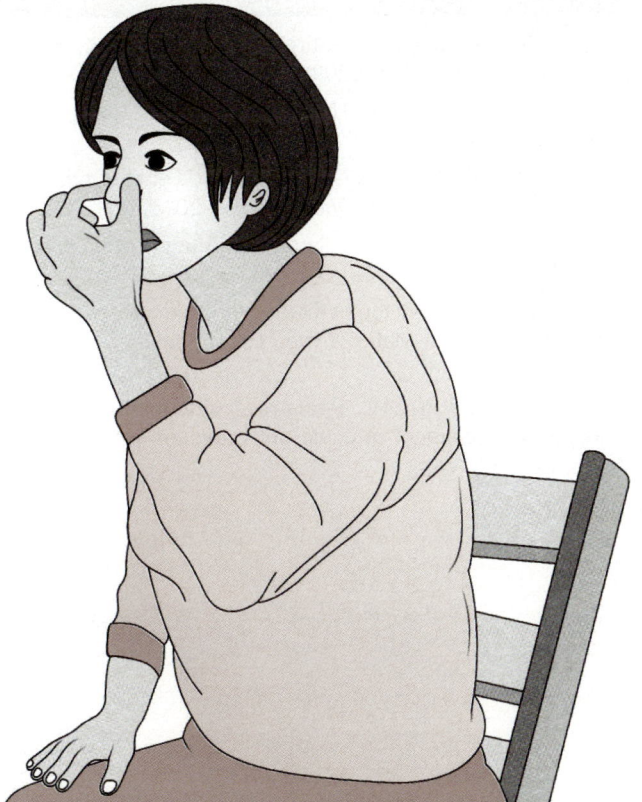

Figure 34.1 The child should be made to sit comfortably, breathe through her mouth and nose kept firmly pinched for at least 5 minutes to stop the bleeding

frequently, an ENT specialist should be consulted for management. To prevent recurrences, nails should be kept trimmed and nostrils kept lubricated with a moisturizing cream.

Drooling

Some normal children continue to drool during infancy without any obvious cause. Drooling occurs either due to excessive production of saliva or because of inability to swallow it. Teething is associated with irritation of gums and increase in drooling of saliva. Drooling is common and persistent in children who are mouth breathers because of blockage of nose and adenoids. Stomatitis and mouth ulcers are associated with increased drooling. Children with mental subnormality and cerebral palsy cannot swallow their saliva and may have persistent drooling throughout childhood.

Tongue-tie

A fold or frenulum on the under surface of tongue fixes it at the base of the oral cavity. When frenulum is too thick or tight it is called tongue-tie. The condition is often wrongly and over diagnosed by the grandmother when the child has some feeding difficulty or delay in the development of speech.

Tongue-tie should be diagnosed when child is unable to protrude the tongue beyond the lips or he is unable to lick his upper lip or touch the roof of oral cavity (palate) with tip of the tongue. The presence of a midline notch at the tip of tongue due to traction of frenulum is diagnostic. *Tongue-tie is never a cause for difficulty in feeding or delay in the development of speech.* Nevertheless, the child with a tongue-tie may lack clarity in speech due to inability to clearly pronounce certain alphabets (N,L,T, D, Th, etc.) which need free mobility of tongue. The genuine tongue-tie may be snipped before one year of age by a pediatric surgeon under anesthetic cover.

White Tongue

The presence of milk crusts or uniformly white furred tongue in the first few weeks of life is normal and does not need any treatment. There is no need to make any special efforts to clean the tongue of an infant. It should not be confused with thrush.

Thrush

There are discrete white patches with red margins over the tongue, buccal mucosa and gums. It is caused by *Candida albicans* which is transmitted commonly through feeding bottles but at times from mother's vaginal tract or nipple of her breast. Oral thrush may

34

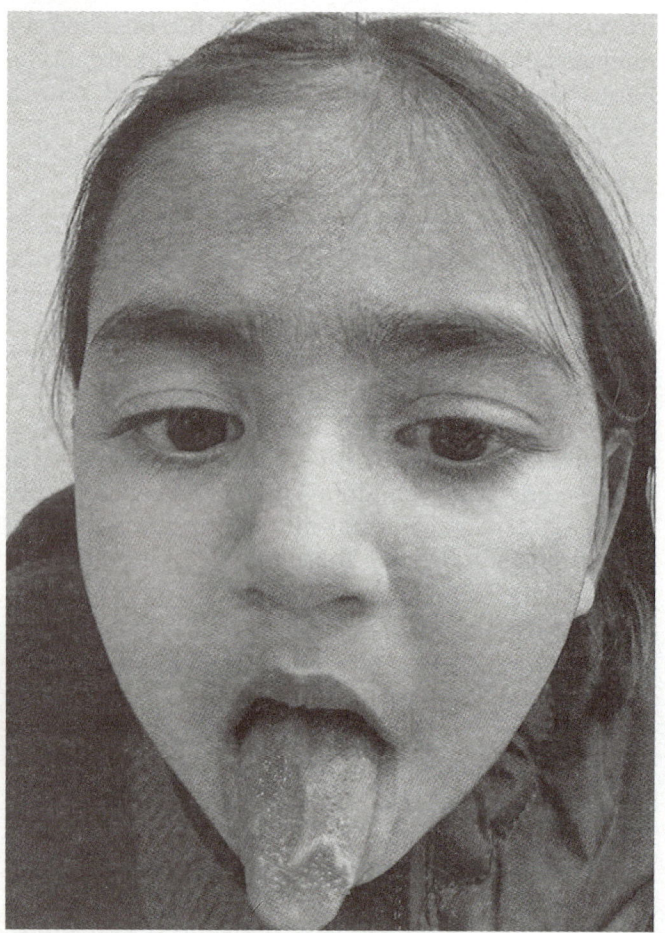

Figure 34.2 Typical appearances of geographical tongue

Geographical Tongue

The presence of bizarre shapes and patterns of grey-white areas on the dorsum (upper surface) of tongue with advancing, slightly elevated margins resembling like a map may be seen in some children **(Figure 34.2)**. The shape and pattern of the map may change from time to time but it is of no significance. It does not cause any discomfort to the child and no treatment is required.

Aphthous Ulcers

Some children are prone to develop recurrent crops of painful ulcers in the mouth. The etiology is usually viral (Herpes simplex) and more than one family member may be affected. Ulcers with angry-red margins develop over the tongue, inner surface of lips and gums. They are extremely painful and cause drooling and difficulty in eating. Regular brushing of teeth (without causing injury to the gums), maintenance of strict oral hygiene and use of antiseptic mouth washes are effective to prevent their recurrence. Local application of an antiseptic-cum-anesthetic gel provides symptomatic relief. Paracetamol may be given if pain and discomfort are marked.

cause feeding and swallowing difficulty. Local application of 0.5% aqueous solution of gentian violet or antifungal lotion containing nystatin or clotrimazole after each feed gives prompt relief. The mother should also receive appropriate treatment if there is any evidence of fungal infection of vagina or breast. When thrush is recurrent, persistent and wide spread involving esophagus, infant should be evaluated for congenital or acquired immunodeficiency disorder.

BIBLIOGRAPHY

Greiner AN, Hellings PW, Rotiroti G, Scadding GK. Allergic rhinitis. *Lancet* 2011, 378 (9809): 2112–2122.

Heikkinen T, Jarvinen A. The common cold. *Lancet* 2003, 361(9351): 51–59.

Ilechukwu GC, Ilechukwu CGA, Ulbesie AC, et al. Otitis media in children: Review article. *Open J Pediatr* 2014, 4: 47–53.

Plaut M, Valentine MD. Clinical practice: Allergic rhinitis. *N Engl J Med* 2005, 353(18): 1934–1944.

Sacko BH. Ear, nose and throat diseases in paediatric patients at a secondary hospital in Mali. *Online J Otolaryngology* 2015, 5(4): 35–42.

Steinbach WJ, Sectish TC. Pediatric resident training in the diagnosis and treatment of acute otitis media. *Pediatrics* 2002, 109(3): 404–408.

Common Eye Problems

Developmental Aspects

Developmental defects of eyes are evident soon after birth and they produce a variety of cosmetic abnormalities like microphthalmia (small eyes), buphthalmos (glaucoma with large cornea), white reflex (cataract, retinoblastoma), ptosis (lid drop), squint (crossed eyes), colobomas (absence of a component of the eye), amblyopia and visual abnormalities. Watering of eyes or epiphora due to blockage of nasolacrimal duct (channel that drains the tears from eyes into the nose) is a common problem in newborn babies. Due to unhygienic conditions, sharing of towels or handkerchiefs, cultural practice of putting *kajal* and *surma* in the eyes, children are more prone to develop conjunctivitis. They are more vulnerable to develop nutritional deficiencies and deficiency of vitamin A is known to cause serious damage to the eyes leading to blindness. Oxygen therapy in preterm babies (<34 weeks), especially when it is not properly monitored, may result in development of retinopathy of prematurity (ROP) which may lead to retinal detachment and blindness. Premature babies should be given the lowest concentration of oxygen to maintain arterial oxygen tension (paO$_2$) between 60 and 80 mm Hg and oxygen therapy should be stopped when it is no longer required. Children are prone to develop serious eye injuries due to sharp objects like pencils, arrows, darts or by explosive crackers. Assessment of visual acuity is difficult in children and demands use of special charts (different objects or shapes), indirect ophthalmoscopy and study of visual-evoked responses (VER).

RETINOPATHY OF PREMATURITY (ROP)

Retinopathy of prematurity, which was previously called as retrolental fibroplasia (RLF), is characterized by proliferation of small retinal blood vessels due to a variety of causes. The condition is by and large limited to preterm babies with birth weight of less than 1500 g or gestational age less than 32 weeks. The overall incidence of ROP varies between 35 and 60% in babies weighing less than 1500 g. The leading cause of ROP is hyperoxia or high oxygen tension in the arterial blood. Other risk factors include exposure to bright light, apneic attacks, vitamin E deficiency, anemia, acidosis, blood transfusion, patent ductus arteriosus and prolonged assisted ventilation. Hyperoxia leads to vasoconstriction of retinal vessels followed by neovascularization with proliferation of vascular or glial cells, arteriovenous shunt formation and retinal damage due to scarring. ROP is emerging as one of the leading causes of preventable blindness in children.

All infants with a birth weight of <1500 g or gestational age of less than 32 weeks should be screened by a pediatric ophthalmologist with indirect ophthalmoscopy in the NICU. According to International classification of ROP, the severity of disease is assessed by (i) area of retina involved, (ii) stage of disease (stage 1–5) and (iii) plus and threshold disease. The prognosis for vision is hopeless when infant presents with leukocoria or white pupillary reflex.

Prevention

Oxygen should be considered as a potentially toxic drug in preterm babies and should be given only when indicated. It should be used in the lowest ambient concentration to maintain paO$_2$ between 50 and 70 mm Hg and arterial oxygen saturation (SaO$_2$) between 90 and 93%. Oxygen therapy should be stopped when there is no valid indication for its administration.

Treatment

Early detection of ROP is important so that avascular peripheral retina can be touched with trans-scleral cryopexy to prevent further spread of the disease. Laser photocoagulation therapy is preferred and has replaced cryotherapy in many centers. The aim of treatment in to ablate the entire avascular retina up to ora serrata.

EPIPHORA

Watering of eyes from one or both the eyes is called epiphora. Tears from the eyes are drained into the nose through a channel called nasolacrimal duct. When nasolacrimal duct is blocked due to debris, there may be persistent watering from one or both the eyes without any redness or conjunctivitis and dacryocystitis. The blockage can be relieved by proper massage of the nasolacrimal duct. Mother should massage the duct with her thumb and index finger by exerting gentle but firm pressure (several times in a day) over the lacrimal glands followed by massage of both ducts by firmly sliding them downward along the outer surface of the nose. At the inner canthi of eyes, the lacrimal sacs or tear glands should be pressed firmly. This will facilitate expulsion of any debris and restore the patency of duct in most cases. If infection occurs, it can be treated by local instillation of antibacterial eye drops. When epiphora persists despite effective massaging, the duct may need surgical probing by an ophthalmologist after 3 to 6 months of age. When repeated probing fails to relieve epiphora, reconstructive surgery (dacryocystorhinostomy) is done.

CONJUNCTIVITIS

Ophthalmia neonatorum may occur because of transmaternal infection due to *N. gonorrhoeae* if prophylaxis eye care is not practiced in endemic areas. Other causative pathogens for conjunctivitis include *S. aureus*, *Pseudomonas aeruginosa* and *Chlamydia trachomatis*. Gonococcal ophthalmia manifests during 2–5 days of life and is characterized by purulent conjunctival discharge with marked chemosis. Mother may give history of gonorrhea during pregnancy. Gram stain of purulent discharge shows characteristic intracellular Gram-negative diplococci. It is treated by frequent irrigation of eyes with normal saline and administration of a single dose of ceftriaxone 50 mg/kg (up to maximum of 125 mg) intramuscularly. Non-specific bacterial conjunctivitis is treated by frequent irrigation of eyes and instillation of chloramphenicol or broad spectral antibiotic drops. Chlamydial conjunctivitis is best treated with oral administration erythromycin (50 mg/kg/d q 6 hr) for 2 weeks which prevents subsequent development of chlamydial pneumonia.

Infection of eyes may develop due to viral or bacterial infection in later childhood. Infection may occur if mother is putting kohl or soot (*surma* or *kajal*) in the eyes or when baby rubs his eyes with dirty hands. When baby towel is not kept clean or is shared by other family members, it is a potent source of infection. The eyes become red and swollen with watery discharge which later becomes thick like pus. There is itching and pain in the eyes. There may be stickiness of eyelids on waking up in the morning. Keep the eyes clean by washing them repeatedly with cotton soaked in boiled water. Local cleaning and instillation of antibacterial eyes drops or ointment are advised. Eye drops are convenient and should be put in the eyes every 1–2 hourly during the day time while ointment is applied at night as it provides prolonged effect. Avoid application of kohl and soot on the eyelids because of risk of infection and lead toxicity.

Allergic conjunctivitis may occur in some children in summer months due to exposure to pollens and dust. The condition may occur in association with allergic rhinitis or hay fever. There is profuse watery discharge with redness and itching in both eyes. The condition is managed by cold compresses and topical administration of eye drops containing cromoglycate or ketorolac tromethamine and oral antihistamines. Steroid containing ophthalmic drops and ointment should be avoided and taken only under the guidance of an ophthalmologist.

Phlyctenular keratoconjunctivitis may develop in one or both eyes due to allergic response to tubercular bacilli, *beta Hemolytic streptococci* and several other antigens and allergens. There is a small, yellowish or brown nodule with a leash of blood vessels located at the corneal limbus either in one or both the eyes. The condition is treated by eliminating the underlying cause and topical instillation of cromoglycate or ketorolac tromethamine eye drops and at times corticosteroids under the guidance of an ophthalmologist.

STYE (Hordeolum)

Stye is an inflammation of the eyelid caused by infection or blockage of the oil glands or follicle of the eye lashes. This may occur due to rubbing of eye with dirty hands or as a result of run down condition of the child who may get frequent styes. There is localized swelling, pain and redness at the margin of the eyelid. Warm fomentation or compresses with cotton soaked in warm water containing a pinch of boric powder provides relief to pain and swelling. Antibiotic eye drops and ointment would control the infection. Frequent hand-washing with soap and water and splashing of eyes with tap water on coming home from school or playground helps to keep the eyes clean and free from infection. Handkerchiefs and towels should not be shared. Chalazion or meibomian cyst should not be confused with stye.

CHALAZION (Meibomian cyst)

Chalazion is a small 2–8 mm fluid-filled cyst in the eyelid. The tiny meibomian gland, located under the inner surface of the eyelid, produce oily fluid to lubricate the eye. If the gland gets blocked, a fluid-filled swelling appears in the eyelid. When it becomes chronic or inflamed, a granulomatous nodule develops. There is a firm, flat, painless nodule on the bulbar conjunctival aspect of the lid adjacent to the tarsal plate. It may cause mild pain, discomfort and irritation with an urge for itching. It may become large and unsightly due to superadded infection. Most cases recover spontaneously by maintenance of local hygiene, avoidance to touch the eye and hot compresses with cotton pad soaked in warm water. Massage of the cyst after hot compresses may facilitate drainage of the cyst. Massage should be done with clean fingers or sterile cotton pads. There is no role of antibiotics in an uncomplicated case of chalazion. In chronic and recalcitrant cases, minor surgery can be done to excise the cyst under local anesthesia.

XEROPHTHALMIA

It is characterized by bilateral lusterless dry appearance of the conjunctiva and cornea, which occurs due to vitamin A deficiency. The condition is common in malnourished children and is precipitated by an attack of measles or persistent diarrhea. It is an important cause of preventable blindness in children in developing countries.

Clinical Features

Initial symptom is poor dark adaptation or night blindness which is difficult to evaluate in under-3 children. Bulbar conjunctiva becomes dry and wrinkled with bitot spots which are foamy chalky-white triangular deposits at the inner or outer fornices of the eyes. As the disease progresses, there is marked xerosis and wrinkling of cornea followed by keratomalacia, i.e. softening of cornea which may lead to ulceration. At this stage recovery occurs by formation of scar resulting in blindness.

Treatment

Vitamin A is administered through intramuscular route (25,000 iu <6 months, 50,000 iu 6–12 months and 100,000 iu >12 months) in two doses 24 hours apart followed by another dose after 15 days. Eyes should be managed under the supervision of an ophthalmologist by instillation of artificial tear solutions and antibacterial eye drops 4–6 times in a day and use of antibiotic ointment at night. In children with keratomalacia, atropine eye ointment is instilled and eye is protected with a sterile pad and bandage.

The underlying and predisposing conditions are managed appropriately and child is encouraged to take calorie-dense nutritious diet containing vitamin A rich foods like green leafy vegetables, carrots, papaya, pulses, eggs, milk and milk products. Timely immunizations should be provided to prevent common childhood illnesses.

PTOSIS

Drooping of upper eyelid may be congenital or acquired because of involvement of the levator palpebrae muscle by trauma or nerve damage due to meningitis. In severe ptosis, the lid covers the pupil and child is unable to see from the affected side leading to amblyopia or "lazy eye" **(Figure 35.1)**.

The condition is treated by surgical correction. In mild congenital cases when vision is not obstructed, surgery is delayed till 4 to 5 years of age. In severe cases, early surgery is done to prevent amblyopia. In acquired cases, surgery is delayed for 6 months or so to look for spontaneous recovery.

35

SQUINT (Strabismus)

When two eyes are not well aligned and they look in different directions and are unable to focus properly it is called squint. Squint or crossed eyes may be

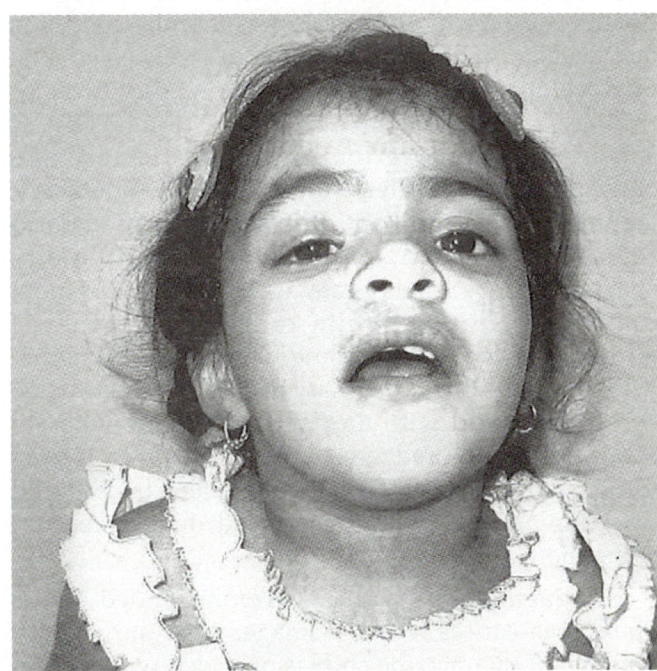

Figure 35.1 Congenital ptosis on the right side. The defect can be rectified surgically after the age of 2–3 years

35

concomitant due to defective vision or paralytic because of paralysis of extraocular muscles. Transient squint is common in early infancy but usually disappears spontaneously by 3–4 months. When squint is associated with roving eye movements, it suggests that baby has defective vision. It is more common in premature and low birth weight babies. When squint persists beyond 6 months or child develops squint in early childhood, an ophthalmologist should be consulted for evaluation and management.

Amblyopia or "lazy eye" is managed by intermittent occlusion or covering of the normal eye so that child is encouraged to use the amblyopic eye. Refractive error is corrected by use of spectacles. Eye exercises and at times surgery is recommended for treatment of weak extraocular muscles.

ASTIGMATISM

Astigmatism occurs due to irregularity in the curvature of cornea (central black or brown part of eye) and lens. It leads to distortion of vision. The child may "frown" or squint to get a clearer vision. He may hold the book too close to his eyes to read. It leads to "eye strain", headache and eye fatigue. The child must be evaluated by an ophthalmologist. The child would feel comfortable on wearing cylindrical glasses or contact lenses.

CATARACT

Cataract or opacification of lens is a senile condition and usually occur in old people. But rarely congenital or developmental cataract may be seen at birth or infancy due to intrauterine infection (TORCH infections), intrauterine hypoxia, galactosemia, chromosomal disorders, type 1 diabetes mellitus, cretinism, eye injury, and prolonged use of steroids **(Figure 35.2)**. Congenital rubella syndrome is characterized by triad of cataract, deafness and patent ductus arteriosus. White reflex or "cat's eye" appearance is seen in infants with retinoblastoma. White opacity in the papillary area is best seen when eye is examined with an ophthalmoscope wherein instead of normal "red reflex", the white opacity is seen. Congenital cataract is usually bilateral. Child should be examined for other associated developmental anomalies.

Treatment Early surgery is recommended before amblyopia causes retinal damage. After surgery for removal of cataract, the child is provided with contact lens or spectacles to treat hypermetropia. Intraocular placement of lens is possible even in children.

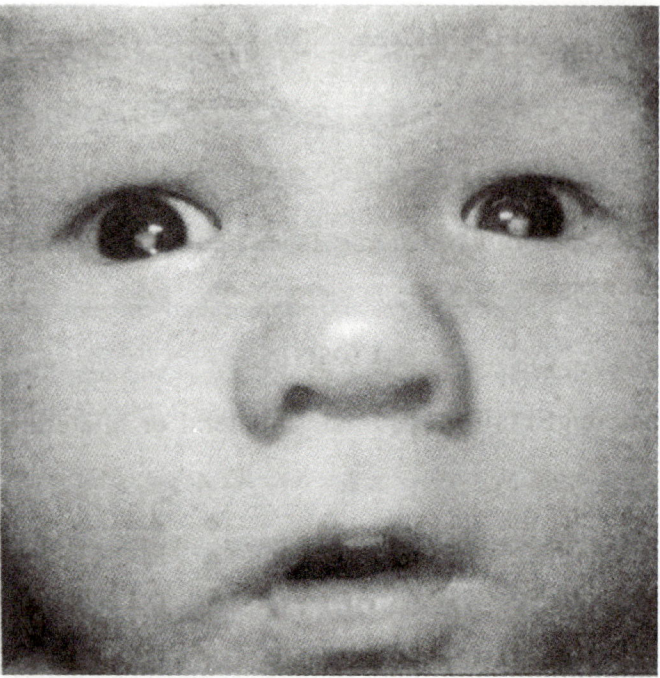

Figure 35.2 Cataract of both eyes due to congenital rubella syndrome

Postoperative nursing care includes topical antibiotics, sedation to prevent crying and administration of antiemetic drugs to prevent vomiting and increase in intraocular pressure.

COLOR BLINDNESS

Color blindness occur in boys as it is inherited as an X-linked (sex-linked) disorder. Girls in general have a better color sense and they do not suffer from color blindness. It is an uncommon disorder, affecting about 8% of boys who cannot distinguish between red and green colors, instead they see them as shades of gray. The condition occurs due to dysfunction of cone photoreceptors in the retina and is diagnosed by using Ishiharas chart. The condition imposes a handicap and is considered as a disqualification for joining certain professions where it is important to distinguish between different colors. There is no specific therapy for the disorder.

Role of a Nurse for Management of Common Eye Problems

- Identifying various predisposing conditions known to cause eye disorders by proper assessment for making nursing diagnosis.
- Proper positioning, restraining and holding the child during examination and various procedures.
- Health education to the family for prevention of eye infections and trauma to the eyes. Advising the

mother against hazards of instillation of kohl or soot in the eyes.

- Guidance to the family for prevention of spread of eye infection from the affected child to others by hand washing and not sharing towel and handkerchief.
- Irrigation of eyes with sterile normal saline and instillation of eye drops and ointment and use of eye shield or occlusive patch.
- Providing relief against discomfort, pain and exposure to bright light.
- Assisting the mother to look after the daily routines and activities of the child like bathing, dressing, eating and toilet needs.
- Providing emotional support to the family by reducing fear and anxiety by giving proper explanation, reassurance and guidance.
- Guidance to the child and family when patient is visually handicapped to prevent accidents and injuries. Orientation for day-to-day activities like bathing, toilet needs and intake of food.
- Support to the family for long-term rehabilitation, education in a special school for visually handicapped

(Braille language), information regarding special help groups, agencies and organizations catering to their special needs.

BIBLIOGRAPHY

Ahmad K. WHO launches international program to combat childhood blindness. *Lancet* 2002, 359: 2258.

American Academy of Pediatrics, American Association for Pediatric Ophthalmology and Strabismus, American Academy of Ophthalmology. Screening examination of premature infants with retinopathy of prematurity. *Pediatrics* 2006, 117(2): 572–576.

Arabi EM, Kelly RJ, Carrim ZI. *Brit Med J* 2010, 341: c4044. doi: 10.1136/bmj.c4044.

Gilbert C, Foster A. Childhood blindness in the context of vision 2020–the right to sight. *Bull world Hlth Org* 2001, 19: 227–232.

International Committee for Retinopathy of Prematurity. The international classification of retinopathy of prematurity revisited. *Arch Ophthalmol* 2005, 123(7): 991–999.

Nirmalan PK, Sheeladevi S, Tamilselvi V, et al. Perception of eye diseases and eye care need of children among parents in rural south India: The Kariapatti Pediatric Eye Evaluation Project (KEEP). *Indian J Ophthalmol* 2004, 52 (2): 163–167.

Rahi JS, Sripathi S, Gilbert CE, Foster A. Childhood blindness in India: causes in 1318 blind students in 9 states. *Eye* 1995, 9: 545–550.

35

Musculoskeletal Disorders

The developmental anomalies most commonly affect the muscles and joints and are discussed in **Chapter 29** dealing with Birth Defects. They include polydactyly, syndactyly, bowed legs, knock knees, flat feet, club feet, in-toeing, out-toeing, toe walking, calcaneovalgus deformity and genu recurvatum.

CONGENITAL DISLOCATION OF HIPS (CDH)

The condition is now called 'developmental' dysplasia of the hip (DDH) which may be associated with a number of abnormalities like immature hip, mild acetabular dysplasia, dislocatable hip and subluxated hip, which may progress to frank dislocation. The incidence of DDH varies from 10 to 35 per 1,000 live born infants. The dislocation is bilateral in about 30 to 40% of cases. The exact etiology is unknown. The condition is more common among first born, post-term or large infants and female babies delivered following breech presentation. The prolonged gestation is associated with increase in the maternal hormones which may account for the laxity of the hip joint. Other risk factors include oligohydramnios, congenital torticollis, club feet and metatarsus adductus. The increased frequency of hip abnormalities in the family members of the affected children is suggestive of genetic predisposition of CDH.

Examination of Hips

The infant is placed supine on a firm surface and both the hips are flexed at right angles to look for alignment of both knees. On the side of dislocation, the knee will be at a lower level due to posterior displacement of femoral head (Galeazzi test). Instability or developmental dysplasia of hip/s is best elicited by a modified Ortolani and Barlow maneuvers. The infant lies supine with legs facing the examiner. One hip is tested at a time. For examination of left hip, the examiner steadies the infant's pelvis between the thumb of left hand which is placed on the symphysis pubis while fingers are placed under the sacrum, **(Figure 36.1)**. The left thigh is flexed by keeping the knee bent. It is grasped by examiner's right hand by placing index and middle fingers over the greater trochanter and thumb on the inner side of the thigh opposite the lesser trochanter. Two maneuvers are performed. In the first maneuver, the examiner assesses whether hip is dislocated or not. By maintaining backward pressure on the femur, hip is abducted in an attempt to relocate the displaced femoral head back into the acetabulum (Ortolani test). If the head is felt to slip back into the acetabulum, with or without a palpable or audible clunk, it confirms the presence of dislocation. If dislocation is ruled out, the second maneuver is performed to assess 'dislocatability' of hip. Backward and lateral pressure is exerted by slightly adducting the thigh to dislocate the femoral

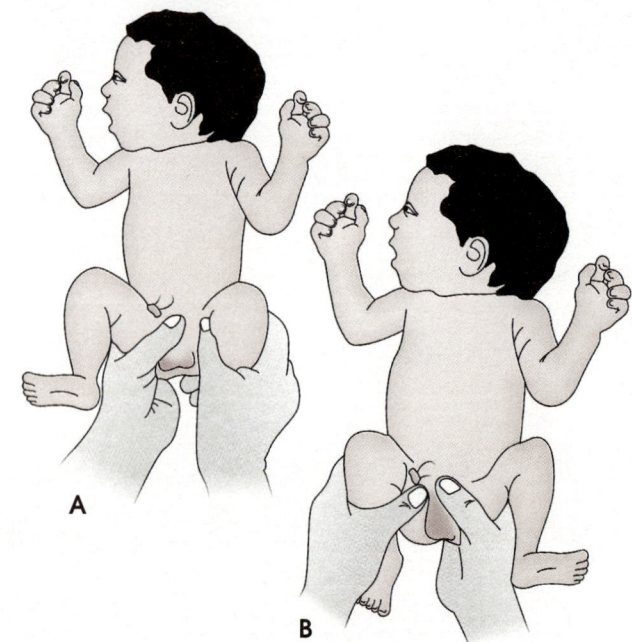

Figure 36.1 Examination for congenital dislocation of hips. Each hip is tested separately. (A) Examination of left hip and (B) shows position for examination of right hip. See text for details

head. If the femoral head is felt to move backward over the rim of acetabulum, with or without a palpable or audible clunk, the hip is said to be dislocatable (Barlow sign). The right hip is examined by reversing the role of examiner's hands. The routine examination of hips of all infants by Ortolani-Barlow maneuver is essential for early diagnosis of DDH.

Diagnosis

The limitation of abduction is not generally seen during neonatal period because it occurs due to shortening of adductors in infants with relatively long-standing dislocation. The femoral pulse may not be readily felt on the affected side. At times asymmetry of skin creases over buttocks or labia and shortening of leg may offer clue to the diagnosis. The X-rays should be taken with both hips extended and legs held in 45° abduction and full internal rotation. The femoral head is displaced upwards and laterally on the affected side **(Figure 36.2)**. On the normal side, the upward projection of longitudinal axis of femur crosses the spine at the lumbosacral junction. If the hip is dislocated, a similar projection of the long axis of the femur passes above the bony edge of acetabulum and crosses the lumbar spine at a higher level. The conventional skiagrams of hips may not show any abnormalities. Ultrasound examination of hip joints provides diagnostic information after one month of age. There is high incidence of false-positive reports during newborn period. Dynamic assessment of stability of the hip on real-time multiplanar ultrasonography with a 7 MHz linear transducer is useful for the diagnosis of DDH.

Treatment

Early management is essential for optimal functional recovery. The legs are maintained in the position of abduction and external rotation by the use of von Rosen splint **(Figure 36.3)**. The Pavlik harness has been effectively used to treat classical cases of CDH by keeping the hips flexed and abducted (frog position). The recovery is generally complete in a period of about 3 to 4 months. In teratologic type of CDH, femoral head does not relocate into acetabulum on flexion and abduction and Ortolani sign is absent. In unilateral cases, there is shortening of leg and asymmetry of the gluteal folds. These infants are best treated by loop traction, adductor tenotomy, open reduction, use of modified Denis Browne splint followed by physiotherapy.

DISORDERS OF MUSCLES

Locomotor difficulties are common due to musculoskeletal disorders which may occur due to general debility, electrolyte disturbances (especially due to hypocalcemia and hypokalemia), muscular dystrophies and neuromuscular disorders.

Floppy Child

Floppy child has marked hypotonia of all the muscles. The spontaneous limb movements are poor and there is excessive range of passive movements at various

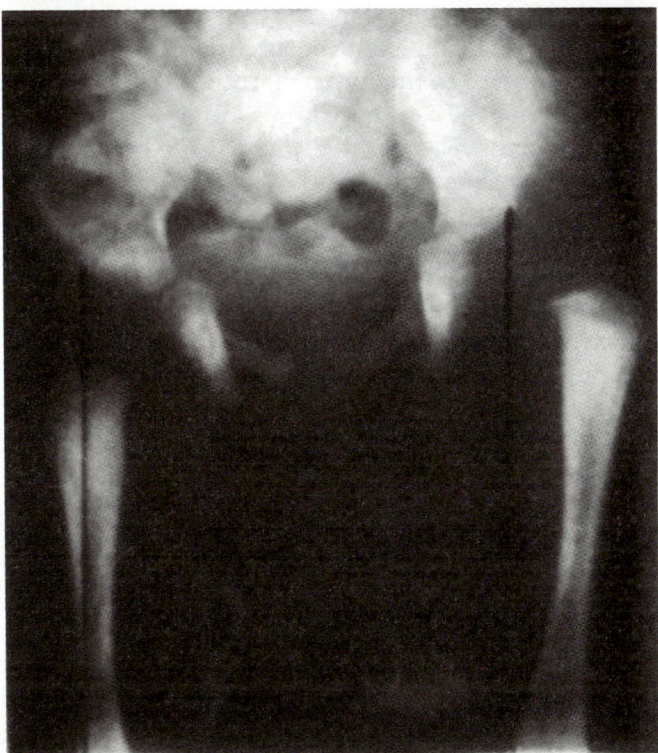

Figure 36.2 Congenital dislocation of hip on left side. The femoral head is displaced upwards and laterally

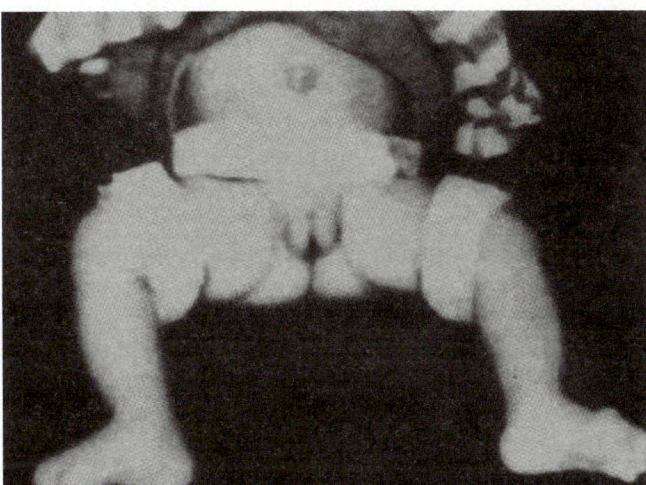

Figure 36.3 Infant restrained with indigenously fabricated von Rosen splint to maintain both hips in abduction and rotation

36

36

joints, and limbs can be placed in bizarre and unusual positions. There may be associated facial weakness, ptosis, and ophthalmoplegia. They are prone to feeding difficulties, frequent respiratory infections, and delay in achieving motor milestones. The salient causes of hypotonia and floppiness include diseases of the CNS (atonic cerebral palsy); spinal cord (spinal muscular atrophy or poliomyelitis); peripheral nerves (acute polyneuropathy or Guillain-Barre disease or congenital neuropathy); myoneural junctions (myasthenia gravis or infantile botulism); or arthrogryposis multiplex congenita and miscellaneous causes such as protein-energy malnutrition, cretinism, Down syndrome, rickets, cutis laxa, and Prader-Willi syndrome.

Limping Child

Abnormalities of gait and limping may occur from a variety of disorders of muscles, bones, joints and ligaments. The gait should be assessed after fully exposing the legs and feet and without wearing shoes and sandals. Ask the child to walk away from you, turn around after walking few meters and walk back towards you. It is best to watch the gait of the child when he or she is not aware that his gait is being observed. Limping occurs due to discomfort, pain and disability due to a variety of causes which are listed in **Box 36.1**. Limping should be classified into two broad groups, painless or associated with pain.

Treatment

The child should be handled with tact and common sense. Pain and discomfort should be relieved by administration of paracetamol (15 mg/kg/dose q 6–8 hr) and ibuprofen (10 mg/kg/dose q 6–8 hr). At times,

---

Box 36.1   **Causes of limping in children**
1. **Trauma** Sprain of ankle, splinter in the foot, contusion or traumatic periostitis, tight fitting shoes, etc.
2. **Osteochondrosis** Involvement of femoral capital epiphysis, tibial tubercle, patella, metatarsal and tarsal bones.
3. **Arthritis and osteomyelitis** Transient synovitis, slipped femoral epiphysis, arthritis, bursitis, and osteomyelitis involving joints of lower limbs.
4. **Neurological disorders** Peripheral neuropathy, muscle weakness or paralysis, spinal cord injury or tumor.
5. **Neoplaster diseases** Leukemia, sarcoma and metastasis from neuroblastoma.
6. **Miscellaneous conditions** Leg length inequality, tight tendo-Achilles, inguinal or iliac lymphadenitis, muscular dystrophy, polymyositis and conversion disorder or hysteria.

---

change of footwear helps. The underlying condition should be identified and managed appropriately under the expert guidance of a pediatric neurologist or orthopedic surgeon.

Muscular Dystrophies

Muscular dystrophies are genetically determined primary disorders of muscles. They are characterized by progressive weakness, hypotonia, delayed motor milestones, and sluggish or absent deep tendon jerks. Depending on the type of muscular dystrophy, the involvement may be generalized or localized to limbs (proximal muscles are affected more than distal), girdle muscles (pelvic or shoulder), and face (ptosis, inability to close the eye or whistle, ophthalmoplegia) with or without associated involvement of cardiac muscles and CNS. Serum creatine phosphokinase (CPK) is grossly elevated. The EMG shows short duration and small amplitude of motor unit potentials. Muscle biopsy is diagnostic by virtue of characteristic histopathological changes on light microscopy, immunocytochemistry, and electron microscopy.

The clinical features of most muscular dystrophies are summarized in **Table 36.1**; but Duchenne muscular dystrophy (DMD), being the most common, is described in detail. Apart from hereditary causes of myopathies, other causes of myopathies that are acquired include endocrinal (thyrotoxicosis, hypothyroidism, steroid induced, and hyperaldosteronism), metabolic (episodic potassium related periodic paralysis, malignant hyperthermia, and glycogen storage disease) and inflammatory myopathies (dermatomyositis; polymyositis; viral, parasitic, and bacterial myositis; and so on).

Duchenne Muscular Dystrophy

Duchenne muscular dystrophy or pseudohypertrophic muscular dystrophy is an X-linked recessive disorder, which is characterized by rapidly progressive muscular wasting disorder, resulting in early confinement to wheel chair and death by the age of 20 years. Becker muscular dystrophy (BMD) is a milder form of the same disease with later onset and slower progression. The incidence of DMD is 1 in 3500 male births, which is five times higher than BMD.

The gene responsible for DMD and BMD is located on the short arm of the X chromosome, at band Xp21. The DMD gene is responsible for production of dystrophin, a high molecular weight cytoskeletal protein, which is normally present in skeletal muscles, smooth muscles, brain, peripheral nerves, and several other tissues. The patients with DMD or BMD have no or little functional dystrophin in various tissues.

Table 36.1 Salient features of muscular dystrophies

Type	Inheritance	Age at onset	Predominant involvement	Characteristic features
Duchenne	X-linked recessive	2–5 y	Pelvic girdle	Pseudohypertrophy of calf muscles, mental subnormality, cardiac involvement, and rapidly progressive
Becker	X-linked recessive	8–10 y	Pelvic girdle	Pseudohypertrophy of calf muscles, pes cavus
Emery-Dreifuss	X-linked recessive or autosomal dominant	5–15 y	Biceps, triceps and peroneal muscles	Contractures, cardiomyopathy, and arrhythmias
Limb girdle	Autosomal recessive or autosomal dominant	10–30 y	Pelvic and shoulder girdle (inability to raise the hands above shoulders or comb the hair)	None
Facioscapulo-humeral	Autosomal dominant	12–15 y	Face (inability to whistle or close the eyes firmly), shoulder, and upper arms	Facial appearance, winging of scapula, asymmetric involvement and deafness
Congenital	Autosomal recessive	Newborn period	Generalized	CNS involvement, mental retardation
Myotonic dystrophy	Autosomal dominant	Any age	Face (ptosis, ophthalmoplegia sternomastoids, and girdle muscles	Myotonia (delayed muscular relaxation), mental retardation, and cardiomyopathy

Abbreviations: CNS, central nervous system; y, year.

Clinical Features

In classical DMD, early motor development is normal. The symptoms usually start after 2 years with unsteady clumsy gait with frequent falls. The gait becomes waddling with compensatory lumbar lordosis. The child has difficulty in climbing upstairs and may use the support of railing or the wall. When asked to rise from a squatting position, the child demonstrates classical Gower sign. The child squirms or turns to the side and lifts up the trunk by supporting its weight on the arms by placing his hands on the floor. The child gradually stands up by making a great effort as if climbing on its body by taking support with its hands at the ankles, knees, and then thighs. The hypertrophy of calf muscles is observed after the age of 4 to 5 years. The hypertrophy of muscles is due to fibrosis (pseudohypertrophy) and characteristically involves calf muscles, glutei, deltoids, serratus anterior, brachioradialis and tongue. Sternal head of pectoralis major and supraspinatus are atrophied and child has difficulty in raising the hands above the shoulders. The condition shows relentless progression with weakness and wasting affecting proximal lower extremity muscles more profoundly. The functions of distal muscles are preserved much longer. Eventually, all the muscles atrophy; and contractures develop at the ankles, knees, hips and elbows. Death occurs because of respiratory infections, respiratory insufficiency and cardiomyopathy. Female carriers are asymptomatic, but 5 to 10% may show some degree of asymmetric muscle weakness and hypertrophy of calf muscles.

Cardiac involvement starts at around 10 years of age by development of fibrosis in the posterior basal portion of the left ventricular wall. Congestive heart failure and cardiac arrhythmias are precipitated by intercurrent infections. Involvement of gastric musculature may lead to acute episodes of vomiting, abdominal pain and distension because of acute gastric dilatation. Mental retardation occurs because of absence of dystrophin in the brain. One-third of children with DMD have an intelligence quotient below 75. There is marked heterogeneity of clinical manifestations and course of illness with a wide spectrum ranging from a mild to very severe or disabling disease.

Diagnosis

The clinical picture of DMD is characteristic and an established case with hypertrophy of calf muscles can be easily diagnosed. The serum CPK enzyme is grossly elevated especially in early stages even before the onset

36

of clinical manifestations. The levels of CPK may fall during advanced stage of the disease. Serum CPK levels may be raised in two-thirds of carrier females. Serum CPK level in DMD or BMD rises because of leakage of CPK from the muscle fibers due to damage to the sarcolemmal membrane.

- *Echocardiography* and ECG should be monitored periodically for identification of cardiomyopathy.
- *Electromyography* is rarely needed unless elevations in serum CPK levels are minimal. The amplitude and duration of motor unit potential is decreased, whereas the frequencies of polyphasic potentials are increased.
- *Histopathology* of muscle fibers shows diffuse changes of degeneration and regeneration. During the advanced stage, muscle is almost replaced by fat and collagen tissue. In contrast, muscular atrophy secondary to neurological diseases shows bundles of degenerated muscle fibers interspersed with normal muscle fibers.
- *Immunohistochemistry* reveals absence of dystrophin in DMD and patchy dystrophin staining in children with BMD.
- *Gene deletion* can be identified by multiplex PCR studies. Antenatal diagnosis can be made on chorionic villus samples by PCR or linkage studies using cancer antigen repeat markers.

Management

The child should be encouraged to remain active by daily walking, climbing stairs and cycling. Physiotherapy and graded physical exercises are useful to maintain muscle strength. The period of active walking can be prolonged by fitting leg braces when child is finding it difficult to walk. Contractures should be prevented by doing regular stretching exercises. Subcutaneous tenotomy of Achilles tendon may be done to relieve severe contracture. Prolonged immobilization should be avoided at any cost because it hastens deterioration in muscle function and progress of disease.

- *Cardiorespiratory care* should be provided by prompt treatment of intercurrent respiratory infections, congestive cardiac failure and by regular breathing exercises and yogic pranayams.
- *Supportive care* Prognosis should be explained with due sensitivity and compassion to both the parents. The child should be given nutritious balanced diet with restricted calories and fats to prevent obesity, which may adversely affect ambulation. Adequate calcium intake should be provided, to prevent osteoporosis. Scoliosis is prevented by use of tight-fitting orthotic braces.

- *Drug therapy* The role of drugs is controversial. Prednisolone given in a dose of 0.75 mg/kg/d for 10 days in a month reduces the rate of progression of the disease. The drug may be continued as long as the child is ambulatory. Deflazacort, oxandrolone, calcium channel blockers, Ql0, and vitamin E have been used with variable success. There is hope that in the near future, the disease may be cured by newer technologies such as myoblast transplantation, gene therapy, and protein upregulation.

SKELETAL DISORDERS

A large number of conditions can affect the bones including nutritional disorders (vitamin D deficiency or rickets), injuries with or without fracture and infections (osteomyelitis due to bacterial or tubercular infection).

Rickets (Vitamin D deficiency)

Apart from bones, vitamin D is essential for a large number of physiological processes to maintain optimal health. Subclinical vitamin D deficiency is now recognized as a pandemic, affecting more than half of the world's population. Rickets is a disease of growing bones and occurs in children with vitamin D deficiency. It primarily affects bones, skeletal muscles, and sometimes the nervous system. It occurs because of deficiency of vitamin D (cholecalciferol), which is a naturally occurring steroid. It can be formed in the skin by irradiation of 7-dehydrocholesterol with ultraviolet B light in the wavelengths of 280 to 305 nm. It is also known as "sunshine vitamin." Exposure to sunlight for 20 minutes every day is sufficient for the body to synthesize enough vitamin D to meet daily requirements. The endogenous production or availability of vitamin D_3 is reduced in the absence of sunlight and in dark-skinned individuals. The dietary sources of vitamin D_3 include fortified foods (milk and milk products, vegetable oil, breads, and juices), fish, cod liver oil, and egg yolk. Ultraviolet B irradiation of ergosterol in plants and yeast produces vitamin D_2 (ergocalciferol), which is also a potent antirachitic substance but is not available commercially as a supplement.

Vitamin D Metabolism

Vitamin D (cholecalciferol) is converted in the liver to biologically inactive but stable 25(OH)D (calcidiol) by hepatic microsomal 25-hydroxylase. This metabolite circulates in the plasma with a transport protein and is used as the marker of vitamin D status. It is further hydroxylated in the kidneys to calcitriol or 1,25-dihydroxyvitamin D (1,25 $(OH)_2$ D) by the action of mitochondrial 1-α-hydroxylase **(Figure 36.4)**. The physiological effects of 1,25 (OH)$_2$ D include (i) increased calcium absorption from the gastrointestinal tract, (ii) improved reabsorption of calcium from renal tubules, and (iii) calcium deposition in the bones. Like vitamin D$_3$, vitamin D$_2$ is further metabolized in the liver and kidneys to form its active metabolite. Apart from vitamin D, calcium absorption is enhanced by the acidic pH in the gut, dietary lactose, and when calcium and phosphate are consumed in a ratio of 2:1.

Biochemical consequences of vitamin D deficiency

Vitamin D deficiency leads to a decrease in the serum calcium level, which stimulates the release of parathyroid hormone (PTH). Parathyroid hormone tries to maintain serum calcium level by (i) mobilizing calcium from bones, (ii) promoting synthesis of 1,25 (OH)$_2$D in the kidneys which in turn increases absorption of calcium from intestines, and (iii) reducing excretion of calcium by the kidneys. Parathyroid hormone reduces renal tubular reabsorption of phosphates leading to phosphaturia. These homeostatic changes tend to maintain serum calcium level while the serum phosphate level falls. This leads to low calcium × phosphorus product, which is a characteristic feature of active rickets. In extreme cases, even serum calcium level may fall when compensatory mechanisms fail. Serum alkaline phosphatase level increases because of increase in the osteoclastic activity in the bones.

Rickets may occur in exclusively breastfed babies because breast milk is a poor source of vitamin D (0.5 to 10 i.u./dL) there is a high prevalence of vitamin D deficiency during pregnancy and lactation. Vitamin D deficiency may occur in infants fed with cow's milk or unfortified formula feeds. Rickets may also occur because of gastrointestinal malabsorption and hepatic and renal disorders. Phytates in the dietary cereals may bind calcium (magnesium and iron as well) in the gut to form phytin, thus compromising calcium absorption. Anticonvulsant therapy with phenytoin and phenobarbitone may interfere with metabolism of vitamin D. Glucocorticoids appear to have effects that are antagonistic to vitamin D for calcium absorption. The risk factors for development of vitamin D deficiency are listed in **Box 36.2**.

Clinical Features

Early Rickets

Congenital rickets may occur if the mother has subclinical vitamin D deficiency with compensatory hyperparathyroidism. The characteristic sign of

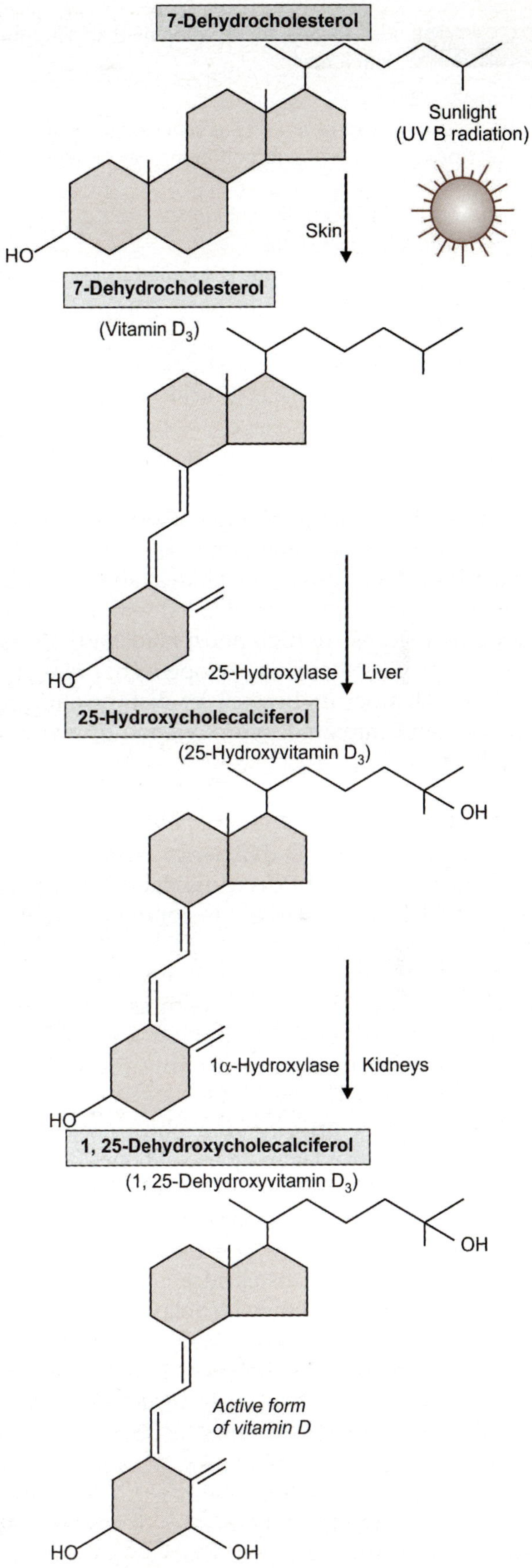

Figure 36.4 Vitamin D metabolism

| Box 36.2 | Risk factors for development of vitamin D deficiency |

- Female gender
- Insufficient sun exposure, skin pigmentation, overcrowding, overclothing, atmospheric pollution, use of sunscreens, and genetic factors.
- Lack of vitamin D supplementation.
- Poor socioeconomic status
  □ Lack of intake of vitamin D fortified foods, fish, cod liver oil, and eggs.
- Diseases
  □ Obesity, inflammatory bowel disease, cystic fibrosis, celiac disease, chronic renal failure and epilepsy.
- Medications
  □ Corticosteroids, anticonvulsants and rifampin.

congenital rickets is craniotabes (softening of skull bones). When the occipital bone is pressed firmly, it gets depressed and gives a feel like a table tennis ball. Tetany is common if the infant is fed with unmodified cow's milk (because of high phosphate load). Preterm babies are prone to develop osteopenia of prematurity or rickets. This occurs because of dietary phosphate deficiency and impaired hydroxylation of vitamin D in the liver.

Classical Rickets

The classical vitamin D-deficiency rickets manifest most commonly in children between the age of 6 months and 2 years. Rickets is common in chubby children who are actively growing. Children with PEM may manifest rickets during recovery when they are actively growing. The clinical features are produced by enlargement of costochondral junctions or ends of long bones, osteoporosis, softening of bones, and skeletal deformities.

- *Skull* is square-shaped and shows bossing or prominence of frontal and parietal bones because of subperiosteal deposition of osteoid. When bossing is marked, the head looks large and square and may give an appearance of "hot-cross-bun." Anterior fontanel is large and its closure is delayed beyond 18 months. Dentition may be delayed.
- *Chest* shows "rachitic rosary" with "beading of ribs" because of enlargement of costochondral junctions. There is visible and palpable swelling of costochondral junctions on both sides of sternum, giving an appearance of a rosary of beads. Sternum may project forward (pigeon breast). There may be depressions or sulci on both sides of lower chest at the level of attachment of diaphragm (Harrison groove) because of softening of ribs. A similar

appearance of lower chest (without costochondral beading) may be seen in children with recurrent respiratory infections, bronchial asthma, and congenital heart disease.

- *Long bones* show enlargement of ends, softening and deformities. There is enlargement and swelling of wrists **(Figure 36.5)** and ankles. The shafts of long bones of lower limbs may develop various curvatures and deformities leading to genu varum (bowed legs), genu valgum (knock knees), and coxa vara (widening or abduction of hips).
- Spinal deformities, such as dorsolumbar lordosis, kyphosis, or scoliosis, may occur because of laxity of spinal ligaments.
- *Stature* may be grossly affected by spinal and lower limb deformities. Pelvic outlet may be narrowed down by forward displacement of the sacral promontory and deformities of pelvic bones leading to difficulties in child birth later in life.
- *Non-skeletal manifestations* of rickets include sweating, muscular hypotonia, hair loss, protuberant abdomen or pot belly, and recurrent respiratory infections. Iron-deficiency anemia is also commonly associated. Tetany may occur rarely.

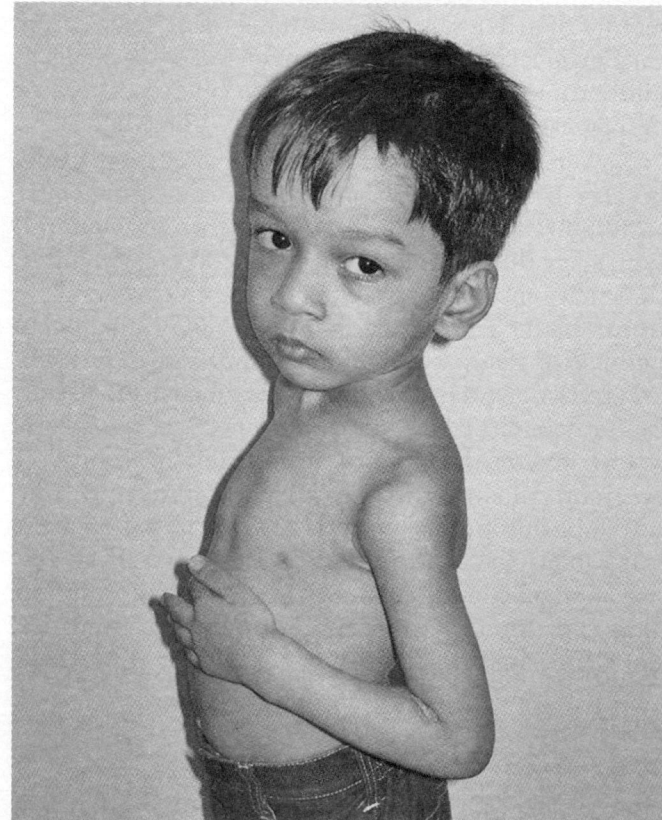

Figure 36.5 Widened wrist with pigeon-shaped chest in a 3-year-old boy with vitamin D deficiency rickets

Laboratory Investigations

Serum calcium is usually normal (9 to 11 mg/dL), phosphate is usually reduced (<4 mg/dL), and alkaline phosphatase is elevated (>500 i.u./dL). The normal plasma calcium despite diminished intestinal absorption of calcium (because of vitamin D deficiency) is explained on the basis of compensatory increased parathyroid activity, which mobilizes calcium from the bones and also causes hypophosphatemia because of phosphaturia. A plasma calcium phosphorus product (mg/dL) above 40 excludes vitamin D-deficiency rickets, whereas a value below 30 indicates active rickets. Serum phosphate level is normal in vitamin D-dependent rickets and metaphyseal dysostosis, whereas it is elevated in renal osteodystrophy. Elevated alkaline phosphatase level is a sensitive indicator of active rickets but may be elevated in primary hyperparathyroidism, obstructive jaundice, fractures, metastatic bone disease, and the "battered baby" syndrome. Plasma 25(OH)D level is usually low while PTH level is increased. Plasma 25(OH)D level of less than 20 ng/dL (50 nmol/L) is suggestive of vitamin D deficiency, whereas a level between 21 and 29 ng/mL suggests vitamin D insufficiency. However, these tests are not routinely required for the diagnosis of rickets. Skiagram of wrists or knees shows characteristic radiological findings. The normally smooth and convex ends of bones become splayed out with metaphyseal fraying and "cupping" **(Figure 36.6)**. The distance between the epiphysis and diaphysis is increased because the metaphysis consists largely of non-opaque osteoid tissue. The periosteum may be raised because of laying down of osteoid tissue while shafts of bones may become decalcified and curved. During healing following administration of vitamin D, a line of preparatory calcification appears near the diaphysis followed by appearance of calcification in the irregular osteoid at the frayed ends of bones.

Differential Diagnosis

Congenital rickets may be confused with hypophosphatemic rickets, which is characterized by defective calcification of the membranous bones of skull, wide sutures, cutaneous dimples, failure to thrive, hypercalcemia, and low alkaline phosphatase. Some healthy toddlers may show physiological bowing of the legs. The ends of bones may be broad in those with osteochondrodystrophy, but they have no other clinical or biochemical features of rickets. Rickets may occur because of malabsorption (celiac disease, fibrocystic disease of the pancreas), hepatic (cholestatic disorders) and renal (renal tubular acidosis, Fanconi syndrome, renal osteodystrophy) causes. These should be excluded on the basis of history, physical examination, and laboratory investigations.

Treatment

Vitamin D_3 is administered in a weekly oral dose of 60,000 i.u. (1 mg calciferol = 40,000 i.u.) for 10 weeks. Alternatively 600,000 i.u. of vitamin D can be given orally or through deep intramuscular injection as a single dose. Radiological healing (zone of calcification) and biochemical improvement are seen within 3 to 4 weeks. The above dose may be repeated if therapeutic response is incomplete. Maintenance doses of vitamin D_3 400 units (10 µg) per day are continued after the process of healing has started. The infant should be given adequate amount of calcium in the diet (600 mg calcium per day or 600 mL of milk). Calcium supplements are not needed once serum 25(OH)D level is normalized. In children with rickets because of renal or hepatic causes, it is preferable to use calcitriol or 1,25 $(OH)_2$ D (0.05 µg/kg/d). Weight-bearing on the legs may be restricted till complete radiological healing has occurred. Skeletal deformities usually disappear over a period of time and osteotomy is rarely required. Children should be encouraged to play outdoor for adequate exposure to sunlight. If there is any underlying gastrointestinal, hepatic (cholestasis), or renal (renal tubular acidosis, Fanconi disease, and renal osteodystrophy) disease, it should be diagnosed and appropriately managed. When two mega doses of vitamin D (600,000 i.u. each dose) fail to elicit any biochemical or radiological response, the child should be investigated for refractory rickets.

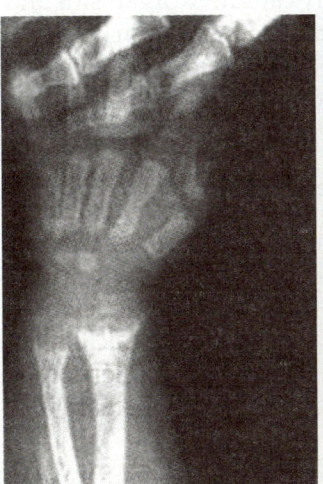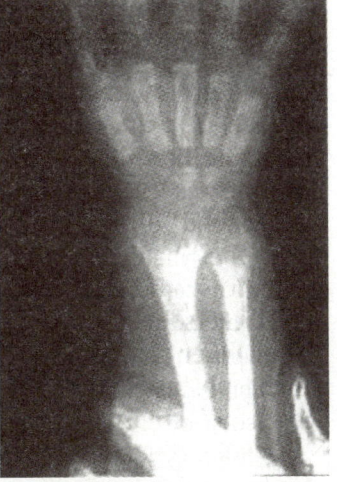

Figure 36.6 Note the typical cupping and rarefaction of metaphyseal ends of both the radius and ulna because of active rickets

36

Non-skeletal health benefits of vitamin D

Calciotropic effects of vitamin D on intestines, bones, and kidneys have been well known since ages. Recent evidence suggests that vitamin D has a beneficial effect on a large number of body tissues and metabolic processes to maintain sound health. Vitamin D receptors have been identified in more than 30 body tissues including intestines, liver, kidneys, heart, lungs, brain, muscles, skin, pancreas and various immune cells. Moreover, apart from kidneys, enzyme CYP27B1 (which helps in conversion of 25(OH)D into biologically active 1,25(OH)$_2$D has been found in various tissues of the body. The non-skeletal autocrine pleiotropic effects of vitamin D are independent of regulation of serum calcium, phosphorus and PTH levels and are not controlled by the feedback-endocrine loop mechanism. There is evidence to suggest that vitamin D exerts beneficial effects on a large number of body organs to maintain optimal health and well-being. Vitamin D is credited with potent antioxidant effects to prevent free radical damage and promote cellular differentiation to protect against auto-immune diseases and carcinogenesis. The long-term health benefits of vitamin D are listed in the **Box 36.3**.

OSTEOMYELITIS

Bones are relatively avascular and their infection is uncommon. Osteomyelitis may occur at any age, and common predisposing factors include trauma or septicemia. It may occur due to pyogenic, tubercular, fungal or parasitic infection. It usually affects the long bones at their metaphyseal region but involvement of small bones of hands and feet may occur due to tubercular and fungal infections.

The most common causative pathogens include *Staphylococcus aureus*, which is responsible for acute hematogenous infection. Other causative organisms include *Group B Hemolytic streptococci, H. influenzae type b, Pseudomonas aeruginosa* and *E. coli* especially in neonates and infants.

Clinical Features

Acute osteomyelitis is characterized by high grade fever with or without chills, localized pain, swelling, tenderness, erythema and warmth. History of preceding injury is reported by 50% of patients. There may be symptoms and signs of generalized sepsis. It may be associated with arthritis, contracture, pathological fracture or leg-length discrepancy. The infection may become chronic and intractable due to inadequate treatment and lack of drainage of underlying pus. Involvement of small joints of hand (dactylitis) is suggestive of tubercular infection and several other conditions which are listed in **Box 36.4**.

Diagnosis

History of preceding trauma or infection, with local symptoms and signs of inflammation and bony tenderness are highly suggestive. Complete blood count shows leukocytosis with predominance of polymorphonuclear leukocytes and elevated markers of infections like C-reactive protein, calcitonin and erythrocyte sedimentation rate. Blood culture and culture of material obtained on drainage of pus, bone aspiration or biopsy are useful to identify causative organisms and their sensitivity to various antibiotics. Skiagrams, computed tomography scan or MRI of the affected bone are useful to identify the extent and severity of disease process.

Box 36.3 Non-skeletal health benefits of vitamin D

- **Autoimmune diseases**
  - □ Reduced risk of type 1 diabetes mellitus, rheumatoid arthritis, bronchial asthma, multiple sclerosis, systemic lupus erythematosus, inflammatory bowel disease and psoriasis.
- **Malignant disorders**
  - □ Decreased risk of malignant disorders such as colorectal cancer, breast cancer, prostate cancer and leukemia.
- **Heart disease**
  - □ Reduced risk of hypertension and coronary artery disease.
- **Better control of type 2 diabetes mellitus and neuropathic pain**
- **Neuropsychological functioning**
  - □ Better cognition, reduced risk of depression and affective disorders
- **Infections**
  - □ Reduced risk of periodontal diseases, respiratory tract infections and tuberculosis.

Box 36.4 Common causes of dactylitis in children

1. Juvenile rheumatoid arthritis
2. Acute lymphoblastic leukemia
3. Sickle cell disease
4. Tuberculosis
5. Syphilis
6. Chikungunya
7. Psoriasis
8. Blistering distal dactylitis due to streptococcal, staphylococcal or fungal infections.
9. Sarcoidosis
10. Reiter's disease

36

Management

Therapy demands close monitoring and nursing care because prolonged therapy and follow-up are required. Antibiotic therapy is started by parenteral administration of amoxicillin, or cloxacillin and amikacin. The choice of antibiotics may be modified on the basis of culture and antibiogram. After about one week of intravenous administration of antibiotics, the therapy should be continued orally for at least 4–6 weeks. Tubercular and fungal infections should be managed by administration of appropriate antibiotics. Supportive and symptomatic management include use of analgesics and antipyretics, immobilization of affected limb, wound care and drainage of abscess. The child must receive adequate hydration and nutritious high-protein diet. Surgical interventions include drainage of abscess, sequestrectomy and bone grafting. During recovery, gradual ambulation, physiotherapy, and use of orthotic devices are mandatory to prevent deformities and disability.

FRACTURES

Children are prone to injuries with risk of sprain and fractures because they are ebullient and restless, and take part in aggressive sports activities. Most fractures are closed and greenstick in nature in children. In young children with history of repeated physical injuries and fractures, the possibility of child abuse by parents should be ruled out. Epiphyseal growth plate may be affected in 15 to 30% of fractures in children, leading to permanent shortening of affected limb. Refer to **Chapter 45** on Accidents, Poisonings and Animal bites for details.

Osteogenesis Imperfecta

It is an autosomal dominant disorder which is characterized by osteoporosis and excessive fragility of bones. There is frequent occurrence of fractures on minor trauma leading to deformities of limbs with poor healing of fractures. The associated features include blue sclerae, conductive deafness and lax ligaments. According to severity of disease, there are four subtypes. Almost 50% cases may die in utero while osteogenesis imperfecta tarda manifests during adolescence or later in life.

Treatment

These patients need tender nursing care on a firm bed and soft pillows with close supervision of daily activities of living. Adequate nutrition with supplements of vitamins D (calcitonin) and magnesium oxide may reduce the risk of fractures. Fractures should be managed by prompt immobilization. Surgical correction of deformities is done later in life during adolescence.

DISEASES OF JOINTS

A number of diseases are associated with arthritis which is characterized by fever, localized pain, warmth, redness, tenderness and limitation of movements. Depending upon the severity of onset and duration of symptoms, arthritis is classified into three types **(Box 36.5)**.

Transient Synovitis

It is a self-limiting arthritis which is characterized by sudden onset of fever, pain in the hips (observation hip), thighs and/or knees following an upper respiratory catarrh. Administration of nonsteroidal anti-inflammatory drugs (NSAIDs) is followed by prompt relief.

Septic Arthritis

There is involvement of a single large joint during the course of sepsis in young infants. There is sudden onset of fever with inflammatory signs and restricted or painful movements at the affected joint. The common etiologic agents in infants include Gram-negative organisms, *E. coli.*, *S. proteus*, *Haemophilus influenzae type b*, *Pseudomonas aeruginosa*, while in older children *Staphylococcus aureus* and *Streptococcus pneumoniae* are

36

> **Box 36.5** **Classification of arthritis**

Acute arthritis (<2 weeks)
- Transient or 'toxic' synovitis
- Septic arthritis
- Rheumatic fever
- Arthritis associated with Kawasaki disease and Henoch-Schonlein disease

Subacute arthritis (2–6 weeks)
- Ractive arthritis
- Arthritis associated with systemic lupus erythematosus, dermatomyositis, polyarthritis nodosa and brucellosis
- Bone pains and arthritis associated with acute leukemia and neuroblastoma
- Sickle cell disease

Chronic arthritis (>6 weeks)
- Juvenile idiopathic arthritis
- Ankylosing spondylitis
- Tubercular arthritis
- Legg-Calvé-Perthes disease
- Psoriasis

the leading pathogens. Complete blood count shows leukocytosis with predominance of polymorphonuclear leukocytes, elevated C-reactive protein and calcitonin. Ultrasonography, magnetic resonance imaging and radionuclide scans provide useful diagnostic clues. A diagnostic arthrocentesis is useful to identify pathogens and their antibacterial sensitivity pattern. The condition is managed by drainage of pus, local immobilization and administration of appropriate antibiotics through intravenous route for one week followed by oral therapy for a period of 3–4 weeks.

Acute Rheumatic Fever

It is an immune-mediated disorder that occurs after 2–4 weeks of a throat or skin infection by Group A β-*Hemolytic streptococci* (GABHS). The classical features of acute rheumatic fever appear after 10 to 14 days of streptococcal throat infection which is either unrecognized or inadequately treated. There is acute onset of polyarthritis with involvement of large joints such as knees, ankles, elbows and wrists. There is marked inflammatory signs of fever, pain and swelling of joints and marked limitation of movements. Polyarthritis may be migratory in nature, i.e. resolution of pain and discomfort in the affected joints within 2–3 days, followed by pain and swelling in the newly affected joints. Two major or one major and two minor criteria should be present along with the presence of essential criteria (evidences of recent streptococcal throat infection) for making the diagnosis of acute rheumatic fever. The diagnostic criteria for acute rheumatic fever are given in **Chapter 39**.

Treatment

Bed rest and good nursing care are essential for recovery. Salicylates are useful for treatment of polyarthritis without carditis. Aspirin is gives in a dose of 100 mg/kg per day in four divided doses after meals for 2 to 3 weeks. The dose is then tapered to 50 to 60 mg/kg per day and given for a total duration of 12 weeks. Antacids may be co-administered to prevent gastric irritation. The involvement of joints recovers promptly without any sequelae but the major concern in patients with acute rheumatic fever is the risk of development of carditis and involvement and damage to the valves of the heart. These children need close monitoring and management with corticosteroids to prevent the sequelae of carditis. In the absence of carditis, penicillin prophylaxis is given for 5 years or up to the age of 18 years. In patients with carditis or RHD, penicillin prophylaxis is continued lifelong or at least up to the age of 40 years.

Juvenile Rheumatoid Arthritis (JRA)

The American College of Rheumatology (ACR) has defined JRA as arthritis without any obvious cause, involving joints with an onset below the age of 16 years and persisting for at least 6 weeks. The other terms include juvenile chronic arthritis and juvenile idiopathic arthritis. It is the commonest rheumatic disorder in children. The sex ratio appears to be almost equal in India unlike the West, where the disease is more common in girls. Juvenile rheumatoid arthritis and adult-onset rheumatoid arthritis (RA) appear to be two distinct clinical entities.

Etiopathogenesis

Juvenile rheumatoid arthritis is an autoimmune disease affecting genetically susceptible individuals. Studies have shown that human leukocyte antigen (HLA)-DR5, HLA-DR6, HLA-DR8 and HLA-A2 are associated with early-onset oligoarthritis (especially in boys); HLA-B27 in relation to late-onset oligoarthritis (especially in girls); and HLA-DR1, HLA-DR4 and HLA-DW4 to rheumatoid factor (RF)-positive polyarthritis.

The etiopathogenesis of JRA, like other autoimmune diseases, remains an enigma. Several environmental triggers such as viral infections (rubella and parvovirus B_{19}), *Mycobacterium tuberculosis, Mycoplasma pneumoniae,* trauma and psychological stress have been linked to the onset of disease. There is formation of antigen-antibody complexes with consumption of complement. The immune complexes get deposited in the synovium of the joint/s with activation of T lymphocytes, which release various inflammatory markers. The cytokine profile of three main types of JRA is distinctive. In polyarthritis, there are increased levels of IL-1α; oligoarthritis is associated with elaboration of IL-1β and TNF-α, whereas systemic-onset JRA has increased antinuclear (ANA) and antismooth muscle antibodies. The classical rheumatoid factor (RF) is usually negative in the serum because it may be tagged (especially with immunoglobulin A [IgA] component) with the circulating or fixed immune complexes.

Clinical Presentation

On the basis of initial presentation, three main types of JRA are recognized, namely systemic onset, pauciarticular (four or fewer joints) and polyarticular (five or more joints).

Systemic onset Approximately 20% of the children with JRA may have an acute onset with high-grade fever and toxemia that may precede the joint manifestations by several weeks or months. Systemic-onset JRA (Still disease) may occur at any age and is slightly more common in boys. The fever is intermittent and high grade with characteristic two peaks in a day. It may be accompanied with an evanescent salmon-colored macular skin rash with central clearing on the trunk. The presence of cutaneous hypersensitivity response to superficial scratch on the skin (Koebner phenomenon) is common. There is generalized lymphadenopathy and mild hepatosplenomegaly. Other systemic manifestations include pericarditis, pleuritis, and interstitial lung disease. *Macrophage activation syndrome* is a rare complication of systemic-onset JRA. It is characterized by fever, drowsiness, anemia, thrombocytopenia, lymphadenopathy, hepato-splenomegaly and markedly elevated hepatic enzymes. The diagnosis is confirmed on liver biopsy and bone marrow examination. The condition is treated with corticosteroids and cyclosporine. Systemic-onset JRA is an important cause of pyrexia of unknown origin and responds to administration of salicylates and non-steroidal anti-inflammatory drugs (NSAIDs). Antinuclear antibodies may be positive, but rheumatoid factor (RF) is usually negative.

Pauciarticular or oligoarticular onset It is the most common mode of onset of JRA wherein four or less number of large joints are involved in an asymmetrical manner, joint swelling is more dominant than pain. Two subtypes are seen.

1. **Type I** It is more common in preschool girls and manifests with the involvement of knees, ankles and elbows. Small joints of hands and feet are usually spared. Iridocyclitis is seen in 25% of the patients on slit lamp examination. It is usually asymptomatic at onset but may progress to blindness.

2. **Type II** It also involves large joints but is more common in boys older than 8 years. Many children are HLA-B27 positive and a proportion of these patients progress to develop ankylosing spondylitis in adult life. They are also prone to develop iridocyclitis, which is usually benign in nature. Antinuclear antibodies are usually absent.

Polyarticular onset Almost one-third of the patients have involvement of five or more joints. There is involvement of both large and small joints of the hands and feet. Hip involvement never occurs at onset, joint pain is usually out of proportion to the degree of joint swelling. Fever, malaise, anorexia, anemia, and weight loss are common. On the basis of RF results, two subtypes are identified.

1. **Rheumatoid factor positive** This subtype is similar to adult-onset JRA and affects older children or adolescents. Arthritis is symmetrical, severe, and deforming and usually involves the metacarpo-phalangeal and interphalangeal joints of the hands **(Figures 36.7** and **36.8)**. Cervical spine and temporo-mandibular joints may be affected. The presence of rheumatoid nodules over the extensor surfaces of the elbows and tendo-Achilles indicates severe disease. Uveitis may occur in 5% of the patients.

2. **Rheumatoid factor negative** This subtype may occur at any age and is usually less severe and without any rheumatoid nodules. The knees, wrists, and hips are most commonly affected, whereas small joints of the hands and feet are rarely involved.

Differential Diagnosis

A number of diseases with polyarthritis and dactylitis may be confused with JRA. The list includes Reiter disease, hemophilic arthropathy, acute lymphoblastic leukemia, polyarticular tuberculosis, pyogenic arthritis,

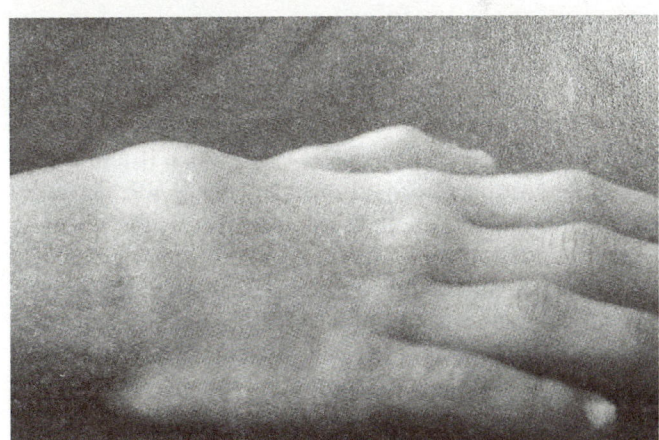

Figure 36.7 Acute inflammation of wrist and proximal interphalangeal joints

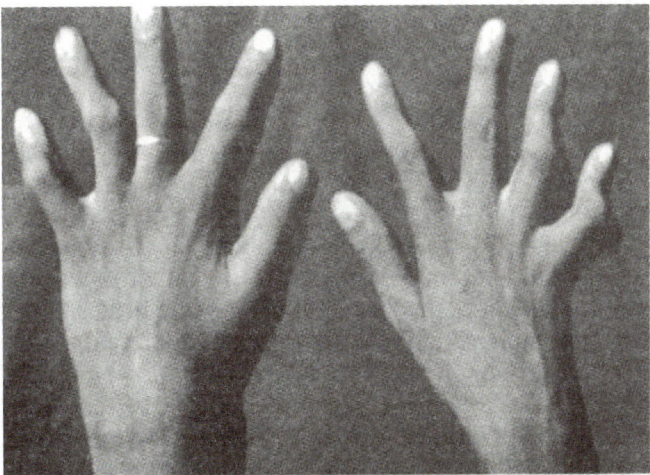

Figure 36.8 Claw-like hands because of deformities in a long-standing case of polyarthritis juvenile rheumatoid arthritis

fungal arthritis, sickle cell dactylitis, chikungunya, congenital syphilis, psoriatic arthropathy and sarcoidosis.

Laboratory Investigations

The diagnosis of JRA is, by and large, based on clinical assessment, and investigations are done to assess the activity of disease process and guide prognosis. Complete blood count may show low hemoglobin level and leukocytosis with preponderance of polymorphs and thrombocytosis. Anemia occurs because of anorexia, chronic inflammation, and GI bleeding as a consequence of the side effects of NSAIDs. Anemia is a good marker of severity of the disease, hemoglobin level of 5 to 7 g/dL indicates longstanding disease process, whereas hemoglobin level higher than 9 g/dL suggests a well-controlled disease. Acute lymphoblastic leukemia may have dactylitis and can be differentiated from JRA by petechiae, thrombocytopenia, lymphocytosis, and lymphoblasts. *When corticosteroid therapy is contemplated in a child with JRA, bone marrow examination should be done to rule out ALL.* Erythrocyte sedimentation rate is grossly elevated and is a good marker for the activity of disease process. Rheumatoid factor and antinuclear antibodies (ANAs) are usually negative; but when present, they indicate adverse outcome. Plain radiographs of affected joints are usually normal during initial stages but may be repeated during the course of disease process for the assessment of erosive changes. Synovial fluid aspiration may be needed in monoarticular disease to exclude infective process. Smear and culture studies for pyogenic organisms and acid-fast bacilli (AFBs) would be negative.

Management

Non-steroidal anti-inflammatory drugs Non-steroidal anti-inflammatory drugs are the mainstay for treatment of JRA. Naproxen (15 to 20 mg/kg/d every 12 hours) and ibuprofen (35 to 45 mg/kg/d every 6–8 hours) are the most commonly used drugs. Non-steroidal anti-inflammatory drugs should be given after meals and coadministered with antacids to reduce GI side effects. Response to therapy is usually slow, and treatment must be continued for 4 to 6 weeks before a decision to switch over to another NSAID is taken.

Disease-modifying antirheumatic drugs (DMARD) When arthritis does not respond to a reasonable trial of NSAIDs, use of DMARD is recommended. Oral weekly administration of methotrexate (10 to 15 mg/m²/wk) has revolutionized the management of JRA. The drug is given on empty stomach and can be continued for years along with NSAIDs. Children are able to tolerate methotrexate better than adults, and there are fewer side effects. Periodic testing of liver functions is mandatory because hepatic fibrosis is the dreaded side effect. Once remission is achieved and the child is stable, methotrexate is tapered off to the minimum effective dose and then gradually stopped.

Corticosteroids Prednisolone (1 to 2 mg/kg/d every 8 hours) is given as an adjunct therapy for the t reatment of severe unremitting polyarthritis, systemic-onset disease (with pericarditis, myocarditis, pleuritis, or interstitial lung disease), and rapidly progressive disease. Oral steroids are usually given as a bridge therapy for a few weeks while awaiting the clinical response to NSAIDs/DMARDs. Intra-articular injection of triamcinolone hexacetonide may be given to patients with pauciarticular JRA as a useful adjunct to DMARD therapy. Local instillation of steroids in the eyes is recommended for the treatment of iridocyclitis under the supervision of an ophthalmologist.

Cytotoxic agents In children with severe erosive disease, unresponsive to methotrexate, cyclophosphamide, azathioprine, and cyclosporine A may be given a trial.

Newer modalities There is evidence to suggest that dietary omega 3 fatty acids, fish oil, and docosahexaenoic acid are credited to provide therapeutic benefit to several autoimmune disorders including RA by inhibiting the synthesis of prostaglandins and leukotrienes. Etanercept (a recombinant soluble TNF receptor p75 fusion protein) and infliximab (a monoclonal antibody) that are targeted against TNF-α have been found to be effective in patients with refractory arthritis.

Follow-up and Prognosis

Children and their families need psychosocial support and counseling because of the chronic disabling nature of the disease. The child should be encouraged to lead a normal life and attend the school. Balanced high-protein diet with supplements of calcium, vitamin D, and iron should be given. Physical therapy helps in relieving pain (local heat, wax baths, infrared exposure, and diathermy), maintenance of posture and joint mobility, improves muscle strength, and prevents deformities and contractures. Night splints are useful to provide rest and prevent deformities. Occupational therapist can help in rehabilitation and for planning career goals of a severely affected child. Girls aged younger than 6 years with ANA-positive pauciarticular JRA should be screened by slit lamp examination every 3 months for early identification of iridocyclitis.

Children with other forms of JRA should be screened by an ophthalmologist once at the time of initial diagnosis and then once a year. Children with pauciarticular JRA type II may develop spondylitis and sacroiliitis later in life especially if they are HLA-B27 positive. Patients with seropositive polyarticular JRA have a disease pattern similar to adults with RA and may develop erosive and disabling disease if not treated aggressively. In systemic-onset JRA, early age of onset, persistent fever, and thrombocytosis are associated with poor prognosis. Almost 50% of the patients with systemic-onset JRA undergo remission with minimal residual joint involvement, whereas others may develop progressive arthritis or have recurrent episodes of systemic disease.

Children with HLA-DR4 are likely to have severe or persistent arthritis. Children with JRA should be followed for their linear growth and shortening or lengthening of a limb. Joint deformities and contractures may cause severe functional disability. Severe involvement of temporomandibular joint may lead to micrognathia. Secondary amyloidosis is a dreaded irreversible complication and should be monitored by periodic testing for proteinuria and hypoalbuminemia.

Systemic Lupus Erythematosus

It is a multisystem autoimmune disease characterized by chronic inflammation of blood vessels and connective tissues. The disease is triggered by altered T cells, which activate or stimulate B cells to produce autoantibodies against a variety of self-antigens with formation of immune complexes with the help of complement.

Clinical Manifestations

Systemic lupus erythematosus (SLE) is characterized by a variety of manifestations because of involvement of several body systems. The disease is more common among girls with female to male preponderance of 4:1 before puberty and 8:1 in adult life. It is characterized by typical malar rash with characteristic butterfly pattern on the face **(Figure 36.9)** due to increased photosensitivity. There may be painless oral and mucocutaneous lesions with non-erosive arthritis involving two or more joints. During the course of disease there will be progressive involvement of various body organs including kidneys, brain, heart, lungs and hematologic system. Children are more likely to have severe manifestations with poor prognosis.

Diagnosis

The hematologic abnormalities include leukopenia, lymphopenia, thrombocytopenia, coagulation abnormalities and Coombs-positive hemolytic anemia. The diagnostic immunoserology include presenec of antinuclear

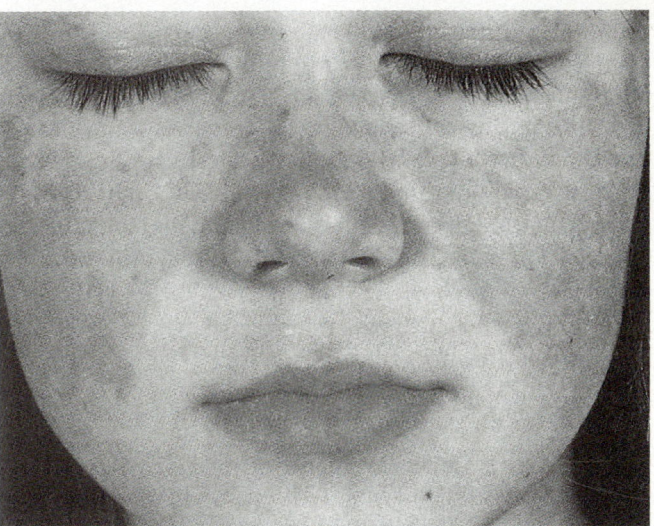

Figure 36.9 Typical butterfly malar flush in a 14-year-old girl with systemic lupus erythematosus

antibodies or anti double-stranded deoxyribonucleic acid (anti-ds DNA) antibodies, antismooth muscle or anti-sm antibodies, antiphospholipid antibodies and anticoagulant antibodies. Serum complement level is reduced. In drug-induced SLE, antihistone antibodies are usually present. Anti-RO antibodies may be transferred from the affected mother to her infant leading to development of complete heart block.

Management

Supportive treatment If patient is taking any of the drugs (anticonvulsants, sulfonamides, isoniazid, hydralazine, or antiarrhythmic agents) that is known to induce SLE, the drug should be stopped. In view of chronic multisystem involvement, the child should be provided a balanced nutritious diet. Protein intake is guided by the involvement of liver and kidneys. Salt intake is restricted if there is hypertension. Infections should be identified early and treated aggressively. Sunscreen lotions (sun protection factor 15–30) should be applied to the exposed parts of the body three to four times per day. Arthritis usually responds to NSAIDs.

Immunosuppressive therapy Glucocorticoids are most useful and form the mainstay of therapy. Prednisolone is started in a dose of 1 to 2 mg/kg/d and gradually tapered depending on the disease activity. In most cases of SLE, daily or alternate-day prednisolone (2.5 to 5.0 mg/d) is continued for several years. When child is in remission, hydroxychloroquine (5 to 6 mg/kg/d) can be started and steroids further tapered.

Life-threatening complications (nephritis, central nervous system and cardiac complications) are treated with pulses of methylprednisolone and cyclophosphamide (750 mg/m^2 once a month through intravenous

36

administration). Intravenous immunoglobulins have been successfully used for the treatment of lupus nephritis, serositis, and thrombocytopenia. In a severe case of SLE unresponsive to corticosteroids, other immunosuppressive agents such as azathioprine, methotrexate, cyclosporine, and cyclophosphamide are tried singly or in various combinations. Patients not responding to the conventional immunosuppressive agents can be given a trial of mycophenolate mofetil, which is a new biological agent. The long-term outlook of SLE has improved with aggressive immunosuppressive therapy.

Juvenile Dermatomyositis

It is an immune-mediated inflammatory myopathy characterized by typical skin manifestations with focal areas of myositis resulting in progressive weakness of proximal muscles. The immune response is triggered by a viral infection in a susceptible child having genetic marking on chromosome 6, DQA1*0501, and DRB1*0301.

Clinical Features

The average age of onset is 6 to 7 years, and girls are affected more often than boys. The onset is insidious with low-grade fever, fatigue, arthralgias, and weight loss. Skin rash appears on sun-exposed areas with the development of characteristic periorbital violaceous (heliotrope) erythema of the eyelids. Rash occurs on other exposed areas like limbs with appearance of hypertrophic reddish-pink papules (Gottron papules) over the skin overlying metacarpals and proximal interphalangeal joints giving an appearance of alligator skin. There is focal myositis involving the muscles of limbs. Gower sign may be positive. Dysphonia, hoarseness, and aspiration may occur because of the involvement of the muscles of upper airways. Dysphagia, abdominal pain, and GI motility disorder are common. The condition should be differentiated from other connective tissue diseases such as scleroderma, SLE, mixed CTDs, acute poliomyelitis, and muscular dystrophies.

Diagnosis

There is elevation in the serum levels of muscle-derived enzymes, that is, creatine kinase and aldolase. In chronic cases with wasting of muscles, muscle enzymes may be normal or reduced. Magnetic resonance imaging of the limbs using T2-weighted images with fat suppression can localize the active sites of disease for undertaking diagnostic muscle biopsy and electromyography.

Treatment

All children with juvenile dermatomyositis should be advised to use sunscreen creams and given supplements of calcium and vitamin D. If there is dysphagia or incoordination of swallowing, the child should be given soft semiliquid nutritious diet. In severe cases, pulse doses of methylprednisolone 30 mg/kg are given IV daily for 3 days, followed by every 2 to 3 days/wk till inflammation subsides as evidenced by fall in the erythrocyte sedimentation rate. This is followed by low-dose oral prednisolone (0.5 mg/kg/d) daily or on alternate days on a long-term basis. Physiotherapy and occupational therapy is done by passive stretching of muscles and active movements of various joints.

Legg-Calvé-Perthes Disease

It is characterized by avascular necrosis of femoral head, usually affecting children between 5 and 10 years of age. The etiology is unknown but condition is associated with hypercoagulable state with deficiency of protein C or protein S. There is increased hereditary predisposition with bilateral involvement in 10% cases. The commen manifestations include sudden onset of pain in the hip with a limping gait. The diagnosis is confirmed by isotope bone scans and magnetic resonance imaging. The treatment is supportive and symptomatic. The disease is relentlessly progressive and in advanced cases femoral varus osteotomies and containment splints are required.

SPINAL ABNORMALITIES

The spinal abnormalities may be congenital or develop subsequently due to defective posture, carrying heavy load (school bag), softening and collapse of vertebrae because of rickets, infection of vertebrae (syphilis, tuberculosis), trauma, primary malignancy or metastatic deposits in the spine, ankylosing spondylitis and Scheuermann disease.

Kyphosis (Hunchback) is characterized by increased roundness of back or there may be increased angulation or gibbus formation when there is localized infection or malignancy. In lordosis, there is anterior curvature of lumbar spine and child develops a swaddling or duck-like gait. Scoliosis is suspected when there is lateral or side-to-side curvature of the spine. It is usually associated with two curves, the primary abnormal curve and a compensatory curve in the opposite direction. Most cases of scoliosis are due to spinal developmental defects like hemivertebrae and wedge vertebrae. Neuromuscular causes include muscular paralysis, cerebral palsy, post polio paralysis and myopathies. Scoliosis may occur due to rickets, fracture of spine, chronic pulmonary disorders (collapse of lung or empyema), defective posture, visual defects, sciatica and leg-length discrepancy.

Evaluation is done by taking a detailed history and conducting a thorough physical and neurological examination. When spinal deformity becomes less prominent or disappears on forward bending (Adam test), it can be managed by supportive measures and physiotherapy. Imaging studies and myelogram may be required in severe cases. Most cases are managed by braces (orthotic devices), yoga, exercises and physiotherapy. Surgical correction (posterior spinal fusion) is done for stabilization of spine when physical measures are unable to achieve the desired cosmetic results.

BIBLIOGRAPHY

Anthony KK, Schanberg LE. Pain in children with arthritis: A review of the current literature. *Arthritis Rheum* 2003, 49(2): 272–279.

Bushby K, Finkel R, Birnkrant DJ, et al. Diagnosis and management of Duchenne muscular dystrophy. *Lancet Neurol* 2010, 9: 77–93.

Chikanza JC. Juvenile rheumatoid arthritis: therapeutic perspective. *Paediatr Drugs* 2002, 4(5): 335–348.

D'cruz DP, systemic lupus erythematosus. *BMJ* 2006, 332(7546): 890–894.

Holick MF, Chen TC. Vitamin D deficiency: Worldwide problem with health consequences. *Am J Clin Nutr* 2008, 87(4): S1080–S1086.

Metules T. Duchenne muscular dystrophy. *Rev Neurol* 2002, 65(10): 39–44.

Rathi N, Rathi A. Vitamin D and child health in 21st century. *Indian Pediatr* 2011, 48(8): 619–625.

Singh M. Causes of limping in children. In: Pediatric Clinical Methods. Singh M (Ed), *New Delhi, CBS Publishers and Distributors Pvt Ltd*. 5th Edition, 2015, p173.

Singh M, Floppy neonate. In: Care of the Newborn. *New Delhi, CBS Publishers and Distributors Pvt Ltd*. Revised 8th Edition, 2016 p 442.

Stichweh D, Arce E, Pascual V. Update on pediatric systemic lupus erythematosus. *Curr Opin Rheumatol* 2004, 16(5): 577–587.

Gastrointestinal and Liver Disorders

ACUTE DIARRHEA

Diarrhea is one of the most common ailments in young children and account for 15% of all deaths of under-5 children. It is defined as passage of liquid or watery stools which are usually passed more than 3 times in a day. A recent change in the consistency or character of stools is more important than the number of stools. The diarrheal stools may be greenish in color and often have a strong offensive smell. Diarrhea (enteritis) is often preceded by vomiting (gastritis) as the infection travels from the stomach to the intestines, a conditon which is often referred to as acute gastroenteritis. When there is passage of blood and mucus or pus in stools the condition is called as dysentery. It is usually associated with abdominal colic, tenesmus (frequent urge to pass stools) and fever.

Causes

Breast fed babies are protected against development of diarrhea because breast milk is free from contamination and it contains several protective agents. Bottle fed babies are more prone to suffer from bacterial diarrhea unless strict precautions are taken to maintain the sterility of the feeding bottle and rubber teat. Feeding with a cup and spoon is associated with lower risk of development of diarrhea. Most episodes of diarrhea start when infant is weaned to semisolid diet unless strict personal hygiene and environmental sanitation is maintained. During weaning, infant must be given safe drinking water (preferably filtered or boiled) which is a common source of infection. The diarrheal episodes may occur throughout the year but they are more common during summer and monsoon because of further shortage and contamination of water and proliferation of house flies. Bacterial pathogens need hot and humid climate for their growth and proliferation. Bacterial diarrhea is more common in undernourished weak children living in poor hygienic conditions. Viral diarrhea may occur in healthy infants during fall and winter along with symptoms of cough and cold. In young infants (below 3 months) and malnourished children, diarrhea may be a manifestation of life-threatening septicemia (blood-borne infection). In older children, parasitic infections (*Giardia lamblia* and *E. histolytica*) may cause diarrhea or dysentery. Prolonged antibiotic therapy may be associated with antibiotic-related diarrhea or fungal superinfection. Presence of oral thrush (white patches in the mouth) is suggestive of fungal infection.

Clinical Features

There is sudden onset of vomiting followed by loose watery stools. Vomiting usually disappears in a day or so. The severity of disease process is variable and frequency of bowel motions may vary from 4 to 5 or more than 50 in a day. The motions may be watery or semiloose with or without blood and mucus. The stools may be green in color and foul smelling. Fever may or may not be present. The child is irritable and cranky due to thirst and is often keen to drink water. *Crying*

Nursing Tip

In an infant with diarrhea, crying is more often a signal of dehydration and not intestinal colic. Administration of ORS is followed by prompt resolution of crying.

should not be considered as a sign of intestinal colic and it usually disappears when child is given water or ORS to drink. Acute diarrhea is usually self-limiting and resolves in 2–3 days time.

Assessment of Dehydration

Based on weight loss, The American Academy of Pediatrics classified dehydration into mild (3–5% fluid deficit), moderate (6–9% fluid deficit) and severe (10% or more fluid deficit). Due to non-availability of accurate weight record of children in developing countries, WHO has simplified the assessment of dehydration by community health workers on the basis of 4 key clinical signs **(Box 37.1)**.

37

Box 37.1	WHO classification of dehydration

Two of the following signs (severe dehydration)

- Lethargic or unconscious
- Sunken eyes
- Not able to drink or drinking poorly
- Skin pinch goes back very slowly

Two of the following signs (some dehydration)

- Restless, irritable
- Sunken eyes
- Thirsty and drinks eagerly
- Skin pinch goes back slowly

Not enough signs to classify some dehydration

- No dehydration

Complications

Occurrence of vomiting and passage of frequent watery stools is associated with risk of development of deficiency of water (dehydration) and salts (electrolytes) in the body. Abdominal distension may occur due to lactose intolerance, paralytic ileus and hypokalemia. Seizures may occur due to electrolyte imbalance, sagittal sinus thrombosis or associated encephalitis. Acidosis is characterized by rapid deep breathing (Kussmaul breathing). If fluids being lost are not adequately replaced, the child may shrivel and dry up (like a plant without water). The child may become irritable and cranky due to thirst because he cannot express his needs. Due to dehydration, the eyes may look hazy and sunken, sweat and tears usually disappear and mouth becomes dry. The skin may become dry and inelastic. When you pinch the skin of abdomen or chest and release it, it immediately spreads out to original shape in a healthy child. In a dehydrated child, the pinched skin remains folded and takes much longer to assume its original shape **(Figures 37.1A and B)**. Urine output is one of the most reliable indicators of hydration status. When dehydration sets in, child passes small quantity of high-colored urine or may even stop passing urine. *When no urine is passed for 6 hours or more in an infant and for 12 hours in an older child, it is suggestive of renal shutdown.* Acute renal shutdown may occur due to hypovolemia and hemolytic uremic syndrome (HUS) as a consequence of shigella dysentery. In a child with acute diarrhea, a close watch on urine output should be maintained. When an accurate weight record of the child is maintained, sudden weight loss during an episode of acute diarrhea gives a correct estimate of degree of dehydration or water loss.

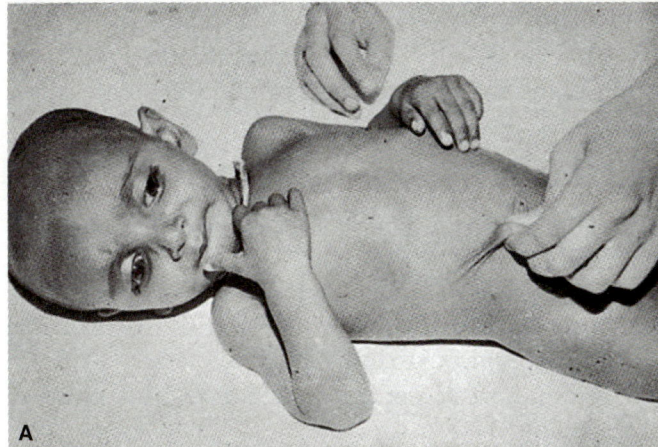

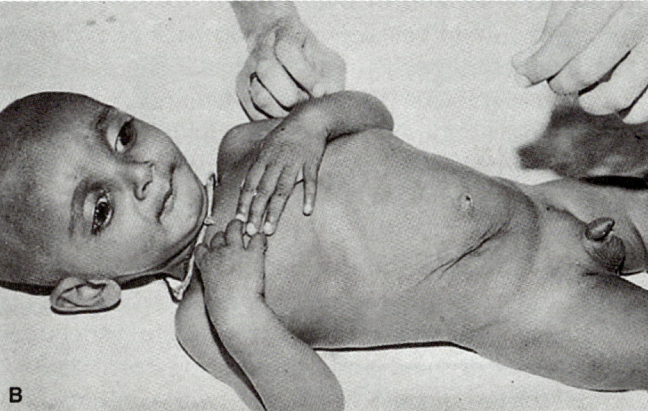

Figures 37.1A and B Method for elicitation of skin turgor. The abdominal skin is pinched, lifted and released (A). When skin turgor is lost due to dehydration (or marasmus) it takes several seconds before the pinched skin assumes its unwrinkled appearance (B). Note the sunken eyes of the child

Investigations

In most cases of acute diarrhea, no investigations are needed. It is futile to order stool culture because stools do contain a number of bacteria and culture will come out as positive. Isolation of *E. coli* from stools is of no significance unless specialized tests are conducted to find out whether these *E. coli* are friendly or pathogenic. When a diarrheal episode continues for more than 4–5 days, routine and microscopic examination of stools may be done to exclude any parasitic infection (*Giardia lamblia*, *E. histolytica*). When a diarrheal episode becomes persistent and prolonged (>2 weeks) and child continues to lose weight, investigations should be undertaken to exclude development of secondary lactose intolerance (stool pH <5 and presence of reducing substance). In children with severe dehydration, serum electrolytes and acid-base parameters should be checked.

Management

Based on the severity of dehydration, WHO recommend three plans for management of children with acute diarrhea.

Plan-A for no dehydration

The mother is counseled to follow four rules of home treatment.

1. Give extra home-made fluids and ORS to replace on-going losses of water and electrolytes through vomitings and diarrheal stools.
2. Continue breastfeeding or whatever milk child is receiving.
3. Give supplements of zinc.
4. Mother should be asked to report back after 5 days if diarrhea is persisting or earlier if there are any danger signs like irritability or lethargy, persistent vomiting, abdominal distension, inability to accept ORS, oliguria, fever or blood in stool.

Plan-B for some dehydration

The child should be given liberal amounts of home-made fluids and low-osmolarity WHO ORS to correct dehydration and replace on-going losses. Breastfeeding should be continued and dehydration corrected by administration of ORS 75 mL/kg over a period of 4 hours. During this period no solid food should be given. Mother should be asked to report back if purging rate is high (> one stool/hr) or there is persistent vomiting (> 3 times/hr) or if there are any danger signs as listed under plan-A.

Plan-C for severe dehydration

The child should be admitted to the hospital and treated promptly with intravenous rehydration with Ringer lactate or normal saline (0.9% sodium chloride solution). Hydration status should be assessed every 1–2 hours and intravenous therapy adjusted accordingly (refer to details under intravenous rehydration). When child is able to drink, ORS should be started along with intravenous therapy which is gradually weaned off. No solid food is offered till dehydration is corrected. Depending upon the hydration status, the child is promoted to plan-A or plan-B.

Home Treatment

Most diarrheas are self-limiting and emphasis should be placed on replacement of fluids and electrolyte losses and maintenance of nutrition rather than on the frequency and quality of stools. Whatever child is losing (through vomiting and diarrheal stools) must be replaced to prevent dehydration, and electrolyte disturbances.

Acute diarrhea is indeed a "flush out" response on the part of the body to eliminate toxins and pathogens from the gut. The "flush tank" of the body should be kept full by replenishing the fluids and electrolytes lost in the vomiting and stools. Breastfeeding should be continued and child given frequent sips of extra plain water. Oral rehydration solution (ORS) is ideal for replacement of fluid and electrolyte losses due to acute diarrhea in all age groups. *Commercial ORS is available in sachets of 6 g (for making 200 mL) and 30 g (for making 1000 mL).*

ORS can be prepared at home by taking 2-finger-and-thumb pinch of table salt (half a teaspoon) and 4-finger scoop of sugar (4 level teaspoons) and by adding few drops of lemon juice in one liter of safe drinking water. The properly formulated ORS should taste like tears. A variety of other home-made fluids like *rice-congee* (Box 37.2), barley water, weak tea, *lassi*, butter milk or *chaaj*, *moong dal* soup, coconut water, etc. can be used with equal efficacy. Infact extra plain water along with breast milk (or other milk if bottle fed) and other gut-friendly foods are equally efficacious. *However, aerated soft drinks, fresh or canned undiluted fruit juices should not be given to a child with diarrhea.*

Preparation of ORS A variety of ORS preparations are available in the market but only those conforming to reduced osmolarity WHO–ORS composition should be used (Table 37.1). The instructions printed on the

> **Key Message**
>
> Oral rehydration solution (ORS) is the greatest advance of 20th century and it has served as a savior to save millions of children throughout the world.

Box 37.2 Preparation of rice-congee

- Take one fistful (30–35 g) of raw rice. Clean and wash with water
- Boil rice in 6 glasses (one glass = 200 mL) of drinking water in a clean pot on a slow fire for 10–15 minutes till rice become soft and rise to the surface.
- Add one level teaspoonful (4 g) of common salt while boiling. Do not add any sugar. Cummin seeds (*Jeera*), cinnamon or cardamom may be added for a mild flavor, if child likes it.
- Keep it covered and store in a cool place. Offer 3–4 teaspoonfuls at a time as often as the child accepts. For an older infant, rice can be mashed in *congee* and fed to the child. Give sips of plain water in-between the *rice-congee* feeds.
- *Rice-congee* can be stored and used up to 12 hours. To avoid wastage, 500 mL of *congee* can be prepared for young infants by taking one-half of the recommended ingredients.

Table 37.1 Composition of reduced osmolarity WHO-ORS

Constituents	Quantity (g/L)
Glucose, anhydrous	13.5
Sodium chloride	2.6
Potassium chloride	1.5
Trisodium citrate dihydrate	2.9
Total weight	20.5

Osmolarity	mOsm/L
Glucose, anhydrous	75
Sodium	75
Chloride	65
Potassium	20
Citrate	10
Total osmolarity	245

sachet for reconstitution should be followed. To avoid risk of contamination, a small sachet (6 g) should be reconstituted in 200 mL or a glass of water. If one liter of ORS is prepared with 30 g sachet, it should be properly covered and stored in a fridge or at room temperature and used within 12 hours. The water for reconstitution should be safe drinking water (boiled, filtered or RO water). *The prepared ORS should never be reboiled.*

Administration of ORS The child should be given frequent sips of ORS with the help of a spoon. Large gulps of ORS with a cup or glass may lead to vomiting. Give sips of ORS every 5–10 minutes or so. In one large watery stool, child usually loses about one cup of fluids which should be replaced by giving that much additional ORS. Give extra fluids to drink every time a child passes a loose motion. When a child has frequent watery stools, ORS must be continued throughout night, otherwise child may get dehydrated. When child has already developed signs of some dehydration, additional ORS (50–100 mL/kg body weight) should be given in 4–6 hours. ORS should be stopped when diarrhea is controlled.

Some children may not like the taste or flavor of ORS and may refuse to take it. When a child with acute diarrhea does not accept ORS and he is not dehydrated, the child may be given plain water and home-available fluids and food. *When a dehydrated child refuses to accept ORS due to lethargy, toxemia, abdominal distension or persistent vomiting, he should be admitted to the hospital for intravenous fluid therapy.*

Dietary Advice

The child with acute diarrhea should never be starved. Breast feeding should be continued because breast milk is usually the only food that a sick child continues to accept. The formula-fed infant may be given undiluted milk once child is fully hydrated. Rice-lentil gruel (*khichadi*), yoghurt, egg white, boiled and mashed potatoes, and banana are well tolerated by a child with diarrhea. These foods are known to improve the consistency of stools, maintain good nutrition of the child and reduce the risk of development of chronic or protracted diarrhea. *Fruit juices both fresh and canned and cola drinks should be avoided due to risk of aggravation of diarrhea and abdominal distension.* There is recent evidence to suggest that half-diluted natural apple juice can serve as a useful ORS.

The problem of lactose intolerance in acute diarrhea is rare and is often over diagnosed. It should be looked for when diarrhea persists beyond 14 days. It is diagnosed by finding stool pH of less than 5.0 on two occasions and by the presence of reducing substance in stools in a concentration of greater than 1.0 percent. The child may be given lactose-free or soy-based milk. Milk-cereal mixture (dalia, sago, kheer) and yoghurt may be gradually introduced and are tolerated better than liquid milk. Most infants with secondary lactose intolerance can be promoted to normal milk diet within 2–3 weeks.

Role of antibiotics Most cases of acute diarrhea are self-limited and antibiotics have no role. Indiscriminate use of antibiotics may lead to emergence of resistant strains of pathogens and elimination of friendly and protective bacteria of gut. Antibiotics should be used when child has invasive diarrhea with fever, mucus or blood in stools and presence of pus cells in the stools. Co-trimoxazole, nalidixic acid, norfloxacin or ofloxacin or ciprofloxacin are useful.

Role of antidiarrheal agents It is important to understand the mechanism and cause of diarrhea before using unnecessary medications. Diarrhea occurs due to entry of a dangerous germs or by release of toxins of germs which makes the gut leaky to wash away or flush out the pathogens and their toxins from the body. It is, therefore, not desirable to stop this flushing mechanism which may actually delay the process of recovery. The superficial lining of intestines is also washed away during an episode of acute diarrhea. The immune mechanism of the body takes one or two days to eliminate the germs and repair the damage caused by toxins. Once all the harmful products are flushed out of the intestines and the intestinal lining is replaced by the normal growth of intestinal cells, the diarrhea stops. The availability of essential nutrients from the breast milk and other foods, facilitates the process of recovery and intestinal repair. Zinc supplements have been shown to promote recovery from acute and persistent diarrhea and is currently recommended for routine use.

37

It is given in a dose of 10 mg/d in infants between 2 and 6 months and 20 mg/d in children above 6 months for 10–14 days. The role of pre and probiotics is controversial. Racecadotril is recognized to reduce fluid losses but its use is controversial. Antimotility agents may reduce the purging rate but the offending germs and toxins will continue to stay in the gut leading to prolongation of illness and delayed recovery. Antibiotics have no role in the treatment of viral diarrhea. Instead, antibiotics may kill the friendly bacteria of the intestines which are known to provide protection to the gut against outside invaders. Thus at times antibiotics may actually prolong and delay recovery from an episode of diarrhea. Therefore, ORS indeed is the "real medicine" for treatment of acute diarrhea.

Danger Signs in a Child with Diarrhea

Most children with acute diarrhea can be managed at home with proper emphasis on ORS and intake of food. Diarrhea is likely to continue for at least 2–3 days despite any medication and during this period fluids and electrolytes should be replenished by administration of home-available fluids or ORS and intake of soft gut-friendly foods. The children with following manifestations and complications may require hospitalization and administration of intravenous fluids:

- Young infants (<3 months) and severely malnourished children.
- High purge rate (>10 mL/kg/hr) and persistent vomitings (>3 times/hr).
- Inability to drink ORS or take feeds.
- Lack of improvement or worsening of dehydration despite adequate ORS therapy for 8 hours.
- Severe abdominal distension.
- Severe dehydration and/or shock.
- Renal shut down (no urine for >6 hours in an infant and 12 hours in an older child).
- Convulsions or altered sensorium.
- Persistent diarrhea (>2 weeks) with malnutrition.

Intravenous Rehydration

Children with severe dehydration, persistent vomiting or abdominal distension and shock are started on rapid intravenous infusion of Ringer's lactate with 5% dextrose or normal saline with 5% dextrose. Initial bolus of 30 mL/kg is administered during first 30–60 minutes followed by 70 mL/kg over next 3–5 hours. The child should be assessed every 15–30 minutes for tissue perfusion, pulse volume and blood pressure. Additional intravenous fluids are given to correct

dehydration, replace on-going fluid losses in stools (10 mL/kg) and vomitings (5 mL/kg) and to provide maintenance fluid requirements. The calculation and administration of fluids and electrolytes in a one year old infant with severe dehydration, metabolic acidosis and hypokalemia is shown in **Table 37.2**. Potassium is added to the intravenous fluids as soon as the urine flow is established. ORS (5 mL/kg/hr) should be started as soon as the child can take orally even while getting intravenous fluids.

Role of a Nurse for Prevention of Future Attacks of Diarrhea

- Promotion of breast feeding as long as feasible (may be up to 2 years).
- Ensure intake of clean and safe water for drinking.
- If child is bottle fed, ensure proper sterility of the feeding bottle and rubber teat. It is preferable and safer to feed with a cup and spoon rather than a feeding bottle.
- Avoid use of a dummy nipple or pacifier and teething ring due to potential risk of contamination.
- Sipper should not be used for administration of water or milk.
- Ensure strict personal hygiene and washing of hands with soap and water.
  - □ after cleaning the potty of the baby
  - □ before preparing food and
  - □ before feeding the baby.
- Ensure that hands and toys of baby are kept clean. The nails should be kept trimmed and clean.
- Ensure that stools of the child are properly disposed off immediately after evacuation.
- Oral rotavirus vaccine is available, which is given in two doses (monovalent) or three doses (penta-valent) 4 weeks apart, starting at the age of two months.

Several do's and don'ts for prevention and treatment of acute diarrhea in children are listed in **Box 37.3**.

BACILLARY DYSENTERY

Dysentery is characterized by passage of blood and mucus in the loose stools due to infection of the colon. It is much more common in children than amebic dysentery. It is caused by four strains of shigella species (*S. dysenteriae*, *S. flexneri*, *S. boydii* and *S. sonnei*). Invasive diarrhea by enterohemorrhagic *E. coli*, salmonella and *Campylobacter jejuni* may produce a similar clinical picture. There is sudden onset of bloody diarrhea with

Table 37.2 Calculate the fluid and electrolyte requirements of one year old, 10 kg infant having severe dehydration (15%), acidosis and hypokalemia

Deficit fluid	15% dehydration
	$150 \times 10 = 1500$ mL
Daily maintenance	$120 \times 10 = 1200$ mL

Total requirements in 24 hours = 2700 mL

Administer one-half (1400 mL) of the above amount in first 8 hours and remainder in the next 16 hours.

First hour 30 mL/kg = 300 mL of Ringer's lactate solution (or 0.45% saline in 5% dextrose)

$$= 300/60 = 5 \text{ mL/minute}$$
$$= 5 \times 20 = 100 \text{ drops/minute}$$

(Alternatively divide mL/hour by 3 to get drops/ minute, i.e. 300/3 = 100 drops/minute)

Next 7 hours give 1100 mL, i.e. 157 mL/hour of Ringer's lactate = 157/3, i.e. 52 drops/min.

Next 16 hours give 1300 mL, i.e. 81 mL/hour of 0.18% saline in 5% dextrose = 81/3, i.e. 27 drops /minute

On-going losses Calculate fluid losses through vomiting and stools every 4–6 hours and replenish with N/2 dextrose-saline solution. For each diarrheal stool and vomiting provide additional fluids to the extent of 10 mL/kg and 5 mL/kg respectively. The commonest cause of persistence of dehydration is lack of adequate replacement of concurrent losses of fluids.

Moderate acidosis 3 mL of 7.5% sodium bicarbonate/kg, i.e. $3 \times 10 = 30$ mL

15 mL is given during first hour and the rest during next 7 hours

Give calcium gluconate 50 mg/kg following correction of acidosis to prevent post acidotic tetany

Hypokalemia Potassium 4 mEq/kg = 40 mEq to be administered only when urine flow is established. Correct slowly over 24 hours. Do not exceed concentration of 40 mEq/L.

Box 37.3 Some do's and don'ts regarding diarrhea

Do's

- Ensure exclusive breastfeeding up to 6 months and continue breastfeeding along with complementary feeds as long as feasible.
- Ensure strict measures of personal hygiene during the process of weaning. Protect cooked foods from flies and cockroaches.
- Give clean and safe drinking water.
- Ensure proper use of comode and potty for disposal of stools of the child
- Keep the hands and toys of young children clean.
- Start home-available fluids or ORS (WHO formulation) at the earliest if diarrhea occurs.
- Continue breastfeeding and offer other easily digestible foods during diarrhea.
- You should be able to assess the hydration status of the child with diarrhea.

Don'ts

- Avoid use of a pacifier (dummy nipple), teething rings and sipper due to risk of contamination and development of diarrhea.
- Do not starve the child with diarrhea.
- Do not give aerated soft drinks, fresh or canned fruit juice to a child with diarrhea.
- Do not continue to give ORS once diarrhea stops.
- Do not give any antidiarrheal medicines or antibiotics without the prescription of a doctor.

fever, abdominal pain and tenesmus (ineffectual urge to pass stools). It may be complicated by dyselectrolytemia and hemolytic uremic syndrome with life-threatening renal dysfunction. Other complications include malnutrition, anemia, hypoproteinemia, shigella encephalopathy, arthritis, rectal prolapse and Reiter's syndrome.

Treatment

The symptomatic treatment includes administration of oral rehydration solution (ORS), antiemetic, antipyretic and antispasmodic agent. Home-based ORS like rice *congee*, *dal ka paani* (lentil soup), butter milk (*chaaj*) and coconut water are well tolerated and provide nutrition. Breastfeeding should be continued and child should be given light diet like rice-dal gruel (*khichadi*), egg white, yoghurt and banana. The specific antibacterial agents include cotrimoxazole, nalidixic acid and ciprofloxacin (15 mg/kg/dose twice daily for 3 days). In refractory and severe cases, ceftriaxone 50–100 mg/ kg/d IV or IM for 3–5 days is curative.

Prevention

Infection can be prevented by promotion of breastfeeding, improving standard of personal hygiene, environmental sanitation and consumption of safe drinking water and food. No vaccine is available for prevention of bacillary diarrheas.

37

CHOLERA

Cholera is caused by *Vibrio cholerae* and occurs in outbreaks especially when there are congregations of people like fairs, *Kumbh mela* and *Haj* pilgrims or following natural calamities like floods and earthquakes. Epidemics may occur due to overcrowding, lack of adequate sanitation and non availability of safe drinking water. Cholera is spread through water contaminated with feces. The patient is contagious for 3 days before the onset of symptoms and 7–10 days during the course of illness.

Clinical Features

After a short incubation period of 1–3 days, the disease manifests with abrupt onset of severe and voluminous (up to 10 liters/stool) watery diarrhea. Stools have characteristic rice-water appearance. Vomiting is usually present. If fluid losses are not corrected promptly, the patient develops severe dehydration, hypovolemic shock, metabolic acidosis, renal shutdown and death. The diagnosis is suspected when there is an outbreak of cholera, rice-water appearance of stools and identification of *V. cholerae* on hanging-drop preparation or culture of stool.

Treatment

Early, prompt and aggressive rehydration with oral rehydration solution (ORS) or through intravenous route as described under acute gastroenteritis is life saving. Drugs have been shown to shorten the severity and duration of diarrhea and reduce the infectivity of the patient. A single dose of either ciprofloxacin (10 mg/kg) or doxycycline (6 mg/kg), or norfloxacin 5.0–7.5 mg/kg twice a day for 3 days have been shown to be effective.

Prevention

The currently available cholera vaccine is not very effective and provides protection for a short duration of 3–6 months. It is given to pilgrims visiting *Haj* or *Kumbh mela* but has no role in routine immunization. Ensuring safe environmental sanitation, high standard of personal hygiene and safe drinking water are more important to prevent and control the spread of cholera. Boiling of water or chlorination (chlorine content 0.2–0.5 mg/L) readily kill *V. cholerae*. Proper disposal of excreta, washing of hands before handling and while eating food, avoiding intake of exposed and cold or uncooked foods, cut fruits or fruit juices sold by the road side vendors are effective to prevent outbreaks of cholera.

FOOD POISONING

Food poisoning may be caused by germs or their toxins or by intake of some poisonous foods like wild variety of mushrooms. Intake of stale food especially in summer and consumption of cut and exposed fruits from road-side food *dhabas* and hawkers may lead to food poisoning. Food poisoning epidemics are known to occur during community meal programs or religious festivals and marriage or birthday parties.

All the members of the family or community who had taken the offending food would manifest symptoms of food poisoning. The symptoms may occur within few hours if they are due to toxins or may take 2 to 3 days if food is contaminated with pathogenic bacteria. There is cramp-like pain in abdomen with severe vomiting and watery diarrhea. The symptoms may be catastrophic leading to sudden development of cold extremities with circulatory collapse or shock. The principles of management are the same as highlighted under acute gastroenteritis. The emphasis is placed on early administration of home-available liquids and ORS. Due to explosive nature of the illness, many patients need referral to a hospital for administration of intravenous fluids.

VOMITING

Vomiting is a common symptom in children due to a variety of causes. It is very frightening for the parents though most of the time it is either due to benign (non-serious) causes or is a self-limiting disorder. Some children are more prone to vomiting on a minor pretext like a bout of coughing, during temper tantrum or after a feed or following administration of a medication.

Benign causes Regurgitation of curdled milk may occur due to improper technique of feeding (bottle feeding, lack of burping), forced feeding or over feeding. These children continue to have a satisfactory weight gain. Some infants may vomit following a bout of cough due to any cause. Administration of certain medications may be associated or followed by vomiting.

Serious causes Persistent regurgitation of milk feeds or vomiting from early infancy may occur due to gastroesophageal reflux. In normal children, regurgitation of stomach contents is prevented due to the presence of a sphincter at the junction of esophagus (food pipe) and stomach. In some children, gastroesophageal junction is lax or lacks a sphincter leading to regurgitation of feeds despite effective burping. The regurgitated feeds may be aspirated into the lungs with frequent episodes of aspiration pneumonia or wheezing. These children tolerate thickened feeds better. Vomiting is commonly the initial or sole symptom of acute gastroenteritis and food poisoning. Vomiting is a common symptom of a systemic infection (like sepsis) and may occur due to infection and inflammation of any organ of the abdomen. The triad of fever, headache and vomiting is suggestive of brain infection (meningitis) but may occur because of a nonspecific acute viral infection. Persistent and forceful green colored vomitings in association with abdominal distension and constipation is suggestive of an obstruction in the intestines beyond ampulla of Vater. Nausea, vomiting and anorexia are common early symptoms of viral hepatitis.

Treatment

The child with vomiting should be encouraged to take sips of water or milk (not gulps with a glass) immediately after the bout of vomiting. If vomiting is related to administration of a drug, it is best to withhold it. Children with gastroesophageal reflux respond to administration of thickened feeds and by restraining them in a propped-up position in a special chair after every feed. When vomiting is persistent or there are associated symptoms (like fever, headache, abdominal pain, constipation, distension, etc.) suggestive of a serious cause, appropriate investigations should be done to identify the cause. Metoclopramide (0.2 mg/kg/dose) or domperidone (0.2 mg/kg/dose) or ondansetron hydrochloride (2–4 mg/dose) are useful to provide symptomatic relief. Vomiting may at times lead to dehydration due to non-acceptance or intolerance of oral rehydration solution (ORS). The child would need intravenous fluid therapy for rapid correction of dehydration and electrolyte disturbances.

HYPERTROPHIC PYLORIC STENOSIS

The condition is characterized by increased thickening of the circular muscles of the pylorus of the stomach. This leads to obstruction of the lumen of pylorus with reduced passage of stomach contents into the duodenum. The condition is developmental in nature but may occur after prolonged use of erythromycin as a prokinetic agent in newborn babies.

Clinical Features

The condition is more common in first-born male infants. It is characterized by persistent and projectile vomiting having onset during first month of life. The vomiting is non-bilious or milk-colored (unlike distal duodenal obstruction when vomiting is green or bilious). The infant looks perpetually hungry and constipation is usually present. Weight gain is poor. Physiological jaundice may be prolonged in some infants.

There is no abdominal distension but visible peristaltic waves may be seen moving from left to the right in the upper abdomen. Careful palpation of the upper abdomen in a quiet child may reveal a firm nodule like the shape and size of an olive or breast nipple due to hypertrophy of circular fibers of the pylorus. The diagnosis can be confirmed on ultrasound examination or upper GI barium study.

Nursing Care

1. Correct fluid and electrolyte abnormalities before surgery. Associated metabolic alkalosis (due to loss of hydrochloric acid from stomach) should be treated.
2. Stop oral feeds and do a stomach wash with normal saline to reduce edema of the gastric wall.
3. The operative procedure is called Ramstedt's pyloromyotomy. The thickened muscles of pylorus are divided along the length of pylorus till the mucosa is seen.
4. After surgery, oral feeds are withheld for 18–24 hours till bowel movements are established. When baby is able to tolerate clear fluids, milk feeds are started and gradually increased in volume.

GASTROESOPHAGEAL REFLUX DISEASE (GERD)

There is laxity or transient episodes of relaxation of gastroesophageal sphincter. The condition is more common during early life (neonates especially preterm babies) and it improves as the child grows. There are frequent episodes of regurgitation after feeds despite adequate burping. The associated symptoms include failure to thrive, irritability and unexplained crying with arching of body at night. Aspiration of stomach contents may cause episodes of choking and gagging which may lead to occurrence of laryngitis (hoarseness), otitis media and wheezing. The condition improves as the child grows and disappears by 2 years of age. The diagnosis can be confirmed by technetium radionuclide scintiscan and 24 hours esophageal pH monitoring.

Nursing Care

The baby should be nursed in a semi-upright position at 45 degrees specially after feed and during sleep. Right lateral and prone positioning also reduces the risk of regurgitation. The feed should be thickened with a rice-based cereal. Prokinetic drugs (domperidone, metoclopramide), H_2 blockers (ranitidine) and proton pump inhibitors (omeprazole, lansoprazole) are useful to provide relief and improve growth.

37

Adequate nutrition should be ensured and growth parameters monitored. In intractable cases, not responding to medical therapy, Nissen fundoplication is recommended. Mother should be provided guidelines for burping, positioning and emotional support.

CELIAC DISEASE

Celiac disease or gluten-enteropathy is a genetic disorder due to intolerance to wheat gliadin. It is associated with mucosal damage to the small bowel.

Clinical Features

The clinical manifestations usually start during 6 months to 2 years of age when wheat products are introduced in the diet. There is anorexia, irritability, vomiting, chronic or recurrent diarrhea, abdominal distension, rectal prolapse, anemia, failure to thrive and stunting. The stools may be loose, foul smelling, bulky and greasy in appearance. Extra intestinal features include iron deficiency anemia, osteoporosis, rickets, cirrhosis, and delayed puberty.

Diagnosis

There are evidences of fat malabsorption and nutritional anemia. Elevation of serum antiendomysial 1gA antibodies, tissue transglutaminase IgA antibodies (tTG IgA) and characteristic histopathological changes of global villus atrophy on jejunal biopsy are diagnostic. These laboratory abnormalities return back to normal on gluten-free diet.

Nursing Care

The child is advised to take gluten-free diet by strictly avoiding intake of wheat, rye and barley. All foods and products containing aforementioned cereals (like bread, biscuits, cake, pastry, etc.) should be avoided throughout life. Rice, corn, oats, pearl millet (*bajra*), finger millet (*ragi*) and Bengal gram are well tolerated and substituted for wheat. Detailed guidelines for choosing gluten-free diet are given in **Box 37.4**. The clinical response to gluten withdrawal is dramatic and is evident within 2–3 weeks. The symptoms gradually disappear and growth velocity is resumed.

CONSTIPATION

Passage of infrequent hard stools is called as constipation. In Indian culture, constipation is believed to be the root cause of many ills due to accumulation of toxins in the body though there is no scientific basis for it. Infants fed on cow's milk or a formula are often constipated due to formation of casein curds in stools.

Box 37.4   **Gluten-free diet**

- **General guidelines**
  - All sources of gluten should be excluded from the diet.
  - Gluten is present in wheat, barley and rye, which should be strictly avoided throughout life.
  - Avoid beverages containing malt such as various health drinks and barley water.
  - Read the contents of the packaged food items and avoid them if they contain *gluten. When in doubt, avoid giving it to the child.*
  - Whenever parents go out they should carry gluten-free snacks or food items with them.

- **Permitted food items**
  - Rice, *bajra*, *jowar* (sorghum), ragi, corn flour, arrowroot, tapioca (Shimla aloo), *makki* (corn), sago, *besan*, *singhare ka atta* (water chestnut flour), *chirwa*, *murmura* (puffed rice), rice noodles and soy flour. Breads and other preparations such as *dosa, idli*, rice *uthapam, vada, pakoras, khichadi* and *papads* can be made from gluten-free cereals and lentils.
  - All pulses, lentils, *kabuli chana* (chickpeas), Bengal gram and soybeans.
  - Milk and milk products (except *burfi, jalebi, gulab jamun* and other *mithais* and sweets).
  - Butter, oil, and ghee.
  - All vegetables and fruits including dry fruits and nuts.
  - Eggs and non-vegetarian food items prepared without use of *atta, maida* or bread crumbs.

- **Chapattis (breads) can be made with following mixes**
  - Rice flour + soy flour (2:1)
  - Rice flour + *besan* (3:1)
  - Corn flour + *besan* (3:1)
  - *Kala chana* flour + *besan* (3:1)
  - *Makki ka atta*
  - *Bajra ka atta*
  - *Singharey ka atta*
  - *Kuttu ka atta* (buck wheat)
  - *Besan*
  - *Ragi* flour
  - *Oats* flour

- **Dessert options**
  - Home-made desserts are safe and there are a variety of options such as caramel custard, fruit cream, rice *kheer*, sago *kheer*, *makhana kheer*, carrot *halwa*, *besan laddo*, fruits in sugar syrup, *shrikhand*, sweet curd, jelly, *rasgulla* and ice cream or *kulfi*. Packaged desserts, snacks and sweets should be avoided unless the package insert clearly mentions that the food items are gluten-free.

The constipation often responds by giving extra sugar, honey and fresh fruit juice to the baby. The use of laxatives should be avoided in infants.

Causes

In older children, constipation is often due to intake of low-fiber diet and lack of intake of enough fluids. Intake of certain medications (opioids, iron, NSAIDs, etc.) and high grade fever may be associated with poor intake of food and constipation. Severe constipation (obstipation) due to dietary and psychological reasons is common around 2 years of age. The stools become dry and hard and are difficult to evacuate The passage of hard and dry stools may cause injury to the lining of anal canal leading to slight bleeding and formation of a fissure or ulcer. The condition becomes self-perpetuating as child refuses to sit on a potty because evacuation is associated with discomfort and pain. Instead, when there is pressure for evacuation, the child stands in a corner and tries to "withhold" stools and does not relax or let go. In some children, it is a phase of psychological development where the child "refuses to part with anything belonging to him including his stools". The child is rebellious and refuses to do anything that pleases his parents. The situation becomes from bad to worse and evacuation is achieved only by insertion of glycerine suppository or by giving rectal enema. At times, the semi-liquefied stools may trickle out spontaneously around the hard stools (encoparesis) staining the underpants and giving the wrong impression that the child has developed diarrhea.

Intractable constipation dating back to birth may occur due to congenital narrowing of anal canal or lack of proper neural development in the colon and rectum (Hirschsprung's disease). Constipation in association with delayed neuromotor development and general lethargy, poor activity and coarse features of the face is highly suggestive of deficiency of thyroid hormone (cretinism).

Treatment

Early treatment of constipation prevents the development of self-perpetuating psychological constipation. The child should be encouraged to take extra fluids, sugar, honey, butter, *ghee*, fruits, fruit juices, green leafy vegetables, salads, lentils and high fiber cereals. Fruits like papaya, guava, citrus fruits, dates, apricots and figs are particularly useful. Formula feeds, rice, white bread, yoghurt, pomegranate, apple and banana should be avoided due to their potential risk to cause constipation. Gentle massage of abdomen and navel may help by improving the tone of abdominal and intestinal muscles. Judicious modification of diet and use of milk of magnesia, osmotic agents (lactulose which imbibes water into gut) and prokinetics (drugs which improve the gut motility) are effective. The child

should not be scolded and instead provided with emotional support and tension-free atmosphere to ensure relaxation of his body, mind and sphincters.

RECTAL PROLAPSE

There is abnormal descent or prolapse of rectal mucosa through the anus after defecation. The condition is mostly seen in infants and preschool children. The precipitating factors include straining due to constipation, persistent bloody diarrhea, laxity of rectal sphincter due to spina bifida, rectal ulcer and irritation due to infestation with thread worms and trichuris trichiura. Rectal prolapse is common in children with celiac disease. The rectal sphincter and muscles are weaked due to loss of ischio-rectal fat because of malnutrition. Child passes blood stained stools and prolapsed rectum is visible as bright red glistening mass protruding through the anus.

Nursing Care

The predisposing conditions like constipation, diarrhea, worm infestation, ulcerative colitis and celiac disease should be treated. The prolapsed rectum should be manually pushed back after defecation. Dietary advice should be given to improve the nutritional status. Sitz baths are useful to strengthen perineal muscles. The child is made to sit in a plastic basin containing warm water and asked to contract (as if trying to stop urination or defecation) and relax the perineal muscles for 5–10 minutes three times in a day. In a severe case the buttocks can be strapped after reduction of the prolapse. Injection of sclerosing agent into the submucosa of rectum and surgical repair (rectopexy) are rarely needed in children.

HIRSCHSPRUNG'S DISEASE

There is absence of the ganglion cells in the rectosigmoid junction leading to ineffective peristaltic movements at the affected site. At times disease may affect multiple segments of gut or a long segment of the intestines. There is intractable constipation with dilatation of the proximal part of colon. The condition is also known as congenital megacolon.

Clinical Features

The constipation is severe and dates back to birth with delayed passage of meconium. There is intractable chronic constipation (obstipation) with progressive distension of abdomen, failure to thrive and marasmus. The abdomen is distended with visible loops of persistalsis and palpable fecoliths in the left iliac region.

37

Episodes of enterocolitis may cause intermittent diarrhea with passage of putrid or foul smelling stool. Rectal examination shows empty rectum and withdrawal of finger results in explosive passage of stool and wind.

Diagnosis

Skiagram of abdomen in erect position may show air-fluid levels with markedly dilated large gut. Barium enema shows narrow rectum with markedly dilated sigmoid colon and retention of barium enema for 2–3 days. Rectal biopsy is diagnostic and shows absence of ganglion cells in the myenteric plexus. Anorectal pressure studies are helpful in the diagnosis.

Treatment

Child is prepared for surgery by evacuation of the feces by bowel wash and correction of any fluid and electrolyte abnormalities. The aganglionic segment of the gut is excised followed by end-to-end anastomosis. Depending upon the site and extent of aganglionosis, the surgical procedure may be done in two or three stages of colostomy.

Nursing Care

1. The passage of first meconium should be looked for and recorded in all newborn babies.
2. Barium enema is done without any preparatory bowel wash as it may distort the anatomy of rectosigmoid junction and transition zone may be missed.
3. Before surgery, thorough rectal wash is done with normal saline. Rectal wash with plain water is dangerous and may cause water intoxication.
4. Care of the colostomy stoma should be explained to the mother to prevent excoriation of the surrounding skin. She should be explained about emptying of pouch, prevention of peristomal skin excoriation and change of pouching system or care of reusable ostomy bag.
5. The family should be psychologically prepared for long-term follow-up and given nutritional advise for treatment of malnutrition.

VIRAL HEPATITIS

Acute viral hepatitis is the commonest cause of jaundice in children. Hepatitis due to hepatitis A, B and E viruses is the most common in our country. Hepatitis A and E infections occur through feco-oral route (by taking contaminated water, milk or food) while hepatitis B and hepatitis C are transmitted through blood (through injections, transfusion of blood or blood products and from infected mother to her baby). Hepatitis may also occur due to drugs, toxins, autoimmune and genetic disorders.

Clinical Features

The common clinical features include fever, loss of appetite, nausea, vomiting, passage of high colored urine, jaundice and pain in the right upper abdomen. Liver is enlarged and tender and spleen may be just palpable. It is difficult to differentiate between hepatitis A and B on clinical examination.

Diagnosis

Viral hepatitis is diagnosed clinically while laboratory investigations are done to identify the etiologic agent and assess the severity of the disease process. Hepatitis A may lead to acute hepatocellular failure while hepatitis B may cause a chronic hepatic disease and may lead to development of hepatocellular carcinoma in adults.

Treatment

There are no specific medicines and treatment is supportive and symptomatic. Most cases recover spontaneously. Child should be encouraged to take unrestricted balanced nutritious diet. Patient should be advised to take high carbohydrate diet with fresh fruit juices and seasonal fruits. Multivitamins are useful and should be given. There are no specific hepatoprotective drugs and tonics. Physical activity should be allowed depending upon the condition of the patient. In general, hepatic transaminases (SGOT and SGPT) levels have poor prognostic utility. Prolongation of prothrombin time and marked elevation of serum bilirubin (> 14 mg/ dL) are associated with poor outcome. For prevention of viral hepatitis, refer to **Chapter 18**.

ACUTE LIVER FAILURE

Acute liver failure is characterized by hepatic encephalopathy and congulopathy within 12 weeks of onset of liver disease. The commonest cause of acute liver failure in children is viral hepatitis especially due to Hepatitis A virus and Hepatitis E virus singly or dual infection. Other causes include metabolic disorders, drug-induced (antitubercular drugs, paracetamol, sodium valproate, phenytoin sodium, nimesulide, etc.), and toxins like mushroom poisoning, rodenticide and Reye syndrome.

Clinical Features

There is sudden onset of fever, loss of appetite, nausea, vomiting, upper abdominal discomfort, passage of high colored urine and jaundice. Bleeding manifestations

Nursing Alert

Sudden shrinkage in the size of liver or dramatic drop in the level of transaminases without any evidence of clinical improvement are ominous and suggestive of impending hepatic encephalopathy.

with prolonged prothrombin time are suggestive of severe liver dysfunction. Hepatic encephalopathy and cerebral edema manifests with progressive alteration of consciousness leading to drowsiness, stupor and coma. Children with persistent vomiting, shrinking liver size, sudden fall in transaminases or extremely raised level of transaminases and markedly prolonged prothrombin time are at an increased risk to develop hepatic encephalopathy. These patients are at an increased risk to develop septicemia. Metabolic alterations (hypoglycemia, hypokalemia, metabolic acidosis) and multi-organ dysfunction especially renal failure are terminal events. The case fatality rate may be as high as 80% and liver transplantation provides hope for the future.

Nursing Care

1. *Monitoring.* Vital signs, pulse oximetry, level of consciousness, intake and output should be closely monitored. Biochemical monitoring is done by regular estimation of serum electrolytes, glucose, prothrombin time, liver function tests, serum creatinine and acid-base parameters.

2. *Supportive care.* Insert nasogastric tube for gastric decompression, feeding and administration of oral medications. Establish IV line for administration of 10% dextrose and electrolytes. Adequate calories are provided while protein intake is restricted to 0.5 g/kg/day. Micronutrients like vitamin B complex, vitamin C, vitamin E and zinc are given. Injection vitamin K is recommended to improve prothrombin time. Associated bacterial infection is treated with appropriate antibiotics. Hepatotoxic drugs should be stopped.

3. *Protocol for hepatic encephalopathy*
   - Raise head end by 30°–45° and maintain head in neutral position.
   - Administer intravenous N/5 saline in 10% dextrose with potassium chloride.
   - Lactulose 0.5 mL/kg/dose 4 times in a day through a NG tube. Bowel wash if patient is constipated.
   - Mannitol 20% 3–5 mL/kg/dose iv slow bolus every 4–6 hours for 6–8 doses.
   - Broad spectrum antibiotics, vitamin K, ranitidine, and phenytoin sodium to control seizures.
   - Liver transplantation in an intractable case before multi-organ dysfunction sets in.

BIBLIOGRAPHY

Acharya SK, Madan K, Dattagupta S, Panda SK. Viral hepatitis in India. *Natl Med J India* 2006, 19(4): 203–217.

Bhatnagar S, Bhandari N, Mouli UC, Bhan MK, IAP National Task Force: Status report on management of acute diarrhea. *Indian Pediatr* 2004, 41(4): 335–348.

Dienstag JL. Hepatitis B virus infection. *N Engl J Med* 2008, 359(14): 1486–1500.

Green PHR, Cellier C. Celiac disease. *N Engl J Med* 2007, 357(17): 1731–1743.

Hahn SK, Kim YJ, Garner P. Reduced osmolarity oral rehydration solution for treating dehydration due to diarrhea in children: Systematic review. *Brit Med J* 2001, 323(7304): 81–85.

Palson J, Lee Woy. AASLD Position Paper: The management of acute liver failure. *Hepatology* 2005, 40: 1179–1197.

Rudolph CD, Muzur LJ, Liptak GS, et al. Pediatric gastroesophageal reflux clinical practice guidelines. *J Pediatr Gastroenterol Nutr* 2001, 32: S1–S31.

Sood A, Midha V, Sood N, Avasthi G, Sehgal A. Prevalence of celiac disease among school children in Punjab, North India. *J Gastroenterol Hepatol* 2006, 21(10): 1622–1625.

37

Respiratory Diseases

COMMON COLD
(Upper or Acute Respiratory Infection)

Refer to **Chapter 34** for details.

SWINE FLU

Swine flu is caused by influenza A (H1N1) or H1N1 influenza 09 virus. After a pandemic of swine flu in 2009, there have been sporadic epidemics. Droplet or air-borne infection occurs through contact with infected humans or by handling infected pigs. Infection does not occur by eating pork. There may be history of travel to an epidemic area or contact with a patient diagnosed to have swine flu.

Clinical Features

The symptoms are similar to seasonal flu and characterized by high-grade fever, chills, headache, nasal discharge (coryza), and cough. The fever may resolve for a day and then return back (bimodal fever or camel hump fever) with more severe symptoms of fever, cough and toxemia. The diagnosis is confirmed by examination of nasopharyngeal swab by real-time reverse transcriptase polymerase chain reaction (rRT – PCR) or virus isolation. A fourfold or greater rise in H1N1-specific neutralizing antibodies is also diagnostic.

Treatment

Most patients recover spontaneously and are treated on an ambulatory basis with paracetamol, fluids, hot soups and antibiotics to control any superadded bacterial infection. The utility of specific antiviral agents (oseltamivir, zanamivir) is controversial, but they do reduce the period of infectivity and risk of cross infection to other family members. High-risk children (<5 years with underlying cardiac and/or respiratory disease and immunocompromised children) and patients with severe manifestations like high-grade fever, toxemia, respiratory difficulty, blood-tinged sputum, inability to feed or cyanosis (SaO_2 <90%) should be admitted to the hospital.

Prevention

Seasonal cum swine flu vaccines (Vaxigrip, Vaxiflu, Influvac) are available. Two doses are given 4 weeks apart (single dose in children above 9 years) followed by boosters once a year after the rainy season. Every year a new batch of vaccine is marketed by incorporating latest strains of flu viruses prevalent in the population.

STRIDOR

Stridor refers to audible noisy breathing due to partial obstruction of larynx or the trachea. When there is associated hoarseness, the disease is likely to be located in the larynx. Stridor is more common in infants because of relatively narrow airways and common occurrence of oronasal abnormalities like enlarged adenoids, tonsils and small mandible. Stridor may occur due to congenital malformations (laryngomalacia, atresia, webs or cysts), infections (viral, bacterial), laryngospasm (tetany), angioedema (anaphylaxis) and inhalation of a foreign body. The common conditions causing stridor are described below.

Laryngomalacia

It is characterized by congenital softness or easy collapsibility of eryepiglottic folds or epiglottis in general. It usually manifests at the end of first week of life as inspiratory stridor, which is low pitched and fluttering in character. The stridor is intermittent and aggravated by excitement, crying, feeding or change of position of the baby. These infants are more prone to develop gastroesophageal reflux, aspiration of feeds and respiratory tract infections. There is no specific treatment, and condition disappears spontaneously between 6 and 12 months of age. The infant should be nursed in a position with minimal stridor.

Viral Croup

Viral croup or acute laryngotracheitis is the most common cause of acute upper airway obstruction in children. It occurs mainly in preschool children with peak incidence during 6 months–3 years of age. There is sudden onset of fever with inspiratory stridor (croup), barking cough, hoarseness of voice or cry, and variable degree of respiratory distress. The symptoms are worse at night and aggravated by agitation, anxiety and crying. The anteroposterior skiagram of neck may show characteristic subglottic tracheal narrowing (steeple sign).

Humidified air (moist air or steam), paracetamol and adequate fluids are useful supportive measures. Corticosteroids are recommended in all children with croup. A single oral or intramuscular dose of dexamethasone 0.5 mg/kg is given. Nebulization with racemic epinephrine (0.5 mL in 2.5 mL normal saline) alongwith steroids provides prompt relief. Oxygen may be required if there is hypoxia ($SaO_2 < 90\%$). Intubation and tracheostomy are not required for management of children with croup.

Acute Spasmodic Laryngitis (Croup)

Acute viral inflammation of larynx with a reactive spasm produces sudden onset of barking cough, respiratory distress with noisy breathing or croup with each inspiration. Swelling or edema of larynx may occur due to viral infection, allergic reaction (anaphylaxis), exposure to cold, inhalation of irritant fumes or due to a foreign body.

Clinical Features

Preschool children with a strong familial predisposition are likely to be affected. The onset is sudden like a bolt from the blue especially on a chilly winter night. The child develops sudden difficulty in breathing, barking cough, feeling of suffocation and loud croaky inspiratory stridor. There are marked suprasternal and substernal retractions with labored breathing. Fever is usually absent or mild but sweating may be profuse due to release of catecholamines. The severity of attack diminishes within few hours but relapses are known to occur.

Diagnosis

The diagnosis is usually based on characteristic clinical findings. Lateral skiagram of neck may show swollen larynx with obliteration of glottis. Direct laryngoscopy is not required and should be avoided due to risk of laryngospasm. When required to rule out epiglottitis, the procedure should be performed in the operation

theater so that emergency tracheostomy may be done if needed as a life-saving procedure. Croup must be differentiated from laryngeal diphtheria, foreign body inhalation, acute bacterial laryngitis or epiglottitis and laryngospasm due to tetany.

Treatment

The treatment is supportive and symptomatic. The child must be nursed in high humidity and given oxygen. Hot steam can be provided with electric kettle or cold steam can be given with a nebulizer in a croupette or tent. Nebulization of racemic epinephrine (0.5 mL in 2.5 mL normal saline) provides prompt relief. The child should be closely watched for respiratory distress and cyanosis so that timely tracheostomy is done when it is indicated. A single dose of dexamethasone 0.5 mg/kg IM may be given but its role is doubtful. There is no role of antibiotics, expectorants, bronchodilators and antihistamines. Most children with spasmodic croup do not require any tracheostomy. Endotracheal intubation and tracheostomy may be life saving in patients with epiglottitis, laryngeal diphtheria and foreign body impaction in the glottis or trachea.

ACUTE EPIGLOTTITIS

Acute infection of epiglottis (most commonly caused by *H. influenzae* type b) is a life-threatening disease, usually affecting children aged between 2 and 6 years. At times, other pathogens such as *S. pneumoniae*, *S. aureus*, *H. influenzae* non-b type, and *Haemophilus parainfluenzae* may be involved. The incidence of this disease has become rare in the West because of routine use of *H. influenzae* type b vaccine. There is marked inflammation and edema of epiglottis, aryepiglottic folds and adjacent structures causing severe occlusion of the airway.

Clinical Features

The onset is abrupt with fever, sore throat, toxicity, dysphagia, drooling and inspiratory stridor with retractions of chest wall. To reduce the severity of airway obstruction, classically the child sits with its mouth open, tongue protruding with drooling of saliva (doggy stance), and neck hyperextended. The epiglottis is swollen and beefy-red in appearance. Retropharyngeal abscess produces identical clinical features, but dysphagia is more marked and epiglottis is normal.

Diagnosis

Oral examination without a spatula confirms the diagnosis by visualizing swollen cherry-red epiglottis. In an uncooperative child, throat should be examined

38

in the operation theater because of risk of reflex laryngospasm and total airway obstruction, which can be handled by emergency tracheostomy. Blood examination shows polymorphonuclear leukocytosis, and blood culture may yield causative pathogens. Lateral skiagram of neck shows enlarged epiglottis as a "thumb sign". Other conditions that may cause inspiratory stridor, such as viral croup, bacterial tracheitis, and aspiration of foreign body, should be considered in the differential diagnosis.

Treatment

Epiglottitis is a life-threatening emergency and need expert nursing care. The child should be closely monitored for severity of airway obstruction and adequacy of oxygenation so that timely endotracheal intubation or tracheostomy is done. Many strains of *H. influenzae* type b have become resistant to ampicillin. The antibiotics of choice include amoxicillin–clavulanic acid, cefuroxime axetil, ceftriaxone, or chloramphenicol, which are given through IV route in adequate doses. *Haemophilus influenzae* type b vaccine (in conjunction with triple antigen schedule) provides effective protection against various diseases caused by *H. influenzae*.

PNEUMONIA

Pneumonia is an acute inflammation of one or both lungs. It is a leading cause of mortality in children accounting for 18% of under-5 mortality rate (U5MR). In young children, both lungs are usually involved (bronchopneumonia or double pneumonia). When a lobe of a lung is affected, it is called lobar pneumonia. It may be caused by bacteria, viruses or fungi. The common bacterial pathogens include pneumococci, streptococci, *H. influenzae* type b and *S. aureus*. It is commonly preceded by cough and cold, and may occur as a complication of measles and whooping cough. Pneumonia may follow inhalation of a foreign body and aspiration into the lungs.

Clinical Features

The usual symptoms are fever, cough and rapid breathing. Breathing rate is fast with visible movements of alae nasi of nostrils and retractions or inward drawing of lower ribs with each breath. Age-related cutoff for fast breathing are shown in **Table 38.1**. A grunting sound may be audible with each expiration in small babies. The expiratory grunt is produced due to partial closure of glottis in an attempt to increase end expiratory pressure in the alveoli so that gas exchange continues even during expiration. In severe

Table 38.1 Age-related cutoffs for fast breathing

Age	Breaths/min
<2 months	≥60
2–12 months	≥50
1–5 years	≥40

Note: Breathing rate should be checked when child is quiet and not crying or restless. Auscultation of chest for crepitations or crackles has low sensitivity.

cases, cyanosis may develop. The child may be irritable or cry excessively due to chest pain and oxygen lack. When breathing difficulty is marked, the child is unable to take his feeds. Auscultation of chest shows diffuse rales on both sides of chest. In lobar pneumonia there is localized bronchial breathing and crepitations.

Severity of pneumonia According to integrated management of childhood illnesses (IMCI) protocol by WHO, pneumonia is classified into 4 groups **(Box 38.1)**. All infants with pneumonia below the age of 2 months are classified as severe and admitted to the hospital.

Diagnosis

There is polymorphonuclear leukocytosis, elevation of erythrocyte sedimentation rate (ESR) and C-reactive protein (CRP). Skiagram of chest shows diffuse bilateral patchy infiltrates. In lobar pneumonia there is a large opaque opacity due to consolidation of a lobe of the lung. In staphylococcal pneumonia, there is formation of thin-walled blebs (pneumatoceles) in the lungs. Pneumatocele may rupture causing sudden respiratory distress due to development of pneumothorax. This is often followed by development of empyema (purulent pleural effusion).

Treatment

When an infant with pneumonia is crying excessively, he should never be given a sedative because it will depress breathing efforts. He may need admission to a

---

Box 38.1 Assessment of severity of pneumonia

Lethargic or unconscious, inability to drink or breastfeed, cyanosis, seizures and severe respiratory distress (RR >70/min) or gasping (**Very severe pneumonia**)

Lower chest indrawing without any signs of very severe pneumonia (**Severe pneumonia**)

Fast breathing but without chest retractions and no signs of severe or very severe pneumonia (**Non-severe pneumonia**)
No signs of pneumonia (**Cough and cold, no pneumonia**)

Children with severe or very severe pneumonia should be admitted to the hospital.

hospital for administration of oxygen **(Box 38.2)**. Pneumonia is a serious condition and should be managed immediately with an appropriate antibiotic. Give paracetamol to relieve fever and pain. The child must be given plenty of fluids (because water is lost through breath due to rapid breathing) and nutritious diet. The position of the child should be changed frequently to facilitate drainage of tracheo-bronchial secretions. Cough suppressants should be avoided. Most cases of pneumonia in children can be treated on the out-patient basis by administration of co-trimoxazole or amoxycillin (25 mg/kg/dose twice daily) or erythromycin and its derivatives like azithromycin or roxithromycin. In resistant or serious cases, second line drugs like combination of amoxycillin with clavulanic acid, cefaclor and cefuroxime axetil may be used. Oral antibiotic therapy is given for 5–7 days while parenteral therapy in serious cases is given for 7–10 days. Staphylococcal pneumonia is treated by giving antibiotics for atleast 2 weeks. Empyema is treated by chest drainage and administration of antibiotics for 3 weeks. Bronchopneumonia in infants below 2 months is treated like septicemia with a combination of intravenous amikacin and cefotaxime or ceftriaxone therapy. In critically ill children with impending respiratory failure, timely assisted ventilation is life saving.

Role of a Nurse

- Monitor the vital signs, arterial blood gases (ABGs), input and output.
- Maintain warm, humid and well-ventilated environment.
- Keep the child comfortable in head up position and maintain good personal hygiene.
- Control fever with paracetamol and tepid water sponging.
- Administration of oxygen (SaO$_2$ <90%) and periodic suctioning of air passages.

Box 38.2 Indications for hospital admission

- Infants below 2 months.
- Severely malnourished child.
- Respiratory rate above 60/min.
- Chest indrawing, grunting and/or head nodding.
- Inability to take oral feeds.
- Marked restlessness and crying or drowsy and depressed infant.
- Cyanosis (SaO$_2$ <90%).
- Lack of improvement after 2–3 days of ambulatory treatment.

- Ensure adequate hydration and nutrition. Breastfeeding and oral feeds are continued if child is able to accept. In critically sick children, nasogastric feeding or intravenous fluid therapy is recommended.
- Ensure timely administration of antibiotics, brochodilators and other prescribed medications.
- Safeguard against the risk of nosocomial infection.
- Provide chest physiotherapy and postural drainage of secretions in the respiratory passages.
- Provide age-appropriate play material and recreational facilities to reduce anxiety and boredom.
- Provide general guidance, health education and emotional support to the family.
- At the time of discharge, give guidelines for follow-up, home care, avoidance of harmful cultural practices and need for administration of any missed vaccines.

EMPYEMA THORACIS (Pyothorax)

Empyema thoracis is defined as collection of pus in the pleural cavity while clear transudate in the chest cavity is called pleural effusion. Empyema may occur following underlying pneumonia, bronchiectasis or lung abscess. Hepatic or subphrenic abscess may burst into pleural cavity. Penetrating chest injury or esophageal perforation or surgical procedure may be followed by pyothorax. The common causative organisms are *Staphylococcus aureus*, *H. influenzae*, streptococci and anerobic organisms.

Clinical Features

The child develops high grade fever, chest pain, shortness of breath, rapid breathing and cough. When there is basal pneumonia, abdominal pain, distension and ileus may occur. In cases of chronic empyema and lung abscess, foul breath, weight loss and clubbing of nails are seen. Chest examination shows stony dullness on percussion, poor air entry and displacement of mediastinum (trachea and heart) to the opposite side. When pus breaks into subcutaneous plane of chest it is called empyema necessitans. There is a soft cystic swelling in the intercostal space which can be reduced by pressure.

Nursing Alert

In a child with pneumonia, sudden chest pain, respiratory difficulty and cyanosis are suggestive of rupture of a pneumatocele with development of pyopneumothorax. The doctor must be informed without any delay.

38

Diagnosis

Skiagram of chest in erect posture (sitting or standing) shows collection of fluid in the pleural cavity. Ultrasonography can identify collection of fluid or pus and any loculations and associated liver abscess. Aspiration of pus or thoracocentesis is diagnostic. The aspirate should be sent for biochemistry, cytology, Gram staining, culture for pyogenic organisms and acid fast bacilli.

Treatment

Because *Staphylococcus aureus* is the most common causative organism, parenteral cloxacillin and gentamicin is administered as the initial antibiotic of choice. Depending upon the culture and sensitivity report or response to therapy, antibiotic therapy can be modified. Antibiotics are continued for at least 3–4 weeks or even longer till pyothorax is completely resolved. Child should be encouraged to take nutritious balanced diet with supplements of vitamins and minerals.

Intercostal drainage A thick-bored intercostal tube is inserted at 6th intercostal space in the midclavicular line and connected to under water seal in a closed system for continuous drainage of pus **(Figure 38.1)**. Instillation of fibrinolytic agent into the pleural cavity

> **Nursing Tip**
>
> *Excessive crying in a child with pneumonia is due to hypoxia. Never give a sedative to quieten a child with pneumonia. Oxygen administration is life-saving and would promptly relieve irritability and crying.*

is associated with faster recovery. If lungs fail to expand and there is marked pleural thickening, decortication is done.

Nursing Care

1. Vital signs should be monitored.
2. General supportive care is provided for relief of fever and pain by administration of paracetamol. Oxygen is administered if SaO_2 is less than 90%. Child is encouraged to take a balanced nutritious diet.
3. *Care of thoracotomy tube*
   - A sterile collecting bottle with savlon should be used and kept below the level of the patient. It should be changed daily or earlier if it gets filled. Dressing should be changed daily. Drainage is usually continued for atleast one week.
   - The tube should be watched for movements of the column of pus. When there are no movements of

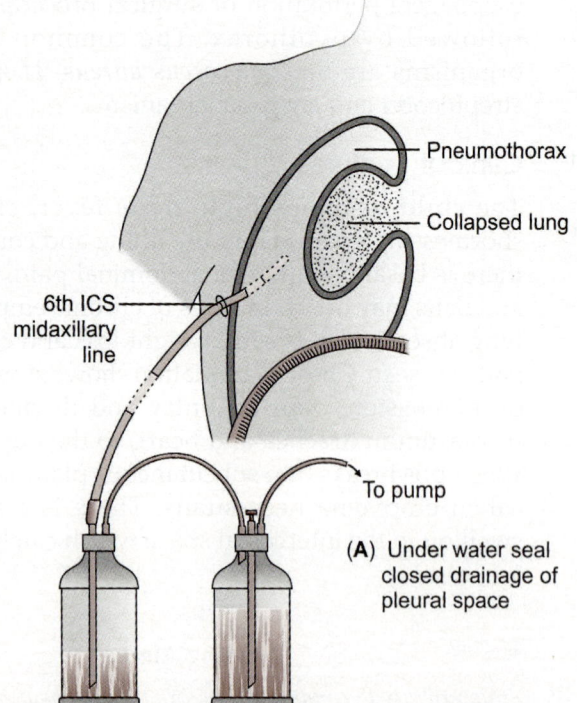

6th ICS midaxillary line

Pneumothorax

Collapsed lung

To pump

(A) Under water seal closed drainage of pleural space

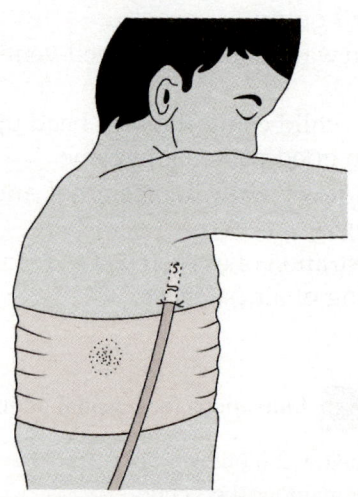

(B) Occlusive chest wall dressing for open pneumothorax

Figure 38.1 Underwater seal drainage is essential to avoid entry of atmospheric air into the pleural cavity. Gentle constant negative pressure of 5–10 cm H_2O facilitates the drainage of air and pus (A). In open pneumothorax following chest trauma, the chest wall should be dressed tightly to seal the external wound (B)

the column of the fluid, the tube should be milked towards the drainage bottle or changed.

- The amount of pus drained daily should be recorded.
- The tube should be clamped whenever the child is being moved for nursing care.
- Before removing the chest tube, it should be clamped for a couple of hours to watch whether any pus reaccumulates in the chest. The tube should be removed when drainage of pus is minimal or nil.

4. *Chest physiotherapy*

- Maintain lung expansion by asking the child to blow a whistle or inflate a balloon. Postural drainage and gentle tapping of the chest with a cupped hand is recommended if there is underlying abscess. Humidification and bronchodilators may be given to facilitate expectoration of thick viscid secretions.

ACUTE BRONCHIOLITIS

Acute bronchiolitis is usually caused by the respiratory syncitial virus (RSV) though rarely para influenza and influenza viruses may cause the disease. The illness is more frequent during winter months and affects infants between 3 months and one year of age.

Clinical Features

The illness usually begins as a viral upper respiratory tract infection. After 1–2 days, cough becomes prominent and progresses to tachypnea (rapid breathing) followed by dyspnea (difficulty in breathing). Fever is usually mild or absent. The chest is hyperinflated and hyperresonant on percussion due to bilateral obstructive emphysema. There are diffuse high-pitched wheezing sounds and occasional crackles or crepitations on auscultation. Most cases recover within one week but disease may last upto one month in some infants. About 40% infants with acute bronchiolitis may develop recurrent wheezing during first 3–4 years of life.

Diagnosis

Skiagram of chest shows hyperinflation, prominent peribronchial markings and areas of atelectasis. The leukocyte count, is usually normal except when there is associated super added bacterial infection.

Treatment

The management is usually supportive and symptomatic. Infant should be nursed in a prone position with head and chest slightly raised. In critically

Nursing Alert

Restlessness, irritability and excessive crying in a child with respiratory distress is a sign of hypoxia. It is managed by administration of oxygen. Never give a sedative to such a child!

sick children, hydration, oxygenation and acid-base parameters should be maintained within normal range. Oxygen saturation (SaO$_2$) should be maintained above 95%. Antibiotics are given to control superadded bacterial infection. Cold humidification is useful. Nebulized epinephrine (2 mL of 1:1000 solution in 2 mL of normal saline) is recommended during acute stage to relieve dyspnea. Nebulization with 3% saline solution is equally effective. Corticosteroids should be used with caution. Sedatives are contraindicated because restlessness is usually due to hypoxia which responds to oxygen administration.

BRONCHIAL ASTHMA (Wheezy Child)

Wheezing is a musical sound produced while breathing due to narrowing of the air passages of the lungs. The narrowing of air passages may occur due to pressure from outside, obstruction of its lumen or spasm of the bronchial wall (which occurs in bronchial asthma). When proximal or larger airways like trachea and bronchi are affected, the breathing-in (inspiration) efforts become noisy (stridor) and difficult. On the other hand, obstruction or spasm of distal airways or bronchioles leads to difficulty and prolongation of breathing-out (expiration) efforts with audible rhonchi (wheezing). The chest may remain constantly inflated (emphysema) because air cannot be completely expelled out of the lungs due to narrowing or spasm of the distal airways.

Etiology

Asthma is characterized by recurrent episodes of breathing difficulty and wheezing in a child who has an inherited susceptibility to manifest atopy or allergy to a variety of environmental allergens. The antigen-antibody reaction in the air passages leads to release of histamine which causes spasm of the muscles of bronchioles. The family history of asthma or allergic disorder is common among close relatives. Bronchial asthma is usually caused by allergens which are inhaled into the air passages. The commonly inhaled allergens include dust, dust mites, pollen of flowers or weeds, mould, cockroaches, hair or dander of pet animals. Food allergens are uncommon cause of bronchial asthma and they include artificial colors (chiclets, soft drinks, juices,

38

ketchup, jam, sweets, etc.) and food preservatives. Allergy to fresh fruits and vegetables is rare but is well documented with dry fruits or nuts especially if they are contaminated with moulds.

Viral infections and certain drugs (especially aspirin and non-steroidal anti-inflammatory drugs) may trigger an attack of asthma. Exercise, exposure to cold and emotional stress of examination may precipitate an attack of asthma in susceptible children. The attack of asthma may be triggered and aggravated by environmental pollution (dust, automobile exhaust, smog, fire crackers, etc.), smoke (over crowding, poor ventilation, cigarette smoking by parents), cooking odors, air freshners, perfumes, *agarbati*, soaps, cosmetics, insect sprays and mosquito repellents. During the last decade, the incidence of asthma has almost doubled among urban children due to increasing pollution, smoke and smog in the cities. The asthmatic attacks in some children may be seasonal because change of season may be associated with activation of a viral infection or dissemination of allergenic pollen particles. When disease becomes more severe, the manifestations may become persistent or perennial throughout the year.

Clinical Features

There may be genetic background or family history of bronchial asthma, recurrent episodes of common cold and sneezing, eczema or drug allergy. The child may show personal manifestations of atopy, i.e. eczema, urticaria, hay fever, food allergy and drug allergy. The usual story is that child gets frequent attacks of viral or allergic colds (cough, watering of nose and eyes, itching of nose, sneezing and redness of eyes) which is followed by breathing difficulty, intractable cough and wheezing. The cough is persistent, spasmodic and worse at night or early morning. The breathing is fast with marked retractions of chest wall. Breathing-out (expiration) is more difficult and often prolonged. Wheezing is best heard when ear is brought close to the chest wall (over the front or back) of the child. In severe cases wheezing may be audible from a distance. In some children wheezing may be minimal and can be easily missed. When cough is persistent, spasmodic, and worse at night and triggered by bouts of crying or laughing, it is desirable to give a trial of bronchodilator medicine even when there is no obvious wheezing. *It must be remembered that all wheezing is not due to asthma and asthma can occur without obvious wheezing.*

Course of the Disease

About two-thirds of asthmatic children have mild and episodic asthmatic attacks while 20–25 percent have persistent and moderately severe asthmatic symptoms.

About one-third of children out grow their asthma by 5 years and one-half are free from asthmatic attacks by 8 years of age. Only 10 percent of affected children continue to have their asthmatic attacks during adolescence and later in life. However, it is difficult to identify those children who are likely to spontaneously out grow their asthmatic tendency.

Treatment

There are a number of drugs which provide symptomatic relief when child has an acute attack of asthma. The parents must identify the earliest trigger or evidence of attack because hospitalization can be avoided if therapy is administered without delay. The use of peak flow meter to assess lung capacity is useful for early identification of an attack of bronchial asthma **(Figure 38.2)**. A number of bronchodilators like salbutamol, terbutaline, theophylline and steroids are available which can be administered either orally or by inhalation. Inhalation therapy is preferred because of its greater efficacy and lower incidence of side effects. Depending upon the age of the child, several modalities are available for inhalation therapy **(Table 38.2)**. There

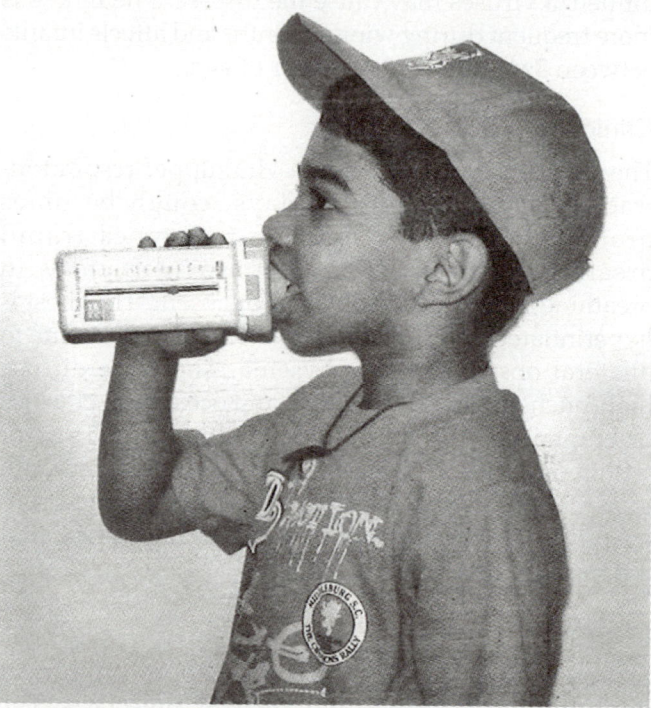

Figure 38.2 Method for recording peak expiratory flow rate (PEFR) with a mini-Wright peak flow meter. The child is asked to stand, take a deep breath in and then forcefully breathe out through the peak flow meter. The best of three values is taken and compared with the child's personal best taken during remission. When child's PEFR is less than 80% of his personal best or predicted PEFR, he needs bronchodilator therapy

Table 38.2 Modes of inhalation therapy in children of different ages

Age	Recommended device
0–2 years	Nebuliser with mask, MDI* with a mask, aerochamber with a mask
2–5 years	MDI with a spacer
5–8 years	Rotahaler, MDI with a spacer
> 8 years	MDI, Rotahaler

*MDI, Metered dose inhaler

is a wrong belief that inhalers are habit forming but they may become ineffective if canister is empty or when they are used without due regard for correct procedure. Electrical nebulizer device can be used for nebulization of bronchodilators (salbutamol, levo-salbutamol, ipratropium bromide and betamethasone). Nebulization can be done with oxygen (hospital) or with room air (home). Procedure is usually completed in 10–12 minutes. A mask (to cover nose and mouth) should be used for effective nebulization in preschool children while an older child is able to inhale the medicine through her mouth **(Figure 38.3)**. Nebulization is ineffective when nebulizer outlet is merely placed infront of the nose of the child. In ambulatory or home setting, multidose inhaler (MDI) can be used for administration of bronchodilators and steroids. Young children cannot coordinate their breath for effective inhalation. It is preferable to use a spacer for effective delivery of inhaler medications to preschool and uncooperative children **(Figure 38.4)**. The correct method for use of a nebulizer and MDI device and their maintenance is summarized in **Box 38.3** and **38.4**. The management protocol and algorithm for treatment of an acute attack of bronchial asthma is shown in **Figure 38.5**.

There is no role of antibiotics or cough expectorants in most cases. Drinking of warm water helps to relieve the bouts of coughing. Antihistaminics should be avoided during an acute attack of asthma as they dry up the secretions in the airways and worsen the cough. Non-steroidal anti-inflammatory drugs (NSAIDs) especially aspirin should be avoided in patients with bronchial asthma as they are known to aggravate bronchial reactivity and worsen wheezing in susceptible children. Paracetamol is the antipyretic of choice in asthmatic children having fever.

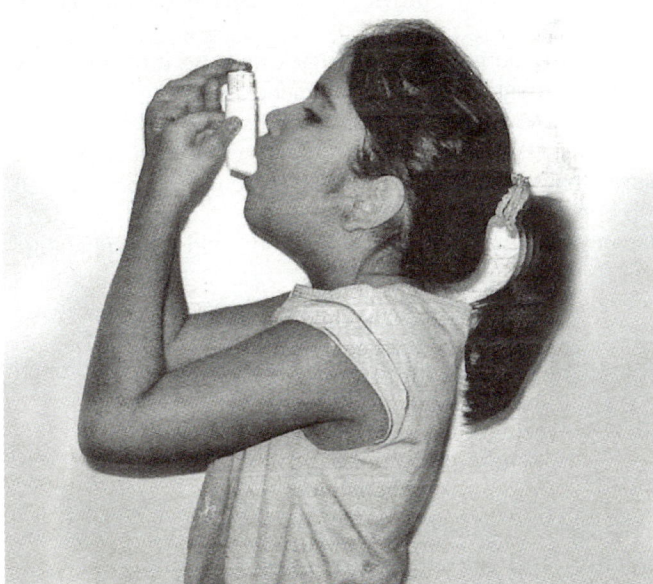

Figure 38.3 Method for using a metered dose inhaler (MDI) device. The child is asked to take a deep breath out, mouthpiece of the MDI is tightly grasped with lips. The actuator of the inhaler is pressed while child simultaneously takes a deep breath to inhale the aerosol. With some guidance and instructions, most school-going children can cooperate and coordinate their breath to effectively inhale the medication directly without using the spacer device

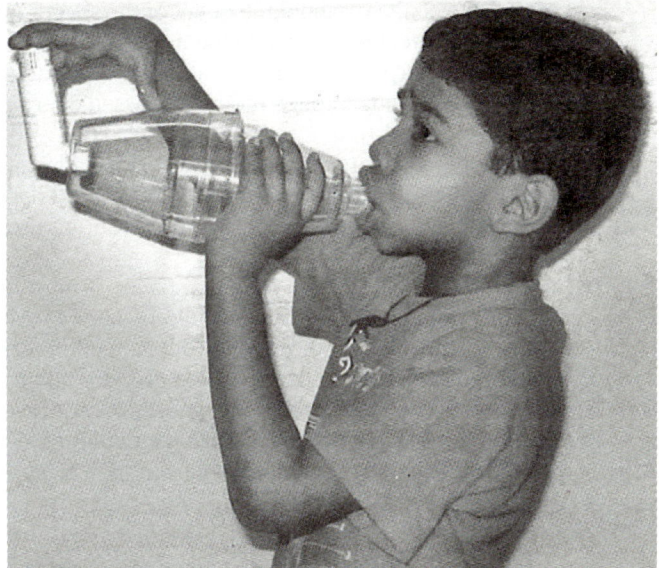

Figure 38.4 In preschool children, metered dose inhaler (MDI) is used with a spacer device. The child firmly grasps the oral piece of the spacer with his lips and MDI device is attached to the other end of the spacer. When MDI device is pressed, aerosole of the medicine is distributed in the spacer. Child is asked to take regular deep in-breaths through his mouth while constantly and firmly grasping the spacer with his lips. The child is asked to exhale through his nose and inhale through his mouth. In a matter of 15–30 seconds most of the aerosol is inhaled. In toddlers and infants, a mask is affixed to the spacer for effective use of MDI

38

Box 38.3   **Correct use of a nebulizer**

1. It is preferable to use central oxygen source or oxygen from a cylinder at a rate of 6–8 liters/min to nebulize the drug during an acute attack. However, if oxygen is not available, compressed air can be used. Face mask or mouth device is used depending upon the age and cooperation of the child.
2. The drug volume should be at least 3 mL. If residual volume (volume after nebulisation is over) is more than 1 mL, a larger amount of drug volume should be prepared. Three doses of the drug should be nebulized after every 20 minutes during first hour of therapy.
3. Patient should be instructed to inhale from his mouth. Although it may be difficult to control breathing pattern during an acute attack but deep and slow breathing is advocated.
4. Drug should be nebulised over a period of 8–10 mintues. If the procedure is taking longer than 10 minutes either chamber is malfunctioning or supply of compressed air/oxygen is defective.
5. A good mist formation suggests that the procedure of nebulization is satisfactory.

Cleaning the Nebulizer

It is preferable to use either a disposable or separate nebuliser chamber for each patient. However, if that is not possible, cleaning the nebuliser and tubings thoroughly in-between patients is mandatory. A light detergent can be used followed by plain water to wash the equipment. 1% vinegar solution can be used for overnight immersion to disinfect the nebulizer and tubings. After sterilization and before next use, the nebuliser should be run dry for a few minutes.

Box 38.4   **Correct use of MDI with a spacer**

1. Multi- or metered-dose inhaler (MDI) without a spacer device is not advocated in under-5 children because of poor hand-lung coordination. A spacer device preferably with a mask is a must while using MDI in preschool children. Children above 5 years of age can hold the outlet of the spacer in their mouth (without a mask) and are asked to breath-in through the mouth and breath-out through the nose.
2. Drug is held in suspension after actuation for a period of at least 10 seconds in the holding chamber.
3. A slow deep breathing through mouth is advised after actuation of the MDI and it provides better delivery of drug into the lungs.
4. Breath holding after a deep slow breath is not advocated, particularly during an acute attack because it may be very uncomfortable or impossible. Continuous slow and deep breathing through mouth is recommended.
5. Two puffs should be used every 10 minutes during first hour of therapy. In between puffs, child should receive oxygen therapy.
6. While using a commercially available spacer, it must be ensured that the patient is able to operate the valve with each inspiration. The click of the valve should be audible with each breath.
7. A smaller volume (250 mL) spacer for younger children and a larger volume (750 mL) spacer for older children is preferable. However, a large volume spacer can be used for all age groups.
8. Indigenously fabricated spacer is as good as a commercial device in treating an acute attack. Absence of valve infact makes it easier to use in younger and sicker children.
9. MDI with a spacer is as good as a nebulizer. However, 4–6 doses of MDI are equivalent to one dose administered through a nebulizer.
10. The spacer should be washed with a detergent every week and air dried.

Prevention

In children with persistent and severe bronchial asthma, sodium cromoglycate or steroids can be given prophylactically through inhalers on a long-term basis. In children with seasonal asthma, prophylaxis can be given for a short term basis at the onset of adverse season. In addition, the body resistance of the child should be boosted against infections and allergy by intake of balanced nutritious diet and micronutrients which are known to be credited with anti-infective, anti-allergic and antioxidant capabilities such as docosahexaenoic acid (DHA), vitamin A, vitamin C, vitamin D, zinc, calcium and selenium. Yoga and breathing exercises help to improve the vital capacity of lungs.

Identification of trigger factors and possible allergens and their elimination can provide curative relief to a child with bronchial asthma. The parents should be extremely vigilant to identify various factors and situations which lead to wheezing. In susceptible children in whom an attack of allergic cold is followed by wheezing, bronchodilator therapy should be started without any delay.

38

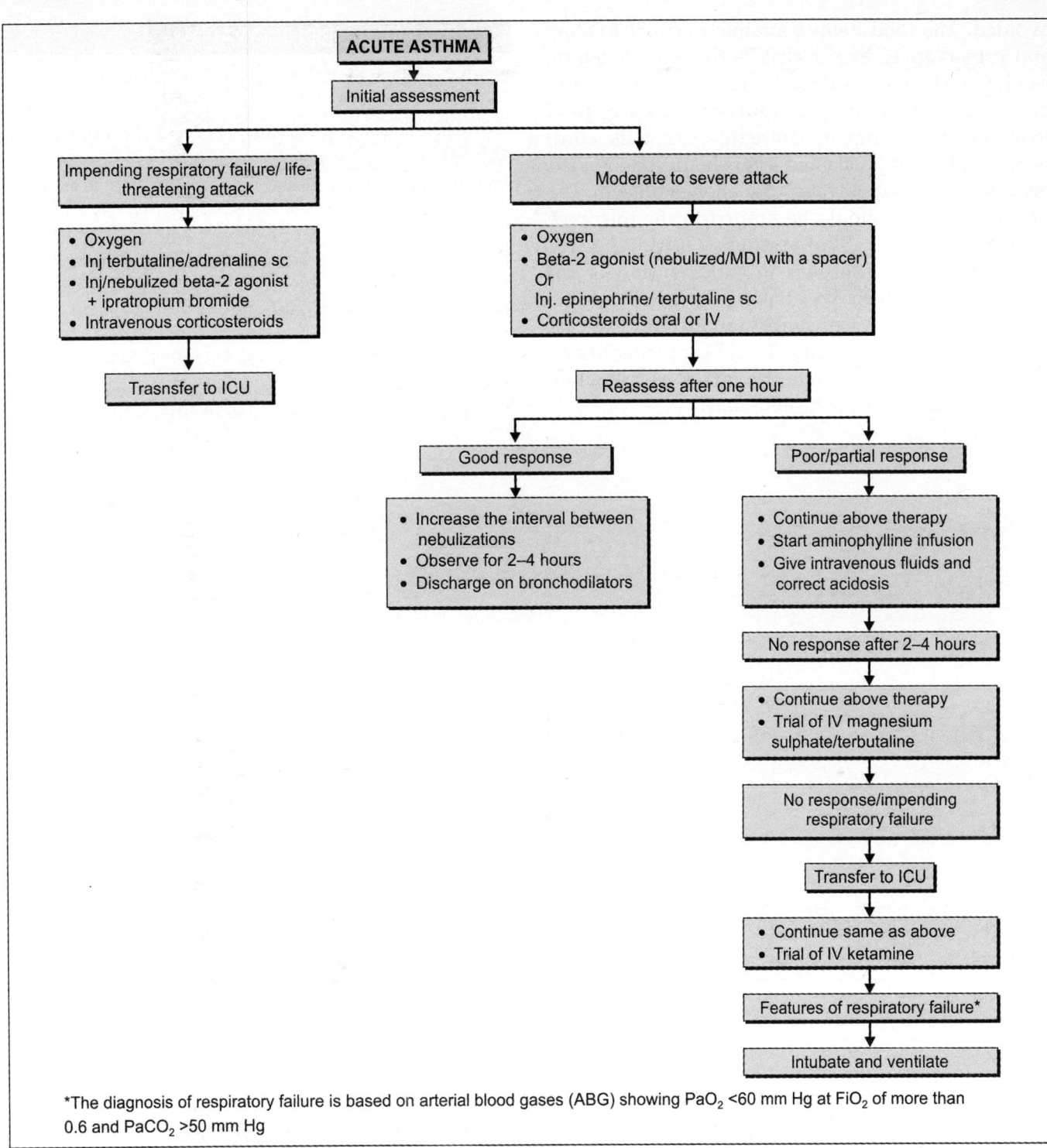

ACUTE ASTHMA

Initial assessment

Impending respiratory failure/ life-threatening attack
- Oxygen
- Inj terbutaline/adrenaline sc
- Inj/nebulized beta-2 agonist + ipratropium bromide
- Intravenous corticosteroids

Trasnfer to ICU

Moderate to severe attack
- Oxygen
- Beta-2 agonist (nebulized/MDI with a spacer) Or Inj. epinephrine/ terbutaline sc
- Corticosteroids oral or IV

Reassess after one hour

Good response
- Increase the interval between nebulizations
- Observe for 2–4 hours
- Discharge on bronchodilators

Poor/partial response
- Continue above therapy
- Start aminophylline infusion
- Give intravenous fluids and correct acidosis

No response after 2–4 hours

- Continue above therapy
- Trial of IV magnesium sulphate/terbutaline

No response/impending respiratory failure

Transfer to ICU

- Continue same as above
- Trial of IV ketamine

Features of respiratory failure*

Intubate and ventilate

*The diagnosis of respiratory failure is based on arterial blood gases (ABG) showing PaO$_2$ <60 mm Hg at FiO$_2$ of more than 0.6 and PaCO$_2$ >50 mm Hg

Figure 38.5 Algorithm for management of an acute attack of asthma

The environment of the child especially bedroom should be kept dust free and well ventilated. Avoid use of carpets and heavy curtains. Instead of brooming, vacuum cleaner should be used. The filter of airconditioner should be cleaned frequently. The home should be kept free of dust mites (expose linen and bed clothes to sunlight once a week), cockroaches and other insects. Pets and stuffed toys should preferably be avoided. Children with asthma should avoid smoky, stuffy, over crowded and polluted places. The use of insect sprays, strong perfumes, *agarbati*, and mosquito repellents should preferably be avoided. The food items containing artificial colors and preservatives like chiclets, soft drinks, ketchup, candies, pickles, canned foods and juices, etc. should be avoided. According to Ayurvedic system, food items which are slimy in nature (like rice, milk, curd, banana, okra, colocasia and *arbi*) should be avoided because they can aggravate production of phlegm. The physical activity should be limited to the tolerance level of the child. Skin testing is unreliable for identification of allergens in children and is not routinely undertaken. The attacks of bronchial asthma can be reduced by constant vigilance and use of common sense. The parents should try to identify all the triggers which initiate the attack of bronchial asthma so that they can be eliminated.

BIBLIOGRAPHY

British Guidelines for the Management of Asthma. *Thorax* 2003, 58 (supple 1): S1–S94.

Cherry JD. Clinical practice: croup. *N Engl J Med* 2008, 358(4): 384–391.

Harmanci K, Bakirtas I, Degim T. Oral montelukast treatment of preschool-aged children with acute asthma. *Ann Allergy Asthma Immunol* 2006, 96(5): 731–735.

Kabra SK, Lodha R. Long-term management of asthma. *Indian J Pediatr* 2003, 70(1): 63–72.

Reijonen T, Korppi M, Pitkakangas S, et al. The clinical efficacy of nebulized racemic epinephrine and albuterol in acute bronchiolitis. *Arch Pediatr Adolesc Med* 1995, 149(6): 686–692.

Tibballs J, Watson T. Symptoms and signs differentiating croup and epiglottitis. *J Paediatr Child Health* 2011, 47(3): 77–82.

Cardiovascular Disorders

FETAL AND NEONATAL CIRCULATION

The heart assumes its normal four-chambered shape at the end of six weeks of intrauterine life. The oxygenated blood from placenta is returned by way of umbilical veins, which enter the fetus at the umbilicus and join the portal vein. Most of the umbilical venous blood (oxygenated blood) is by-passed through low resistance portal vein to the inferior vena cava and enters the right atrium. In the right atrium, blood flow is divided into two streams by the inferior margin of septum secundum. Most of the oxygenated blood enters left atrium through foramen ovale. There it mixes with the small amount of blood returning from the lungs (which have no ventilatory role in the fetus) via pulmonary veins and is pumped from left ventricle for distribution to the coronaries, brain and upper extremities.

The deoxygenated blood from superior vena cava enters the right atrium and directly traverses through tricuspid valve to enter the right ventricle. The right ventricle pumps out blood into the pulmonary trunk. A small amount of this blood enters the pulmonary circulation, the rest passes through the ductus arteriosus into the descending aorta for distribution into lower extremities. The elevated pulmonary vascular resistance in fetal life is responsible for this physiological right-to-left shunt through ductus. During fetal life, no more than 10% of combined right and left ventricular output perfuses through the lungs while placenta receives more than 50% of the cardiac output to perform the ventilatory role **(Figure 39.1)**.

After birth, with first breath, pulmonary vascular resistance rapidly falls, resulting in increase in pulmonary blood flow. The clamping of cord is followed by sudden increase in systemic vascular resistance due to loss of low resistance placental circulation. The pressure relation between the aorta and pulmonary trunk are reversed, resulting in left-to-right shunt through ductus arteriosus. However, ductus

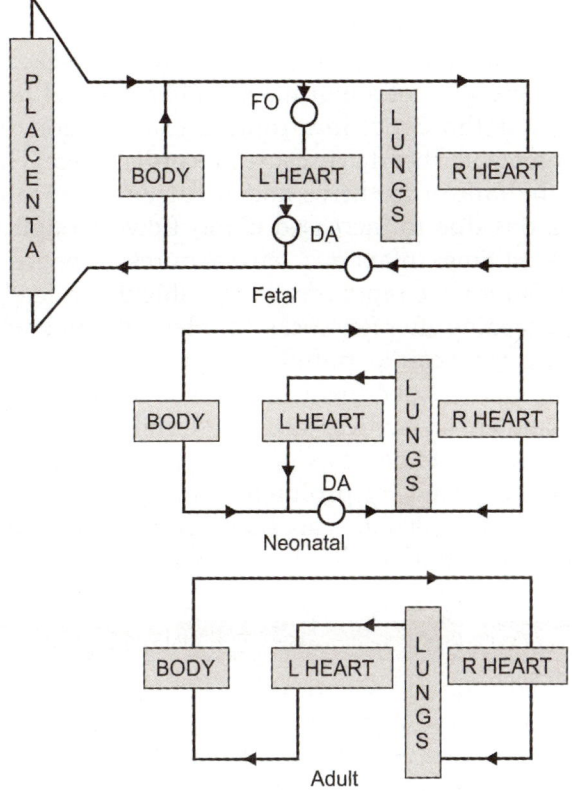

Figure 39.1 Diagrammatic representation of fetal, neonatal (transitional) and adult circulation

FO, foramen ovale; DA, ductus arteriosus; L heart, left heart; R heart, right heart

rapidly constricts on exposure to oxygen and by the end of 72 hours it is functionally closed in term babies. The pulmonary vascular resistance continues to fall over several weeks and lowest pulmonary pressure is achieved around 8–12 weeks of age when most left-to-right shunts become functional and symptomatic.

Heart diseases mainly fall into two broad groups; congenital and acquired. Congenital heart diseases are caused by developmental defects of the heart while acquired heart diseases are mainly due to rheumatic fever and myocarditis.

CONGENITAL HEART DEFECTS

Congenital heart defects occur in around 1% of live births. The common causes include maternal and fetal infections during first trimester (rubella, mumps), teratogenic effects of drugs taken during early pregnancy, maternal diabetes mellitus, maternal dietary deficiencies and genetic factors (Down syndrome). In almost 90% cases no cause is found. Common causes of congenital heart diseases are listed in **Table 39.1**.

Clinical Features

Acyanotic heart diseases are more common and majority of cases are due to left-to-right shunt. There is no cyanosis and many a times heart defect is picked up by the presence of a murmur (rumbling sound heard with a stethoscope) in a routine examination. The enlargement of heart may cause precordial bulge. There may be failure to thrive and recurrent respiratory infections due to increased blood flow through the lungs. At times infant may have features of congestive heart failure like rapid breathing, difficulty in feeding (stops feeding after few sucks), marked sweating while feeding, tachycardia, puffiness of face and swelling of feet or sacral region (because infant is mostly lying in bed) and enlarging liver size. These children are at an increased risk to develop infective endocarditis which is characterized by prolonged unexplained fever, anemia, mild splenomegaly subtle bleeding manifestations (hematuria, splinter hemorrhages under the nail

Table 39.1 Classification of congenital heart diseases

A. *Acyanotic*

- Left-to-right shunt
  - □ Patent ductus arteriosus (PDA)
  - □ Atrial septal defect (ASD)
  - □ Ventricular septal defect (VSD)
- Obstructive lesions
  - □ Aortic valvular stenosis (AS)
  - □ Pulmonary stenosis (PS)
  - □ Coarctation of aorta (COA)

B. *Cyanotic*

- Right-to-left shunt with decreased blood flow through lungs
  - □ Tetralogy of Fallot (TOF)
  - □ Tricuspid atresia
- Mixed blood flow with increased blood flow through lungs
  - □ Transposition of great arteries (TGA)
  - □ Total anomalous pulmonary venous drainage

bed, hemorrhages in retina as Roth spots) and mild clubbing of nails.

Cyanotic heart defects (blue baby) are less common and occur if the blood does not pass through the lungs or there is mixing of blood between the right and left chambers of the heart. The child may have blue lips, tongue and finger and toe nails. The ends of fingers may become rounded and bulbous with clubbing of nails (thick and curved). Chronic hypoxia leads to polycythemia (rise in red blood cell count and hematocrit) as a protective response. Cyanotic heart defects with decreased flow of blood through lungs (tetrology of Fallot and pulmonary stenosis) may have typical history of anoxic or hyper-cyanotic spells with crying, worsening of cyanosis, rapid breathing and squatting. These children generally do not develop congestive heart failure. Cyanotic heart defects with increased pulmonary blood flow (transposition of great arteries or TGA) are not prone to develop anoxic spells but are more likely to manifest recurrent chest infections, congestive heart failure and plethoric lung fields.

Skiagram of heart and ECG provide supportive evidences of congenital heart defect but 2-D echocardiography and Doppler study are confirmatory and provides definitive diagnosis of underlying cardiac malformation.

Nursing Care

1. Provide emotional support to the family and prepare the child and family for prolonged follow-up and surgery or interventional cardiac procedure.
2. Arrange for financial support with the help of a medical social worker, if required by the family.
3. Monitor physical growth, neuromotor development, early features of congestive heart failure and level of exercise intolerance. Provide guidance to the family for level of activity allowed for the child.
4. Mother should be advised to reduce the episodes of avoidable crying or fussing by the infant by anticipating his needs, feeding promptly when hungry, looking after toilet needs, and keeping the infant comfortable. Bouts of crying due to hyper-cyanotic spell should be treated as outlined in **Box 39.1**.
5. Advise the mother to provide frequent small feeds without tiring the baby. In bottle fed babies, provide high caloric density feeds with reduced water and sodium intake. Iron supplements should be started as soon as weaning foods are given.
6. Prophylactic antibiotics should be given before any invasive procedure (genitourinary instrumentation

> **Box 39.1** **Treatment of hypercyanotic spell**
>
> - Place the child in a knee-chest position.
> - Provide humidified oxygen through a face mask or head box @ 6–8 liters/min.
> - Give injection morphine 0.1–0.2 mg/kg sc and propranolal 0.1 mg/kg iv stat followed by 1.0 mg/kg/day orally in 2 divided doses.
> - If arterial blood gases (ABG) show metabolic acidosis, administer sodium bicarbonate 7.5% solution 1.0 mL/kg diluted 1:1 in distilled water slowly iv over 10 minutes.
> - Correct anemia* by packed cell transfusion and start the child on oral supplements of iron.

* Hemoglobin may be normal but RBCs will be small in size and hypochromic on peripheral blood smear examination.

and dental workup) to prevent occurrence of infective endocarditis.

7. Prevent exposure to respiratory infections, teach about importance of personal hygiene and ensure up-to-date immunization status by administration of optional vaccines like *H. influenzae* type b, influenza vaccine, and pneumococcal vaccine. Explain the importance of early treatment of fever by prompt administration of paracetamol because fever causes tachycardia with increased risk of cardiac decompensation

8. Provide nursing care to a critically sick child with congestive heart failure.

    i. Monitor vital signs, arterial oxygen saturation (SpO_2), fluid intake and output, and body weight.

    ii. Elevate head by 45° to reduce the pressure of viscera on diaphragm and lungs. Prevent kinking of airways by keeping the head slightly extended.

    iii. Keep the nose and oral cavity free of secretions and prevent risk of aspiration. Abdominal distension should be relieved by decompression.

    iv. Provide oxygen therapy as indicated.

    v. Ensure timely administration of all medications and watch for their adverse effects. Prevent occurrence of nosocomial infections by practicing strict barrier nursing. Feeding and nutrition should be supervised.

RHEUMATIC FEVER

Rheumatic fever is a post-infective disorder that affects the joints, the heart and other parts of the body. The common age of occurrence is between 5 and 14 years. The disease occurs when Group A beta hemolytic

> **Nursing Tip**
>
> *Acute streptococcal pharyngitis usually occurs after the age of 2 years and is characterized by high grade fever, sore throat (without cough and coryza), markedly enlarged and inflamed tonsils with pus points or follicles. It must be treated by administration of penicillin or amoxycillin or erythromycin in appropriate doses for a period of atleast 10 days to prevent occurrence of rheumatic fever and acute glomerulonephritis.*

streptococcal infection of the throat has been inadequately treated or not treated at all. After about 2 weeks of sore throat, the child develops high grade fever, with pain or swelling in several joints. The joint pain jumps or migrates from one joint to the other after every couple of days. The commonly affected joints include wrists, elbows, knees and ankles. Subcutaneous nodules may appear over the bony prominences like elbows, shin, occiput and spine. A transient erythematous rash (erythema marginatum) over the trunk may be seen in children with fair skin. Chorea may occur especially in adolescent girls. Initially child is observed to become clumsy followed by typical jerky, purposeless, incoordinated choreic movements. Patient is unable to keep her tongue out.

The main danger of rheumatic fever is that it can affect and damage the heart. Carditis is a serious manifestation and may permanently damage the valves of the heart. Cardiac involvement is characterized by tachycardia, chest pain, dilatation of the heart, presence of pericardial rub and murmurs. In serious cases, when congestive heart failure occurs, the child looks sick and pale with rapid breathing and palpitations of heart. The child may develop puffiness of face and swelling of feet. Patient may have difficulty in walking and gets easily tired.

Diagnosis

The diagnosis is made on the basis of Duckett Jones essential, major and minor criteria listed in **Table 39.2**. Two major or one major and two minor criteria should be present alongwith presence of essential criteria for making the diagnosis of acute rheumatic fever.

There is leukocytosis, raised erythrocyte sedimentation rate (ESR) and C-reactive protein. The elevation of antistreptolysin O titer (ASO) or antideoxyribonuclease-beta (anti-DNase-β) titers in response to preceding streptococcal infection are mandatory before making the diagnosis of acute rheumatic fever. In patients suspected to have carditis, ECG, echocardiography and X-ray chest should be taken.

39

Table 39.2 Criteria for making the diagnosis of acute rheumatic fever

- **Essential criteria**
  - □ Evidences of recent (within 45 days) streptococcal infection except in case of rheumatic chorea[a]
  - □ History of streptococcal sore throat or scarlet fever
  - □ Positive throat culture for group A streptococci
  - □ Antistreptolysin O titer of >333 units in children and >250 units in adults
  - □ Antideoxyribonuclease-β titer (anti-DNase-β) of >1:60 units in preschool children, >1:480 units in school children, and >1:340 units in adults
- **Major criteria**
  - □ Polyarthritis
  - □ Carditis
  - □ Chorea
  - □ Subcutaneous nodules
  - □ Erythema marginatum
- **Minor criteria**
  - □ Fever
  - □ Polyarthralgia
  - □ Elevated polymorphonuclear leukocytes, erythrocyte sedimentation rate, and C-reactive protein
  - □ Prolonged PR interval[b] on electrocardiogram

[a] In chorea, the interval between streptococcal infection and chorea may be of several months and therefore no evidences of previous streptococcal infection may be found.

[b] Upper limit of PR interval: 3 to 12 years 0.16 second, 12 to 14 years 0.18 second, >15 years 0.20 second.

Nursing Care

The residual streptococcal throat infection must be treated with an appropriate antibiotic. Bed rest and salicylates are used for relief of joint pains. Corticosteroids are recommended for treatment of carditis. The patient with chorea should be provided with padded railings in the bed to prevent any injury. Handwriting of the patient should be monitored to assess the progress of disease. Sleeping pulse rate should be recorded to assess recovery from carditis.

The child should be under careful observation and follow-up by a pediatrician and pediatric cardiologist. Recurrence of rheumatic fever can be prevented by administration of long acting penicillin (6,00, 000 units <6 yr and 12,00,000 units >6 yr) every 3 weeks IM for several years. In the absence of carditis secondary prophylaxis given for 5 years or up to the age of 18 years. In patients with carditis or rheumatic heart disease, penicillin prophylaxis is continued lifelong or at least up to the age of 40 years. When valves of the heart are permanently damaged the child may need a surgical correction later in life.

CONGESTIVE HEART FAILURE (CHF)

Congestive cardiac failure may occur due to a variety of cardiac and non-cardiac disorders. The heart is unable to maintain satisfactory cardiac output to meet the metabolic needs of the body (systolic failure) or is unable to receive blood into the ventricles during diastole (diastolic failure). The common causes of CHF include congenital heart disease, rheumatic heart disease, myocarditis, severe anemia and hypertension (Table 39.3).

Clinical Features

There is easy fatigability, anorexia, palpitation (unpleasant feeling of heart beats), cough and breathlessness.

Table 39.3 Common causes of heart failure on the basis of age at onset

- **Fetal causes**
  - □ *Anemia* Erythroblastosis (Rh-isoimmunization), fetomaternal transfusion, *parvovirus B-19* infection (hydrops fetalis), and hypoplastic anemia.
  - □ *Arrhythmias* Supraventricular tachycardia, ventricular tachycardia, and complete heart block.
- **First 48 hours**
  - □ *Premature infants* Fluid overload, patent ductus arteriosus (PDA), bronchopulmonary dysplasia, and hypertension.
  - □ *Full-term infants* Asphyxial cardiomyopathy, systemic atrioventricular fistula, viral myocarditis, polycythemia, sepsis, hypoglycemia, hypocalcemia, complete heart block, congenital thyrotoxicosis, and fluid overload.
- **First week of life** Critical aortic/pulmonary atresias or stenosis, hypoplastic left heart syndrome, transposition of great vessels with intact ventricular septum, obstructed total anomalous pulmonary venous connection, coarctation of aorta, and Ebstein anomaly.
- **Second week of life** Large ventriculoseptal defect, AV septal defect, large PDA, unobstructed total anomalous pulmonary venous drainage, truncus arteriosus, single ventricle, and tricuspid atresia.
- **1 to 2 months of life** Large left-to-right shunts, transposition and malposition complexes, endocardial cushion defects, anomalous left coronary artery from pulmonary artery, aorta-pulmonary window.
- **Older children and adolescents** Rheumatic heart disease, palliated, postoperative or complicated congenital heart disease, cardiomyopathies, arrhythmias, corrected transposition of great arteries, truncus arteriosus, hypertension, severe anemia, and Kawasaki disease.

39

Initially child gets easily tired and breathless on walking or going upstairs. In severe cases, child is dyspneic even at rest and may have orthopnea (dyspneic or uncomfortable while lying down in bed and feeling better on sitting up). The systemic venous congestion is manifested by elevated jugular venous pressure (JVP), edema feet (puffiness of face and sacral edema in infants), tachycardia, cardiomegaly, enlarging liver size and rales or crepitations at the bases of lungs.

Management

Good nursing care, bed rest in a semisitting position with a back rest and administration of oxygen provides comfort. Child should be given a balanced nutritious diet with sodium restriction. Parenteral administration of diuretics (furosemide 1–2 mg/kg) and digitalis are life saving decongestive measures. Effective digitalization should be achieved in 24–48 hours depending upon the severity of CHF. In rapid digitalization, one-half of the total dose is given stat, one-fourth after 4–8 hours and remaining one-fourth after 8–16 hours. Total digitalizing dose is 0.04–0.06 mg/kg in infants. Daily maintenance dose is 1/5th to 1/3rd of the digitalizing dose. Patients with myocarditis should be given 2/3rd of the digitalizing dose due to greater risk of digitalis toxicity. Children with pulmonary edema should be given morphine (0.05–0.2 mg/kg SC) or pethidine (1–2 mg/kg 1M). Intercurrent infections should be treated with an appropriate antibiotic. Anemia should be treated with slow transfusion of packed red blood cells. The stepwise guidelines for treatment of cardiac failure are summarized in **Box 39.2**.

> **Box 39.2** **Stepwise guidelines for the treatment of cardiac failure**
>
> - **Step 1** Rest, propped up position, humidified oxygen, and nutritions diet with sodium restriction.
> - **Step 2** Start digoxin and diuretics. It is better to use furosemide alone with potassium supplements.
> - **Step 3** Add angiotensin-converting enzyme (ACE) inhibitor. If not acceptable because of cough, change to angiotensin receptor blocker.
> - **Step 4** Add isosorbide dinitrate if ACE inhibitors or angiotensin receptor blockers are not tolerated. Do not use hydralazine because it has been shown to increase the mortality.
> - **Step 5** In the presence of inadequate response especially when the patient has tachycardia, start carvedilol.
> - **Step 6** Consider use of once or twice weekly infusion of dobutamine and add carnitine as a supplement.
> - **Step 7** Consider stem cell therapy and cardiac transplantation in selected cases.

HYPERTENSION

Hypertension is uncommon in children but is being increasingly recognized due to rising incidence of obesity in adolescent children. Blood pressure should be taken when child is at rest and relaxed and by using an appropriate size of the cuff to cover two-thirds of the upper arm (refer to **Chapter 49**). The normal range of blood pressure values in children is shown in **Table 39.4**.

Unlike adults where most cases of hypertension are essential or idiopathic, in children hypertension is usually secondary to an underlying cause. The common causes include renal disease (glomerulonephritis, pyelonephritis, dysplastic kidneys), renal artery stenosis, coarctation of aorta, aorto-arteritis, pheochromocytoma, collagen vascular disease, Cushings syndrome and corticosteroid therapy. Essential hypertension may occur in association with obesity.

Clinical Features

Most cases are asymptomatic and manifest with clinical features of the underlying disease process which is causing hypertension. Patients may manifest with features of CHF or hypertensive encephalopathy.

Treatment

Diuretics like thiazides and salt restriction are advised to all children. The useful antihypertensive drugs for children include beta blockers (propranol), ACE inhibitors (enalapril) and calcium channel blockers (amlodipine besylate). The underlying cause of hypertension should be identified and appropriately managed by medical therapy and surgical intervention.

INFECTIVE ENDOCARDITIS

The infection of the endocardial lining of the heart occurs when there is underlying cardiac disease (congenital or acquired), at the sites of prosthetic valves and palliated congenital heart disease. Endocarditis may also occur following a surgical procedure or percutaneous intervention. Endocarditis usually occurs following bacteremia because of focus of infection or as a consequence of an invasive procedure like tooth

39

Table 39.4 Average blood pressure values in children (mm Hg)		
Age	Systolic	Diastolic
1–3 months	75 ±5	50 ±5
4–12 months	84 ±5	65 ±5
1–8 years	95 ±5	65 ±5
7–14 years	105 ±5	65 ±5

extraction, catheterization, endoscopy and surgical procedure. The common bacterial pathogens causing infective endocarditis include *Streptococcus viridans, Staphylococcus aureus, Streptococcus faecalis* and rarely Gram-negative organisms.

Clinical Features

Infective endocarditis should be seriously considered in any patient with unexplained fever of 5–7 days who is known have an underlying heart disease. Fever is moderate in severity with chills and rigors, night sweats, malaise, loss of appetite and weight loss. The underlying cardiac condition may worsen with development of a new murmur, change in the character of murmur, and onset of cardiac failure. Other features include pain in the muscles and joints, petechiae, Osler nodes (tender nodules over finger tips), clubbing, splinter hemorrhages under nail bed, enlargement of spleen and microscopic hematuria. Fundus examination may show oval shaped hemorrhages (Roth spots).

Diagnosis

The positive blood culture is the gold standard for the diagnosis of infective endocarditis. Three samples of 10 mL blood should be collected with due aseptic precautions at every 30 minutes interval for culture studies. Peripheral blood examination may show polymorphonuclear leukocytosis and microscopic hematuria on urine examination. Both M-mode and 3D echocardiography are useful for identification of vegetations.

Treatment

After taking blood samples for culture, empirical parenteral antibiotic therapy should be started while awaiting for culture report. The patient is started on intravenous penicillin (10–20 million units/d q 6 hr), amikacin (30 mg/kg/d q 8 hr) and vancomycin (60 mg/kg/d q 8 hr). Depending upon the response to empiric therapy and blood culture report, appropriate antibiotic therapy is continued for at least 4–6 weeks to achieve cure and prevent relapse.

Prophylaxis

Patients with known congenital or rheumatic heart disease should be promptly treated with antibiotics whenever they have intercurrent infection. Various procedures like dental extraction, endoscopy, and catheterization should be performed under strict aseptic precautions. Amoxicillin (25 mg/kg oral) and gentamicin (20 mg/kg IM) is given one hour before the procedure, followed by at least two more doses after the procedure.

CHRONIC CONSTRICTIVE PERICARDITIS

Constrictive pericarditis is mostly caused by tuberculosis in India, less commonly it may follow pyogenic and autoimmune pericarditis or may be idiopathic. There is encasement or constriction around the heart, which restricts filling of both the ventricles.

Clinical Features

The onset is insidious with fever, easy fatigability, breathlessness and nocturnal dyspnea. Pulse is fast and low volume and there may be pulses paradoxus. There are evidences of passive venous congestion namely engorged neck veins, gross enlargement of liver, ascites and pleural effusion.

Investigations

The ECG shows low voltage and nonspecific ST and T-wave changes. Skiagram of the chest shows normal sized heart with ragged or shaggy borders and prominent superior vena cava shadow merging with the right atrium. Fluoroscopy shows reduced cardiac contractions.

Treatment

Antitubercular therapy is given for 9 months as per standard protocol, especially when there are additional clinical or laboratory markers of tuberculous infection. Surgical decortication is the treatment of choice to relieve myocardial constriction. Surgical intervention is done after 6 weeks course of antitubercular therapy.

MYOCARDITIS

Myocarditis is usually caused by a viral infection due to ECHO, Coxsackie B, rubella, herpes simplex and influenza viruses. Rarely diphtheritic myocarditis may occur after one week of onset diphtheria. The onset is usually abrupt with fever, marked tachycardia, cardiomegaly, muffled heart sounds and congestive cardiac failure. Arrhythmias and conduction disorders may occur. The electrocardiogram shows low voltages and nonspecific ST and T wave changes. Chest X-ray shows cardiac enlargement with pulmonary venous congestion.

Treatment is symptomatic and supportive. Digoxin should be used with caution, preferably in half to three quarters of the standard dose. Corticosteroids are of doubtful utility and should preferably be avoided. Angiotensin converting enzyme (ACE) inhibitors are a useful adjunct. The utility of intravenous immunoglobulins (IVIG) is not proven. Prognosis is guarded.

39

BIBLIOGRAPHY

Baddour LM, Wilson WR, Bayer AS, et al. Infective endocarditis: Diagnosis, antimicrobial therapy and management of complications. *Circulation* 2005, 111(23): 394–433.

Chaturvedi V, Saxena A. Heart failure in children: clinical aspects and management. *Indian J Pediatr* 2009, 76(2): 195–205.

Ramakrishanan S, Kothari SS, Bahl VK. Heart failure: definition and diagnosis. *Indian Heart J* 2005, 57(1): 13–20.

Saxena A, Kumar RK, Gera RP, et al. Working Group on Pediatric Acute Rheumatic Fever and Cardiology Chapter of Indian Academy of Pediatrics. Consensus guidelines on pediatric acute rheumatic fever and rheumatic heart disease. *Indian Pediatr* 2008, 45(7): 565–573.

Saxena A. Working Group on Management of Congenital Heart Disease in India. Consensus on timing of intervention for common congenital heart diseases. *Indian Pediatr* 2008, 45(2): 117–126.

Seikaly MG. Hypertension in children: an update on treatment strategies. *Curr Opin Pediatr* 2007, 19(2): 170–177.

Shrivastava S. Rheumatic heart disease: Is it declining in India? *Indian Heart J* 2007, 59(1): 9–10.

39

40

Genitourinary Disorders

Developmental Aspects

Each kidney is composed of approximately one million nephrons, each consisting of a glomerulus and renal tubule. The fetal kidneys are lobulated in shape and ascend from the pelvis to their normal position between 6 and 9 weeks of gestation. The kidneys can be visualized on antenatal ultrasound examination by 12–13th week. Glomerular filteration begins around 5–9 weeks of gestation by production of urine which is voided in the amniotic sac. The amniotic fluid is predominantly composed of fetal urine and oligo-hydramnios (reduced quantity of amniotic fluid) may occur due to fetal oliguria or anuria. Tubular function contributes to urine formation at 14 weeks of gestation. The proximal tubules reabsorb up to 80% of the glomerular filtrate. Almost 65% of sodium is reabsorbed in the proximal tubules through several active transport mechanisms. Distal tubules and collecting ducts are responsible for urinary acidification, concentration and regulation of sodium balance. Exchange of potassium and hydrogen ions for sodium takes place in the distal tubules under the influence of aldosterone. Antidiuretic hormone (ADH) mediates absorption of water in the collecting tubules to regulate water balance. The kidneys help in the regulation of acid-base balance by controlling the excretion of bicarbonate and carbonic acid (H^+ ions). Renal function continues to improve during first two years of life, at the end of which, various parameters of renal function approach adult values.

URINARY TRACT INFECTION

Urinary tract infection (UTI) may not produce any specific symptoms and is often missed in young children. It is usually caused by *E. coli* but may occur due to other Gram-negative bacteria. It is more common in girls than boys due to ascending infection from vulva. In infants, the incidence of UTI is identical in children of both sexes because it occurs as a consequence of septicemia. Intractable and persistent constipation may predispose to development of UTI by stasis of urine due to compression of bladder because of loaded rectum. Boys with a nappy rash and inflammation of foreskin have an increased risk of UTI. Associated developmental defects in the genitourinary system may predispose to the development of recurrent urinary tract infections. In a boy when urinary stream is narrow or child strains while passing urine and there is dribbling of urine in the end, it is suggestive of bladder neck obstruction.

Clinical Features

There is sudden onset of fever with feeling of chills and shivering. In infants, urinary symptoms are either absent or difficult to identify. *Therefore, whenever a young child has fever without any obvious cause, UTI should be seriously considered*. Infection may involve the kidneys (pyelonephritis) or remain limited to the urinary

---

Practical Tip

Many neonates and infants cry before passing urine due to discomfort of a full bladder. They become quiet and dazed while passing urine and start crying again after voiding due to wet diaper. This should not be considered as dysuria or an indication of UTI.

---

bladder (cystitis). Difficulty or smarting (dysuria) while passing urine and frequency of micturition occur in cystitis. In pyelonephritis, there is fever with chills and rigors with discomfort and tenderness at the renal angles.

Diagnosis

Diagnosis is confirmed by finding pus cells in the urine and growth of pathogenic bacteria in a properly collected sample of urine. The sample for urine examination and urine culture must be collected before starting antibiotic therapy. Genital area should be washed with soap and water before collection of urine sample. A "clean catch" mid-stream sample of urine should be collected straight into a sterile bottle. A urinary sample obtained with a collection bag is not suitable for culture studies. A reliable urine sample for culture can be obtained by percutaneous suprapubic aspiration or urethral catheterization. The colony count of 10^5 (100,000 colonies/mm^3) is considered as diagnostic of urinary infection. Detailed radiological and radionuclide studies should be undertaken to identify any congenital malformations or evidences of structural damage to the kidneys.

Treatment

Infants with UTI are likely to have pyelonephritis and are treated with parenteral ceftriaxone and an aminoglycoside. Older children are treated with oral cefixime or amoxycillin or norfloxacin for 7 days. The antibiotic may be changed on the basis of culture report. Child is encouraged to take plenty of fluids. The child should be followed closely for development of reinfection. When recurrent UTI is associated with obstructive uropathy, surgical correction is advised. Long-term prophylaxis with cotrimoxazole or cephalexin is given in recommended doses if there is associated vesicoureteric reflux. The girls must be taught to wash the bottom (after each urination and defecation) from front-backwards to prevent the risk of contamination of vulva with stools.

ACUTE GLOMERULONEPHRITIS (AGN)

It occurs in school going children following an acute infection of the throat or skin with Group A *beta hemolytic streptococci*.

Clinical Features

The common manifestations include development of puffiness around eyes, edema feet and oliguria with "smoky" or tea or cola colored urine or frank hematuria. Blood pressure is usually elevated. *Transient hypertension in children is most commonly due to AGN.* At times the illness is so mild that there is only microscopic hematuria. Rarely, AGN may manifest with sudden onset of hypertensive encephalopathy and congestive cardiac failure with headache, breathlessness, convulsions and coma.

Diagnosis

Urine examination shows proteinuria, hematuria, hyaline or RBC casts. Blood urea and serum creatinine are usually elevated while lipid profile is normal. The level of complement C_3 is usually low. Antistreptolysin O (ASLO) titer in the blood may be elevated as an evidence of preceding streptococcal infection.

Treatment

Treatment is symptomatic and supportive. Penicillin or amoxicillin is given for 7 days to eradicate any residual streptococcal infection. Blood pressure should be monitored closely and treated with an appropriate anti-hypertensive drug like hydralazine, nifedipine or furosemide. Protein intake is restricted if there is azotemia (elevation of blood urea and creatinine). Intake of sodium, potassium and fluids should be restricted until urine flow is established and blood urea returns back to normal. AGN is a benign self-limiting condition and most children recover without any sequelae. The best indicator of resolution of disease is return of C_3 level to normal. Microscopic hematuria and mild proteinuria may persist for 6–12 months in some children.

NEPHROTIC SYNDROME

It is characterized by generalized edema (anasarca), massive proteinuria (>2g/d), hypoproteinemia (serum albumin <2.5 g/dL) and hypercholesterolemia (serum cholesterol >200 mg/dL). Most cases are idiopathic (without any cause) nephrotic syndrome and are called "minimal change nephrosis". It is an antoimmune disease with frequent remissions and relapses. Disease is most common during 1½ to 5 years of age. It is more common in boys than girls.

Clinical Features

There is gradual onset of swelling starting as puffiness of face and spreading to the whole body. Puffiness is most common in the morning when child gets up and becomes less when he is up and about. During next few days, there is generalized swelling including development of ascites (anasarca) and marked swelling of genitals. There is fall in urine output. There is no fever and blood pressure is usually normal.

Diagnosis

Urine examination shows massive proteinuria (3 to 4+) and hyaline casts. Serum albumin is grossly reduced while serum cholesterol is elevated. Kidney function tests are usually normal. Serum electrolytes may show hyponatremia, hypokalemia and hypocalcemia. Serum complement is usually normal. Kidney biopsy is done when disease is unresponsive or resistant to steroid therapy.

Treatment

Nephrotic syndrome is a chronic disease of kidneys and child should be under the care of a pediatric nephrologist. Child is given drugs, which promote excessive excretion

40

of urine (diuretics) and corticosteroids. Daily predni-solone therapy (2 mg/kg/day q 6–8 hr) is given during 4–6 weeks followed by 1.5 mg/kg on alternate days once remission has occurred for the next 4–6 weeks. These children are prone to intercurrent infections which should be treated with appropriate antibiotics. In patients with intractable or steroid resistant nephrotic syndrome and frequent relapses, methyl-prednisolone, levamisole, cyclophosphamide and cyclosporine have been tried with success. Angiotensin-converting enzyme (ACE) inhibitors such as enalapril (0.2 mg/kg) can be given as an adjunct to reduce proteinuria.

The child should be given a diet containing high quantity of proteins like milk and milk products, *dals*, *chana* (chickpeas), lentils, soybeans, eggs, meat and fish. Extra intake of protein is required to replenish the loss of protein in the urine. Supplements of calcium, vitamin D and zinc should be given. The child needs long term treatment and follow-up because disease is known to have remissions and relapses. Urine should be examined at home regularly for severity of protein loss with the help of uristix or albustix testing strips. The parents should maintain a careful account of the child's treatment, report of urine tests and his general health and symptoms. The child must attend regular school as soon as the swelling disappears. When child is taking prednisolone, live vaccines like measles, mumps, rubella (MMR), oral polio vaccine and chickenpox should not be given. They can be given after 3 months of stopping prednisolone. The frequency of relapses decreases as child grows and complete cure occurs between 12 and 18 years of age.

Nursing Care

In view of the chronic nature of the disease, with frequent remissions and relapses, the nurse has an important role to provide supportive care to the child and family.

1. Provide guidance and emotional support to the family.
2. Education of the parents for promotion of personal hygiene, prevention of intercurrent infections and maintaining health record of the child including regular urine examinations with uristix strips.
3. Nutrition education to the mother to promote intake of high protein and low salt diet.
4. Family should be told about the need for giving pneumococcal vaccine to a child with nephrotic syndrome. Live vaccines (measles, MMR, OPV, chickenpox) should not be given to a child receiving prolonged high dose steroid therapy.
5. Ensure compliance regarding administration of medications, and encouraging physical and play activity and social interactions of the sick child. The normal siblings should not be neglected.
6. Monitoring physical growth and development of the child and the side effects of the corticosteroid therapy.
7. The child must attend regular school as soon as remission is achieved. When child is unable to attend school, home tuition should be provided.
8. Parents should be told about the importance of early treatment of intercurrent infections and indications for hospitalization of the child.

HEMATURIA

Hematuria is uncommon in children, may be microscopic or grossly blood-tinged urine. The common glomerular causes of hematuria include post streptococcal acute glomerulonephritis (AGN), rapidly progressive glomerulonephritis (RPGN), chronic glomerulonephritis and hereditary nephritis. The nonglomerular causes include urinary tract infection (especially cystitis), cystic kidneys, renal stones, vascular malformation, tumor or trauma to the urinary system.

Clinical Features

A detailed history is taken to assess the severity of hematuria, whether it is first episode or recurrent in nature and any associated symptoms of urinary tract infection, glomerular disease (edema, oliguria and hypertension), urolithiasis (colicky renal pain, dysuria and suprapubic pain), trauma and intake of nephro-toxic drugs. Asymptomatic gross hematuria may occur because of chronic glomerulonephritis, IgA-nephropathy, hydronephrosis, Wilm' tumor and arteriovenous malformation in the kidneys. Family history may be positive in Alport syndrome (associated with deafness) and urolithiasis.

Investigations

Urine examination is done for proteinuria, microscopic hematuria, crystaluria and casts. Complete blood count (CBC), sickle cell screen, renal function tests, ASLO titer and C_3 level should be checked. Ultrasonography of kidneys and urinary tract is a useful non-invasive investigation. Urine analysis of first-degree relatives is done to exclude hereditary conditions.

Treatment

Treatment is supportive and symptomatic depending on the underlying cause. Antibiotics are given for treatment of urinary tract infection. The child should

40

be monitored for physical growth, blood pressure, deafness and urinalysis. Surgery is required for removal of a tumor and renal stone. When hematuria is persistent or recurrent and there are clinical evidences of primary or secondary glomerular disease, a renal biopsy should be taken.

Non-retractable Foreskin

The foreskin (prepuce) is not retractable at birth in almost all newborn babies. Even by one year of age, foreskin is not retractable in up to 50 percent of boys. This does not cause any problem or difficulty in passing urine. Ballooning of prepuce during micturition is normal in infancy. There is no need to retract the foreskin during 1–2 years of age. After 2 years, efforts may be made to gently retract the foreskin while bathing the baby. Nappy rash should be prevented or promptly treated to prevent scarring of the prepuce. The boys should be explained to retract their foreskin and wash the penis with soap and water during bathing.

Circumcision Circumcision (surgical excision of foreskin) has been practiced from times immemorial (over 6000 years) as a religious ritual. However, till recently there was no justification on medical grounds for undertaking routine circumcision. Nature has supreme wisdom and if God has created foreskin there must be a good reason and justification. It is a cruel practice to circumcise a baby without anesthetic because babies do feel pain and they have a memory for unpleasant experience. Circumcision should not be done just because child is having a long foreskin and for relief of enuresis or masturbation. If nappy rash is neglected in boys, it may lead to scarring and narrowing of the prepucial orifice. The condition can be treated by a minor procedure of dilatation of the orifice. When there is recurrent formation of pus at the tip of the penis (balanitis) or recurrent episodes of urinary tract infection due to phimosis (non-retractable prepuce), circumcision is indicated. The procedure should be done by a pediatric surgeon under proper anesthetic cover. There is recent evidence to suggest that there is reduced risk of HIV, urinary tract infection, carcinoma penis, sexually transmitted genital ulcer and carcinoma cervix (among spouse) in circumcised males.

CONGENITAL ABNORMALITIES

Congenital abnormalities or developmental defects of genitourinary system are common and can be picked up on antenatal ultrasonography. They are usually asymptomatic except when complicated by stasis, infection and renal dysfunction. The common correlates of underlying renal malformations include oligo-hydramnios, single umbilical artery, chromosomal abnormalities and hemihypertrophy. Abnormalities may be seen at any site in the renal system namely kidneys, ureter, bladder and urethra. The location, nature and severity of abnormalities can be diagnosed by ultrasonography, radioimaging studies (CT scan and MRI), micturiting cystourethrography (MCU) and radionuclide scans.

Renal Agenesis

There is non-formation or absence of kidney due to failure of development of ureteric bud or mesenchymal blastema. It may be unilateral or bilateral, and is usually associated with oligohydramnios because amniotic fluid is principally contributed by fetal urine. Renal agenesis is associated with Potter facies which is characterized by squashed face (due to oligohydramnios), receding chin, low-set ears, epicanthal folds with antimongoloid slant of eyes **(Figure 40.1)**. Most of the affected babies are stillborn, but those born alive, develop severe respiratory distress due to associated pulmonary hypoplasia. Other associated internal malformations include single umbilical artery, esopha-geal, duodenal, colonic and anal agenesis and Meckel's diverticulum.

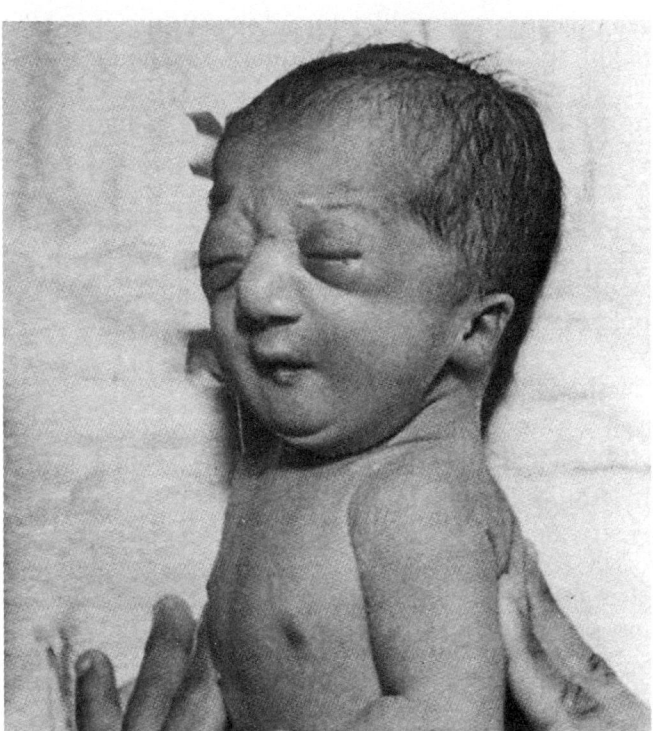

Figure 40.1 Potter facies showing receding chin, low-set ears and prominent skin folds below the eyes

40

Renal Dysplasia

Renal hypoplasia and dysplasia with multicystic kidneys is a rare life-threatening malformation. Bilateral renal dysplasia is not compatible with life and affected children are either stillborn or die soon after birth. Multicystic dysplastic kidneys may be associated with encephalocele, eye abnormalities, cleft palate, congenital heart defects and polydactyly (Meckel's syndrome). The common complications include urinary tract infection, hypertension and chronic renal failure. Nephrectomy is indicated if affected kidney is non functional and associated with hypertension and pyelonephritis or renal mass is causing respiratory difficulty.

Horseshoe Kidney

It is a rare abnormality which is picked up accidentally on ultrasound examination and intravenous pyelography. Two kidneys are fused with each other in the midline at their lower poles due to fusion of ureteric buds. These kidneys are more likely to develop complications and are more susceptible to develop Wilms' tumor.

Polycystic Kidneys

There are two distinct variants of polycystic kidneys namely infantile type (autosomal recessive inheritance) and adult type (autosomal dominant inheritance). There is progressive dilatation of specific regions of the nephron due to adverse hereditary metabolic factors. The infantile type presents with palpable bilateral nodular cystic masses with hypertension and progressive renal failure. There may be associated abnormalities in several other organs of the body like hepatic fibrosis and/or dilated bile ducts. Renal transplantation is the only hope for these children. The adult variant is usually associated with anemia, polyuria, renal osteodystrophy and hypertension.

Obstructive Uropathy

The common causes of enlarged palpable kidneys in children include multicystic or polycystic kidneys and hydronephrosis due to obstructive uropathy. The obstruction may occur at the pelvi-ureteric junction(s), vesico-ureteric junction, posterior urethral valve and stenosis of urethral meatus. The obstruction of the urinary tract produces dilatation above the site of lesion and a retrograde rise in hydrostatic pressure causing structural and functional damage to the kidneys. Hydronephrosis may be unilateral or bilateral, produce either a single mass in the flank or two masses one in each flank.

Bladder neck obstruction due to posterior urethral valve is characterized by presence of three masses, i.e. distended urinary bladder in the suprapubic region and two enlarged kidneys in the flanks. Ascites may occur due to leakage of urine because of rupture of pelvis, calix or ureter. Urethral obstruction may be associated with prune-belly syndrome which is characterized by flabby abdominal wall due to congenital absence of abdominal musculature (Figure 40.2). It is associated with evidences of gross dilatation of whole urinary tract and kidneys, alongwith undescended testis and a large flaccid penis due to grossly dilated urethra. Other congenital malformations such as pulmonary hypoplasia, malrotation of gut and imperforate anus may be associated. Like most other renal malformations, obstructive uropathy is more common among male infants.

Treatment The obstructive uropathy should be considered as an emergency and urgent action should be taken to identify the cause and relieve the obstruction to prevent damage to the kidneys due to retrograde pressure. Catheter evacuation of bladder should be attempted with due aseptic precautions. If catheterization fails, emergency suprapubic cystostomy and nephrostomy is done. Associated urinary tract infection should be identified and managed with appropriate antibiotics. The outcome is good if obstruction is identified early and managed promptly.

Abnormalities in the Location of Urethral Meatus

These abnormalities are usually seen in boys.

Epispadias

The urethral opening is located on the dorsal aspect of penis. It may be associated with exstrophy of bladder and ambiguous genitalia. The pubic bones are widely separated. In girls there may be bifid clitoris.

Surgical correction is difficult and done in 3 stages. First stage operation is done around one year of age for elongation of penis and correction of chordee

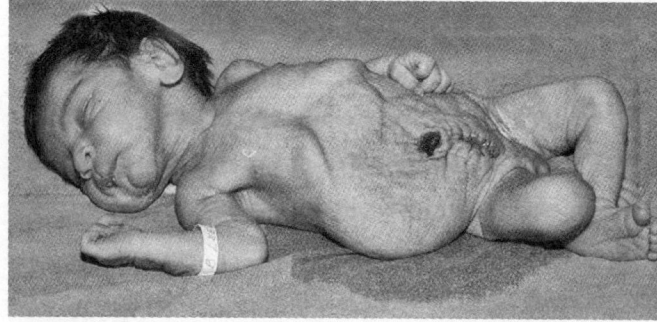

Figure 40.2 Prune-belly syndrome. Note large flaccid phallus

40

(curvature of penis). Second stage surgery is done for urethroplasty after 6 months to one year of chordee correction. Bladder neck reconstruction, cystoplasty and correction of vesico-ureteric reflux (VUR) are done at 4–5 years of age.

Hypospadias

The urethral opening is located on the ventral surface of penis. It is classified on the basis of site of urethral opening, i.e. glandular (glans penis), penile shaft and penoscrotal region or perineal. It is usually associated with downward curvature (chordee) of the penis. The boy is unable to void urine while standing. The commonly associated anomalies include undescended testis, inguinal hernia and upper urinary tract abnormalities. If untreated, it is associated with sexual inadequacy and infertility.

Surgical correction is done is stages. Meatotomy is done at any age after birth. Chordee correction and advancement of prepuce is done between 6 months and one year. Urethroplasty is done at 1½ – 2 years of age. The surgical repair should be completed before the child joins play school.

Nursing Care

1. Provide tender loving care to the child and emotional support to the family for long-term management and follow-up.
2. Ensure timely surgical repair, essential preoperative and postoperative management.
3. Inculcate concept of personal hygiene, environmental sanitation and healthy lifestyle.
4. Essential vaccines should be administered at appropriate ages.
5. Child should be provided with emotional support to prevent anxiety and stress due to genital abnormalities.
6. The goal of surgery is to ensure that child grows to become a healthy confident adult with normal looking genitalia, without any difficulty in sexual intercourse and normal fertility.

Undescended Testis (Cryptorchidism)

The testes are retractable and get easily pulled up if scrotum is touched with cold hands. In premature and small babies, testes may be undescended at birth but gradually descend to the scrotum within a couple of weeks. Around 1.0 percent boys may have undescended testis by first birthday. The scrotal sac may be small and underdeveloped on the side of undescended testis. The testis may be located in the groin or inside the abdomen. The undescended testis

poses serious psychological embarrassment to the child and is associated with markedly increased risk of development of cancer. There is no role of hormonal treatment. Surgery (orchiopexy) is recommended to bring down the testis in the scrotum at the age of one year. When testes are undescended on both the sides, it is likely to be associated with a serious developmental or a chromosomal disorder.

Ectopia Vesicae (Exstrophy of Bladder)

There is deficiency of lower anterior abdominal wall and absence of anterior wall of the bladder. The glistening reddish posterior wall of urinary bladder is exposed with a constant leakage of urine. The pubic bones are widely separated. It is associated with epispadias (urethral opening is located over the dorsal aspect of penis) in a male infant and bifid clitoris in the female. Radioimaging studies, ultrasonography, intravenous pyelography and urodynamic evaluation is done to assess the severity of anomaly and associated malformations.

The defect is closed and cosmetically repaired by a skilled pediatric urologist in several stages. Bladder is closed immediately after birth, preferably within 72 hours. The epispadias is tackled at one year and procedure to achieve urinary continence is done around 4 years of age.

Nursing Care

1. Provide emotional support to the family and allay any feelings of anger, anxiety and guilt.
2. Explain the need for multistaged surgical procedures and a prolonged follow-up. Give advise about the optimal nutrition and vaccinations.
3. Prevent hypothermia and risk of nosocomial infections.
4. Cover the exposed bladder mucosa with a sterile wet gauze piece to prevent dribbling of urine and protect the skin around the margins of bladder from excoriation.
5. Prevent contamination of bladder wall or surgical wound with fecal matter.

40

ACUTE RENAL FAILURE (Acute Kidney Injury)

Acute renal failure (ARF) or acute kidney injury (AKI) is defined as abrupt onset of decline in renal functions with sustained rise in blood levels of urea and creatinine. There may be oliguria (urine output <0.5 mL/kg/hr) or anuria (urine output less than 400 mL/m^2/day) and rarely normal urine output, i.e. non-oliguric ARF.

Causes

The etiology of ARF may be pre-renal, intrinsic renal or postrenal

1. *Prerenal failure* Hypovolemia due to dehydration, blood loss, diabetic ketoacidosis, burns, septicemia, congestive heart failure and asphyxia.
2. *Intrinsic renal failure* Acute tubular necrosis (may follow hypovolemia), glomerulonephritis, hemolytic uremic syndrome, intravascular hemolysis, tumor lysis syndrome, drugs and toxins like aminoglycosides, radionuclide contrast, NSAIDs, amphotericin B, diethylene glycol, and methanol.
3. *Post-renal failure* Posterior urethral valve, urethral stricture, ureteral obstruction, and neurogenic bladder.

Clinical Features

There may be features of underlying predisposing cause of ARF which is followed by abrupt onset of oliguria or anuria. There may be history of persistent vomiting, diarrhea, burns, blood loss, drug intake, and sepsis or

Nursing Alert

Acute renal failure is usually associated with reduced or absent urine output. But at times urine output may be normal (non-oliguric ARF) especially when ARF is due to nephrotoxic drugs, asphyxia or sepsis.

asphyxia. Renal perfusion is reduced by preceding dehydration, hypotension or shock. In obstructive uropathy, there is sudden cessation of urine with dilated urinary bladder and enlarged kidneys. There is progressive elevation of blood urea and serum creatinine levels with hyponatremia (sodium <130 mEq/L), hyperkalemia (potassium > 6.0 mEq/L) and metabolic acidosis (base excess greater than 10 mmoles/L).

Investigations

Complete blood count and peripheral blood smear should be examined for microangiopathic hemolysis (deformed RBCs or burr cells), thrombocytopenia and reticulocytosis as a marker of hemolytic uremic syndrome (HUS). Urine must be examined for proteinuria, RBCs and casts. Ultrasonography is done to evaluate urinary system for any structural abnormalities and calculi. Kidney function tests, electrolytes and acid-base parameters should be checked. Electrocardiogram may show evidences of potassium and calcium toxicity on the heart. Skiagram of chest is useful for diagnosis of pulmonary edema.

Nursing Care

1. *Supportive care* Maintain strict fluid intake and output chart, vital signs and biochemical abnormalities. Intake of any nephrotoxic drug is immediately stopped. Urine should be collected with a condom in boys and urine collection bag in girls. The fluid intake is restricted to daily insensible water losses (300–400 mL/m²), urine output and any extra renal fluid losses. Potassium containing fluids should not be given till adequate urine output is established. Acidosis is treated by administration of sodium bicarbonate. A diet with adequate calories but restricted protein and fluid intake is recommended. A diet containing 0.8–1.2 g/kg of protein in infants and 0.6–0.8 g/kg in older children is given. Intercurrent nosocomial infection is treated with appropriate antibiotics which are not toxic to the kidneys. Dopamine in low doses (1–3 µg/kg/min) may be given to improve renal perfusion.

2. *Treatment of complications* Life-threatening complications should be identified early and managed effectively **(Table 40.1)**. Electrocardiogram is taken to monitor abnormalities in potassium and calcium and an X-ray chest for any evidences of pulmonary edema.

3. *Specific therapy* Intravenous methylprednisolone is given to patients with crescentic glomerulonephritis, lupus nephritis and interstitial nephritis. In children with obstructive uropathy, catheterization or vesicotomy in posterior urethral valves or percutaneous nephrostomy in bilateral obstruction of pelviureteric junction is performed.

4. *Dialysis* Dialysis can be done with a variety of modalities like peritoneal dialysis, intermittent hemodialysis or continuous hemofilteration. Indications for initiating dialysis include severe or persistent hyperkalemia (serum potassium > 7 mEq/L), fluid overload (pulmonary edema), uremic encephalopathy, severe unresponsive metabolic acidosis, hyponatremia or hypernatremia.

PERITONEAL DIALYSIS

Intermittent peritoneal dialysis (IPD) is done to facilitate recovery of children with acute renal failure but continuous ambulatory peritoneal dialysis (CAPD) is used in patients with end-stage renal disease till a suitable donor is identified for renal transplant. Peritoneal dialysis is commonly performed in children because it is an easy procedure, does not require any sophisticated technology, can be performed in patients with hemodynamic instability, and is effective in children of all ages including neonates.

Table 40.1 Treatment of complications of acute kidney injury

Complication	Treatment
■ Fluid overload	Fluid restriction
■ Pulmonary edema	Oxygen, furosemide 2–4 mg/kg iv
■ Hypertension	Sodium nitroprusside 0.5–8.0 µg/kg/minute, furosemide 2–4 mg/kg iv, nifedipine 0.3–0.5 mg/kg oral or sublingual
■ Metabolic acidosis	Sodium bicarbonate 2–3 mEq/kg iv over 15–30 min
■ Hyperkalemia	Calcium gluconate (10%) 0.5–1.0 mL/kg over 5–10 minutes iv, salbutamol 5–10 mg by nebulization
■ Hyponatremia	Fluid restriction, 6–12 mL/kg of 3% saline over 30–60 minutes if there are seizures or sensorial changes
■ Hyperphosphatemia	Phosphate binders like calcium carbonate or acetate, aluminium phosphate
■ Severe anemia	Transfusion of packed red blood cells 3–5 mL/kg

Indications

1. Severe and persistent hyperkalemia (serum potassium >7 mEq/L).
2. Fluid overload with pulmonary edema.
3. Uremic encephalopathy.
4. Severe metabolic acidosis (base excess of greater than 15 mmol/L).
5. Severe hyponatremia (serum sodium >160 mEq/L).

Procedure

1. Strict aseptic precautions should be taken by wearing surgical gloves and using surgical drapes.
2. Most centers use a stiff catheter and a trocar for insertion of catheter in the peritoneal cavity as a bedside procedure. Thick catheters can be kept in situ for 48–72 hours, beyond which risk of injury to the viscera and infection is very high. When prolonged or repeated peritoneal dialyses are required, it is preferable to use soft silastic (Tenchkhoff or Cook's) catheters. The catheter is placed in the peritoneal cavity either surgically or with the help of a guide wire.
3. The composition of dialysate solution depends upon the condition of the patient. The commercially available dialysate solutions are lactate based with a dextrose concentration of 1.7%. In patients with fluid overload, the concentration of dextrose is increased to 2.5–3% to facilitate ultrafilteration. The fill volume for each cycle varies between 30 and 50 mL/kg and initial cycles are repeated after every 20–30 minutes. It is important to maintain an accurate record of volume of each indwell infused and drain or outflow retrieved as an estimate of efficacy of dialysis. After 10 cycles, if potassium levels are normal, 2–3 mEq/L of potassium chloride is added to the dialysis fluid. Patients who are sick and have severe lactic acidosis are dialyzed using a bicarbonate containing dialysate. The dialysate effluent should be checked for clarity, cell count and culture. Biochemical parameters should be checked before and after completion of the procedure.

Complications

1. Peritonitis
2. Blockage of catheter with reduced drainage of effluent. Catheter is milked or its position altered till free flow is established.
3. Bleeding and perforation of the bowel or bladder especially when a thick catheter is used.

Ambulatory Peritoneal Dialysis

In chronic renal failure with end-stage renal disease ambulatory peritoneal dialysis is performed till arrangements are made for renal transplant. Ambulatory peritoneal dialysis can be performed either manually; (continuous ambulatory peritoneal dialysis, CAPD) or with the help of an automated device (continuous cycling peritoneal dialysis; CCPD). In CAPD, parents are taught to connect the dialysate bag and manually cycle the dialysate from the bag into the peritoneal cavity and then back to the bag after every 20–30 minutes. Every day 3–5 cycles are performed to maintain renal function parameters within normal range. CCPD is more convenient and it involves automatic cycling of dialysate by a cycler machine at night when child is sleeping. The procedure is less cumbersome, does not interrupt the daily routine of the child or parents and has a better compliance.

Role of a Nurse

1. Nurse should monitor the vital signs, hydration status, fluid intake and urine out put and changes in the body weight.

40

2. Provide emotional support and compassionate care to the child and her family. Anxiety and stress should be reduced.
3. Child should be kept busy by indoor age-appropriate play activities, interactive games and by reading books.
4. Prevent risk of intercurrent infections, identify them early and treat promptly if they do occur.
5. Assist the family to maintain good personal hygiene, provide skin care and adequate nutrition with restricted intake of proteins.

WILMS' TUMOR

Wilms' tumor or nephroblastoma is the most common mixed embryonal neoplasm of the kidney. The age of onset is usually below 5 years. There is increased association of Wilms tumor in children with congenital anomalies such as aniridia, hemihypertrophy, and Beckwith-Wiedemann syndrome.

Clinical Features

It usually presents with enlargement of abdomen due to asymptomatic abdominal mass. The tumor is smooth, firm, movable or blottable, palpable bimanually (both hands) and does not cross the midline. The associated

> **Practical Tip**
> *Whenever there is a solid tumor in the abdomen or pelvis of a child, it should be considered as malignant unless proved otherwise.*

symptoms include fever, anorexia, vomiting, anemia, abdominal pain, hematuria and hypertension. The tumor commonly metastizes in the lungs and liver. It should be differentiated from other causes of flank or abdominal masses such as neuroblastoma, hydroneph-rosis, multicystic kidney, duplication of gut, mesenteric cyst and non-Hodgkin lymphoma.

Investigations

Laboratory studies should include complete blood counts (CBCs), urinalysis, kidney and liver function tests. Unlike neuroblastoma, plain skiagram of abdomen does not show any calcification. Computed tomography (CT) scan and magnetic resonance imaging (MRI) are diagnostic and can assess the extent of disease and metastasis in the liver. Skiagram of chest should be taken to exclude metastases in the lungs.

Treatment

The standard modalities of treatment include surgical excision, chemotherapy and radiotherapy depending upon the stage of the disease. Many surgeons prefer preoperative chemotherapy (actinomycin D and vincristine for 4 weeks) inorder to reduce the size of tumor so that it can be excised more effectively. Post operative chemotherapy is provided by administration of actinomycin D, vincristine and adriamycin. Radiotherapy is given when residual tumor is present after surgery. When early and aggressive management protocol is followed, more than 90% patients of Wilms' tumor are curable.

Nursing Care

1. A comprehensive nursing process should be drafted including a complete protocol of chemotherapy, radiotherapy and follow-up. There should be an atmosphere of hope and optimism. The family should be advised to join the cancer support group.
2. Provide tender loving care to the child and emotional support to the family to allay their anxiety and stress. Family should be told that early and effective treatment of childhood cancer is associated with good chances of cure so that optimism, hope and faith are kept alive.
3. Give advice regarding importance of personal hygiene and environmental sanitation as these children are immunocompromised and are prone to develop intercurrent infections. Orodental hygiene should be maintained to prevent fungal infection.
4. During therapy, child should be isolated and nursed in a sterile environment. Wearing a mask can reduce the risk of droplet infections. Barrier nursing should be practiced to prevent nosocomial infections.
5. Child should be encouraged to take high protein nutritious diet of his liking. Adequate hydration should be maintained during chemotherapy for effective excretion of waste products.
6. Family should be mentally prepared for occurrence of several adverse effects of chemotherapy including baldness and lack of sexual fertility.
7. Social and financial support should be provided with the help of a medical social worker because of the exorbitant cost of chemotherapy.
8. Family should be told about the need for prolonged medical treatment and follow-up and likelihood of repeated hospitalizations for parenteral chemotherapy and treatment of intercurrent infections.
9. Child should be encouraged to participate in indoor play activities and continue with his studies by coaching classes at home.

40

10. Maintain up-to-date schedule of immunizations. The administration of live vaccines should be postponed till chemotherapy is completed.

11. Healthy siblings should not be neglected. They need proper attention and care to prevent feelings of envy, jealousy and rivalry. The whole family should be encouraged to work as a close-knit unit with active involvement and participation of every member to jointly face the challenge with courage and fortitude.

BIBLIOGRAPHY

Bagga A. Nephrotic syndrome in children. *Indian J Med Res* 2005, 122(1): 13–28.

Dai B, Liu Y, Jia J, Mei C. Long-term antibiotics for prevention of recurrent urinary tract infections in children: a systematic review and meta-analysis. *Arch Dis Child* 2010, 95(7): 499–508.

Dickson PV, Sims TL, Streck CJ, et al. Avoiding misdiagnosing neuroblastoma as Wilms tumor. *J Pediatr Surg* 2008, 43(6): 1159–1163.

Eison TM, Ault BH, Jones DP, Chesney RW, Wyatt RJ. Post streptococcal acute glomerulonephritis in children: clinical features and pathogenesis. *Pediatr Nephrol* 2011, 26(2): 165–180.

Fischbach M, Edefonti A, Schroder C, Watson A. The European Pediatric Dialysis Working Group. Hemodialysis in children: general practical guidelines. *Pediatr Nephrol* 2005, 20: 1054–1066.

Gulati A, Bagga A, Gulati S, Mehta KP, Vijayakumar M. Indian Society of Pediatric Nephrology. Management of steroid resistant nephrotic syndrome. *Indian Pediatr* 2009, 46(1): 35–47.

Norman ME. An office approach to hematuria and proteinuria. *Pediatr Clin North Am* 1987, 34(3): 545–560.

Ricci Z, Cruz D, Ronco C. The RIFLE criteria and mortality in acute kidney injury: A systematic review. *Kidney Int* 2008, 73: 538–546.

Vijayakumar M, Kanitkar M, Nammalawar BR, Bagga A. Indian Society of Pediatric Nephrology. Revised statement on management of urinary tract infections. *Indian Pediatr* 2011, 48(9): 709–717.

40

Hematologic Disorders

NUTRITIONAL ANEMIA

Anemia is defined as low level of hemoglobin in the blood, either because there are too few red blood cells or because there is too little hemoglobin in each cell or both.

Causes

The most common cause of nutritional anemia is iron deficiency. It is a common condition in infants and adolescents. The iron stores are adequate at birth in term neonates and breast milk provides enough iron up to 6

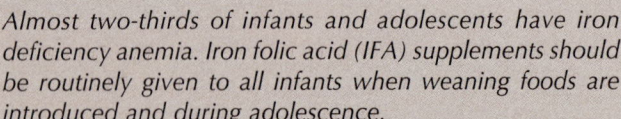

Nursing Alert

Almost two-thirds of infants and adolescents have iron deficiency anemia. Iron folic acid (IFA) supplements should be routinely given to all infants when weaning foods are introduced and during adolescence.

months of life. Prolonged milk feeding without complementary semisolid iron-containing foods is the commonest cause of iron deficiency anemia. During weaning when complementary feeds are deficient in iron, infants are likely to develop anemia. Parasitic infections such as malaria and worm infestation (especially hookworm) and frequent respiratory and gastrointestinal infections further aggravate iron deficiency. Dietary deficiency of folic acid and vitamin B_{12} cause a different type of anemia (megaloblastic) but it is commonly associated with iron deficiency. Other important causes of anemia include blood loss (especially excessive menses in adolescent girls), breakdown of red blood cells inside the body (hemolytic anemia especially due to thalassemia major) and blood cancer (leukemia).

Clinical Features

The child looks pale (some fair skinned children may look pale without anemia). Pallor is seen on the face, bulbar conjunctiva, palms and tongue. The child may be lethargic, irritable and have poor appetite. The child

may like to eat inedible objects like clay and mud (pica). The child may not be playful and active due to easy fatigability. Anemic children are more susceptible to develop frequent infections. Iron deficiency during early life has been shown to slow neuromotor development, cause attention deficit hyperactivity disorder and reduce learning capacity. Anemic children are prone to develop breath holding spells and febrile seizures. Anemia is diagnosed by estimation of hemoglobin. Hemoglobin level of <11.0 g/dL in preschool children and <12.0 g/dL in school-going children is suggestive of anemia. Hemoglobin level below 5 g/dL is labeled as severe anemia while a level between 5 and 10 g/dL as moderate anemia.

Laboratory Investigations

Hemoglobin level falls (<11.0 g/dL) and peripheral blood smear shows microcytic hypochromic RBCs with anisocytosis (different sizes) and poikilocytosis (different shapes) of RBCs and red cell distribution width of greater than 15%.

The biochemical indicators of iron deficiency, in order of their appearance, include fall in serum ferritin (<10 mg/mL), serum iron (<30 mg/dL), transferrin saturation (<15%), rise in total iron binding capacity (TIBC >350 mg/dL), and elevated free erythrocyte porphyrin (>2.8 mg/g of hemoglobin). Prussian blue staining of bone marrow shows absence of hemosiderin which is an earliest marker of iron deficiency.

Prevention and Treatment

Delayed clamping of cord at birth is associated with maternofetal transfusion with reduced incidence of early-onset iron deficiency anemia. After 6 months, when complementary feedings are started, child should be given foods rich in iron. Cereals, pulses, legumes, jaggery, dark green leafy vegetables, certain fruits (banana, apple and pomegranate) and egg yolk are good sources of iron. Non-vegetarian foods (especially muscle, blood and liver) are excellent sources of iron, which is more readily absorbed. Iron absorption is enhanced by intake of vitamin C-rich foods (citrus fruits, sour vegetables).

Medicinal iron may be given for prevention (1–2 mg/kg/d elemental iron) and treatment (3–5 mg/kg/day elemental iron) of iron deficiency anemia. Following iron therapy, reticulocyte response is observed within 3–4 days, evidenced by rise in hemoglobin by 1.0 g/dL per week. The causes of poor response to hematinic therapy are listed in **Box 41.1**. Iron therapy must be continued for at least 2 to 3 months to correct anemia and build up the body stores of iron. However, some children may not tolerate medicinal iron and may develop either constipation or loose motions. The child taking iron supplements may develop black staining of teeth and pass black colored stools. The child should be asked to take a crunchy fruit (apple, pear) or given water after intake of iron tonic to prevent staining of teeth. Iron-dextran complex can be given by deep intramuscular injection when oral iron is not tolerated. In children with severe anemia (hemoglobin <5 g/dL), packed red blood cell transfusion is given slowly after administration of furosemide to prevent circulatory overload.

MEGALOBLASTIC ANEMIA

Megaloblastic anemia occurs due to folic acid deficiency which may coexist with iron deficiency. Common causes of folate deficiency in children include intake of goat's milk, chronic diarrhea, malabsorption, recurrent infections, intake of anticonvulsants (phenytoin, mysoline) and antifolinic acid (methotrexate, pyrimethamine). In hemolytic anemia with marked compensatory erythropoiesis, relative folic acid deficiency may occur.

There is pallor, irritability, anorexia and failure to thrive. There is an increased pigmentation on the back of hand especially over interphalangeal joints or knuckles. Tremors and neuromotor retardation may occur when there is associated vitamin B_{12} deficiency.

| Box 41.1 | **Causes of poor response to hematinic therapy in iron deficiency anemia** |

- Wrong diagnosis. Patient may be having thalassemia trait or other nutritional deficiencies (vitamin B_{12}, folic acid)
- Poor compliance with therapy.
- Use of H_2 blockers or proton pump inhibitors that cause achlorhydria.
- There may be on-going blood loss, hemolysis or infection.
- Malabsorption state, e.g. celiac disease, giardiasis, *H. pylori* infection.

Peripheral blood smear shows macrocytic normochromic red blood cell morphology suggestive of megaloblasts and large sized polymorphonuclear leukocytes with hypersegmented nuclei. Neutropenia and thrombocytopenia may be present.

It is preferable to treat nutritional anemia with a formulation containing a combination of iron, folic acid and vitamin B_{12}. The daily therapeutic dose of folic acid and vitamin B_{12} are 0.5–1.0 mg and 1.0–5.0 μg, respectively. Folic acid supplements are recommended in children suffering from chronic hemolytic anemia or receiving drugs (phenytoin, pyrimethamine) which are known to cause folic acid deficiency.

THALASSEMIAS

Beta-thalassemia (Mediterranean anemia, Cooley's anemia) is a form of hereditary anemia where patient cannot form enough amount of normal adult type of hemoglobin, and instead fetal hemoglobin is formed. Both the parents carry the defective gene and they usually hail from west Pakistan. The disease is more common in certain communities namely Lohana, Khoja, Agarwal, Bhanushali, Bania, Neobuddhist, Sindhi and Jains. There is suppression of β-chains with overproduction of α-chains of hemoglobin. The disease is common in countries wherever Alexander the Great and his forces went and conquered. It is the commonest form of chronic hemolytic anemia in children.

The carriers of defective gene (parents of patients with thalassemia major) are designated to have thalassemia trait (thalassemia minor) and they have no symptoms or mild anemia. When both the parents have thalassemia trait, there is 1:4 chance that their child may have thalassemia major. The child appears normal at birth but develops gradually increasing severity of anemia between 3 months and 2 years of age. Anemia does not respond to any drugs and as the disease progresses there is gradual enlargement of liver and spleen. There is bossing or prominence of frontal and parietal bones of skull with a flattened vertex giving an appearance of hot-cross bun. The face assumes a typical appearance with prominent forehead and cheeks, depressed bridge of the nose and prominent cheek bones (hemolytic facies) due to erythroid hyperplasia in the bone marrow. The teeth may get malformed, crowded and protrude out (rodent facies). In advanced cases when iron chelation therapy is unsatisfactory, these children our likely to have short stature, delayed sexual maturation, or hypogonadism, endocrinopathies, cirrhosis, congestive heart failure, respiratory and renal insufficiencies.

41

Diagnosis

Peripheral blood smear shows grossly reduced hemoglobin, microcytic hypochromic anemia with anisocytosis and normoblasts or nucleated RBC's or erythroblasts. Reticulocyte count is raised. Hemoglobin electrophoresis shows markedly elevated fetal hemoglobin, some elevation of hemoglobin A_2 and reduced hemoglobin A. Serum iron and ferritin levels are markedly raised due to iron over load.

Thalassemia minor (beta-thalassemia trait) or carrier state is characterized by mild anemia (with or without mild splenomegaly) which is unresponsive to iron supplements. Hemoglobin is low (8–10 g/dL), RBC distribution width (RDW) is normal, RBC count is normal or elevated and RBCs are microcytic and hypochromic. Serum ferritin level is either normal or raised. Hemoglobin electrophoresis shows elevation of hemoglobin A_2 (HbA_2) with normal level of fetal hemoglobin.

Treatment

During premarital counselling, the would-be-couples can be screened for thalassemia trait, if they belong to a high ethnic group for thalassemia. If only one of the potential parents is carrying thalassemia trait, there is no risk of transmission of thalassemia major to the offsprings.

The patient with thalassemia major needs repeated blood transfusions along with administration of drugs to eliminate excess iron. Efforts are made to maintain hemoglobin level between 10–12 g/dL to ensure normal physical growth and prevent adverse effects of hyperplasia of bone marrow. Iron chelators (desferrioxamine 25–50 mg/kg/day over 8–12 hr) are usually given as continuous subcutaneous infusion with the help of a mini-infusion pump. Iron chelation therapy is started after 10–12 blood transfusions and given for 5–6 nights every week. Oral iron-chelating agent, deferiprone (DFP) is available and given in a dose of 75–100 mg/kg/d in 2–3 divided doses. Serum ferritin level should be maintained between 1000 and 2000 ng/mL. The patient should not be given any iron supplements but is given replacements of folic acid. When packed cell transfusion is required more often than every 2 weeks to maintain hemoglobin level above 10 g/dL, it indicates presence of hypersplenism. Splenectomy is useful to reduce the demand for blood transfusion but the procedure should be delayed beyond the age of 6 years because earlier splenectomy is associated with increased risk of pneumococcal infections and sepsis. The disease can be cured by a complicated and expensive procedure of bone marrow or stem cell transplantation. When both the parents are known to have thalassemia trait (as diagnosed on the basis of premarital counseling or because they have earlier given birth to a child with thalassemia major), it is advised to under go specialized antenatal screening tests for the diagnosis of the disease in their unborn baby during 10–18 weeks of pregnancy by doing a chorionic villus biopsy. If baby in the womb is found to be suffering from thalassemia major, the mother is offered the option of undergoing an abortion on medical grounds.

SICKLE CELL ANEMIA

Sickle cell disease is an uncommon hemoglobinopathy which is limited to tribal population. It occurs due to deletion of B-globin gene on chromosome 11 where valine is substituted for glutamic acid on the B-polypeptide chain. The erythrocytes get deformed into sickle-shaped cells especially under conditions of anoxia and acidosis. The sickle cells adhere to each other and may block the capillaries at various sites leading to ischemic manifestations (sequestration crises) in any organ of the body.

Clinical Features

The usual symptoms include chronic anemia with enlargement of liver and spleen (which may regress or shrink in size because of repeated infarctions), mild jaundice, non-healing leg ulcers and delayed onset of puberty. Sickle cell crises produce acute episodes of abodominal pain and body aches because of involvement of bones (metacarpals of hands producing dactylitis) and joints with worsening of anemia and jaundice. Complete blood count (CBC) shows anemia, leukocytosis and thrombocytosis. Diagnosis is confirmed by demonstration of sickling on peripheral blood smear and hemoglobin SS (HbSS) on electrophoresis.

Treatment

Treatment is symptomatic and supportive. Hydration and use of safe analgesics are the mainstays of treatment during pain crises. Oxygen should be administered to relieve hypoxia. Intravenous rehydration and blood transfusion are recommended for treatment of aplastic crisis and acute sequestration crisis. These children should be given pencillin prophylaxis during first 5 years of life and effectively immunized against pneumococci, meningococci and *Hemophilus influenzae type b*. They are given lifelong folate supplements. Hydroxyurea, a cytotoxic agent is credited to increase HbF, which can reduce the episodes of sequestration crises and may be tried in children above 5 years of age.

41

APLASTIC ANEMIA

Acquired aplastic anemia is uncommon but causes life-threatening anemia because of immune-mediated global depression of all the hematopoietic elements not only in the bone marrow but in all other extramedullary sites (lymph nodes, liver and spleen) leading to pancytopenia. The predisposing factors may include certain viral infections (parvoviruses, Epstein-Barr virus, hepatitis B, C and D), exposure to ionizing radiation, intake of certain drugs (chloramphenicol, oxphenyl butazone, analgin, sulfonamides, quinacrine, cimetidine, phenytoin and carbamazepine) and chemicals like DDT, benzene, arsenicals and certain heavy metals such as gold.

Clinical Features

There is progressive and intractable anemia with clinical features because of leukopenia (intercurrent infections) and thrombocytopenia (ecchymoses and bleeding manifestations). Despite severe anemia, there is absense of any enlargement of lymph nodes or hepatosplenomegaly. It should be differentiated from idiopathic thrombocytopenic purpura (ITP), acute leukemia, and paroxysmal nocturnal hemoglobinuria (PNH).

Laboratory Investigations

There is pancytopenia with low RBC count, leukopenia, neutropenia, and thrombocytopenia in the peripheral blood. Reticulocyte count is low. Bone marrow aspiration may be dry and bone biopsy shows marked hypocellularity of all the hematopoietic elements.

Treatment

The disease carries high morbidity and grave prognosis. Patient should be provided with excellent supportive and nursing care. The risk of infection should be reduced by ensuring adequate personal hygiene, frequent washing of hands with soap and water and daily bath. Intercurrent infection should be identified early and treated promptly with broad spectrum antibiotics and metronidazole. Packed red blood cell transfusion is given to maintain hemoglobin above 8 g/dL. Bleeding manifestations because of thrombo-cytopenia should be treated with administration of single donor platelets to maintain platelet count above 20,000/mm^3. The definitive therapy include immunosuppression with antilymphocyte globulins or equine antithymocyte globulin and cyclosporine. Various hematopoietic growth factors (G–CSF) have been used with variable results. Corticosteroids have limited therapeutic utility. Androgens provide variable results. Bone marrow or stem cell transplantation from an HLA-matched sibling or unrelated donor is curative.

BLEEDING DISORDERS

Bleeding disorders may occur due to a vascular defect, reduced level or abnormal function of platelets or a coagulation disorder **(Table 41.1)**.

Clinical Features

Platelet deficiency or defects usually manifest as petechiae, i.e. pin point hemorrhagic spots in the skin while vascular defects are characterized by ecchymoses, i.e. large patches of hemorrhages under the skin. Petechiae and ecchymoses should be differentiated from maculopapular erythematous skin rash which can be blanched by application of pressure while petechiae or ecchymoses cannot be blanched. Coaguoltion disorders usually manifest by frank bleeding which may be external (visible) or it may be internal (occult or non visible) in various viscera including brain.

The usual clinical features include petechiae, ecchymoses, generalized bruises, subcutaneous hematomas, hemarthrosis (bleeding into the joint), and bleeding from various body orifices (nose, oral cavity, anus, vagina). Internal bleeding may occur in any viscera or body cavity including central nervous system leading to development of features of raised intracranial tension (headache, vomiting, papilledema), seizures and coma. Excessive bleeding may lead to hypovolemia and circulatory collapse (cold extremities, rapid thready pulse, fall in blood pressure). The child

---

Table 41.1 Common causes of bleeding disorders

- **Platelet disorders**
  - Thrombocytopenia (<100,000/mm^3): Septicemia, viral hemorrhagic fever (dengue fever), disseminated intravascular coagulation, aplastic anemia, immune thrombocytopenia, hemolytic uremic syndrome, drug-induced, leukemia, etc.
  - Platelet function disorders (thrombocytopathy) which may be congenital or acquired.
- **Coagulation disorders**
  - Vitamin K deficiency (hemorrhagic disease of the newborn).
  - Inherited disorders (hemophilia)
  - Acquired disorders (liver disease, DIC)
- **Vascular disorders**
  - Henoch-Schonlein purpura, collagen vascular disorders.

41

with bleeding manifestations should be classified into two groups.

1. *Sick child* Bleeding manifestations in a critically sick child is suggestive of septicemia, viremia, disseminated intravascular coagulation (DIC), liver dysfunction, collagen vascular disorder and hemolytic uremic syndrome (dysentery, hemolysis and renal failure).

2. *Well child* Bleeding manifestations in a well child is suggestive of hereditary coagulation disorder, vitamin K deficiency (hemorrhagic disease of the newborn), drug-induced thrombocytopenia or immune thrombocytopenia (ITP). Hemophilia is limited to boys (X-linked disorder) and is characterized by recurrent episodes of bruising, subcutaneous hematomas, hemarthrosis following minor day-to-day injuries. Family history of a bleeding disorder may be positive.

DISSEMINATED INTRAVASCULAR COAGULATION (DIC)

In a large number of life-threatening conditions like septicemia, hypoxia, hypothermia, burns, shock, malignancy, and collagen vascular disease, DIC may set in. Neonates especially preterm babies are more susceptible to develop DIC. The condition is characterized by intravascular coagulation which is associated with increased consumption of platelets and plasma clotting factors (consumptive coagulopathy) leading to widespread bleeding manifestations.

Clinical Features

The child is critically sick with features of underlying predisposing condition. The child usually has circulatory collapse with generalized bleeding manifestations from various sites including injection and venepuncture sites. Petechiae, GI bleeding, and hematuria may occur. There is multi-organ dysfunction with paralytic ileus, hepatic and renal dysfunction.

Laboratory Investigations

There is thrombocytopenia and global depression of all the coagulation factors with prolongation of prothrombin time (PT), activated prothrombin time (APTT), and thrombin time (TT). There is an increased level of fibrin degradation products (FDPs) and D-dimers. There is microangiopathic hemolytic anemia as evidenced by presence of fragmented, distorted or shrunken RBCs with spherocytes and schistocytes.

Role of a Nurse

The child needs care in the pediatric intensive care unit under the supervision of specialized nurses. There is a need for close monitoring and life support interventions to maintain fluid and electrolyte balance, correct acidosis, support circulatory system and other vital organs. Specific treatment and appropriate antibiotics are administered to manage the underlying predisposing condition/s. Venepunctures and invasive procedures should be kept to the bare minimum. Coagulation factors are replaced by administration of fresh frozen plasma (FFP 10–15 mL/kg every 12–24 hours), or cryoprecipitate, platelet concentrate and packed red blood cells. Platelet count should be maintained above 50,000/mm³ while fibrinogen level should be kept above 75 mg/dL. Heparin may be given to reduce the severity of bleeding and thromboembolic complications. Exchange blood transfusion is done in a desperate situation. The child needs intensive nursing care while family needs emotional support.

IDIOPATHIC THROMBOCYTOPENIC PURPURA

Idiopathic or immune thrombocytopenic purpura (ITP) is the most common acquired bleeding disorder which is of unknown etiology. Thrombocytopenia occurs due to increased destruction of the antibody-coated platelets by the reticuloendothelial cells in the spleen. Most cases (>80%) recover spontaneously within 6 months (acute ITP). When condition persists beyond 6 months, it is labeled as chronic ITP.

Clinical Features

Acute ITP affects preschool children of both sexes, while chronic ITP occurs in school going children and is more common in females. Onset is usually acute without any known predisposing factors. Thrombocytopenia occurs due to increased destruction of the antibody coated platelets by the reticuloendothelial cells in the spleen. Most cases have asymptomatic petechiae or ecchymoses with severe thrombocytopenia (platelets <20,000/mm³). Mucosal bleeding spots on the lips, buccal mucosa and palate may be seen. Visceral bleeding or intracranial hemorrhage are rare. There is no anemia, enlargement of lymphnodes, liver and spleen. Peripheral smear does not show any abnormalities except thrombocytopenia.

Diagnosis

Bone marrow shows a large number of 'lazy' megakaryocytes (precursors of platelets) with poor "budding" and reduced production of thrombocytes

41

or platelets. Bone marrow examination is essential to exclude conditions like aplastic anemia, leukemia, tumor cell infiltration and other myelodysplasias.

Treatment

In acute ITP, no specific treatment is advised if platelet count is above 20,000/mm^3. General supportive care includes avoidance of trauma and participation in aggressive sports. When platelet count falls below 20,000/mm^3 or there are active bleeding manifestations, either corticosteroids (prednisolone 2 mg/kg/day for 3–4 weeks), intravenous immune globulins (IVIG 1.0 g/kg daily for 2 days) or platelet transfusion are given.

Splenectomy may be considered in children with severe chronic ITP who are not responsive to steroids or IVIG and bleeding manifestations are intractable, severe or recurrent. The risk of intracranial hemorrhage is high when platelet count falls below 5,000/mm^3. Splenectomy should be delayed till child is at least 5 years old because of high risk of pneumococcal infections in preschool children.

Role of a Nurse

1. Family should be reassured because most cases of acute ITP recover spontaneously. Unnecessary fear due to low platelets should be allayed.
2. Physical activity of the child should be guarded to prevent bleeding due to trauma. Intramuscular injections should be avoided.
3. Adolescent girls should be given guidance for possibility of excessive menstrual flow.
4. Pneumococcal vaccine should be given before splenectomy.
5. After splenectomy, penicillin prophylaxis is advised until adulthood to prevent occurrence of pneumococcal infections.
6. Family should be advised to seek early medical attention whenever there is a febrile illness.

HEMOPHILIA

Hemophilia is an X-linked genetic disorder wherein boys suffer with bleeding manifestations while girls are carriers of defective gene without any symptoms. There is a deficiency of clotting factors such as Factor VIII (Classical hemophilia) or Factor IX (Christmas disease). It is characterized by excessive bruising and prolonged bleeding in boys following a minor injury. Excessive bleeding may occur at the time of routine circumcision or bleeding may occur from the umbilical stump. Bleeding into the joints (hemarthroses) leads to swelling, pain and deformity. Hemophilia is a lifelong disease without any cure.

Diagnosis

Easy bruising, spontaneous episodes of bleeding or excessive bleeding following mild trauma in a boy with a positive family history are highly suggestive of hemophilia. These children have normal platelet count and bleeding time. The clotting time and activated partial thromboplastin time (APTT) are prolonged. The deficiency of factor VIII and IX can be identified by specific assay or by conducting mixing studies with normal plasma and adsorbed plasma.

Treatment

Affected children should be protected against injuries and advised to wear protective guards over the major joints. Bleeding manifestations can be controlled by local application of pressure, ice packs and elevation of limb. Paracetamol is a safe analgesic-antipyretic for relief of joint pains and fever. Administration of plasma concentrate (cryoprecipitate) and factor VIII (antihemophiliac globulin 25 units/kg every 12 hours for two doses) are life saving to stop active bleeding. Vaccines should preferably to given orally, intradermally or subcutaneously with a small needle. Surgical procedures, whether minor or major, should be undertaken only after infusing clotting factors. The blood components should be procured from a reliable blood bank who is credited to collect blood from voluntary donors and is equipped with facilities to screen the blood for hepatitis B, C and HIV viruses.

Role of a Nurse

1. The family should be explained about the need for constant supervision at home and school to prevent injuries.
2. Advise the parents regarding the need for wearing a helmet and protective padding gears over the joints during sports or play activity.
3. The child should not participate in contact sports like football, hockey, boxing and wrestling. He can participate in individual sports like swimming, cycling, golf, squash, table tennis, lawn tennis and badminton.
4. Intramuscular injections should be avoided and all vaccines should be administered subcutaneously.
5. Avoid intake of aspirin and NSAID due to risk of aggravating bleeding. Paracetamol, morphine and pethidine are safe for relief of pain.
6. The child should be effectively vaccinated against hepatitis B because he is likely to receive frequent transfusions of blood and blood products.
7. The family should be provided guidance for genetic counseling. When mother is a carrier of hemophilia

41

gene, 50% of her sons are likely to suffer from hemophilia, while 50% of daughters will be carriers. When father is suffering from hemophilia, then all the daughters will be carriers while all the sons will be normal.

8. It is possible to make antenatal diagnosis of hemophilia at 18–20 weeks of gestation. When fetus is found to be hemophiliac, medical termination of pregnancy can be advised to the family.

LEUKEMIAS

The commonest cancer in children is acute leukemia. The other common sites of cancer in children include brain, lymphoid tissue, kidneys and embryonal tissue. Depending upon the types of white cells involved, leukemia may be acute lymphoblastic or myelocytic. Acute stem cell or lymphoblastic leukemia is more common and carries good prognosis. The common symptoms are unexplained fever, bone pains, progressive anemia, bleeding manifestations, loss of appetite and progressive anemia, enlargement of lymph nodes, liver and spleen. The outcome of acute leukemia in children is better than adults and cure is possible in over 50 percent of children.

Treatment

The children with acute leukemia are prone to develop serious infections and nutritional deficiencies. Chemotherapy and radiotherapy are known to further depress appetite and immunological system. Efforts should be made to maintain utmost personal hygiene and environmental sanitation at home. Individuals with any infection should not come and visit the child. When child is taken to the hospital, he should preferably wear a mask. Whenever the child develops fever, it is a medical emergency and should be promptly treated with broad spectrum antibiotics. Supportive management includes administration of platelet concentrates and blood transfusion. Corticosteroids and chemotherapy with newer anticancer drugs can achieve remission in most patients. When facilities are available, bone marrow or stem cell transplantation is curative.

Nursing Care

The child should be encouraged to take a balanced and nutritious diet of his choice. He should be given small and frequent meals and snacks of his liking. Vitamins and tonics should not be given unless advised by the physician. The child should be handled with utmost care, compassion and optimism. You should remember that faith and optimism have tremendous healing capabilities and it should be effectively harnessed. The child should not be unnecessarily allowed to suffer from pain and discomfort. Pain should be relieved by use of an effective analgesic.

SOLID TUMORS

Cancer in children is rare and mostly affect the hematologic or lymphoreticular system by causing leukemia and lymphoma. Common solid tumors include brain tumor, neuroblastoma, Wilms tumor,

> **Nursing Alert**
>
> *Children with unexplained bone pains and joint swellings should be investigated for possible lymphoreticular malignancy.*

rhabdomyosarcoma, and bone tumors. Early diagnosis, effective chemotherapy and surgical excision are associated with better outcome and long-term survival and cure in children.

Common Clinical Features

They are related to the site of malignancy. Lymphoreticular or hematologic malignancy is usually associated with progressive anemia, loss of appetite, weight loss, petechiae, bone bones, swelling of joints, lymphadeno-

> **Practical Tip**
>
> *Every solid tumor in the abdomen or pelvis in a child should be considered as malignant unless proved otherwise.*

pathy, and hepatosplenomegaly. Mediastinal mass may produce hoarsness of voice, suffusion of face, engorged neck and chest veins, breathing and feeding difficulties.

Whenever there is a solid tumor in the abdomen or pelvis, it should be considered as malignant unless proved otherwise. Every solid tumor in the abdomen should be promptly investigated by ultrasonography, CT scan or MRI.

Brain tumors manifest with evidences of raised intracranial pressure (intractable morning headache, vomiting, behavioral changes, diplopia or double vision, papilledema), ataxia, incoordination, seizures and focal neurological signs.

Nursing Care

1. Provide tender loving care (TLC) to the child and emotional support to the family to allay their anxiety and stress. Keep the optimism alive as there is a good chance of cure in childhood cancer by early and effective chemotherapy.

41

2. Advise importance of personal hygiene and environmental sanitation as these children are immunocompromised and more prone to develop intercurrent infections. Orodental hygiene should be maintained to prevent fungal infections.

3. During chemotherapy, child should be isolated and nursed in a sterile environment. Wearing a mask can reduce the risk of droplet infections. Barrier nursing should be practiced to prevent nosocomial infections. Family should be mentally prepared for occurrence of several adverse effects of chemotherapy including baldness and sterility.

4. Social and financial support should be provided in view of the exorbitant cost of chemotherapy.

5. Family should be mentally prepared for prolonged treatment and follow-up and need for repeated hospitalizations for parenteral chemotherapy and treatment of intercurrent infections.

6. Child should be encouraged to participate in indoor play activities and continue with his studies by coaching classes at home.

7. A comprehensive nursing process should be drafted including a complete protocol of chemotherapy, radiotherapy and follow-up. There should be an atmosphere of hope and optimism. The family can be advised to join the cancer support group.

8. Ensure adequate nutrition of the child with the help of a dietician.

9. Attempts should be made to maintain up-to-date schedule of immunizations. Killed vaccines, toxoids and recombinant antigen-based vaccines can be safely given to immunocompromised children. The live vaccines such as measles, MMR, chickenpox, oral polio vaccine are contraindicated due to risk of development of vaccine-related diseases. Even siblings of patients should not be given oral polio vaccine because of transmission of vaccine virus to the immunocompromised sick child through orofecal route. Instead inactivated or injectable polio vaccine (IPV) should be given.

10. Healthy siblings should not be neglected and they should be informed and involved in the care of affected child. They need proper attention and support to reduce the feelings of envy, jealousy and rivalry. The whole family should be encouraged to work as a close-knit unit with active involvement and participation of every member to jointly face the challenge with courage and fortitude.

BIBLIOGRAPHY

Chandy M. Management of hemophilia in developing countries with available resources. *Hemophilia* 1995, 1(supple 1): 44–48.

Dubey AP, Parakh A, Dublish S. Current trends in the management of beta thalassemia. *Indian J Pediatr* 2008, 75(7): 739–743.

Galloway MJ, Smellie WS. Investigating iron status in microcytic anemia. *Brit Med J* 2006, 333(7572): 791–793.

Goldsby RE, Mattbay KK. Neuroblastoma: Evolving therapies for a disease with many faces. *Paediatr Drugs* 2004, 6(2): 107–122.

Hershko C. Treating iron over load: The state of the art. *Semin Hematol* 2005, 42(2 supple 1): S2–S4.

Kalapurakal JA, Dome JS, Perlman EJ, et al. Management of Wilm's tumor: Current practice and future goals. *Lancet Oncol* 2004, 5(1): 37–46.

Marsh JC, Ball SE, Cavenagh J, et al. Guidelines for the diagnosis and management of aplastic anemia. *Br J Haematol* 2009, 147(1): 43–70.

Monagle PT, Tauro GP. Infantile megaloblastosis secondary to maternal vitamin B_{12} deficiency. *Clin Lab Haematol* 1997, 19(1): 23–25.

Trantino MD. Recent advances in the treatment of childhood immune thrombocytopenic pupura. *Semin Hematol* 2006, 43: 11–18.

Central Nervous System Disorders

CONVULSIONS (Fits, Seizures)

A seizure or convulsion is a paroxysmal event due to abnormal, excessive and hypersynchronous electrical discharge from a group of neurons in the brain. There is sudden involuntary stiffening or twitching movements of a limb or whole body with or without loss of consciousness. It may be associated with staring look or uprolling of eyeballs. It occurs due to involvement of the brain by a localized or generalized disease process. In children, seizures may occur due to metabolic changes in the body, because of alterations in blood glucose, calcium, sodium or magnesium levels. The salient causes of seizures are listed in **Table 42.1**.

EPILEPSY

When episodes of convulsions occur repeatedly, and there is no underlying metabolic cause or fever, it is called epilepsy. About 3–5 percent children suffer from epilepsy. Epilepsy may be generalized (twitchings of both upper and lower limbs with loss of consciousness) or partial and localized (twitchings of one side of body or one limb with or without loss of consciousness). Most cases of generalized epilepsy are familial in nature while partial epilepsy occurs due to a localized disease process in the brain like birth asphyxia, injury, infection, tumor, granuloma, (tuberculoma, cysticercosis), and vascular malformation. Seizures may be precipitated by

---

Table 42.1 Common causes of seizures

Neonatal period

- Birth asphyxia, birth trauma and hypoxic ischemic encephalopathy.
- Intracranial hemorrhage.
- Transient metabolic conditions: Hypoglycemia, hypocalcemia, dyselectrolytemia, and hypomagnesemia.
- Inborn errors of metabolism.
- Developmental malformations of CNS.
- Infections: Intrauterine infections, meningitis, septicemia, tetanus neonatorum.
- Maternal withdrawal of drugs or substance abuse.
- Pyridoxine dependency.
- Inadvertent injection of local anesthetic into the fetal scalp during pudendal block.

Infants and children

- Simple febrile convulsions.
- Infections: Pyogenic meningitis, tubercular meningitis, aseptic meningitis, encephalitis, encephalopathy, cerebral malaria, Reye syndrome.
- Metabolic causes: Dyselectrolytemia, hypocalcemia, hypoglycemia, hypomagnesemia, inborn errors of metabolism.
- Space occupying lesions: Neoplasm, brain abscess, cysticercosis, tuberculoma.
- Vascular: Arteriovenous malformation, thrombosis, emboli, hemorrhage.
- Miscellaneous conditions: Hypertensive encephalopathy, storage disorders, developmental defects of CNS.
- Drugs and poisons: Fluoroquinolones, phenothiazines, salicylates, organophosphates, methyl phenidate, amphetamine, piperazine salts, caffeine, mefenamic acid, isoniazid, local anesthetics, strychnine, carbon monoxide, and drugs of abuse.
- Epilepsy syndromes
- Idiopathic

fever, sleep deprivation, photic stimulation, over breathing (absence attacks), intake of CNS stimulant drugs (fluoroquinolones, methyl phenidate, chlorpromazine, metoclopramide, theophyllin, amphetamine, piperazine salts, coffein, isoniazid, mefenamic acid, local anesthetics, and drugs of abuse) and due to electrolyte and metabolic disturbances. Epilepsy is a disease and not a curse by nature or possession by an evil spirit.

Types of Epilepsy

Seizures are classified into generalized and partial types.

Generalized seizures The epileptic discharge starts simultaneously from both the cerebral hemispheres right at the time of onset of seizure.

i. *Tonic-clonic seizures (grand mal epilepsy)* There are tonic-clonic twitchings of both upper and lower limbs with loss of consciousness. There may be a loud moan or cry at the onset. Seizures may occur during sleep and when they occur during waking hours, the child may get injured. During the seizure there may be biting of the tongue and incontinence of bladder or bowel. After recovery (post-ictal state), the child may have confusion, fatigue, headache, muscle ache but lacks any memory of the seizure event. Family history may be positive.

ii. *Myoclonic seizures* There is sudden brief jerky contractions of muscles involving a limb or part of a limb, or there may be sudden bending of trunk (salaam seizures or infantile spasms) with momentary loss of consciousness. Seizures are frequent but extremely brief in duration.

iii. *Atonic or akinetic seizures* There is sudden loss of muscle tone leading to "drop attacks".

iv. *Absence attacks (petit mal epilepsy)* These are characterized by brief staring spells, blank look with or without blinking of eyes or fluttering of lips or chewing movements. They occur in school going children and are more common in girls. Electroencephalography (EEG) shows characteristic 3 HZ spike-and-wave discharge.

Partial seizures The seizure discharge is localized to a part or a discrete region of the brain one one side.

i. *Simple partial seizures* There is sudden jerking (tonic-clonic movements) of a part of one side of the face or limbs without any impairment of consciousness. The focal symptoms may be motor, sensory, autonomic or psychic.

ii. *Complex partial seizures* Focal seizures (mostly tonic) with stiffness of limbs, retraction of neck and uprolling of eyes and fluttering of eyelids is followed by loss of consciousness. Temporal lobe seizures are characterized by complex stereotyped motor activity and automatisms in a trance like mental state which may be confused with a psychological disorder.

iii. *Partial seizures with secondary generalization* Seizure starts as a focal phenomenon and slowly progresses to become generalized with loss of consciousness. The march of events (Jacksonian march) is slow and easily discernible. There may be transient paralysis (Todd's paralysis) of the affected limb after the seizure.

Diagnosis

Diagnosis is based on clinical characteristics of seizures because all investigations may be negative. Computerized axial tomography (CT) scan and magnetic resonance imaging (MRI) studies of brain may show underlying brain abnormality causing symptomatic epilepsy. EEG may show abnormality during a seizure but may be normal during inter-ictal period. Metabolic screening should be done to rule out hypoglycemia, hypocalcemia and electrolyte disturbances. Several disorders may be confused with seizures and should be ruled out by meticulous attention to history, observations and relevant laboratory studies (Table 42.2).

Treatment

Most children with epilepsy can lead a normal life under long-term anticonvulsant medications. The goal of therapy is to prevent seizures with minimal side effects of drugs. The drugs are started at the lowest recommended dose which is gradually increased till seizures are controlled or side effects appear. A large majority have normal intelligence and can attend a regular school. Anticonvulsants should never be stopped suddenly as it may lead to repeated seizures. The potentially hazardous activities like swimming and driving should be avoided unless fits are well controlled. When a seizure occurs, loosen the clothes and protect the child against injury. He should be placed on a bed with face turned to one side to avoid choking due to aspiration of secretions or vomiting. Never try to force open the mouth with a teaspoon. Epilepsy is due to disease of the brain and should never be viewed as handiwork of evil spirits. A large number of effective anticonvulsant medications are available (Table 42.3). Over 80 percent of children with epilepsy can be effectively treated with one or more medicines. In a select group of children who do not respond to drugs, surgical treatment has been used with success for control of seizures.

42

Table 42.2 Characteristic features of common conditions mimicking seizures

Condition	Salient features
Syncope	Episode is invoked by Valsalva maneuver, sudden rising from sitting or lying position and acute pain, anxiety or emotional stress especially in adolescent children. The attack may occur because of cardiac arrhythmia. There is transitory loss of consciousness, pallor, dizziness, bradycardia, cold clammy extremities, and tunneling of vision. A brief period (up to 10 sec) of convulsive motor activity may occur when subject remains upright. Headache may occur soon after the syncope.
Psychogenic seizures	The behavior is usually a part of conversion reaction, which occurs in a dramatic way when patient is being watched. There may be side-to-side turing of head, large amplitude shaking movements of limbs, pelvic thrusting, screaming, groaning, moaning, gesturing and so on. There is no injury or loss of consciousness. The abnormal behavior gradually abates when patient is left alone.
Migraine	There may be visual or auditary aura or photophobia followed by unilateral headache. It may be associated with recurrent abdominal pain and cyclical vomiting, light headedness, scalp tenderness, vertigo, and at times alteration of consciousness may occur. Rarely syncope, seizure and confusional state may occur.
Tics	They are stereotyped, awkward, and repetitive movements of a particular part of the body. The common examples of tics are shrugging of shoulders, blinking of eyes, twisting of neck, or attempts at coughing. They usually occur between 8 and 10 years of age and are more common when a child is tense and anxious.
Breath-holding spells	The child gets angry, throws a temper tantrum or gets hurt and cries loudly. After a long uninterrupted cry, the child holds his breath in expiration. The child may become blue and rarely the attack may lead to a seizure. After the spell, the child may start crying again and start asking for the same demand that triggered the attack. Breath-holding spells usually occur in children between 6 months and 3 years of age.
Narcolepsy	There is excessive, uncontrollable, daytime episodes of sleep with disturbed night sleep. There may be sudden weakness or loss of muscle tone (cataplexy). At the onset of sleep, there may be vivid hallucinations or feeling of muscle paralysis.
Drug abuse	Intake of psychoactive drugs may be associated with hallucinations and schizophrenia-like reactions.

Table 42.3 Rational choice of antiepileptic drugs

Seizure type	Anticonvulsant of choice
■ Generalized tonic-clonic seizures (grand mal)	Phenytoin, carbamazepine, sodium valproate, clobazam
■ Partial seizures	Carbamazepine, phenytoin, sodium valproate, clobazam, levetiracetam
■ Absence attacks (petit mal)	Sodium valproate, ethosuximide, clonazepam, topiramate
■ Atonic seizures	Sodium valproate, carbamazepine, clonazepam
■ Myoclonic seizures	Sodium valproate, clonazepam, levetiracetam, nitrazepam, topiramate
■ Infantile spasms	ACTH or prednisolone, sodium valproate, benzodiazepines, vigabatrin, clonazepam, topiramate
■ Mixed type	Sodium valproate, lomotrigine, clobazam, topiramate

Adapted from Singh M, Deorari AK *Drug Dosages in Children*, New Delhi, CBS Publishers and Distributors Pvt Ltd. 9th edition 2015.

A vast majority of children with epilepsy grow up to have normal or even above normal intelligence. Many great intellectuals and leaders like Sir Isaac Newton, Socrates, Alexander the Great, Julius Caesar and Napolean Bonaparte, made outstanding contributions in life despite having epilepsy.

STATUS EPILEPTICUS

When there are repeated seizures over a period of 30 minutes without regaining consciousness it is called status epilepticus (SE). A patient who started having seizures at home and continues to have seizures when reporting to the hospital, should be considered to have SE. Status epilepticus may lead to hypoxia and neuronal damage and should be managed in the pediatric intensive care unit in accordance with a set protocol.

Etiology

Status epilepticus may occur due to any one of the causes of seizures listed in **Table 42.1**. The nature of underlying cause depends on the age of the child. Hypoxic–ischemic encephalopathy, inborn errors of metabolism and congenital malformations of CNS are likely to manifest in infancy.

42

Diagnosis

History should be taken whether it is the first episode of seizure or child is a known case of epilepsy. Identify the antiepileptic drugs being taken and whether there has been any lack of compliance in taking medications. Ask for history of trauma and poisoning. Bradycardia may suggest raised intracranial pressure (ICP). Blood pressure should be checked to rule out hypotension and hypertensive encephalopathy. Fundus should be examined for hemorrhages, chorioretinitis and papilledema.

Laboratory Investigations

Therapy must be started while laboratory studies are being undertaken. Blood sample is taken for complete blood count (CBC), determination of electrolytes, glucose, calcium and magnesium level, liver and kidney function tests, ABG and acid-base parameters, and blood level of anticonvulsant drugs. Peripheral smear should be examined to rule out malaria caused by *Plasmodium falciparum*. When indicated, blood and urine sample should be sent for metabolic and toxicology studies.

Cerebrospinal fluid should be examined to rule out meningitis and encephalitis. Computerized tomography or MRI scan of brain is obtained if (i) seizures are refractory to treatment, (ii) partial or focal nature of seizures, (iii) evidences of raised ICP and (iv) history of head trauma. EEG monitoring in the ICU is useful to exclude herpes encephalitis, monitor response to anticonvulsant therapy, and identify when seizure activity stops.

Nursing Care

1. Patient needs excellent nursing and supportive care in the pediatric ICU.
2. Ensure effective ABC, monitor vital signs and arterial oxygen saturation with a pulse oximeter. Oxygen should be given by nasal prongs or a mask.
3. Establish two intravenous lines, one for administration of fluids, electrolytes and anticonvulsant drugs, and the other for infusion of specific medications and antidotes.
4. Anticonvulsant therapy should be started without delay as per protocol shown in **Figure 42.1**.
5. Fever should be brought down by administration of an antipyretic and hydrotherapy.
6. Metabolic disorders like hypoglycemia, hypocalcemia and dyselectrolytemia should be managed as per standard protocol.
7. The underlying infective disorders like meningitis, cerebral malaria and herpes encephalitis are treated by specific antibiotics, antiviral and antimalarial agents. Administer a specific antidote if indicated.
8. Monitor fluids and electrolytes by maintaining strict intake-output chart by taking into account all the infusates given for administration of anticonvulsant drugs and specific medications.
9. Acidosis should be corrected and fluid restricted if there is hyponatremia caused by syndrome of inappropriate antidiuretic hormone (SIADH).
10. Raised intracranial pressure (ICP) is managed as per standard protocol. Head is kept raised by 15° and nasopharyngeal secretions are sucked periodically. Hypertonic mannitol (0.5–1.0 g/kg) is infused over 30 minutes and may be repeated after every 4 hours up to 4–6 doses.

Prognosis

The overall mortality rate of SE is about 5% and is related to the underlying condition, adequacy and promptness of treatment. Prolonged uncontrolled seizures for more than 45 minutes and septic shock are associated with poor outcome. The long-term neuro-motor sequelae include recurrent seizures, focal neurological abnormalities and mental retardation.

FEBRILE CONVULSIONS

Sudden onset of high grade fever in some children may lead to convulsions. It is most common during 6 months to 3 years of age. They seldom occur after the age of 5 years. Around 5–10% of under-5 children are likely to experience febrile seizures. They occur due to immaturity of brain and are more common in certain families. Children with iron deficiency anemia are at a greater risk to develop febrile seizures. Even before the mother realizes, that the child has fever, he becomes stiff and develops jerky movements or twitchings of upper and lower limbs. There may be uprolling of eye balls, clenching of teeth (with injury to tongue) and loss of consciousness. Most convulsions are of a brief duration lasting for a few seconds to 2–5 minutes. Convulsions usually stop by the time child is taken to the hospital and they do not recur during the course of fever. They can occur again when child gets another episode of fever after couple of weeks or months. After the convulsion, the child may start crying or go to sleep.

Treatment

There is no need to panic or get alarmed because convulsions stop automatically within a brief period. The child should be placed on his back on a bed. The head should be turned to one side so that the secretions in the mouth are drained out and the tongue does not

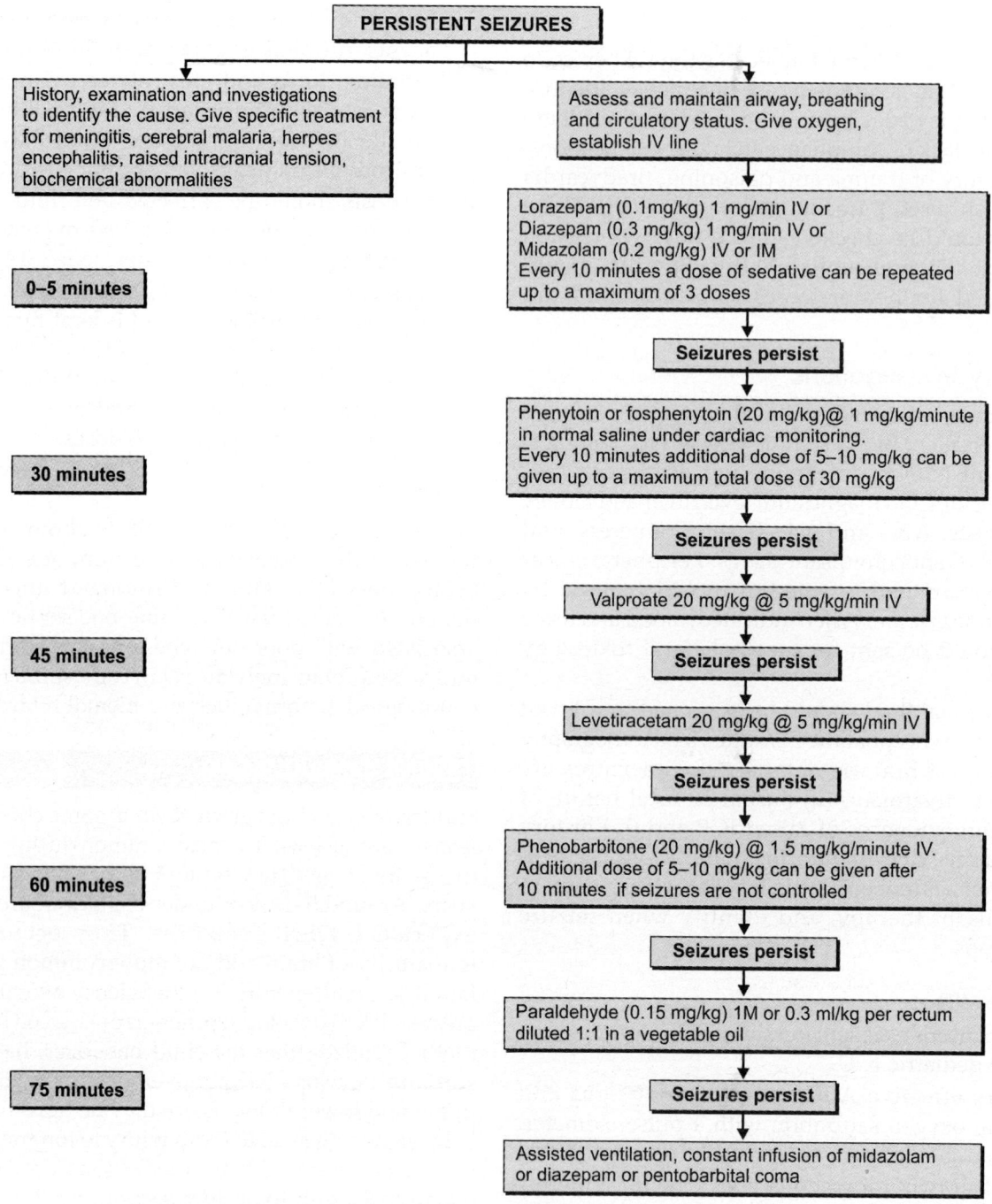

PERSISTENT SEIZURES

History, examination and investigations to identify the cause. Give specific treatment for meningitis, cerebral malaria, herpes encephalitis, raised intracranial tension, biochemical abnormalities

Assess and maintain airway, breathing and circulatory status. Give oxygen, establish IV line

0–5 minutes

Lorazepam (0.1mg/kg) 1 mg/min IV or Diazepam (0.3 mg/kg) 1 mg/min IV or Midazolam (0.2 mg/kg) IV or IM
Every 10 minutes a dose of sedative can be repeated up to a maximum of 3 doses

Seizures persist

Phenytoin or fosphenytoin (20 mg/kg)@ 1 mg/kg/minute in normal saline under cardiac monitoring.
Every 10 minutes additional dose of 5–10 mg/kg can be given up to a maximum total dose of 30 mg/kg

30 minutes

Seizures persist

Valproate 20 mg/kg @ 5 mg/kg/min IV

45 minutes

Seizures persist

Levetiracetam 20 mg/kg @ 5 mg/kg/min IV

Seizures persist

Phenobarbitone (20 mg/kg) @ 1.5 mg/kg/minute IV. Additional dose of 5–10 mg/kg can be given after 10 minutes if seizures are not controlled

60 minutes

Seizures persist

Paraldehyde (0.15 mg/kg) 1M or 0.3 ml/kg per rectum diluted 1:1 in a vegetable oil

75 minutes

Seizures persist

Assisted ventilation, constant infusion of midazolam or diazepam or pentobarbital coma

Figure 42.1 Algorithm for pharmacotherapy of status epilepticus

fall back into the throat, blocking the opening of wind pipe. Do not restrain the child to stop the convulsions and never pour water on his face. No attempt should be made to open his mouth by inserting a spoon.

The temperature should be brought down by switching on the fan and sponging the body with tap water. When child is conscious give paracetamol to bring down the temperature. In an unconscious child, paracetamol and diazepam can be given per rectum. Febrile convulsions do not cause any damage to the brain and they do not occur after the age of 5–6 years. When convulsions are prolonged for more than 10 minutes or child is getting repeated convulsions during a bout of fever (atypical or complex febrile convulsions), he must be investigated for meningitis. When a child is known to suffer from febrile convulsions, parents should be vigilant (not worried) to give him paracetamol and diazepam or clobazam at the earliest evidence of fever. The underlying iron deficiency should be treated which may reduce the frequency of

42

febrile seizures. The condition should not be confused with epilepsy which needs long-term anticonvulsant therapy.

Prognosis

Prognosis of simple febrile convulsions is excellent without any risk of neuromotor disability or death. In case of complex or atypical febrile convulsions, the prognosis depend on underlying cause. In some families, there is an increased risk of development of temporal lobe epilepsy in adult life.

Role of a Nurse in the Care of an Epileptic Child

1. Parents should be explained about the care of the child during an episode of seizure.
2. They should stay calm and protect the child against injury.
3. Do not attempt to restrain the child or try to insert a spoon in the mouth or sprinkle water over face or make him smell a shoe.
4. The child should be put on the bed with head turned to one side to prevent aspiration.
5. Educate the family regarding compliance of therapy and importance of uninterrupted administration of antiepileptic drugs (AEDs). The timings of administration of AEDs should be fixed and not flexible.
6. Nurse should explain the common side effects of antiepileptic drugs being taken by the child.
7. Child should be encouraged to take a nutritious diet with supplements of vitamins especially vitamin D and folic acid.
8. Educate parents and the child regarding avoidance of certain activities that may pose danger to life in the event of an unexpected seizure like swimming and driving motor vehicles.
9. Emphasize the importance of regular follow-up and provide emotional support to the family against any stigma.
10. Drug therapy is tapered or weaned off slowly when patient is seizure-free for 2 years or more. Some children with CNS abnormalities may need life-long anticonvulsant therapy.

PYOGENIC MENINGITIS

Inflammation of the "meninges", the membranes covering the brain and spinal cord, is called meningitis. It may be caused by bacterial (pyogenic and tubercular), viral and fungal infections. Acute pyogenic meningitis is a serious life-threatening disease, may manifest in a couple of hours or days. The typical symptoms include fever, severe headache, vomiting and convulsions. Neck stiffness and dislike for bright light (photophobia) are common. The child may become drowsy or unconscious. In young infants, anterior fontanel (soft spot on the top of the head) becomes tense, bulging and non pulsatile. Skin rash due to small bleeding spots inside the skin (petechiae) may occur in cases of meningococcal meningitis.

Diagnosis

Peripheral blood shows marked polymorphonuclear leukocytosis and elevated CRP. Diagnosis is established by CSF examination which is turbid, pleocytosis with polymorphonuclear cells, high protein and grossly reduced sugar. Direct smear and culture of CSF may reveal the causative organisms. Blood culture may be positive.

Treatment

When child is suspected to have meningitis he must be admitted in the hospital without delay. Early and effective treatment of meningitis is associated with complete recovery. Children with pyogenic meningitis require intravenous administration of a combination of third-generation cephalosporin, cefotaxime (150–200 mg/kg/d q 12 hr) or ceftriaxone (50 mg/kg/d single daily dose) and vancomycin (60 mg/kg/d q 6 hr) and excellent supportive care for a minimum period of 10 to 14 days. Administration of dexamethasone (0.15 mg/kg/dose) 15 minutes before administration of first dose of antibiotic and subsequently every 4–6 hours for 4–5 days reduces the risk of deafness in meningitis due to *H. influenzae type b* (Hib). Anticonvulsants may be required to control seizures. When treatment is delayed or is unsatisfactory, it may lead to permanent brain damage, neuromotor disability and deafness.

Nursing Care

1. Children with pyogenic meningitis need excellent supportive and symptomatic care.
2. Monitor vital signs, input-output chart, level of consciousness and evidences of raised intracranial pressure.
3. Administration of adequate fluids and electrolytes maintains cerebral perfusion. Fluid restriction is indicated if there is hyponatremia because of SIADH.
4. Raised ICP is treated with a standard protocol.
5. Ensure timely administration of antibiotics and anticonvulsants.
6. Prevent risk of nosocomial infection by following aseptic routines, maintenance of orodental hygiene and providing care to the eyes.

42

7. Provide care to the bowels and bladder. Constipation is managed by rectal enema or insertion of glycerine suppository to prevent atony of rectum. Retention of urine is managed by gentle suprapubic pressure or a hot-water bottle.

8. The family should be provided with emotional support to allay their anxiety and stress. She should provide guidance to the family regarding the need for chemoprophylaxis to prevent the disease among the contacts.

Chemoprophylaxis to contacts Patients with meningitis are contagious to close contacts through their oral secretions or respiratory droplets. Chemoprophylaxis is given to all household contacts, staff members and children in the day care center or nursery school, where two or more children have suffered from pyogenic meningitis **(Table 42.4)**.

Prevention

There is no single vaccine to ensure protection against meningitis because it is caused by several bacteria. Hib vaccine provides protection against meningitis due to *H. influenzae type b* and can be administered along with triple antigen. Meningococcal vaccine is recommended to be taken if there is an epidemic of meningococcal meningitis. Pneumococcal vaccine can be given to high-risk children to prevent pneumococcal meningitis. For details regarding these vaccines refer to **Chapter 21**.

TUBERCULAR MENINGITIS

Infants and young children are more likely to have disseminated tuberculosis including tubercular meningitis. Primary site of tuberculosis in the body may or may not be present. Children get infection by a close contact with an adult suffering from tuberculosis. Tuberculosis may involve any organ of the body but tubercular meningitis is relatively common in infants and carries poor prognosis. BCG vaccination does provide protection against disseminated form of tuberculosis and reduces the risk of development of tubercular meningitis.

Clinical Features

Prodromal stage Child gradually becomes irritable, listless with lack of interest in his toys and surroundings. There is loss of appetite and low to moderate grade fever. This stage lasts for 2–4 weeks.

Stage of meningeal irritation Child is febrile with episodes of headache, irritability and vomiting. There is neck rigidity, positive Kernig's sign and opisthotonos (hyperextension of trunk like a bow). Anterior fontanel is bulging and tense. Seizures may occur with alteration in consciousness. Fundus may show papilledema (swelling of optic disk) or optic atrophy with tubercles in the choroid.

Terminal stage This stage is characterized by deep coma, dilated pupils, spasticity of the limbs and recurrent seizures. The child gradually lapses into persistent vegetative state.

Diagnosis

Primary tubercular focus should be identified by doing a detailed physical examination by looking for enlargement of peripheral lymph nodes and hepatosplenomegaly. X-ray chest and Mantoux test should be done. There may be no BCG scar. Mantoux test may be negative because child is critically sick and often immunocompromised. Skiagram of chest may show evidences of miliary tuberculosis or primary pulmonary complex. CSF examination shows straw colored fluid with formation of a coagulum on standing, raised proteins, slightly low sugar (not as low as in pyogenic meningitis) and presence of lymphocytes. Tubercular bacilli may be demonstrated on the smear prepared from the coagulum and on culture studies. CT scan of the brain shows inflammation and exudates in the basilar region with dilatation of ventricles. At times it

Table 42.4 Guidelines for chemoprophylaxis

Disease	Drugs	Age of the contact	Dosage
Haemophilus influenzae type b meningitis	Rifampicin	<1 month	10 mg/kg single daily dose for 4 days
		1 month–12 years	20 mg/kg single daily dose for 4 days
Meningococcal meningitis*	Rifampicin	<1 month	5 mg/kg twice a day for 2 days
		1 month–12 years	10 mg/kg twice a day for 2 days
	Ceftriaxone	<12 years	125 mg single dose IM
		>12 years	250 mg single dose IM
	Ciprofloxacin	Adults	500 mg single dose

*Anyone of the three options for chemoprophylaxis can be used.

may be difficult to differentiate tubercular meningitis from chronic or partially treated acute pyogenic meningitis.

Treatment

Excellent supportive and nursing care is required. Nasogastric feeding is given to provide adequate calories, proteins and micronutrients. Fluid and electrolyte balance should be maintained. Anticonvulsants like diazepam and phenytoin are given to control seizures. Hypertonic mannitol 20% and furosemide may be used to reduce cerebral edema. Specific therapy consists in administration of antitubercular drugs (streptomycin, pyrazinamide, INH and rifampicin) along with corticosteroids to prevent development of adhesions in the subarachnoid space. Prednisolone, streptomycin and pyrazinamide are given for a period of 2 months while INH and rifampicin is continued for 9 months to one year. Prognosis is guarded and depends upon the stage of the disease. The long-term sequelae include paralyses, convulsions, hydrocephalus, mental retardation, deafness and blindness.

ENCEPHALITIS AND ENCEPHALOPATHIES

Encephalitis is defined as inflammation of the brain parenchyma (encephalon) which can cause permanent neurologic disability and death. When there are associated features of meningeal irritation, it is called meningoencephalitis. The term encephalopathy refers to cerebral dysfunction due to toxins, post infectious, (typhoid fever, shigella, Reye syndrome), allergic, hypoxic, metabolic disorders and electrolyte disturbances. The common viruses causing encephalitis in India include Japanese encephalitis, herpes viruses, enteroviruses, measles, mumps and rubella. Encephalopathy may occur following administration of certain vaccines like whole-cell pertussis, rabies, chickenpox, measles and yellow fever.

Clinical Features

The onset is sudden with development of fever, headache, vomiting and progressive alteration of consciousness. There may be marked irritability, agitation, confusion, delirium, stupor and coma. Seizures and neurological deficits are common. Encephalitic features predominate, whereas meningeal signs are minimal or absent. Progressive rise in intracranial pressure because of cerebral edema leads to decerebration, hippocampal herniation and involvement of cardiorespiratory centers.

Laboratory Investigations

Cerebrospinal fluid (CSF) examination shows raised pressure with lymphocytic pleocytosis, elevation of protein and normal or slightly raised glucose level. Detection of specific antigen or antibodies by PCR or ELISA in the CSF provide etiologic diagnosis but these tests are available in advanced centers. Electroencephalographic (EEG) findings are non-specific except in herpes simplex encephalitis (HSE), which is characterized by 2 to 3 Hz periodic lateralized epileptiform discharges. Neuroimaging studies especially MRI are useful to exclude tuberculous meningitis, herpes simplex encephalitis, Japanese encephalitis, acute demyelinating encephalomyelitis (ADEM) and space occupying lesions of brain.

Nursing Care

The mainstay of therapy is supportive and symptomatic care because there are limited options for specific therapy. The child should be admitted in the pediatric intensive care unit (PICU) and therapeutic measures are instituted to protect the brain from further damage.

Supportive Care

1. Monitor vital signs.
2. Maintain adequacy of airway, breathing and circulation (ABC) and internal homeostasis.
3. Input-output charting with maintenance of fluids, glucose, electrolytes and acid-base status within normal range.
4. Control body temperature with a safe antipyretic agent (paracetamol 15 mg/kg/dose every 4–6 hours) and hydrotherapy with tepid water sponging.
5. Seizures are controlled by administration of intravenous lorazepam or diazepam followed by maintenance therapy with phenytoin.
6. Ranitidine is given to prevent stress ulcers in the stomach.
7. Nasogastric tube feeding is started once patient is stabilized and convulsions are controlled.
8. Provide nursing care to the comatosed child.

Measures to Reduce Intracranial Pressure

1. Keep the head raised by 15 degrees.
2. Administer 20% mannitol (0.5 g/kg every 4–6 hours for 4–6 doses) and intravenous furosemide (1–2 mg/kg every 6–8 hours for 4–6 doses).
3. Maintain arterial carbon dioxide tension ($PaCO_2$) between 25 and 30 mm Hg by hyperventilation.
4. There is no role of corticosteroids except in patients with brain tumor and acute demyelinating encephalomyelitis (ADEM).

42

5. Surgical decompression is life saving if there is impending herniation of the brain stem.

Specific Therapy

Antihypertensives are life saving for treatment of hypertensive encephalopathy. Specific chemotherapeutic agents are available for treatment of cerebral malaria, herpes simplex encephalitis, tuberculosis, typhoid, shigella and antidotes for specific toxins and poisons.

Prognosis

Outcome is uniformly bad in all types of encephalomyelitis. There is high case fatality rate and high risk of neuromotor sequelae, among the survivors. The common sequelae include recurrent seizures, spastic paralyses involving one or several limbs, learning disability and mental retardation.

Prevention

Vaccines are available for prevention of several diseases which are associated with encephalopathy, namely tuberculosis, typhoid fever, measles, mumps and rubella, rabies, yellow fever and Japanese encephalitis. Availability of acellular pertussis vaccine has reduced the risk of encephalopathy as a side effect. The risk of Reye syndrome can be reduced by avoidance of use of salicylates in children with viral infections especially chickenpox. Poisoning due to heavy metals and insectisides can be prevented by proper guidance and education to the parents.

THE CHILD WITH COMA

Alteration in sensorium occurs due to dysfunction of cerebral hemispheres, structural lesions, metabolic or toxic effects on the central nervous system. The stages of altered consciousness are summarized in **Box 42.1**. Coma is a life-threatening emergency and is defined as a state of decreased consciousness from which the child cannot be aroused by ordinary verbal, sensory or physical stimuli. The Glasgow Coma Scale (with its modifications in children) is simple and useful to objectively assess the severity of coma (**Table 42.5**).

Causes

The common causes of non-traumatic coma in children are listed in **Table 42.6**. The CNS infections is the leading cause and account for two-thirds of cases.

Clinical Assessment

History should be taken for nature of onset (slow insidious, acute, sudden), associated symptoms, ingestion of drugs or poisons and any trauma. History of fever

Box 42.1   Stages of altered consciousness

Confusion There is inability to think clearly with presence of disorientation for time, place and person.

Drowsy There is reduced awareness or wakefulness and presence of hyperexcitability with irritability, alternating with drowsiness or clouding of consciousness.

Delirium Patient has restlessness, disorientation, hyperactivity, hallucinations and talkativeness.

Obtundation There is increased sleep, reduced alertness with mental blunting.

Persistent vegetative state The patient has complete lack of awareness of self and environment but has periods of wakefulness and sleep. There is no comprehension of language, any speech, voluntary movements, emotional or social interactions.

Stupor or semicoma The child is unresponsive but arousable by vigorous repeated stimuli but lapses back to unresponsiveness when stimulus is withdrawn.

Coma Unresponsive and unarousable by any stimulus.

with vomiting, headache and seizures are suggestive of meningitis, encephalitis and cerebral malaria. Anuria and jaundice are suggestive of renal and hepatic dysfunction. Child should be examined for signs of meningeal irritation, raised intracranial tension and elevated blood pressure. Brainstem reflexes should be checked. Eyes should be examined for size of pupils and fundus examined for papilledema, optic atrophy and retinal hemorrhages. Episodes of flexion and adduction of upper and lower limbs (decorticate posture) are suggestive of high pontine lesions, and bilateral involvement of cerebral hemispheres. When midbrain and medulla are involved, child develops decerebrate rigidity (episodes of hyperextension and inversion of upper and lower limbs with opisthotonos), non-reactive pupils and irregular breathing.

Laboratory Investigations

Complete blood counts, smear for malarial parasites, blood glucose, electrolytes, liver and renal functions, toxicology screen, blood ammonia and lactate level and ABG studies should be obtained. Gastric aspirate should be sent to a poison control laboratory when poisoning is suspected. Urine should be screened for glucose and ketones. Lumbar puncture is done when meningitis or encephalitis is suspected. Neuroimaging studies (CT scan and MRI) are done when there are evidences of trauma, structural lesions, raised ICP and focal neurological deficits. Portable facilities for monitoring EEG and evoked potentials are useful for assessment and prognosis.

42

Table 42.5 Modified Glasgow coma scale

	Eye opening	
Score	>1 y	<1 y
4	Spontaneously	Spontaneously
3	To verbal command	To shout
2	To pain	To pain
1	No response	No response

	Best motor response	
Score	>1 y	<1 y
6	Obeys	Spontaneous
5	Localizes pain	Localizes pain
4	Flexion withdrawal	Flexion withdrawal
3	Flexion abnormal (decorticate rigidity)	Flexion abnormal (decorticate rigidity)
2	Extension (decerebrate rigidity)	Extension (decerebrate rigidity)
1	No response	No response

	Best verbal response		
Score	>5 y	2–5 y	<2 y
5	Oriented and converses	Appropriate words and phrases	Smiles, coos appropriately
4	Disoriented and converses	Inappropriate words	Cries, consolable
3	Appropriate words	Persistent cries and screams	Persistent inappropriate or inconsolable crying or screaming
2	Incomprehensible sounds	Grunts	Grunts, agitated, or restless
1	No response	No response	No response

y; years

Table 42.6 Common causes of non-traumatic coma

- **Infections**
  - ☐ Meningitis (pyogenic, tubercular, fungal)
  - ☐ Encephalitis, acute disseminated encephalomyelitis (viral, vaccinal, post-infectious)
  - ☐ Cerebral malaria
  - ☐ Brain abscess
- **Metabolic conditions**
  - ☐ Diabetic ketoacidosis
  - ☐ Hypoglycemia
  - ☐ Reye syndrome
  - ☐ Hepatic encephalopathy
  - ☐ Acute renal failure
  - ☐ Dyselectrolytemia
- **Drugs and poisons**
  - ☐ Sedatives
  - ☐ Salicylates
  - ☐ Organophosphates
  - ☐ Snake bite, scorpion sting
- **Miscellaneous conditions**
  - ☐ Postictal (status epilepticus)
  - ☐ Hypoxic–ischemic encephalopathy
  - ☐ Space occupying lesions of brain
  - ☐ Demyelinating disorders of CNS
  - ☐ Hypertensive encephalopathy

Management

After initial stabilization in the emergency room, the comatose child should be shifted to the pediatric ICU.

Supportive Care and Monitoring

1. Monitor vital signs, evidences of raised ICP and fluid intake and output.
2. Maintain patency of airways, adequacy of breathing, circulation (ABC) and normal body temperature.
3. Fluids and electrolytes should be provided to correct any abnormalities and maintain adequate tissue perfusion.
4. Raised ICP should be managed by a standard protocol and anticonvulsants given for control of seizures.
5. Adequate nutrition should be maintained by nasogastric feeding. When intravenous therapy is required for more than 3–4 days, total parenteral nutrition is provided.

Specific Treatment

1. Antibiotics for treatment of pyogenic meningitis or sepsis and antitubercular drugs are given when TBM is the likely possibility.

42

2. Acyclovir 10 mg/kg every 8 hours is given intravenously for 10–14 days for treatment of herpes encephalitis.

3. Methyl prednisolone 30 mg/kgIM once daily for 5 days is given to children with acute demyelinating encephalomyelitis (ADEM).

4. Antimalarials are given for treatment of cerebral malaria.

5. Antidotes for specific poisonings and insect bites are life saving.

6. Diabetic ketoacidosis, hepatic encephalopathy, acute renal failure and hypertensive encephalopathy are treated by standard protocols.

7. Surgical decompression is indicated for treatment of brain abscess, subdural effusion, space occupying lesion and transtentorial herniation.

Nursing Care of a Comatosed Child

Depending upon the degree of unconsciousness, the child may be having confusion, delirium, stupor or coma. It is useful to evaluate consciousness by the acronym "AVPU".

A = **A**lert and Awake
V = Responsive to **V**erbal stimuli
P = Responsive to **P**ainful stimuli
U = **U**nresponsive to any stimulus

1. *Maintenance of clear airway* The child is nursed in a lateral or semiprone position with no pillow under the head. The oral cavity and pharynx should be sucked frequently to prevent aspiration. Oxygen should be administered if there is hypoxia.

2. *Vital signs* Vital signs should be monitored as advised by the physician. Involvement of brainstem is associated with marked lability of vital signs. The size of pupils and their response to light should be checked. Evidences of raised ICP should be looked for.

3. *Fluid and electrolyte balance* In comatosed children, fluid restriction is advised due to risk of fluid overload because of inappropriate secretion of antidiuretic hormone (SIADH). A strict input and output chart should be maintained. Accurate collection of urine output with a condom (boys) or a urine collection bag (girls) and at times by an indwelling urinary catheter is recommended.

4. *Ensure adequate nutrition* Basal needs for calories, proteins and micronutrients should be provided by nasogastric feeding. Nutritional supplements can be added in the milk-based feeds. When intravenous therapy is required for more than 3–4 days, total parenteral nutrition (TPN) is advised.

5. *Body sponging and orodental hygiene* The child should be sponged daily and kept tidy, neat and clean. Teeth and oral cavity should be thoroughly cleaned every 8 hourly with gauze soaked in antiseptic mouth wash.

6. *Posture and comfort* Provide a comfortable soft bed with a clean bed sheet. The paralysed limb should be placed in such a position that in the event of incomplete recovery and contracture formation, limb is preserved in most useful or functional position. Lower limbs are kept slightly flexed at hips and knee joints by placing a small pillow under the knees. The feet should be kept at right angles by placing sand bags against the soles or by using right angled splint. Upper limb is kept adducted at the shoulder with forearm flexed at right angle and in semiprone position at the elbow. A splint is used at the back of the wrist to prevent hyperextension of the hand. Fingers are kept in a semiflexed position by placing a soft ball of an appropriate size in the palm and splinting the fingers around it.

7. *Care of pressure sites* Frequent changes of posture and provision of a soft bed helps to prevent pressure sores. It is often forgotten that back of the head is commonly affected by bed sore in children. Mother should be advised to change the position of the child every 1–2 hours. This also helps in the expansion of lungs and facilitates drainage of tracheobronchial secretions.

8. *Care of eyes* In a comatosed child, eyes are partially open and corneal reflexes are usually absent. There is increased risk of dryness of cornea and development of corneal ulcers. Antibacterial eye ointment or protective oily eye drops should be instilled frequently in the eyes. The eyes should be covered with sterile paraffin gauze pads with lids closed.

9. *Care of bladder and bowels* Bladder paralysis may lead to constant dribbling or incontinence of urine. More commonly, there is retention of urine with overflow incontinence. In these children, suprapubic pressure is applied gently every 2–3 hours to evacuate the bladder. Indwelling urinary catheter should be avoided. These children are prone to develop urinary tract infection and hydronephrosis because of stasis of urine and incomplete emptying of bladder.

Bowel paralysis usually leads to constipation and fecal impaction. Gentle massage of the left side of the abdomen from above downwards may help in evacuation of bowel. Glycerine suppository or enema may be required after every 2–3 days. Intake of fruit juice, honey, lactulose and fluids may keep the feces soft to facilitate easier evacuation. Whenever bottom is cleaned, perineum should be thoroughly dried and silicone based cream is applied to provide a protective barrier to the skin.

10. *Physiotherapy* When condition of the child is stabilized, active and passive movements of the limbs should be encouraged. Full range of passive movements should be carried out at all the joints. In children with flaccid paralysis, when muscle pain has disappeared, limbs should be massaged 2–3 times a day, starting from fingers and toes and going upwards. This helps to prevent venous stasis and thrombosis, and improves the tone of the muscles. During follow-up, the child may need orthopedic appliances like calipers, walking aids, special shoes, etc. Surgery may be required for release and correction of contractures.

11. *Management of associated problems* Associated fever, seizures, and raised intracranial pressure would need symptomatic care. Some of these patients may develop neuromotor sequelae like mental retardation, visual and hearing problems, speech defects and behavior disorders, which would need the help and guidance of a number of specialists. Vocational training and occupational therapy may be required to make them useful and productive members of the society.

ACUTE FLACCID PARALYSIS

Acute flaccid paralysis (AFP) is defined as paralysis of acute onset (<4 weeks) with limp, floppy or flaccid limb/s. Muscle tone is diminished as assessed on palpation of muscles or passive movements of joints but sensations are normal. The commonest cause of AFP is acute paralytic poliomyelitis (due to wild virus) or vaccine-related poliomyelitis. The non-polio causes of AFP include Guillain-Barré syndrome, transverse myelitis, and traumatic neuritis (sciatic nerve damage due to wrongly administered gluteal injection). The prevalence rate of non-polio AFP is reported to be around 1:1,00,000 population.

Guillain-Barré Syndrome

It is post-infectious polyneuropathy due to alteration of the protein component of the myelin because of an autoimmune mechanism. The predisposing viral infections include *Epstein-Barr* virus, influenza, measles, mumps, enteroviruses or administration of a neural vaccine for rabies.

Clinical features There is sudden onset of symmetrical paralysis of muscles, which starts from legs and rapidly ascends to involve the muscles of upper limbs, abdomen, chest and face (Landry ascending paralysis). The weakness is more marked in the proximal group of muscles. There is hypotonia, sluggish or absent deep tendon jerks and flexor plantar response. Bilateral facial nerve involvement is common lending to expressionless face, paucity of facial movements and inability to close the eyes firmly. Subjective sensory symptoms like paresthesias and tingling sensations are common. Respiratory insufficiency may occur if intercostal muscles and diaphragm are involved.

Diagnosis The CSF examination shows the characteristic albuminocytological dissociation. There is no pleocytosis, but protein level is grossly elevated. Electromyography (EMG) is normal while nerve conduction studies may show abnormalities of demyelination after 3 weeks of onset.

Treatment The disease is self-limiting with spontaneous recovery in most cases during a period of few weeks to months. Early administration of intravenous immunoglobulins (IVIG) 300–400 mg/kg/day through IV route for 5 days is associated with good response. Plasmapheresis is also a useful therapeutic modality. Assisted ventilation is life-saving if there is paralysis of respiratory muscles. Physiotherapy should be continued till complete recovery takes place.

Acute Paralytic Poliomyelitis

Poliomyelitis is caused by single-stranded RNA viruses of Picornaviridae family and infection may occur with one of the three distinct serotypes, namely 1, 2 and 3. Polio viruses circulate in summer and fall, transmission occurs by close contact, mostly through fecal-oral route. Pregnancy, B cell immunodeficiency, strenuous excercise and intramuscular injection during the incubation period increases the risk of development of paralytic disease. Polio viruses cause neural damage by involvement of anterior horn cells. Because of global launch of pulse polio immunization program, poliomyelitis has become rare and is likely to be eradicated from the world in next 2–3 years.

Clinical features After an incubation period of 7–14 days, the disease starts with fever, malaise, headache, nausea and loss of appetite. Most cases recover spontaneously without any further progression. In some cases, the minor illness is followed by onset of pain and stiffness in the neck with appearance of signs of meningeal irritation. There is neck rigidity, inability

42

to kiss the knees (stiff back), child sits with support of hands which are placed behind the buttocks (tripod sign). The paralytic phase is heralded by muscle pains, tenderness of muscles, flaccidity of neck (head drop) and limbs and absent deep tendon jerks. The distribution of paralysed muscles is characteristically asymmetrical due to patchy involvement of anterior horn cells. Death may occur due to involvement of respiratory muscles and bulbar paralysis. Salient differences between acute paralytic poliomyelitis and GBS are shown in **Table 42.7**.

Diagnosis The diagnosis is usually based on the history and characteristic clinical manifestation of asymmetrical flaccid paralysis. CSF examination shows mild pleocytosis (polymorphonuclear cells for first 1–2 days, followed by lymphocytes) with normal or mild elevation of protein and normal biochemistry. Polio virus can be isolated from the CSF, oropharynx and urine during early stage of illness. EMG abnormalities are observed after 3 weeks of onset of the disease.

Treatment The treatment is supportive and symptomatic. Paracetamol and hot wet packs are useful for relief of muscle pains and spasm. The paralyzed limbs should be placed in a position of maximum comfort and function, with the help of sand bags. Physiotherapy is started once pain and muscle spasms are relieved. Patients with involvement of respiratory muscles demand excellent nursing care to prevent aspiration of pharyngeal secretions and feeds. Timely assisted ventilation is life saving. Prolonged physiotherapy, occupational therapy and orthopedic support are required during follow-up.

AFP Surveillance

The government of India has launched AFP surveillance program to complement national polio eradication program or pulse polio immunization program. It is mandatory that all children under 15 years of age, who manifest with AFP, should be investigated, followed up, classified and reported to the health authorities as per following protocol.

i. Collect 2 adequate stool (8–10 g each) samples, atleast 24 hours apart, preferably within 14 days of onset of paralysis (up to maximum of 60 days of onset). The stool samples should be stored properly under cold chain and sent to WHO approved testing laboratory.

ii. The report of viral isolation from stool samples is likely to take 8 weeks. In the meantime, the outbreak response of providing OPV to all the potential contacts should be operationalized.

iii. The patient should be followed up and classified as follows:

a. *Acute paralytic poliomyelitis* The wild polio virus has been isolated from the stools.

Table 42.7 Salient differences between acute poliomyelitis and Guillain-Barré syndrome (GBS)

Features	Poliomyelitis	Guillain-Barré syndrome
Age	<5 years	All ages
Fever	Common during acute stage	May occur 2–3 weeks before the onset of paralysis
Meningeal signs	May be seen	Absent
Muscle pains and tenderness	Common	Uncommon
Progression	Rapid over 24–48 hours	Slow over a period of 1–2 weeks
Symmetry	Asymmetrical involving one or all the four limbs	Symmetrical, legs affected more than arms
Sensory features	None	Subjective sensory symptoms are common
Cranial nerves	May be involved in bulbar polio	Bilateral facial involvement, ophthalmoplegia and bulbar nerves are involved
Atrophy of muscles	Rapid and evident within 5–7 days	Absent or delayed onset of atrophy
CSF findings	Pleocytosis with mild elevation of protein, polio virus can be isolated	No pleocytosis with significant elevation of protein (albuminocytological dissociation)
Electrophysiology	Acute denervation and reduced action potentials	Reduced conduction velocity of nerves
Treatment	Symptomatic and supportive	IVIG and plasmapheresis are credited to enhance recovery
Prognosis	Poor	Good
Prevention	Oral and injectable polio vaccines are available	None

42

b. *Polio-compatible AFP*
- Stools specimens were inadequate or unsatisfactory (dry, leaking, poorly stored sample, etc).
- Residual muscle weakness was present after 60 days of onset of paralysis or follow-up on day 60 was not done either due to death of the patient or non compliance of the family.
- The "Expert review" believes that the case is most likely to be polio on the basis of available data.

INTRACRANIAL SPACE OCCUPYING LESIONS

The space occupying lesions (SOL) in the brain occur due to brain tumors, infections or inflammatory conditions (brain abscess, inflammatory granulomas due to cysticercosis and tuberculosis, subdural effusion), developmental defects (angiomatous malformation, aneurysm) and intracranial bleeding due to trauma. Brain tumors may be infratentorial (medulloblastoma and astrocytoma of cerebellum, and gliomas of the brainstem) or supratentorial (craniopharyngioma, glioma, ependymoma, and optic nerve glioma). In children, infratentorial tumors are more common and they produce early features of raised intracranial pressure and cerebellar signs.

Clinical Features

There are non-specific clinical features of raised intracranial pressure (ICP) and specific or localizing symptoms depending on the site, size and nature of SOL. The clinical features of raised ICP are shared by non-mass lesions, namely congenital hydrocephalus, meningitis, encephalopathy, cerebral edema and pseudotumor cerebri.

The common symptoms of raised ICP include headache, vomiting and increase in head size. Headache is most severe when patient wakes up and gradually decreases in severity by afternoon or evening. It may be associated with vomiting but there is no nausea. In infants, when sutures are open, there is progressive increase in head size. Anterior fontanel becomes bulging and non-pulsatile and its closure is delayed. Tapping of skull may elicit "cracked pot" sound (Macewen sign) due to separation of sutures. The onset of papilledema is delayed because rise in intracranial pressure is buffered by enlargement in head size. The downward displacement of brainstem may cause damage to 6th cranial nerve with lateral or divergent squint and diplopia (double vision). The stretching of brainstem and medulla causes compression of vasomotor centers leading to bradycardia, cardiac dysrhythmia, irregularity of breathing and elevation of blood pressure.

Focal neurological signs Depending upon the site of SOL, specific and focal neurological signs are seen. Ataxia of trunk (truncal ataxia), unsteady gait, incoordination, hypotonia and sluggish deep tendon jerks are seen in children with medulloblastoma and astrocytoma in the cerebellopontine angle. Isolated sixth nerve palsy has no localizing value because it may occur due to increased intracranial pressure due to any cause. In pontine glioma, multiple cranial nerve palsies are seen. Bulbar paralysis may occur due to involvement of ninth to twelfth cranial nerves or their nuclei. It is characterized by pooling of secretions in posterior pharynx, drooling of saliva, dysphagia, nasal regurgitation, dysarthria and nasal twang. Seizures may occur because of cortical or subcortical lesions, whereas infratentorial tumors may cause decerebrate posturing. Craniopharyngioma and hypothalamic glioma may cause endocrinal abnormalities. Spasticity with motor deficits and exaggerated deep tendon jerks and extensor plantars are seen because of involvement of cerebral hemispheres and spinal tracts.

Diagnosis

Fundus examination is done to exclude optic atrophy (glioma of optic chiasma) and papilledema (raised ICP). Lumbar puncture is contraindicated if there is papilledema because of risk of transtentorial herniation. The diagnosis can be confirmed by radioimaging studies like CT scan or MRI of the brain. Gadolinium-enhanced MRI increases its usefulness for evaluation and follow-up of SOL.

Treatment

Supportive and symptomatic treatment is provided for control of seizures, raised ICP, associated endocrinal abnormalities, risk of aspiration and choking and maintenance of feeding and nutrition. Dexamethasone (0.5 mg/kg every 6 hour IM or IV) is useful to control vasogenic edema before taking the patient for surgery. Depending upon the nature and location of tumor, surgical excision is done with a gamma knife and is followed by cranial irradiation when indicated on the basis of histopathological diagnosis.

BIBLIOGRAPHY

Baumann RJ, Duffner PK. American Academy of Pediatrics. Treatment of children with simple febrile seizures: The AAP practice parameters. *Pediatr Neurol* 2003, 23(1): 11–17.

42

Farinha NJ, Razali KA, Holzel H, et al. Tuberculosis of the central nervous system in children: A 20 years survey. *J Infect* 2000, 41(1): 61–68.

Ferrari S, Toniola A, Monaco S, et al. Viral encephalitis: Etiology, clinical features, diagnosis and management. *Opin Infect Disease J* 2009, 3:1–12.

Karceski S, Moerreli M, Carpenter D. Expert consensus guideline series. Treatment of epilepsy. *Epilepsy Behav* 2001, 2:1–50.

Leven M. The clinical conundrum of neonatal seizures. *Arch Dis Child* 2002, 86: 75–77.

Rose W, Kirubakaran C, Scott JX. Intermittent clobazam therapy in febrile seizures. *Indian J Pediatr* 2005, 72(1): 31–33.

Swartz MN. Bacterial meningitis: A view of the past 90 years. *N Engl J Med* 2004, 351(18): 1826–1828.

Walker DM, Teach SJ. Update on the acute management of status epilepticus in children. *Curr Opin Pediatr* 2006, 18(3): 239–244.

Warviru C, Appleton R. Febrile seizures: an update. *Arch Dis Child* 2004, 89(8): 751–756.

Endocrinal Disorders

INTRODUCTION

Endocrine glands are ductless glands that secrete hormones which have profound physiological and biological effects on physical growth, mental and psychological development, sexual maturation, chemical homeostasis, metabolic and reproductive processes of the body. The hormones or secretions of endocrine glands are directly released into the blood stream. They exert their physiological effects through the receptors and specific binding sites in the target tissues.

The endocrine glands are located deep in the midline of the body. The supreme or master endocrine gland is hypothalamic-pituitary axis that produces growth hormone and controls the functioning of other endocrine glands by a feedback mechanism by production of a variety of trophic hormones. The other endocrine glands from neck downwards include thyroid and parathyroid glands, thymus, pancreas (islet-cells), adrenal gland (located at upper poles of kidneys), and gonads (ovaries and testes). It is interesting that the location of endocrine glands corresponds to various energy fields or *Chakras* that are used in yogic and meditation practices to release hidden potential energy from spinal cord and brain **(Figure 43.1)**.

HYPOTHYROIDISM

Among various hormonal disorders in children, cretinism due to congenital thyroid deficiency is the most common. It may occur due to absence or ectopic location of thyroid gland (which is normally located below Adam's apple infront of the neck) or due to defective production of hormones (thyroid dysgenesis). Cretinism may occur due to deficiency of iodine which is widely prevalent in our country but is a more serious problem in sub-Himalayan region and hilly terrains. Many people in these areas develop enlargement of thyroid gland (goiter). Their children are more likely to suffer from various grades of thyroid deficiency.

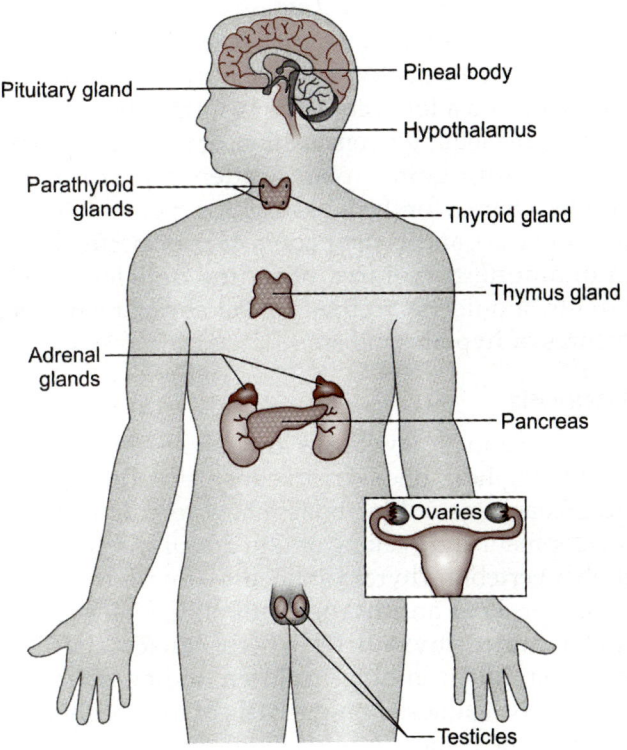

Figure 43.1 Endocrine glands of the body

Clinical Features

Cretinism is difficult to diagnose in newborn period and clinical features become obvious as the child grows. The baby is rather lethargic, does not cry much, sucks and feeds lazily (may not cry for feed) and is constipated. The skin may be dry, cool and mottled and facial features may look coarse. Anterior fontanel is large and cranial sutures are widely open. The physiological jaundice during newborn period may persist longer than the usual duration of 10–14 days. The

Nursing Alert

Cretinism is a preventable cause of mental retardation. Early diagnosis and replacement therapy with thyroxine is curative.

43

developmental milestones are delayed. The first suspicion of cretinism may arise when baby does not give a smile to the social interactions of the mother at 4–6 weeks of age. As the child grows, his skin and hair become rough and dry, and facial features appear more coarse and puffy with a large tongue. Cry and voice are hoarse. Abdomen is distended with an umbilical hernia. Constipation may become worse. Dentition and skeletal maturation are delayed. The child is extremely slow and lazy without any interest in usual play activities. The child looks short and stumpy. *Early diagnosis of cretinism is extremely important because delay in the diagnosis and treatment are associated with permanent damage to the brain with mental subnormality.*

Acquired hypothyroidism may occur during childhood and adolescence. It is suspected by excessive weight gain, lethargy, constipation, bradycardia, mental dullness with goiter, poor academic performance (sudden change for the worse), goiter, poor adolescent growth spurt and constipation. It may occur due to autoimmune thyroiditis or iodine deficiency. The parents should be vigilant to the above mentioned features of hypothyroidism.

Diagnosis

Serum T_3 and T_4 levels are low while TSH (thyroid stimulating hormone) is markedly elevated (>10 µIU/mL). Skiagrams of long bones show retarded osseous development and beaking of 12th dorsal and 1st or 2nd lumbar vertebra. Thyroid antibodies (thyroid antiperoxidase or TPO antithyroglobulins) are elevated in autoimmune thyroiditis which causes acquired hypothyroidism in older children. Iodine deficiency disorder is diagnosed on the basis of low excretion of iodine in the urine.

Treatment

Early diagnosis and prompt replacement therapy with thyroxine prevents mental retardation. The dose of thyroxine is 10–15 mg/kg/day in neonates and 5–10 mg/kg/day in older children. Thyroxine should be taken on empty stomach because its absorption is interfered by food. It is a long acting drug and given as a single dose in the morning. The dose of thyroxine is gradually increased to maintain TSH level within normal range. Biochemical parameters should be

Nursing Alert

Replacement therapy with thyroxine is usually needed life-long. The dose of thyroxine is increased periodically as the child grows because dose is calculated on the basis of body weight.

checked every 4–6 weeks till normal values are achieved, and then they are monitored once in every 6 months. It is recommended that everybody must take iodized salt to prevent development of goiter and occurrence of acquired or late-onset hypothyroidism.

Role of a Nurse

The importance of early diagnosis and prompt treatment should be explained to the parents. Intake of iodized salt should be promoted in the community. Thyroxine is a cheap drug and parents should be told that it must be taken regularly. In congenital hypothyroidism, replacement therapy is required lifelong. The child should be monitored closely for physical growth, mental development, gain in height, improvement in general activity and relief of constipation. It is important to monitor biochemical parameters to ensure that T_3, T_4 and TSH levels are maintained within normal range. Parents need constant emotional support and encouragement because replacement therapy is often needed lifelong.

Neonatal Screening

Congenital hypothyroidism occurs in one in 1100 to 1200 newborns in India and affected children are clinically normal at birth. Screening for hypothyroidism is highly cost-effective and should be done as a routine in all neonates because if thyroxine replacement is delayed, it leads to irreversible brain damage. Cord blood is collected on a special filter paper and screened for TSH by an ultrasensitive radioimmune assay method. Infants with raised TSH (>20 µIU/mL) are recalled after 3–4 days to recheck the blood levels of T_4 and TSH for confirmation of the diagnosis before starting therapy. The replacement therapy must be started within first two weeks of life as a safeguard against brain damage.

HYPERTHYROIDISM (Graves disease)

Thyrotoxicosis due to Graves disease in children is rare and account for less than 5% of patients with hyperthyroidism. It usually occurs by production of thyroid-stimulating autoantibodies because of lymphocytic thyroiditis. The disease occurs mostly in adolescent children and is more common in girls. The common manifestations include restlessness, emotional excitability, sweating, weight loss despite excessive appetite, heat intolerance and tachycardia. Thyroid gland is enlarged, firm and smooth, and a bruit (continuous murmur) may be heard due to increased blood supply. There is bilateral bulging of eyes or exophthalmos with infrequent blinking and a staring look.

43

Diagnosis

The diagnosis is confirmed by finding elevated blood levels of T_3 and T_4, and extremely low levels of TSH. The radio iodine uptake is high, rapid and diffuse. There are elevated levels of thyroid-stimulating immunoglobulins and thyrotropin stimulating antibodies.

Treatment

The condition is treated with oral administration of propyl thiouracil (5–10 mg/kg every 8 hours) or neomercazole (0.5–1.0 mg/kg every 8 hours). When patient becomes euthyroid, the dose of antithyroid drugs is reduced to the minimum. Lugol's iodine (1–2 drops twice a day) is useful to inhibit release of thyroid hormones. Propranolol (2 mg/kg/d every 8 hours), a beta-blocker is given for symptomatic relief of restlessness, tremors and tachycardia. In resistant cases, radiolabeled iodine (^{131}I) ablation is curative. Post irradiation hypothyroidism is treated with supplements of thyroxine.

GOITER

The enlargement of thyroid gland is called goiter. It may be classified as congenital or acquired, sporadic or endemic in populations living in hilly terrains. Goiter may be associated with diminished, normal (euthyroid), or increased thyroid secretions.

Physiological goiter is common during adolescence because of increased demands for thyroxine or relative iodine deficiency. Iodine deficiency in endemic regions is the most common cause of goiter which may be associated with euthyroid state or hypothyroidism. Other causes of euthyroid goiter include puberty goiter, chronic lymphocytic thyroiditis, benign thyroid adenoma, and carcinoma. Goiter with hypothyroidism is commonly seen in children with dyshormonogenesis, iodine deficiency, Hashimoto thyroiditis, intake of antithyroid drugs and goitrogens. Rarely goiter may occur because of a viral or pyogenic infection, cyst, or cancer. A standard clinical staging protocol is used to assess the size of goiter **(Box 43.1)**.

| **Box 43.1** | **Assessment of thyroid size by palpation** |

- **Stage 0** No goiter
- **Stage 1–A** Goiter detectable by palpation but not visible when neck is fully extended.
- **Stage 1–B** Goiter palpable and visible only when neck is fully extended.
- **Stage 2** Goiter is visible when neck is in normal position.
- **Stage 3** Goiter visible from a distance.

Thyroid gland is best examined by standing behind the patient and using fingers of both hands to palpate the gland. Goiter may be diffuse, firm in consistency with a smooth surface, for example, puberty or colloid goiter, iodine deficiency, dyshormonogenesis, Graves disease, Hashimoto thyroiditis, intake of thyroid drugs, or goitrogens. The presence of a single well-circumscribed nodule is suggestive of cyst, adenoma, or cancer. Multiple nodular goiter may be seen in endemic areas because of iodine deficiency and chronic lymphocytic thyroiditis. Goiter with pain and inflammatory signs is suggestive of a viral or bacterial infection.

Investigations

Thyroid status is assessed by measuring levels of T_3, T_4, and TSH. Anti-TPO and thyroxine-binding globulin antibodies are measured to exclude autoimmune thyroiditis. Iodine status is assessed by estimation of urinary iodine excretion. Ultrasound and fine-needle aspiration biopsy is performed when enlargement is nodular or diagnosis is uncertain.

Treatment

Treatment depends on the underlying cause. Puberty goiter and hypothyroidism are treated with supplements of thyroxine. Thyrotoxicosis is managed by antithyroid drugs. Drugs and foods (soybeans, peanuts, cabbage, spinach, peaches) that are known to cause goiter should be stopped. Surgery is indicated in children with an isolated nodule, cyst, and carcinoma or when there is respiratory embarrassment.

DIABETES MELLITUS

Unlike type-2 diabetes mellitus in adults, diabetes is uncommon in children (type-1) but a more serious disease and must be treated by administration of insulin (insulin-dependent). The exact cause of diabetes in children is not known. There may be autoimmune destruction of beta cells of pancreas. It may occur following a viral infection (mumps, coxsackie, cytomegalovirus) of pancreas (a gland which produces insulin and is located deep in the center of abdomen) and is more common in babies fed with cow's milk. There is evidence to suggest that vitamin D supplementation during early childhood may offer protection against the development of type-1 diabetes mellitus. There is no genetic predisposition unlike adult-onset diabetes mellitus. Type-2 diabetes may occur in adolescent children with obesity, metabolic syndrome X, and girls with polycystic disease of ovaries.

Clinical Features

Disease may occur at any age but is more common in a school going child. Due to marked elevation of blood glucose level (because of lack of insulin) there is excessive urination (polyuria), marked thirst (polydypsia) and increased appetite (polyphagia). Despite excessive intake of food, the child remains lean and thin. At times, the disease may manifest as an emergency (without any prior warning symptoms) due to diabetic ketoacidosis or diabetic coma. There may be sudden episode of vomiting, abdominal pain, fever, dehydration, drowsiness or coma.

Diagnosis

The classical triad of polyuria, polydypsia and polyphagia (with failure to thrive) is diagnostic. Fasting plasma glucose level of >126 mg/dL or random plasma glucose level of >200 mg/dL on two occasions is diagnostic. Glycosylated hemoglobin (HbA1c) is elevated and suggests that blood glucose has been raised over a period of time.

Treatment

Type-1 diabetes mellitus cannot be treated by oral drugs. The usual insulin dose is 1.0–1.5 units/kg/day and a combination of intermediate acting (lente) and short acting (regular) human insulin is given 20–30 minutes before breakfast and dinner. The currently available insulins are produced by recombinant-DNA technology. Approximately two-third of the dose is given as lente insulin and one-third as regular insulin (split-mix regimen). Usually two-thirds of total dose is given before breakfast and one-third before dinner. Insulin pen injectors are available for ease of administration. Injections are given subcutaneously and rotated between anterior abdominal wall and anterolateral parts of thighs and arms. The most accurate method of achieving glycemic control is by use of an insulin pump. It utilizes insulin delivery devices to accurately deliver a baseline continuous infusion of insulin coupled with periodic boluses related to food intake and activity level. A nasal spray of insulin or oral insulin are undergoing clinical trials which is likely to simplify the treatment of diabetes.

Role of a Nurse

1. The nurse should work in close collaboration with a pediatrician, health educator, dietician, psychologist and medical social worker.
2. The parents should be educated about the principles of management of a diabetic child.
3. The child and family need constant encouragement, guidance, emotional support and compassionate handling.
4. The importance of timely administration of insulin should be explained to the parents. The risk of hypoglycemia (excessive insulin, fasting, exertion) and diabetic ketoacidosis (infection, missing of insulin, bingeing or overeating) should be explained.
5. The family should be told about various types, strengths, storage and cost of available insulins. The importance of using appropriate disposable syringes, technique, rotation of injection sites or use of insulin pump should be explained to the child and parents.
6. Proper monitoring protocol for examination of urine with uristix, blood glucose with a glucometer, glycosylated hemoglobin (HBA1c), and lipid profile should be provided. Glycosylated hemoglobin is an excellent marker of glucose control over a period of 6–8 weeks and it should be maintained below 8%.
7. The broad principles of dietary management should be explained to the family. A diet plan should be provided with distribution of calories into three major meals and three mid-meal snacks to prevent hypoglycemia. In due course of time, most children can have a flexible lifestyle instead of a rigid diet plan.
8. The importance and advantages of regular exercise and physical activity should be explained. The child should be encouraged to undertake vigorous walking, jogging, cycling, swimming, dancing, and aerobic exercises.
9. The need for early recognition and prompt treatment of intercurrent infection should be explained.
10. The importance of regular follow-up should be explained to the family. Nurse should review the lifestyle and check weight, height, blood pressure and insulin injection sites at each visit.
11. A detailed biochemical and clinical monitoring, atleast once in a year, are recommended to identify and manage any chronic complications of diabetes mellitus. Annual eye checks are important for early diagnosis of diabetic retinopathy.

Complications

Acute complications include intercurrent infection, hypoglycemia and diabetic ketoacidosis. Chronic complications occur due to involvement of blood vessels (micro- and macrovascular pathology) and include diabetic retinopathy, neuropathy and nephropathy. Most of the chronic complications manifest during adult life.

Hypoglycemia It occurs due to administration of high dose of insulin or missing of a regular meal. It is characterized by adrenergic symptoms like sweating, pallor, trembling, uneasiness and tachycardia. When treatment is delayed it progresses to confusion, drowsiness, coma and seizures. The blood glucose level is likely to be less than 60 mg/dL. When hypoglycemia is suspected, child should be immediately given simple carbohydrates like sugar, glucose, honey, candy, fruit juice or sherbet. Coma and convulsions are treated with intravenous administration of 25% dextrose (2–4 mL/kg).

> **Practical Tip**
>
> *In every child with coma or seizures, blood glucose should be tested to exclude hypoglycemia and diabetic ketoacidosis.*

DIABETIC KETOACIDOSIS (DKA)

Diabetic coma may be the first symptom of type-1 diabetes mellitus without any prior warning or may occur in a child who is known to be diabetic. Inadequate insulin intake, intercurrent infection or stress are common precipitating factors. There is sudden onset of abdominal pain, vomiting, fever and progressive loss of consciousness leading to coma. The child has severe dehydration (due to marked polyuria) and deep rapid or acidotic breathing (Kussmaul breathing). Cerebral edema is a dreaded complication. Blood glucose is elevated to >250 mg/dL with ketonemia and metabolic acidosis (pH < 7.3 and base excess > –20 mEq/L). There is hyperosmolality (>350 mOsm/kg), increased anion gap (>12 mmoles/L), and metabolic acidosis. Anion gap is calculated by the formula;

$[Na^+] - [(Cl^-) + (HCO_3^-)]$. Moderate leukocytosis may occur due to stress but severe leukocytosis (>25,000/mm³) is suggestive of associated infection. Urinalysis shows presence of glucose and ketone bodies. It is a life-threatening emergency and managed by following protocol.

1. Start iv infusion with normal saline which is given as a bolus of 20 mL/kg within first hour. After 1 hour, N/2 (0.45%) saline is started and continued till dehydration is corrected.
2. When blood glucose falls below 300 mg/dL, 5% glucose is added to the infusate.

3. Acidosis is corrected by administration of sodium bicarbonate. Potassium is added in the infusate (40 mEq/L) once child has passed urine.
4. Soluble insulin is given as a bolus dose of 0.1 unit/kg IV followed by continuous intravenous infusion at a rate of 0.1 unit/kg/hour. Blood glucose should be checked after every hour and one should try to achieve reduction in blood glucose by 50–100 mg/dL every hour. The dose of insulin is reduced to 0.05 units/kg/hr when acidosis is corrected (pH >7.3) and blood glucose falls below 200 mg/dL. Insulin infusion is discontinued when blood glucose level becomes normal and metabolic acidosis has been corrected. The child is then started on subcutaneous insulin therapy. At this stage, the dose of insulin is 1.0–1.5 units kg/day given in 3–4 divided doses 30 minutes before meals.
5. Antibiotics are given to treat any underlying infection.

Prevention

1. Provide education, guidance and emotional support to the child and family.
2. Explain the need for regular exercise or activity, regular meals and snacks, and administration of insulin.
3. Intercurrent infection should be identified early and managed promptly.
4. Nurse should provide guidance for correct technique of administration of insulin and dangers of overdose and missing the shot.
5. Family should be educated regarding home monitoring of blood glucose with the help of glucose strips and and an electronic device (Accu-chek®). Glycosylated hemoglobin (HbA1c) should be monitored every 3 months and maintained below 8%. It is an excellent marker of adequacy of glucose control over a period of 6–8 weeks.

DIABETES INSIPIDUS

It is a rare disorder which is characterized by passage of large quantities of urine (polyuria) and excessive thirst (polydypsia) to replenish excessive urinary losses of water. Polyuria adversely affects the physical growth, activity, sleep and schooling of the child. These children are prone to develop dehydration and fever.

Diabetes insipdus occurs due to inadequate secretion of antidiuretic hormone (ADH) because of damage to neurohypophysis or hypothalamus by suprasellar tumor, trauma, encephalitis, tuberculoma and histiocytosis. In nephrogenic diabetes insipidus, there is inability of the kidneys to respond to ADH.

43

Diagnosis

The 24-hour urine output ranges between 4 and 10 liters. Urine is dilute with a specific gravity ranging between 1001 and 1005 and osmolality between 50 and 200 mOsm/kg. Computed tomography (CT) or magnetic resonance imaging (MRI) scan of brain may reveal intracranial tumor or tuberculoma.

Treatment

Administration of desmopressin (DDAVP), an analog of ADH is given as a nasal spray in a single or two daily doses of 2.5–10 μg, sublingual or through oral route (50–200 μg every 12 hr). Nephrogenic diabetes inspidus responds to hydrochlorthiazide 0.5–1.5 mg/kg/day as a paradoxical response.

Nursing Alert

It is dangerous to deny or restrict fluids to children with diabetes inspidus.

DISORDERS OF SEXUAL MATURATION

The age of onset of puberty is variable but usually occurs between 10 and 12 years in girls and 12–14 years in boys. It is a unique process triggered by hormonal changes in the body. During adolescence, gonadotropin-releasing hormone (GnRH) is secreted from the medial basal region of the hypothalamus. This is followed by pulsatile release of luteinizing hormone (LH) and follicle-stimulating hormone (FSH) which leads to release of testosterone in boys, and estrogens and progesterone in girls. When peak levels of sex hormones are achieved there is negative feedback to prevent further release of GnRH, FS and LH. The first sign of sexual maturation is enlargement of breasts in girls and testes in boys.

Precocious Puberty

The puberty is considered as precocious if it occurs before 8 years in girls and 9 years in boys. It is associated with appearance of all the secondary sex characters of puberty namely enlargement of breasts, pubic and axillary hair, and menarche in girls and change in voice, appearance of pubic, axillary and facial hair and increase in the size of testes and penis in boys.

Etiology The precocious puberty may be true due to central or CNS causes or pseudoprecocity because of peripheral or gonadal causes. The central precocity occur due to premature activation of hypothalamic pituitary-gonadal axis because of congenital anomalies (hypothalamic hamartomas), tumors or post-infectious conditions. It is more common than peripheral and is more common in girls than boys. The peripheral precocious puberty is more common in boys than girls and is most commonly due to congenital adrenal hyperplasia (CAH). The common ovarian causes include McCune-Albright syndrome, follicular cysts and tumors. Pseudoprecocity may occur because of variations in pubertal development like premature thelarche, pubarche and menarche. Detailed hormonal and imaging studies are needed to identify the cause of precocious puberty.

Treatment In rapidly progressive precocious puberty when menarche occurs before 6 years of age, it is treated by administration of GnRH agonists. They reduce the symptoms of precocity and increase the growth velocity to improve the ultimate adult height. In peripheral precocious puberty, the treatment is directed to the underlying cause. Surgical excision is done for treatment of tumors of ovaries, testes and adrenals. Pineal tumors and hCG-producing suprasellar tumors are treated with radio therapy.

Delayed Puberty

Puberty is considered to be delayed if there is no budding of breasts by 12 years in girls or no increase in the volume of testes by the age of 14 years in boys. The condition is more common in boys than girls. The most common cause of delayed puberty is constitutional delay in boys and Turner syndrome in girls. Most cases of delayed puberty can be classified under constitutional delay in growth and puberty (CDGP), hypogonadotropic hypogonadism and hypergonadotropic hypogonadism. Constitutional delay in growth and puberty is associated with low gonadotropin levels and is characterised by (i) family history of delayed puberty, (ii) delayed bone age, (iii) low or borderline gonadotropins and sex steroids, (iv) absence of micropenis or cryptorchidism and (v) slow initial growth velocity but normal ultimate adult height.

Investigations The endocrinal assessment includes estimation of basal levels of sex hormones (testosterone in boys and estrogens in girls), gonadotropins (FSH, LH and prolactin) and GnRH and hCG stimulation studies. A buccal smear and karyotype is indicated in most cases. Skeletal survey and bone age are useful. Pelvic ultrasound examination should be done in girls. Testicular biopsy may be indicated in boys.

Treatment Children with CDGP need reassurance and counseling. Short-term low dose hormonal treatment with testosterone or estrogens for 3 to 6 months may be given to a psychologically stressed child. Administration of GnRH in pulsatile doses is useful for treatment of hypogonadotropic hypogonadism.

43

Human growth hormone is useful to increase the growth velocity in girls with Turner syndrome. In permanent hypogonadism, long-term replacement therapy with monthly testosterone injections in boys and cyclical estrogen-progesterone therapy in girls is started at the age of around 10 years.

CONGENITAL ADRENAL HYPERPLASIA

In congenital adrenal hyperplasia (CAH), cortical synthesis from cholesterol is affected by deficiency of one of the several enzymes involved in steroidogenesis. It is the most common adrenal disorder in childhood. There is over production of the hormonal precursors proximal to the block and deficiency of the hormones distal to the blocked enzymatic step. The two main variants of CAH include 21-hydroxylase deficiency and 11-β hydroxylase deficiency. There is poor production of cortisol with excessive release of ACTH which leads to excessive production of sex steroids (androgens).

Clinical Features

The female infant is born with features of masculinization of external genitalia. The clitoris is enlarged with fusion of labia giving an appearance of empty "scrotal sacs". There is increased pigmentation of external genitals and areola of breasts. In male infants, CAH does not produce any abnormalities in the external genitals except slight increase in the size of penis. Children with CAH due to 21-hydroxylase deficiency may present with life-threatening salt-wasting syndrome characterized by vomiting, diarrhea, dehydration and vascular collapse with hyponatremia and hyperkalemia in neonatal period or infancy. The diagnosis is difficult in male infants because of lack of any significant genital abnormalities.

Investigations

In salt-wasting type of CAH, serum sodium is low while potassium is elevated. The diagnostic hormonal profile include markedly elevated serum 17-hydroxyprogesterone (17–OHP), lowered serum cortisol, elevated serum levels of dehydroepiandrosterone (DHEAS) and testosterone.

Treatment

Administration of glucocorticoids is the mainstay of treatment in order to replace the deficient cortisol and suppress ACTH oversecretion. Salt wasting crisis is managed by a bolus dose of hydrocortisone 50 mg/m^2 followed by 100 mg/m^2/day in 4 divided doses. Hypertension also responds to physiological doses of corticosteroids (11-β hydroxylase deficiency). During maintenance, hydrocortisone acetate is given in an oral dose of 10–15 mg/m^2/day in 3 divided doses. The daily dose of cortisone is doubled during acute infection. Salt losers are given additional salt (1–3 g/d) and 9-α fluohydrocortisone acetate or fludrocortisone 0.1–0.3 mg per day. Surgical repair of masculinized genitals may be undertaken at adolescence.

BIBLIOGRAPHY

Bajpai A, Kabra M, Menon PSN. Central diabetes inspidus in children: clinical profile and factors indicating organic etiology. *Indian Pediatr* 2008, 45: 463–468.

Bohn D, Daneman D. Diabetic ketoacidosis and cerebral edema. *Curr Opin Pediatr* 2002,14(3): 287–291.

Counts DR, Cutier GB. Pathogenesis and therapy of precocious puberty. *Curr Opin Pediatr* 1992, 4: 674–678.

Daneman D. Type 1 diabetes. *Lancet* 2006. 367(9513): 847–858.

Delange F, de Benoist B, Pretell E, Dunn JT. Iodine deficiency in the world: Where do we stand at the turn of century? *Thyroid* 2001, 11(5): 437–447.

Eugster EA, LeMay D, Zerin JM, Pescovitz OH. Definitive diagnosis in children with congenital hypothyroidism. *J Pediatr* 2004, 144(5): 643–647.

Hughes IA. Congenital adrenal hyperplasia: A life long disorder. *Hormone Res* 2007, 68(Supple 5): S84–S89.

Lee PA, Houk CP, Ahmed SF, Hughes IA. Consensus statement on management of intersex disorders. *Pediatrics* 2006, 118: 488–500.

Madison LD, La Franchi S. Screening for congenital hypothyroidism: Current controversies. *Curr Opin Endocrinol Met* 2005, 12: 36.

Merke DP, Bornstein SR. Congenital adrenal hyperplasia. *Lancet* 2005, 365(9477): 2125–2136.

44

Sexually Transmitted Diseases

Adolescents are highly vulnerable to develop sexually transmitted diseases (STDs) because of unhygienic and unnatural sexual practices, lack of awareness, sexual promiscuity and lack of sex and family life education in school. *It is important to remember that use of oral contraceptives can prevent unwanted pregnancy but not STDs*. Effective use of condom by the male partner is mandatory to prevent occurrence of STDs which are listed in **Box 44.1**. There is a greater need for family life and sex education in India because of early marriages and high incidence of teenage pregnancy. Sexually transmitted diseases are an important cause of serious morbidity, dyspareunia (pain during sexual intercourse), pelvic inflammatory disease (PID), infertility and mortality. Whenever STD is suspected, both the partners should be examined, investigated and treated.

ACQUIRED IMMUNODEFICIENCY SYNDROME (AIDS)

AIDS is a fatal disease caused by human immuno-deficiency virus (HIV). There are two main types of the virus, HIV-1 and HIV-2. The latest estimates suggest that in India 0.36% of adult population is infected by HIV accounting for 2.5 million cases, the third worst affected country after South Africa (5.5 million) and Nigeria (2.9 million). It is estimated that around 10 million children are infected by HIV in the world and they are destined to die within the next 5 years.

Mode of Infection

Children are usually unfortunate victims of HIV infection due to none of their fault. In developing countries, pediatric AIDS account for 20% of all HIV infected cases. Most children get infected by vertical transmission of infection from their HIV-positive mother during pregnancy and delivery. The mother-to-child transmission risk varies between 20 and 35%. There is an additional 10–15% risk of transmission of

> **Box 44.1 Sexually transmitted diseases**
>
> - Bacterial vaginosis and pelvic inflammatory disease
> - *Candida albicans* (yeast infections)
> - Trichomoniasis (Trich) due to *Trichomonas vaginalis*
> - *Chlamydia trachomatis*
> - *Mycoplasma genitalium*
> - Genital herpes simplex virus type 1 and type 2
> - Genital or venereal warts
> - Chancroid (*Haemophilus ducreyi*)
> - Lymphogranuloma venereum (LGV) due to invasive serovars of *Chlamydia trachomatis*
> - Granuloma inguinale (donovanosis) due to *Klebsiella granulomatis*
> - Gonorrhea
> - Syphilis
> - Hepatitis B and C
> - Human immunodeficiency virus (HIV)
> - Human papillomavirus (HPV)

HIV infection through breast milk. Around 80% AIDS infections in children occur during perinatal period and the rest by transfusion of potentially infected blood and blood products to children suffering from hemophilia, thalassemia major and other hemato-oncologic disorders. Transfusion of unscreened blood carries a grave risk of infection. In adolescent children, there is an additional risk of HIV infection by use of infected needles by drug abusers and by indulging in unprotected homosexual or heterosexual activity. There is no risk of transmission of HIV through fomites, physical contact, kissing, droplet infection or mosquito bites.

Clinical Features

HIV-positive mothers have an increased risk of abortion, fetal malnutrition and premature delivery. Rarely, a baby may be born with congenital defects like small box-like head, increased distance between the eyes, flat nose, long slit like eyes and patulous lips. Most babies born to HIV-positive mothers are, however, normal at birth. The manifestations of disease usually appear between 6 and 18 months and most affected children die by 5 years of age. There is profound damage to their body defense mechanisms. These children develop frequent and persistent episodes of unexplained fever, diarrhea, respiratory infections (persistent cough due to lymphoid interstitial pneumonitis), fungal infection of mouth (thrush), tuberculosis, enlargement of lymph nodes, parotid glands, liver and spleen.

They are prone to develop unusual bacterial, viral, fungal and parasitic infections. They are more vulnerable to suffer from *Pneumocystis carinii* pneumonia, disseminated tuberculosis, cryptosporidiosis, toxoplasmosis and CMV infection. Some children may develop AIDS-associated cancer and encephalopathy. Recurrent infections and failure to thrive with varying grades of malnutrition are invariably present.

Diagnosis

Elisa and Western blot tests may be positive in a newborn baby, even in the absence of actual infection, because maternal IgG antibodies against HIV may be passively transferred through the placenta from the mother to her fetus. These passively transferred antibodies gradually wane off and disappear by 15 months of age. When these antibodies persist beyond 15 months, it is indicative of active HIV infection of the infant. Early diagnosis of HIV infection in an infant can be made by demonstration of HIV-specific IgM antibodies, p24 core antigen or demonstration of HIV-DNA by PCR technology. These children manifest defective cell-mediated immunity (reduced number of lymphocytes and CD4 cells with reduction CD4 to CD8 ratio) while their serum immunoglobulin levels may actually be elevated because of occurrence of frequent infections. Anemia, neutropenia (lymphopenia) and thrombocytopenia are common. There may be laboratory evidences of unusual and intercurrent infections.

Treatment

These children need tender, loving care with compassion and concern because they are likely to lose their parent(s) in infancy because of AIDS. They should never be isolated or shunned because they are not contagious (unlike cough and cold) and there is no risk to other babies and care takers who can safely caress, cuddle, kiss and feed them. It is important that the child and family should not be ostracized by the society due to the stigma of AIDS. The child can attend a creche or play school without any risk to other children. However, precautions should be followed for taking and handling specimens of blood and for disposal of used needles and syringes.

A number of antiviral agents are available for treatment of AIDS but they are expensive and have limited efficacy. They can prolong life but are not curative. Breastfeeding is recognized to transmit HIV infection (10–15% risk). But decision for giving or withholding breast feeding should be based on the education, socioeconomic status and risk of bottle feeding in a community or family. When mother opts to breast feed her baby, exclusive breastfeeding poses less risk of maternofetal transmission of HIV virus compared with a combination of breast feeding and formula feed. Child should be given high calorie nutritious diet to prevent intercurrent infections. Maintenance of strict oral hygiene and topical application of antifungal lotion can prevent thrush. Co-trimoxazole is recommended for prophylaxis against *P. carinii*. Intravenous polyvalent immunoglobulins are recommended for long-term administration at intervals of every 3 weeks for boosting humoral immunity. Intercurrent infections should be recognized early and treated promptly. Anti-retroviral drugs are extremely expensive and potentially toxic. They are not curative but slow the progression of disease process. National AIDS Control Organization (NACO) provides anti-retroviral drugs and logistic support which should be sought and harnessed. Mortality due to AIDS is higher in children compared to adults.

Immunizations

Live vaccines (like BCG, oral polio and chickenpox vaccine) should be avoided in children with manifest AIDS (as diagnosed by IgM-specific HIV antibodies and viral studies). Affected children (and their siblings as well) should be given killed or inactivated polio vaccine (IPV). Administration of oral polio vaccine to healthy siblings may infect the child with AIDS. In addition to routinely administered killed vaccines, special vaccines like pneumococcal, Hib and influenza vaccines should be given to all children with HIV infection. When HIV-infected children develop serious viral infections like chickenpox and measles, specific immune globulins may be life saving.

Prevention

Risk of perinatal or vertical transmission of HIV from mother to her baby can be reduced by administration of zidovudine. During pregnancy, starting any time between 14 and 34 weeks of gestation, zidovudine

44

100 mg 5 times/day is given orally. At onset of labor, zidovudine 2 mg/kg is given IV for first hour and then 1 mg/kg/hr till delivery. Neonate is started on oral zidovudine 2 mg/kg/dose every 6 hourly starting at the age of 8–12 hours and continued for 6 weeks. Other strategies and interventions which can reduce the risk of mother-to-child transmission (MTCT) of HIV are listed in **Box 44.2**.

There is no protective vaccine as yet against AIDS. Public health education and crusade should be launched against drug abuse, dangerous sexual practices and risks posed by professional blood donors. Sex and family life education should be imparted to adolescent boys and girls in high schools to spread the message of safe sex (by use of condom) and contraception to control both sexually transmitted diseases and population explosion. Health care providers should follow "universal precautions" as a safeguard against risk of infection from needle stick injuries and handling of blood and body secretions.

CONGENITAL SYPHILIS

Among various sexually transmitted diseases (STDs) during pregnancy, untreated syphilis during pregnancy is associated with almost 100% risk of transmission of infection to the fetus. It is caused by *Treponema pallidum* belonging to Spirochaetceae family.

Clinical Features

Syphilis is a devastating disease and can involve any organ of the body. Fetal and perinatal deaths occur in 40% of affected infants. Early features of congenital syphilis include mucocutaneous rash, presenting with erythematous maculopapular or bullous lesions,

Box 44.2	**Interventions that can reduce the risk of vertical transmission of HIV**

- Providing good nutrition and vitamin A supplements to the mother during pregnancy.
- Avoiding invasive procedures such as amniocentesis, chorionic villus sampling, cordocentesis, fetal scalp pH monitoring and surgical rupture of membranes.
- Elective cesarean section.
- Avoiding surgical rupture of membranes before spontaneous rupture of membranes.
- When vaginal delivery is planned, episiotomy should not be done.
- Vaginal douching with chlorhexidine.
- Taking all possible precautions against accidental or nosocomial transmission of HIV.
- Avoidance of breast feeding and providing guidance for feeding safely with a cup and spoon or *paladay*.

followed by desquamation involving hands and feet. Anemia, thrombocytopenia, jaundice, lymphadenopathy and hepatosplenomegaly may occur. Osteochondritis may lead to pseudoparalysis and swelling over the small joints of hands and feet (dactylitis). There may be persistent blood-tinged discharge from the nose (snuffles) with vertical excoriations over the philtrum (rhagades).

The late manifestations include depressed nasal bridge (saddle nose), anterior bowing of tibia (saber tibia) and abnormalities of permanent teeth (Hutchinson teeth, i.e. peg-shaped or bifid upper incisors and mulberry shaped first molars). Neurological manifestations due to involvement of brain and spinal cord may occur during adolescence. Interstitial keratitis, choroiditis, deafness and clutton joints (painless swelling of knees) are other late manifestations.

Diagnosis

Venereal disease research laboratory (VDRL) and rapid plasma reagin (RPR) are useful tests for screening. *T. pallidum*-specific IgM antibodies can be detected by immobilization test (TPI) and fluorescent treponemal antibody absorption test (FTA-ABS). Definitive diagnosis can be made by demonstration of *T. pallidum* by dark-field microscopy or direct immunofluorescence on specimens taken from skin lesions.

Treatment

Penicillin is the drug of choice for treatment of syphilis. Aqueous crystalline penicillin G (100,000–150,000 unit/kg/d q 12 hr during first 7 days of life and q 8 hr subsequently) is given intravenously for 10–14 days. Alternatively, procaine penicillin G (50,000 units/kg) can be given in a single daily dose intramuscularly for 10–14 days. Ceftriaxone is useful in patients resistant to penicillin.

PREVENTION OF STDs

There is a need for promotion of human values, morality and spirituality or divinity in various teaching institutions of the country. A regular curriculum on family life and sex education should be introduced in all high schools of the country. Young boys and girls should be taught the skills needed for maintenance of sexual hygiene and mothercraft. *It must be understood that oral contraceptives can prevent unwanted pregnancies but they do not provide any safeguards against the development of STDs.* The use of condom by the male partner is useful both for contraception as well as transmission of STDs. Blood and blood products should be effectively screened for various infective agents especially human immunodeficiency virus (HIV), spirochetes (VDRL), malarial parasites, hepatitis B virus (HBV) and hepatitis C virus (HCV) before administration.

Health care professionals (HCPs) should follow "universal precautions" to prevent risk of infection with HIV and HBV from contact with blood and body secretions of patients. In case of inadvertent needle stick injury, recommended protocol for prevention of HIV infection by proper rinsing, oozing of blood and administration of antiretroviral drugs should be followed. Infants born to mothers with HIV are at an increased risk for vertical transmission of infection during delivery and through breastfeeding. The risk can be reduced by administration of antiretroviral therapy. The risk of ophthalmia neonatorum can be reduced by administration of a single shot of ceftriaxone to a baby born to a mother with gonorrhea. The menace of drug abuse should be curbed by proper health education and risk of transmission of HIV and HBV reduced by maintaining proper sterility by using disposable needles and syringes. The risk of HBV and human papilloma virus (HPV) infection can be reduced by timely administration of HBV and HPV (Cervarix and Gardasil) vaccines.

BIBLIOGRAPHY

American Academy of Pediatrics Task Force on Circumcision. Circumcision policy statement. *Pediatrics* 2012, 130: 585–586.

Arnold SR, Ford-Jones EL. Congenital syphilis: A guide to diagnosis and management. *Pediatr Child Health* 2000, 5(8): 463–469.

Havens PL, Water D. Management of the infant born to a mother with HIV infection. *Pediatr Clin North Am* 2004, 51(4): 909–937.

Kaul D, Patel JA. Clinical manifestations and management of pediatric HIV infection. *Indian J Pediatr* 2001, 68(7): 623–631.

Lodha R, Singhal T, Kabra SK. Pediatric HIV infection: Clinical manifestations and diagnosis. *Ann Natl Acad Med Sci* 2000, 36: 75–82.

O'Connor EA, Lin JS, Burda BU, et al. USPSTF: Behavioral sexual risk-reduction counseling in primary care to prevent sexually transmitted infections. *Ann Intern Med* 2014, 161: 874–883.

Workowski K, Berman S. Sexually transmitted diseases treatment guidelines. *MMWR Recomm Rep* 2006, 55(RR 11): 1–94, PMID16888612.

44

45

Accidents, Poisonings and Animal Bites

Children are at an increased risk of accidents and poisoning because of their inherent curiosity, careless attitude and innocence. Children try to learn and explore their environment by pulling, pushing, climbing, poking, probing and touching and mouthing every object that they come across. During their process of learning, the child is at an increased risk to hurt himself. During 6–18 months, children do not understand the meaning of "No" and have a poor memory to learn. Unless closely and constantly watched and supervised, they are likely to sustain accidental injuries and poisonings. During the process of exploration and learning, the child must be provided both with protection and education to modify his behavior. While the child should be protected at all times from burns and scalds, he should be allowed to feel the heat of a cup of tea or a glass of milk or hot iron. When he learns what is hot and it hurts, he would soon listen when he is told not to touch it because it is hot and it will burn.

BURNS AND SCALDS

Scalds

They are more common in children and usually occur when some one is drinking a hot cup of coffee or tea while holding the child in his lap. The child may get burnt while taking steam inhalation or spilling hot water bucket in the bath room. The child may pull a table cloth spilling hot tea or milk over himself. Every effort should be made to prevent occurrence of scalds **(Box 45.1)**.

First aid Pour cold water over the burnt area or place it under running tap so that skin temperature is brought down immediately. Do not apply an ice pack over the burnt site. Give paracetamol to relieve pain. Apply silver-sulfadiazine (silverix™) cream over the burnt area. The child should be taken to the hospital if blisters have formed.

> **Box 45.1** **Prevention of scalds**
>
> - Never leave the child alone in the kitchen and bathroom.
> - Never hold the baby in your lap while drinking anything hot or during cooking.
> - Do not leave the child alone near a hot iron, tea pot and hot water bucket, etc.
> - Do not leave a tray of hot food on the dining table with a hanging table cloth.
> - Always turn the pot handles towards the back of the stove or cooking range so that child cannot reach up and grab them.
> - Be extremely vigilant and careful while giving steam inhalation. It is better to use a facial steamer rather than a cooking utensil with boiling water.

Burns

Burns may occur due to toppling or bursting of kerosene stove or leakage of cooking gas. Children are known to suffer from burns by lighting match sticks. The joyous festival of Diwali is a cause for tragedy in many families every year. The fire crackers stocked in one place may catch fire accidentally. Even an innocuous *phuljari* may cause serious damage to the hand unless proper care is exercised. Extreme care should be taken while lighting fire-crackers like bombs because they can occasionally explode in hand causing extensive damage. Children should celebrate Diwali under the direct supervision of adults. They must wear shoes and put on clothes made of nonsynthetic material like cotton, while playing with fire-crackers. A bucket of water should be kept handy while exploding crackers.

First aid Parents should not panic and remain calm and composed. Wrap the child immediately with a bed cover or blanket and extinguish the flames. The child should not be allowed to run. He can be made to roll on the ground. Pour cold water over the burnt area.

Keep pouring the cold water over the burnt area for 10–15 minutes to reduce tissue damage. Avoid pouring ice cold water if a wide area of skin is affected in a young child. It may lead to extreme lowering of body temperature. Dry the skin with a clean towel and wrap him in a clean white sheet. If burnt area is small, apply silver-sulfadiazine cream. Give paracetamol to relieve pain and discomfort. If burnt area is large or it has affected vital parts like face, hands, genitals or blisters have formed he must be rushed to the hospital (Box 45.2). Do not use cotton to cover the burnt area, as it will get stuck to the damaged skin. Even a small area of full thickness burns may cause severe disfigurement unless it is managed with due care and professional competence. Give sips of plain water or oral rehydration fluid during journey to the hospital.

Prevention

Burns is largely a preventable tragedy. A remarkable decrease in incidence of burns has been observed in developed countries by enforcing legislation and providing education regarding preventive measures. The strategies to prevent burns are summarized in Box 45.3.

Box 45.2   Indications for hospitalization

- Partial thickness burns of greater than 10% of the total body surface area.
- Third degree or deep burns.
- Burns involving face, hands, feet and perineum.
- Electrical or chemical burns.
- Burns associated with other physical injuries or suffocation.

Box 45.3   Prevention of burns

- Never leave a child alone in the kitchen.
- Keep the gas and stove turned off when not in use.
- Keep the match boxes out of reach and out of sight of children.
- Children should play with fire crackers only under the direct supervision of adults.
- Avoid wearing inflammable synthetic fabric like nylon while exploding crackers.
- Never light fireworks inside the house.
- Keep doors and windows of home closed on Diwali night to prevent entry of fire crackers.
- Do not burst crackers near motor vehicles.
- Keep a bucket of water handy while playing with fire crackers.

Chemical Burns

Burns can occur due to contact with strong acids, alkalis, caustic soda and some dyes. Fingers are more likely to be affected. Wash the burnt area under a constant flow of tap water for at least 30 minutes till all traces of chemical is washed away and burning sensation has disappeared. After first aid, child must be taken to the hospital as most chemical burns are rather deep.

Electric Shock

Toddlers love to put their fingers into small holes including electrical sockets (power points). They can get an electric shock by biting into an electrical cord or by poking metal objects like steel rod, fork or knife into an unprotected electrical outlet. Electrical accidents also take place when electrical toys and tools are used incorrectly or when electric current makes contact with water in the bathroom. Every effort should be made to prevent accidental electrocution (Box 45.4).

First aid Switch off the current immediately or remove the plug from the socket. If that is not possible, push the child away from source of current with a wooden stick, broomstick or rolled-up magazine or newspaper. *Never touch the child with your bare hands if he is attached to the source of the current.* Severe electric shocks are fatal. Shock which does not appear to be severe can also cause extensive burns and severe damage to the internal organs especially heart and brain. The victim must be rushed to the hospital immediately, irrespective of the severity of injury at the entry point.

Hospital Management of Burns

The general condition of the child, vital signs, extent and depth of burns and any associated injuries should be assessed. "Rule of five" and "modified rule of nine"

Box 45.4   Prevention of electric shock

- Do not amuse the child by repeatedly switching the light or fan on and off.
- The electrical appliances should always be kept unplugged so that child cannot put them on.
- The electrical sockets should be kept covered with dummy plugs or made inaccessible to the child by blocking them with heavy furniture.
- Avoid using electrical tools and toys near bath tubs and pools.
- Do not buy toys for young children which operate on main electrical supply.
- When constructing a new house, install safety circuits in the wiring. In case of an electric shock, the fuse will blow off automatically.

are used to calculate the extent of burns in children (**Figures 45.1** and **45.2**). In severe burns, the child may be in shock because of loss of plasma from intravascular compartment.

Depth of Burns

The burn injury may be superficial or partial thickness (first and second degree), or full thickness burns involving all layers of skin (third degree).

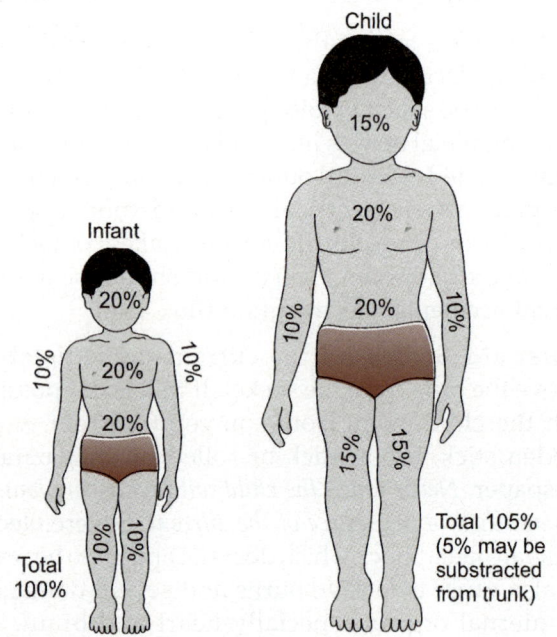

Figure 45.1 Estimation of burn area by "Rule of fives" (Lynch and Blocker 1963)

First degree burns Burn injury involves epidermis and manifests as pink to red discoloration with mild edema. Pain and smarting may last for 48 hours. Healing takes place within 10–12 days without any scarring.

Second degree burns They are further subclassified as second degree partial or deep burns. There is pink or red discoloration of skin with blister formation, exudation and edema. The deep second degree burns may look mottled in appearance and pain may be less or absent. Healing occurs by scar formation and may take 2–3 weeks.

Third degree burns They are full thickness burns involving all the layers of skin and may even burn the fat, muscles and ligaments. The burnt areas do not blanch on pressure and are painless inelastic waxy brown in color. Eschar develops by formation of leathery devitalized tissue. The wound needs surgical debridement, skin grafting and cosmetic repair over a period of several weeks or months.

Treatment

Fluid resuscitation is started immediately according to Parkland formula by providing 4 mL/kg of fluids for each percent of burnt surface area with Ringer lactate during first 24 hours. One-half of the calculated fluids are given in first 8 hours and the rest during next 16 hours. The maintenance fluid requirements can be provided orally. After 24 hours, one plasma volume (5% of body weight) is provided with infusion of colloids for every 15% of burns. Oxygen is given if child

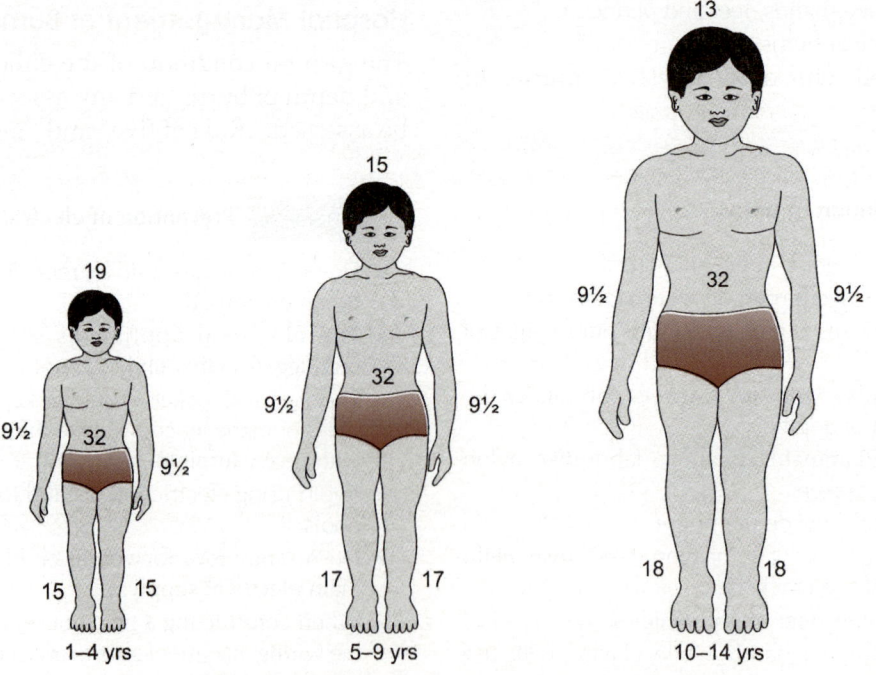

Figure 45.2 Modified "Rule of nines" for pediatric burns

has suffered inhalation burns. Tetanus toxoid or Td should be given as a prophylaxis against tetanus. When status of immunization is uncertain and burns are massive or grossly contaminated, tetanus human globulins are given. Sedation and pain relief is provided by administration of morphine sulfate 0.1–0.2 mg/kg IV or IM. Ketamine in analgesic doses (0.2–0.3 mg/kg) is useful in children during the change of dressings. Enteral nutrition should be built up gradually to provide enough calories, proteins and micronutrients. Nosocomial infection should be controlled by systemic administration of broad spectrum antibiotics to cover *S. aureus* and *P. aeruginosa*. Burnt areas are covered with silver sulfadiazine ointment and dressed with vaseline-soaked sterile gauze. During recovery skin grafting is required for third degree burns to prevent contractures and deformities. Psychosocial rehabilitation should be provided to enable the child to emerge as a hero out of the tragedy and to prevent depression.

Role of a Nurse

1. Provide tender loving care to the child and emotional support to the family to reduce anxiety and stress.
2. Monitor vital signs and maintain airway, breathing and circulation.
3. Assess the location, extent (percent surface area of burn) and depth of burns, and associated skeletal and visceral injuries.
4. Provide fluid resuscitation, maintain input-output chart and ensure urine output of at least 0.5 mL/kg/hr.
5. Isolate the child to prevent nosocomial infection, identify it early and provide effective systemic antibiotics to cover methicillin-resistant *S. aureus* and *P. aeruginosa*. Provide tetanus prophylaxis.
6. Provide calorie dense and high protein oral feeds or through nasogastric route in gradual increments. When enteral feed cannot be given or child is unable to tolerate, parenteral nutrition is provided.
7. Sedation and pain control are provided by giving parenteral morphine sulfate 0.1–0.2 mg/kg 2–3 times in a day. Ketamine in analgesic doses (0.2–0.3 mg/kg) is useful during change of dressings.
8. Wound care and application of silver sulfadiazine cream, sterile vaseline gauze, cotton pad and bandages should be applied with atmost asepsis.
9. Nurse should coordinate surgical procedures like excision, skin grafting, biological dressings, cosmetic surgery, reduction of scarring and contractures by maintaining a liason with a number of specialists.
10. The family needs guidance, motivation and emotional support for prolonged physiotherapy, occupational therapy and psychosocial rehabilitation.

FALLS, BUMPS AND BRUISES

Children are prone to falls and bumps both at home and play ground. Toddlers may fall from the cot unless protected with railings or by placing pillows around the baby. *"Walkers" are notoriously dangerous for causing accidents in children.* They do not help the baby to learn to walk, instead his motivation for independent walking is actually delayed. When children learn to crawl or walk upstairs they need close supervision. Several accidents happen in relation to balcony of the house when it is too short or it is shaky or fragile. Fabrication of sturdy railings over the balcony is useful to satisfy the child's curiosity to have an outside view. The railings should never have horizontal bars because child would climb over them. The vertical bars should be closely placed to prevent the child to squeeze through them. Kite flying on the roof top is notorious for causing serious life-threatening injuries due to *manjha*, falls and accidents. Children also enjoy climbing trees, walls and rocks which should be done under the supervision of an adult.

First aid The accident should be faced without any panic and parents should remain calm and confident. Reassure and caress the child and tell him that everything will be alright. Apply an ice bag over the site of bump for several minutes. It reduces bleeding, swelling and pain. Cold pack applications should be continued during 48–72 hours following the fall or blunt injury. A safe analgesic like paracetamol can be given for relief of pain. Subsequently local application of analgesic cream and hot fomentation helps to reduce pain and swelling.

Fractures (Broken bones)

When injury is severe and fracture is suspected due to inability to move a limb or limb has assumed an odd or bizarre position, the child should be handled gently. The upper limb should be placed in a sling and lower limb should be splinted or both lower limbs tied together by placing soft padding between them. When fracture of neck or spine is suspected, child should not be moved and he should be handled by trained paramedical personnel. The child is placed on a hard surface and lifted carefully without moving him sideways. The injured child should not be given anything to eat or drink after the accident till he has been examined by

45

45

an orthopedic surgeon. Administration of food or fluids to the child would delay correction of his fracture if this has to be done under general anesthesia.

Head Injury

Most head injuries at home are minor. The child cries, may develop a bruise or bump but there are no serious consequences. During first year of life, the baby should not be tossed in the air and head should not be shaken. *When head injury is associated with bleeding from nose or ear, vomiting, temporary loss of consciousness or convulsion, child should be admitted to a hospital for observation and management.*

When none of the above mentioned symptoms of serious head injury are present, the child can be given paracetamol for relief of pain. Avoid use of any sedative, as that would interfere with evaluation of consciousness of the child. Sometimes the effects of head injury become apparent later on after couple of hours when enough blood leaks out of the blood vessels. If child is not feeling his normal self and has become drowsy or refuses to eat or is having headache or vomiting on the next day, he should be evaluated by a neurologist. The presence of a bump or swelling over the head (without other symptoms) may occur due to collection of blood in the scalp and it does not affect the brain. The swelling would disappear spontaneously in due course of time and there is no need to do local fomentation. Every effort should be made to prevent house hold accidents and injuries **(Box 45.5)**.

Box 45.5 Prevention of physical injuries

- The railing of the baby cot should be close enough so that the baby can't entangle his limbs or head.
- The child should not be given toys with sharp edges and projectile toys like guns, pistols, bow and arrows, etc.
- Discourage the child to play with a swinging door.
- Avoid the use of "walkers".
- Do not leave the child on a high chair, table or cot unattended.
- Never allow the child to run with anything dangling out of his mouth.
- Always place a barrier infront of the stairs and gates.
- Discourage children to fly kites from roof tops.
- Never allow the child to play on the street with heavy traffic.
- Never place the child between you and the steering wheel while driving. Infant should be placed in a special baby seat or taken in the lap on the back seat. The child should not stand on the back seat of the car facing the rear window (like a dog!).
- Teach road sense to your child.

DROWNING

Drowning accidents in children commonly occur in bath tubs, buckets, commode, swimming pools, ponds and rivulets. During the monsoons, the roads and streets get flooded with rain water. The open sewers pose a hazard to unsuspecting children playing or wading through the rainwater. Every effort should be made to prevent drowning accidents in children **(Box 45.6)**. The clinical features depend upon duration of submersion in water. Child may be apneic or gasping with cyanosis. There may be mild impairment of sensorium or deep coma and convulsions. There may be respiratory distress with pulmonary edema. The clinical picture may be complicated by cardiogenic shock, acute renal failure and disseminated intravascular coagulation.

First aid

Place the child on his tummy (face down) and clean the mouth of any secretions and debris with a handkerchief. If child is gasping or not having any breathing, cardiopulmonary resuscitation (CPR) should be started immediately. The child should be dried and effectively covered with woolens to prevent hypothermia (fall in body temperature). The child should be taken to the hospital while CPR is continued during the journey.

Management

The child should be admitted to the pediatric ICU. Cardiopulmonary resuscitation and assisted ventilation should be continued till spontaneous breathing is established. The child should be given oxygen to maintain arterial oxygen saturation above 95%. Fluids, electrolytes, acid-base parameters and glucose should be monitored and maintained within the normal range.

Box 45.6 Prevention of drowning

- Never leave the young child alone in the bath tub, water bucket, inflatable pool even for a moment.
- Keep the bathroom door latched and always keep the comode covered with the lid.
- Children should not be left alone near a tube well, pond or lake.
- Children should be taught to swim but they should never be allowed to swim without adult supervision.
- Children with epilepsy should not be allowed to swim.
- Swimming pools should be equipped with safety measures and training in CPR and rescue techniques should be provided to the swimming pool staff.

Fluid restriction and hypertonic mannitol may be required to reduce cerebral edema. Inotropic agents (dopamine and dobutamine) may be required to sustain cardiac output. Antibiotics are usually given to treat superadded bacterial infection. There is no role of corticosteroids.

FOREIGN BODIES, CHOKING AND SUFFOCATION

Children have an uncanny habit of inserting objects into their body holes. They are known to put a safety pin, splinter, crayon, and cotton into their nose, ear or vagina. The child may cry due to pain or develop persistent blood stained discharge from the orifice. Toddlers are notorious for "mouthing" small objects like coins, buttons, peas, ground nuts, beads, button batteries and tablets. The objects may be swallowed or get lodged in the air passages causing sudden bouts of coughing with choking. The child may develop gasping, stridor or difficulty in breathing and may become blue. The child is unable to cry or speak if object is stuck in the larynx. When foreign body lodges in the bronchus, it may lead to unilateral wheezing and recurrent episodes of pneumonitis.

Parents should never put any oil into the nostrils and ears. Instillation of oil in the nostrils may lead to development of severe lipoid pneumonia because oil may trickle into the lungs. Oil in the ear canal often leads to development of fungal infection. However, nasal passages and ear canal can be kept moistened with a cotton wick soaked with coconut or olive oil.

First aid

When an object or insect has lodged in the nostril or ear canal, parents should not make any attempts to remove it unless it is too close to the orifice. Otherwise there is a risk that they may push the foreign body deeper. They should immediately seek the help of an ENT specialist to remove the foreign body. The rounded objects like coins, and beads, when swallowed are passed out automatically in the stools. Repeat skiagram of abdomen should be taken after 4–5 days of ingestion of a foreign body to check whether it has been passed out or not. When a foreign body is lodged in the oropharynx or esophagus, give mashed potatoes or banana to dislodge it.

When a child gets choked or suffocated by a foreign body, do not panic but act immediately. Never try to sweep or recover the foreign body with your fingers. It may get further pushed and impacted in the throat. Instead suspend the infant or small baby upside down

by supporting his chest and abdomen over your left arm or thighs. The child will be hanging with his feet up and his head facing the ground (or preferably over the bed or couch). Slap his back firmly between his shoulder blades with your right hand. Repeat the thumping up to 5 times to dislodge the foreign body. To do the same procedure in an older child, you should sit on a stool or an armless chair. Place the child on his tummy across your thighs with his head down and feet up position **(Figure 45.3)**. Give 4–5 good thumps or blows between his shoulder blades with moderate force. Most of the times, the impacted object may be expelled out and the child will take a sigh of relief. If this procedure fails Heimlich procedure should be performed to raise the intra-abdominal pressure to expel the foreign body **(Box 45.7)**.

The above mentioned procedure should be conducted quickly with a sense of purpose but without panic. If breathing stops or child becomes unconscious, start cardiopulmonary resuscitation (CPR) and rush the child to a hospital.

Prevention The guidelines to prevent choking and suffocation accidents in children are summarized in **Box 45.8**.

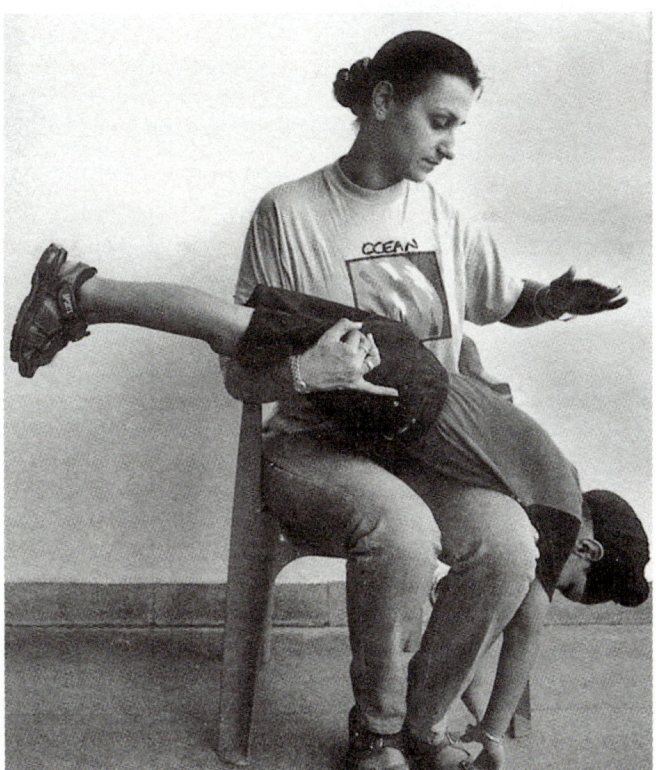

Figure 45.3 Procedure for dislodging foreign body in a child. The toddler is suspended upside down on the arm or legs and thumped firmly on the back between the shoulder blades

45

Box 45.7 Heimlich's maneuver

Toddler

- Place the child on a table or bed in a knee-chest position with head low and hips elevated.
- From behind grasp the upper abdomen with your both hands.
- Exert upward pressure and thrusts with fingers of your both hands.
- This would lead to sudden increase in the pressure inside the chest with popping out of the foreign body.

Older child

- Stand behind the child.
- Put your arms around his body and interlock your hands below his chest cage **(Figure 45.4)**.
- Sharply pull your locked hands up and deep into the child's abdomen. You can give up to 5 upwards thrusts with your hands.
- The resultant sudden increase in pressure inside the chest is likely to push out the foreign body.

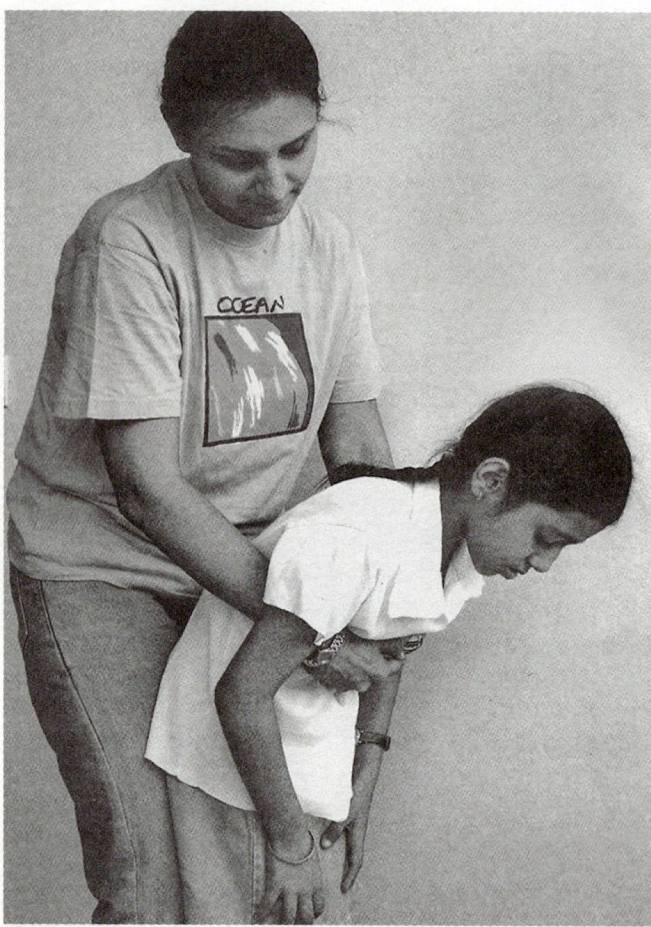

Figure 45.4 Heimlich maneuver. The child is firmly held from behind by interlocking your hands over the centre of the abdomen just below the rib cage. The locked hands are sharply pulled upwards with thrusting movements to raise the pressure inside the abdomen and chest

Box 45.8 Prevention of choking and suffocation accidents

- Children below 2 years should not be given nuts, popcorn, peas, seeds and candies.
- Do not give toys with small, loose or detachable parts.
- Children should not have access to small objects like coins, buttons, safety pins, clips, beads and button cells.
- Do not let the child eat while playing or running. Never tickle or provoke the child to laugh or cry while he is eating.
- Discourage children to play hide and seek by hiding in cupboards or *almirahs*.
- Do not let the child play with an empty plastic bag or talcum powder.
- Do not tie any thread on his neck.
- Do not burn hard coke in a closed room.

ACCIDENTAL POISONING

Poisoning is a common medical emergency in children. Children are at an increased risk to accidentally ingest a number of toxic agents. The commonly ingested poisons include kerosene, insecticides, or agricultural pesticides, rat poison, acids and alkalies, and naphthalene balls. Children in the villages are at risk to eat poisonous seeds, fruits and leaves, the most common being *dhatura* and castor-seed poisoning. Most of the household cosmetics (except nail polish, after shave lotion, depilators and skin color lighteners) are safe and non-toxic. Infants may get choked due to talcum powder. Medicines are now one of the leading causes of accidental poisoning in children and certain safeguards should be taken to prevent them **(Box 45.9)**. Poisoning as a suicide attempt may occur in adolescent children.

The child may have a strong smell of the poison or show burning and discoloration around his mouth. Retching, vomiting, breathlessness and drowsiness are

Box 45.9 Prevention of poisoning due to drugs

- Do not refer to medicines as a "delicious syrup".
- Do not take medicines infront of children.
- Store medicines in a locked up cabinet.
- Do not give medicines in the dark without reading the label.
- The discarded medicines should be sealed in a plastic bag and disposed off in the road-side garbage container.
- Medicines should be dispensed in child-proof foils and containers.

National Poison Information Center at AIIMS can be contacted to verify that the material ingested by the child is poisonous or not and to seek information regarding availability of a specific antidote.

common signs of poisoning. Intake of acid or alkali may cause severe burns over the lips, tongue and food pipe (esophagus) leading to complications later on. Identify the constellation of symptoms and signs (Toxidrome) which may provide useful clues to the likely toxin or poison. History should be taken to identify the name of toxin, amount and time of ingestion. Check the list of drugs being taken by the family members.

First aid

When poisoning is suspected, try to induce vomiting by tickling his throat with your finger. If this fails, give a glass of water containing two teaspoons of salt and repeat tickling the throat with your finger. After vomiting give him a glass of milk or mixture of milk with egg white which helps to dilute and delay absorption of most poisons. In certain situations, it is dangerous to induce vomiting **(Box 45.10)**.

The child may look normal for several hours after having taken the poison. Parents should not take any poisoning episode lightly and whenever they suspect that the child may have taken a poison, he must be taken to the hospital. The empty bottle of medicine must be taken along with to show to the doctor. Every effort should be made to prevent accidental poisoning due to household products **(Box 45.11)**.

Box 45.10 Contraindications to induce vomiting

- Drowsy or unconscious child
- Kerosene
- Petrol
- Cleaning agents and thinners
- Insect sprays
- Camphor
- Furniture polish

Box 45.11 Prevention of poisoning with household products

- The nurse in the Well Baby Clinic should provide guidelines and instructions to parents for prevention of accidents and poisonings.
- Keep cleaning agents, insecticides and rodenticides properly locked in a cupboard.
- Never store kerosene, cleaning agents, acids and alkalies in soft drink or water bottles.
- Keep medicines locked in a cupboard and out of reach of children. They should be kept in containers having child-proof screw caps.
- Cosmetics should be kept out of reach of children.
- Instruct children not to eat wild fruits, seeds and leaves while trekking.

Hospital Management

The general principles of care include (i) prevention of absorption of poisons, (ii) enhanced elimination of poison and (iii) administration of a specific antidote.

Prevention of Absorption of Poison

Dilution Simple dilution of poisons, which have irritant effect on GI mucosa (acids, alkalies, household cleansing agents), can be achieved by administration of water, milk and egg white. In case of medicinal tablets, administration of water or diluting agent is contraindicated as it may increase the absorption of drug.

Induction of vomiting Vomiting can be induced by stimulation of soft palate or pharynx by inserting fingers, administration of syrup ipecac, table salt solution and injection apomorphine. These modalities are rarely practised in hospital setting and has been replaced by gastric lavage. But lavage is contraindicated in children suspected to have poisoning with acids and hydrocarbon agents.

Gastric lavage Gastric lavage is done with a wide-bored orogastric tube with the help of normal saline 15 mL/kg (maximum of 200–400 mL/cycle) and repeated till effluent is clear. It is contraindicated in children with ingestion of caustics and hydrocarbon poisoning.

Activated charcoal It is useful binding agent in all cases of poisoning except iron, cyanide and after oral administration of an antidote. The dose is 1 g/kg mixed in water and given orally or through nasogastric tube. A saline cathartic or sorbitol is administered with each dose.

Whole bowel irrigation Isotonic balanced electrolyte solution containing propylene glycol is administered in a dose of 30 mL/kg/hr through nasogastric tube. It is continued till effluent from rectum is clear. It is useful modality in iron poisoning and intoxication with sustained release or enteric coated preparations.

Enhancing Excretion of the Poison

Diuresis It is useful when toxic agent is excreted primarily through the kidneys. The important prerequisites for giving diuretics include (i) excretion of poison through renal route, (ii) blood pressure is normal and there is no evidence of cardiac or respiratory insufficiency and (iii) renal functions are normal. The diuresis can be induced by intravenous administration of 20% mannitol in repeated doses of 0.5 g/kg to maintain urine output of 6–9 mL/kg/hr.

Osmotic diuretics are preferred agents because they prevent reabsorption of toxins by the renal tubules. Urinary alkalinization is useful for excretion of salicylates and barbiturates, while acidification of urine is associated with excretion of amphetamine, quinine and strychnine.

Dialysis Hemodialysis is useful to treat poisoning with salicylates, paracetamol, chloroquine, chloramphenicol, camphor, propranolol, ethylene glycol, vancomycin and snake bite. Peritoneal dialysis is less effective but can be used for treatment of salicylate poisoning.

Hemoperfusion and hemofiltration They are more effective than hemodialysis but available only in select centers. Hemoperfusion is useful for toxins with low water solubility and with high affinity for the adsorbent viz. carbamazepine, barbiturates and theophylline. Hemofiltration can remove compounds with high molecular weight like aminoglycosides, theophylline, iron, and lithium.

Pharmacological Antidotes

A number of toxins, drugs and poisons can be treated by administration of specific antidotes **(Table 45.1)**. It is desirable that all pediatric ICUs should prominently display charts of specific antidotes with their doses and mode of administration. Nevertheless optimal supportive therapy and nursing care must be provided even when a specific antidote is administered.

Kerosene Poisoning

It is the commonest poisoning in children. When kerosene is stored in a soft drink bottle, a thirsty children is likely to drink it by mistake. Due to unpleasant taste, child is likely to take a few sips but when taken in excess of 30 mL it may prove fatal.

Clinical features There is strong smell of kerosene with irritation of mouth and upper GI tract. It is readily aspirated into lungs producing cough, respiratory distress, cyanosis and fever due to chemical pneumonia. Drowsiness, lethargy, convulsions and coma may occur. Hepatic toxicity and renal damage may occur.

Treatment Gastric lavage is contraindicated due to risk of aspiration of kerosene into the lungs. Supportive management is provided by administration of fluids, electrolytes and oxygen. Antibiotics are given when there is secondary bacterial infection. There is no role of steroid therapy. Children who are asymptomatic and X-ray chest is normal, can be sent home after 6 hours of observation.

Organophosphate Poisoning

Organophosphate compounds are commonly used as agricultural pesticides and often kept at home in the rural areas. The poisoning may occur due to accidental or suicidal ingestion and following absorption through skin.

Clinical features There may be excessive salivation, lacrimation, urination and bowel movements. Exudation of fluid in the bronchi with wheezing may occur. Anxiety, restlessness, confusion, seizures and coma may occur. Respiratory failure due to paralysis of respiratory muscles is common mode of death. Pupils are constricted.

Treatment If the insecticide was in contact with skin or eyes, these areas should be thoroughly washed. Stomach wash is done. General supportive measures should be started after establishing an IV line. Atropine is given in doses of 0.02–0.05 mg/kg/dose every 10–30 minutes till child is fully atropinized. Pralidoxime is a specific antidote for organophosphates. The child should be observed for 24–48 hours after the onset of recovery to ensure that cholinergic signs do not recur as the effect of atropine and pralidoxime wanes off.

ANIMAL AND INSECT BITES

Dog Bite

Pet animals are known to transmit certain diseases to human beings (zoonosis) and dogs often bite strangers and at times even family members. Dog bite is associated with a high risk of transmission of rabies which is invariably a fatal disease. Rabies can also be transmitted through the bites of cats, monkeys, mongoose, jackals and cattle. In India, rats, mice, bandicoots, squirrels and rabits have not been shown to transmit rabies. Children are more likely to have dangerous dog bites on the head, face and neck. Pet animals must be effectively immunized against rabies and other diseases on the advice of a veterinary doctor.

First aid

Wash the wound immediately and thoroughly with soap and running water for 5 minutes. Never apply any turmeric, chilly powder or oil over the wound. You may apply tincture iodine, betadine or any other antiseptic lotion. The wound should be left open without stitching. Rush the child to a doctor without wasting any time. Refer to **Chapter 21** for post-exposure antirabies vaccination. Antirabies serum should also be given when bites are associated with oozing of blood. In case of bite by a pet dog, further vaccination shots may be omitted if animal is normal and alive after 10 days of the bite.

45

Table 45.1 Specific antidotes

Poison	Antidote
1. Acetaminophen (paracetamol) Toxic dose: 150 mg/kg	N-acetyl cysteine 140 mg/kg followed by 70 mg/kg every 4 hours for 68 hours (17 doses) as oral (preferred) solution mixed with fruit juice.
2. Amphetamines Toxic dose: 50 mg	Chlorpromazine 1 mg/kg IM or IV.
3. Atropine	Pilocarpine 2–4 mg orally or 0.25–0.5 mg IM. Physostigmine 1–2 mg IM every 30 min.
4. Belladonna (*dhatura*)	Physostigmine 0.5–2.0 mg IM every 30 min. Neostigmine is ineffective because it does not enter the CNS.
5. Benzodiazepines	Flumazenil IV in incremental doses of 0.1, 0.2, 0.3, 0.5 mg at 1-min intervals until desired effect is achieved.
6. Carbon monoxide	100% oxygen inhalation or hyperbaric oxygen therapy.
7. Cyanide Fatal dose: 200–300 mg	i. Amyl nitrite (vaporal) 0.3 mL inhalation for 15–30 sec after every min. ii. Sodium nitrate 3% solution, 0.33 mL/kg (max 10 mL) slowly IV. iii. Sodium thiosulphate 1.65 mL/kg 25% solution (max 50 mL) at a rate of 2.5–5.0 mL per min IV.
8. Ethylene glycol	Ethanol 10 mL/kg 10% solution IV or 1 mL/kg of 95% by mouth. Maintenance dose is 1.5 mL/kg/hr 10% solution IV or 3 mL/kg/hr 10% solution IV during hemodialysis.
9. Heavy metals I. Mercury i, iii II. Arsenic i III. Lead i, ii, iii, iv	i. British anti-lewisite (BAL) 12–24 mg/kg/day in 6 divided doses IM (BAL or dimercaprol 100 mg/mL, 3 mL amp). ii. EDTA (calcium disodium ethylene diamine tetra acetic acid) 50–75 mg/kg day in 4 div doses IM or IV as 0.2–0.4% solution (200 mg/mL ampoule) iii. D-penicillamine 20–40 mg/kg per day orally for 5 days. iv. Oral thiamine and dimercapto succinic acid (DMSA) is useful.
10. Heparin	1.0 mg protamine sulfate for 100 units heparin as 1% solution IV (10 mg/mL ampoule).
11. Iron Toxic dose: 35 mg/kg	Deferoxamine 15 mg/kg/hr IV infusion. Therapy needed for 12–36 hours till urine color becomes normal (desferal 500 mg/vial).
12. Isoniazid	Pyridoxine 1.0 mg IV for every 1.0 mg of isoniazid upto a maximum of 500 mg if amount of isoniazid ingested is unknown.
13. Methemoglobinemia	Methylene blue 1–2 mg/kg/hr IV 1% solution. May be repeated after 4 hours (10 mg/mL ampoule). Maximum dose is 7 mg/kg.
14. Methyl alcohol	Ethyl alcohol (ethanol) 0.75–1.0 mL/kg IV followed by 0.5 mL/kg every hourly IV as 5% solution in sodium bicarbonate. Alternatively it an be given as 3–4 ounces of of whisky (45% alcohol) every 4 hourly for 1–3 days in adults (Inj ethanol 2 mL ampoule).
15. Morphine, other opiates, semi- and synthetic narcotics (heroin), meperidine, lomotil (diphenoxylate hydrochloride) and pentazocin	Naloxone 0.1 mg/kg IV (max 2 mg). Repeat every 2–3 min till the reversal of toxic effects or a cummulative dose of 10 mg is reached (Inj narcan 0.4 mg/mL).
16. Organo-phosphate poisoning (insecticides which are cholinesterase inhibitors)	i. Atropine 0.02–0.05 mg/kg/dose IV every 15–30 min till signs of atropinization develop. For continuous infusion 0.02–0.08 mg/kg/hour after the initial bolus. ii. PAM or pralidoxime (2-Pyridine aldozime methiodide) 25–50 mg/kg IM or IV as 5% solution over 15–30 minutes. The dose may be repeated after 1–2 hours and then at 10–12 hours intervals if cholinergic signs recur. For continuous infusion 9–19 mg/kg/ hour after the initial bolus of 25–50 mg/kg.
17. Phenothiazine and metoclopra- mide (extrapyramidal reactions)	Diphenhydramine 1–2 mg/kg/IV every 30 min. (Benadryl cap 25 mg; 50 mg; suspension 12.5 mg/5 mL; amp 50 mg/mL; vials 10 mg/mL).
18. Propranolol (beta-blockers)	Atropine 0.01–0.02 mg/kg per dose SC every 5–10 min to achieve full atropinisation. Glucagon 0.25–1.0 mg IM or IV (Glucagon amp 1 mg/mL).
19. Warfarin, dicumarol	Vitamin K 5–10 mg IM or IV (Inj kapilin 10 mg/mL).

Source: Singh M and Deorari AK, Drug Dosages in Children, *CBS Publishers and Distributors Pvt Ltd.,* New Delhi, 9th edition 2015, pp 186–192.

45

Prevention

Children should be sensitized and educated to prevent dog bites (Box 45.12).

Snake Bite

There are over 3500 known species of snakes in the world, only 200 (around 50 in India) are poisonous. Even when bitten by a poisonous snake, 20–50% of victims may have little or no poisoning. There is pain and marked swelling at the site of bite. Children are more likely to die due to snake bite because the same amount of venom is injected into the small body size of the child.

Clinical manifestations depend upon the type of the biting snake. There are neurological manifestations like ptosis, ophthalmoplegia, paralysis of muscles of palate, deglutition and breathing in case of bites by cobra and krait. The bites by vipers and pit vipers are anti-hemostatic leading to circulatory collapse, hemolysis and widespread bleeding due to coagulation disorder. There may be hemoglobinuria with acute renal failure.

First aid

Do not panic because majority of the bites are by non-poisonous snakes. Reassure and keep the child calm and relaxed by moral support. Most victims suffer mostly due to fear and mental shock rather than the snake venom. The bitten limb should be splinted to prevent movements. The child should be lifted and not allowed to walk to reduce absorption of venom. Do not try to suck the venom out as it is usually ineffective. Immobilize the limb and keep it horizontal. *Application of tourniquet above the site of bite is controversial and should be avoided*. Do not apply ice pack over the bite or waste time in rituals and folklore remedies. The child should be rushed to the nearest hospital. The outcome of snake bite depends on how soon the supportive therapy and

specific anti-snake venom (ASV) is given to the victim. A delay of few hours may prove fatal. If the snake has been killed, it should be taken along with to identify whether it is poisonous or non-poisonous.

Treatment

Excellent nursing care and supportive management is life saving. Assess vital signs and ensure adequacy of airway, breathing and circulation. Pain and anxiety should be relieved by administration of morphine. Intravenous Ringer lactate or normal saline should be started to maintain circulation. Tetanus prophylaxis should be provided. Polyvalent antivenom serum is administered intravenously after conducting hypersensitivity skin test. The dose of antivenom in children is the same or even higher compared to adults. Neostigmine and assisted ventilation is life saving when there is paralysis of respiratory muscles. Blood loss should be replenished by administration of fresh whole blood. Role of heparin is doubtful while infusion of fresh frozen plasma and fibrinogen is not recommended because they may perpetuate the bleeding tendency. Shock is managed by rapid infusion of dextrose-saline and use of vasopressors especially dopamine. Broad spectrum antibiotics are given to treat superadded bacterial infection. Mortality due to snake bite is higher in children because they are exposed to much higher dose of snake venom per unit body weight.

Scorpion Sting

Scorpion stings are more common than snake bites in tropical and subtropical countries. They are less likely to be fatal but deaths may occur due to pulmonary edema. There is intense pain, redness and swelling at the site of bite. The systemic features include bradycardia or tachycardia, hypotension, excessive sweating, cold extremities, salivation and lacrimation, and increased urge for urination and defecation due to parasympathetic dysfunction. Pulmonary edema because of myocardial dysfunction may develop after 1–3 hours of the sting. The common CNS manifestations include restlessness, difficulty in swallowing, blurring of vision and involuntary jerky movements or fasciculations.

Supportive measures Vital signs should be monitered. Maintain airway, breathing and circulation. Keep the child in a propped up position and administer oxygen if indicated. Pain should be relieved by use of ice pack, oral paracetamol or NSAID, and local infiltration of 2% xylocaine. Administration of morphine is contraindicated due to risk of arrhythmias. Maintain adequate fluid and electrolyte balance.

Box 45.12	Prevention of dog bites

- Train your dog to be social, friendly and obedient.
- Never leave the young child alone with the dog unsupervised.
- Teach children never to disturb a dog that is sleeping, eating or when caring for the puppies.
- Warn children never to approach a strange dog.
- Always allow a pet dog to see and sniff you before you touch it.
- Instruct children never to stare a dog in the eyes.
- Children should be told not to run past dogs.
- When a stray dog threatens you, never run or stare directly into the eyes. Stay calm, be stoic and ignore the animal.

Specific therapy Prozosin, alpha-1 adrenoreceptor antagonist, is life saving to suppress sympathetic outflow and activate venom-inhibited potassium channels. It should be administered without any delay whenever there are evidences of autonomic hyperactivity. It is available as 1.0 mg tablet and is administered in a dose of 30 mg/kg orally every 3–4 hours till extremities become warm and tachycardia disappears. Hypotension and pulmonary edema are managed by administration of furosemide, inotropes, sodium nitroprusside and assisted ventilation. Administration of atropine, ACE inhibitors and steroids are contraindicated in the treatment of scorpion sting. Monospecific antivenom is sparingly available and may be given to critically ill children with neurotoxicity.

Wasp and Bee Stings

Wasp and bee stings usually cause local pain, itching, stinging sensation and swelling. Rarely, severe hypersensitivity anaphylaxis reaction with urticaria and difficulty in breathing may occur.

First aid Apply bicarbonate of soda (baking soda) dissolved in few drops of water or a drop of vinegar, clarified butter (*desi ghee*) or onion juice over the sting. Local application of soothing lotion (calamine), or anesthetic cream and ice pack reduces irritation and pain. If bee sting is visible, remove it with a tweezer or a blunt knife. In case of multiple bites or severe reaction, paracetamol and an antihistaminic (like phenergan) can be given for relief of pain and itching. In a rare instance of an hypersensitivity reaction, the child should be rushed to a hospital. Anaphylaxis is treated by administration of epinephrine.

ANAPHYLAXIS

It is a rare life-threatening hypersensitivity reaction to a variety of triggers or allergens. It may occur due to intake of certain food items like dairy products, nuts, seafood, eggs, etc. or follow a wasp or bee sting. It may follow parenteral administration of certain drugs like antibiotics, NSAIDs, opioids, vaccines and sera.

Clinical features The onset is dramatic with laryngeal edema, stridor, bronchospasm and air hunger. There may be sudden palpitation, chest pain and shock. Skin manifestations include urticaria, angioedema and itching. Gastrointestinal features include swelling of lips and tongue, nausea, vomiting and abdominal pain. There is feeling of impending doom and child may become drowsy or comatosed.

Treatment Whenever any injection or vaccine is given to a patient, nurse should be prepared to handle this emergency with calmness and confidence. Administration of adrenaline 0.01 mL/kg 1:1000 solution (max dose 0.5 mL) IM is life saving. The dose can be repeated after 5–10 minutes intervals. Administer oxygen and establish an IV line to give methyl prednisolone (1–2 mg/kg) or hydrocortisone hemisuccinate 5–10 mg/kg and diphenhydramine or chlorpheniramine maleate (1 to 2 mg/kg). When a trigger is identified, the patient should be warned to avoid it throughout life.

CARDIOPULMONARY RESUSCITATION (CPR)

Availability of oxygen to the tissues is a fundamental requirement for human survival. The brain of the child may be permanently damaged or child may die if he fails to get oxygen supply for as brief a period as 3 minutes or so. When such a life-threatening situation develops at home, play ground, swimming pool or road side, there is no time to transfer the victim to the hospital and child may die or get permanently brain damaged unless he is immediately resuscitated at the site of accident and during his journey to the hospital. Every adult, therefore, must receive training in basic life-saving techniques and CPR.

Indications for Resuscitation

A child may stop breathing due to choking, smothering, drowning, smoke inhalation, electric shock and poisoning. The common causes of cardiopulmonary arrest in children are shown in **Box 45.13**. He would require mouth-to-mouth breathing to ensure delivery of oxygen into the lungs. If resuscitation is delayed, it would lead to damage to the most vital organs of the body, i.e. brain and heart. The heart may stop beating if there is lack of oxygen supply to the heart for several minutes. At this stage, artificial breathing alone cannot revive the child unless simultaneous cardiac massage

---

Box 45.13 Common causes of cardiopulmonary arrest

- Birth asphyxia
- Anaphylaxis
- Airway obstruction: Foreign body, aspiration, upper airway obstruction, drowning, bronchopneumonia, ARDS.
- Cardiogenic causes: Shock, sepsis, arrhythmias, cardiac failure.
- Central nervous system causes: Meningitis, encephalitis, cereberal edema, raised ICP, space occupying lesion, and persistent seizures.
- Accidents: Trauma, burns, electrocution, drowning and poisoning.

is done to ensure that the oxygen entering into the body through the lungs is being actually delivered to the tissues of the body through circulation by active pumping actions of the heart.

Assessment

Is he conscious? Firmly shake, shout and tap the victim as if trying to awaken him. If there is no response after three attempts, assume he is unconscious.

Is he choked? Sudden choking with difficulty in breathing, coughing and blueness are suggestive of foreign body inhalation. When foreign body completely obstructs the airways, there will be no coughing, crying, or speaking and child would become limp and blue. Refer to page 392 for maneuvers to expel the foreign body. Avoid mouth-to-mouth breathing till foreign body is expelled.

Is he breathing? Look for movements of the chest wall and take your ears close to his nose and mouth or hold a piece of paper infront of his nose and mouth to see whether he is breathing or not. If there is no breathing, give mouth-to-mouth breathing without wasting any time. Never give artificial breathing to a child who is breathing on his own.

Is heart beating? Gently feel the pulse over the front of inner side of elbow (brachial artery in children) and in the neck just below the jaw bone (carotid artery in infants). When pulse is not felt, it means heart has stopped beating. In this situation, give simultaneously both mouth-to-mouth breathing as well as external cardiac massage.

Mouth-to-mouth breathing

1. Place the child on the floor or a hard surface. Clean the mouth of any foreign material, secretions, vomitus or blood with your handkerchief. Gently bend the child's head back with one hand and lift up the chin with the other hand. This is done to lift the tongue so that air passage is cleared at the back of the throat or nasopharynx (**Figures 45.5** and **45.6**).
2. Keep the head tilted backwards with his mouth open and jaw supported with one hand. Pinch both the nostrils with fingers of your hand which is resting on his forehead.
3. Take a deep breath and make a tight seal with your lips around the child's mouth. Breathe out into the child's mouth with sufficient force so that his chest should rise.
4. Take your mouth away and let his chest fall. Take another deep breath, make a tight seal around the child's mouth again and give another breath to the child. Continue giving breaths at a rate of 15–20 breaths per minute till he starts breathing on his own or medical help arrives and takes over.

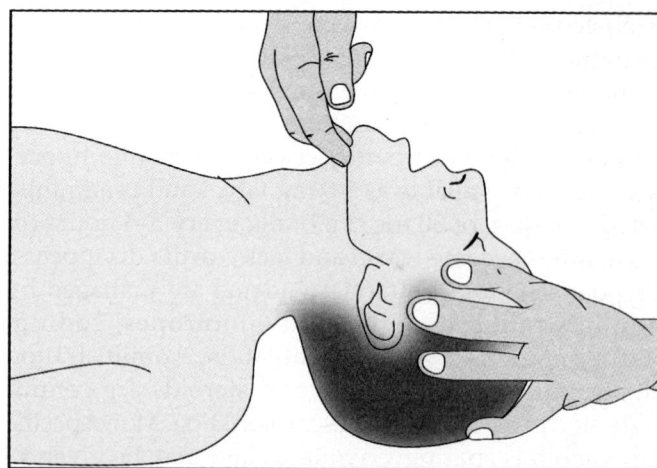

Figure 45.5 Opening the airway by head tilt-chin lift maneuver

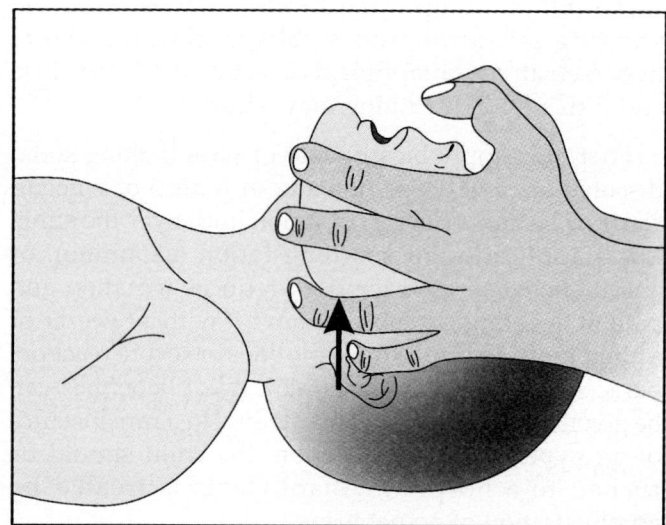

Figure 45.6 Opening the airway with the jaw thrust maneuver

Mouth-to-mouth and nose breathing

In infants below 2 years, mouth and nose are very close to each other. It is, therefore, easier and more practical to breathe into the mouth and nose together. Make a tight seal with your lips to enclose both the nose and mouth of the baby (**Figure 45.7**). The artificial breaths should be given with lesser force but at a faster rate (around 30 breaths/minute).

In hospital setting, bag to mask ventilation is provided which is more effective.

Heart massage (External cardiac massage)

When despite mouth-to-mouth breathing, the child remains blue or markedly pale and you are unable to feel his pulse, it means heart has become extremely weak or stopped beating. In this situation you must provide simultaneously both mouth-to-mouth breathing along with cardiac massage.

1. The child should be lying on the floor on a hard surface.
2. Kneel beside the child. Place heel of one hand over the lower half of the child's breast bone (sternum). The sternum is located in the middle of the chest and extends from the mid-point between the two collar bones (clavicles) from the highest point of chest to the pit of the stomach.
3. Move yourself forwards over the child's body so that your shoulders are directly over his sternum.
4. Keeping your arm straight and without bending it at the elbow, press down on the breast bone.
5. Repeat chest compressions at a rate of about 80–100 per minute without lifting your hands off the sternum.
6. After every five chest compressions, stop and give him one mouth-to-mouth breathing. Continue the cycle of these two combined procedures, i.e. five chest compressions followed by one mouth-to-mouth breathing.
7. If two rescuers are available, one can continue with mouth-to-mouth breathing while the other can provide cardiac compressions. You should temporarily stop doing chest compressions when the other rescuer delivers mouth-to-mouth breathing.
8. As soon as the heart beats are established (as evidenced by easily palpable brachial or carotid pulse), you can stop cardiac massage and continue with mouth-to-mouth breathing till the child starts breathing spontaneously.

Heart massage in infants

In infants below 2 years, chest wall and ribs are softer and cardiac massage can be performed with two fingers as described below:

1. Instead of heel of the hand, two fingers (middle and index) are used for providing chest compressions. In newborn babies, chest can be enclosed by both hands and compressions are provided by both thumbs meeting over the lower part of sternum (Figure 45.8).
2. The chest should be compressed by about ½–1 inch with gentle pressure to avoid injury to the ribs and lungs.
3. The fingers used for chest compressions are placed over the middle of the sternum (at the imaginary line joining the two nipples).
4. The chest compressions are done at a relatively faster rate of 100–120 compressions per minute. Mouth-to-mouth breathing is given once after every five chest compressions as in the case of older children.

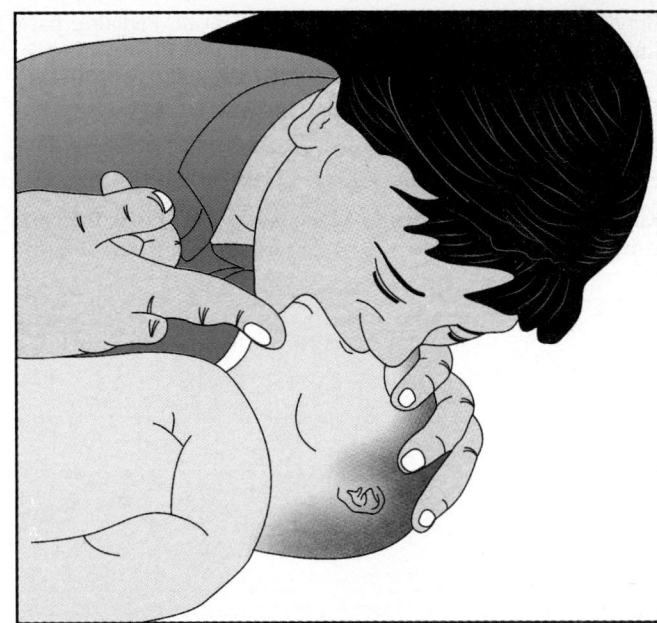

Figure 45.7 Mouth-to-mouth and nose breathing in an infant for resuscitation

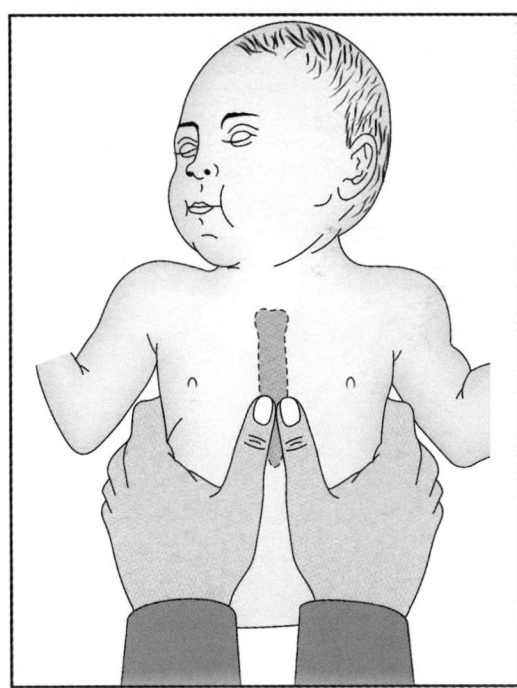

Figure 45.8 Method for cardiac massage with the help of thumbs in case of a newborn baby

BIBLIOGRAPHY

American Academy of Pediatrics Committee on Injury, Violence and Poison Prevention. Prevention of drowning. *Pediatrics* 2010, 126(1): 178–185.

Arnoldo B, Klein M, Gibran NS. Practice guidelines for the management of electrical injuries. *J Burn Care Res* 2006, 27(4): 439–447.

Berg MD, Schexnayder SM, Shameides L, et al. Pediatric basic life support: 2010 American Heart Association Guidelines for Cardiopulmonary Resuscitation and Emergency Cardiovascular Care. *Circulation* 2010, 122 (Suppl 3): S862–S875.

Bryant S, Singer J. Management of toxic exposure in children. *Emerg Med Clin North Amer* 2003, 21(1): 101–119.

Kleinman ME, Chameides L, Schexnayder SM, et al. Pediatric Advanced Life Support: 2010 American Heart Association Guidelines for Cardiopulmonary Resuscitation and Emergency Cardiovascular Care. *Circulation* 2010, 122(Supple 3): S876–S908.

Mahadevan S. Scorpion sting. *Indian Pediatr* 2000, 37(5): 504–514.

Menon PR, Lodha R. Poisoning in children. In: Pediatric Emergencies in Children. Singh M (Ed.) New Delhi, CBS Publishers and Distributors Pvt Ltd. Revised 5th Edition, 2016, p799–822.

45

Community and Social Pediatrics

RIGHTS OF CHILDREN

Children are dependent and at the mercy of their parents and caretakers to safeguard their fundamental rights. The Convention of the Rights of the Child (CRC) of 1989 defines a child as any human person who has not reached the age of 18 years. As far back as 1924, the League of Nations adopted the Geneva Declaration of the Rights of the Child to receive the care for normal development, the right of the hungry child to be fed, the right of sick child to receive healthcare, the right of the backward child to be protected, the right of orphans to shelter and the right to protection against exploitation. The United Nations Convention on the Rights of the Child (UNCRC) defines **Child Rights** as the minimum entitlements and opportunities that

---

Declaration of the Rights of the Child

"The child, by reason of his physical and mental immaturity, needs special safeguards and care, including appropriate legal protection, before as well as after birth".

---

should be offered to every citizen below the age of 18 years regardless of race, national origin, color, gender, language, religion, economic background, birth status, disability or other characteristics. The components of Rights of Children are listed below:

Right to Survival

- Right to be born
- Right to minimum standard of food, shelter and clothing
- Right to live with dignity
- Right to healthcare, safe drinking water, nutritious food, a clean and safe environment, and information to help them to stay healthy.

Right to Protection

- Right to be protected from all sorts of violence
- Right to be protected from neglect
- Right to be protected from physical and sexual abuse
- Right to be protected from dangerous drugs

Right to Participation

- Right to freedom of opinion
- Right to freedom of expression
- Right to freedom of association
- Right to information
- Right to participate in any decision making that involves him/her directly or indirectly

Right to Development

- Right to education
- Right to learn
- Right to recreation
- Right to global development—physical, mental, emotional, social and spiritual.

THE NATIONAL POLICY FOR CHILDREN

India is home to the largest child population in the world. In India, children under the age of 18 years account for 40% total population. Children are supremely important asset and government of India reiterated its commitment to secure the rights of its children by ratifying related international conventions and treaties. The National Policy for Children 1974, recognized that progress for children should find prominent place in national plans for the development of human resources, so that children grow up to become robust citizens, physically fit, mentally alert and morally healthy, endowed with skills and motivation provided by the society. The national policy for children was revised in 2013.

Preamble

- Child is any person below the age of 18 years
- Childhood is an integral part of life with a value of its own.

- Children are not a homogenous group, have multi-dimensional variabilities and needs.
- A long-term sustainable, multisectoral integrated and inclusive approach is necessary for the overall harmonious development and protection of children.

Guiding Principles

1. Every child has universal, inalienable and indivisible human rights.
2. The rights of children are interrelated and interdependent and each one of them is equally important and fundamental to the well-being and dignity of the child.
3. Every child has the right to life, survival, development, education, protection and participation.
4. Right to life, survival and development goes beyond the physical existence of the child.
5. All children have equal rights and no child should be discriminated against on the ground of religion, race, caste, sex, place of birth, social class, language, disability, social, economic or any other criterian.
6. Every child has the right to dignified life, free from exploitation.
7. Safety and security of children is integral part of their well-being in all settings.
8. Family or family environment is most conducive for the all-round development of children.
9. Children are capable of forming views and must be provided a conducive environment and opportunity to express their views.
10. Children's views, specially those of girls, children from disadvantaged and marginalized communities, must be heard in all matters affecting them.

Key Priorities

The following key priorities should be provided to global children at all levels of society without any discrimination.
1. Nutrition, health and survival of children.
2. Education, knowledge and human development.
3. A safe, secure and protective environment for each and every child.
4. Children should be made aware of their rights and they should participate in all the activities for their development.
5. Advocacy, participation and collective action of all stakeholders.
6. Coordination, implementation and monitoring of all activities for the welfare of children.
7. Research, documentation and capacity building for implementation of the National Policy.

8. Resource allocation, financial and managerial, to work for welfare of children at all levels.
9. A comprehensive review of the National Policy initiatives every 5 years by the Ministry of Women and Child Development.

Universal Children's Day The United Nations adopted the Declaration of the Rights of the Child on 20 November 1959 and subsequently adopted the Convention of the Rights of Child on 20 November 1989. The Universal Children's Day is celebrated by all countries on 20 November to promote the commitment to honor the rights of children and to initiate actions to promote the wellfare of the world's children. The day is celebrated to foster global awareness for the benefit of children that have succumbed to violence in forms of abuse, exploitation and discrimination. Apart from Universal Children's Day, many countries celebrate National Children's Day (*Bal Divas*), which is celebrated in India on 14 November, the birth anniversary of the first Prime Minister of the Country, Pandit Jawaharlal Nehru (Chacha Nehru).

THE GIRL CHILD

Girls are the creators of progeny and their health and well-being is closely interlinked with the health and well-being of their children. Healthy and well-informed mothers are likely to give birth to healthy babies and they are in a better position to look after the health and well-being of their children. There is a need to provide equal status and opportunities to girl children throughout their life cycle so that they grow to become healthy, literate, empowered and economically independent adults to look after their own health and well-being of their children. The concept of gender equality means that boys and girls should have equal access to food, health care, education and opportunities in life. In our patriarchial society, the common reasons for gender discrimination include the need for sons to look after the ancestral property and for tilling the land and girls on the other hand are often viewed as a liability because of greater need and responsibility for their upbringing and protection, and the economic burden of dowry. There is a mistaken cultural belief that a son is likely to look after the parents in their old age. But it is a myth rather than reality because daughters in general are

> *"The prevailing sense of despair and despondency at the birth of a female child should be replaced by the awareness and hope that she is the creator and sustainer of progeny".*
>
> — **Meharban Singh**

more caring and concerned to provide comfort and emotional support to the aged parents. The current dismal status and discriminatory practices against girl children are listed below.

Feticide and infanticide It is an unfortunate fact that gender discrimination may begin before birth. Although antenatal determination of fetal sex by ultrasound examination is a criminal offence but there is epidemiological evidence to suggest that it is widely practiced for selective abortion of female fetuses. It is estimated that 100,000 abortions are performed every year in India solely because the fetus is female. The 2011 census data suggest that there is unusually high proportion of male births and male to female sex ratio in our country is skewed in favor of males (1000 boys vs 940 girls). The worst sex ratio (fewer girls) is seen in the affluent urban populations of Punjab, Delhi, Mumbai and Ahmedabad. It is unfortunate that society is indulging in an inhuman practice which is against the dictates of nature and will of God. The Government of India has launched multipronged strategies to curb female feticide, which include legislative measures such as Preconception and Prenatal Diagnostic Techniques (PCPNDT) Act in 2004, advocacy and awareness programs for socioeconomic empowerment of women.

Education Over the years, there has been an increasing trend for girls being sent to schools especially in the urban areas. But nevertheless, of 5 girls who enroll in school, one girl drops out and never completes the primary education. There is data to suggest that under-5 mortality of their children falls by about half for mothers who complete their primary school education. Due to social, economic and cultural reasons, girls are often denied secondary education. In a recent survey by UNICEF, it was found that only 40% of girls in the developing world attend secondary school. Educated girls are likely to have better status and say in society, more empowerment, economic independence, greater freedom to take decisions about their marriage and reproductive life. They are likely to have better nutrition and health status with delay in the birth of their first child and better spacing, health and well-being of their children.

Child marriages and teenage pregnancy The child marriages have been banned by the Sarda Act in 1929 during British regime. The Child Marriage and Restraint Act (Amendment) 1978 fixed the legal minimum age of marriage as 21 years for boys and 18 years for girls. However, child marriages are still rampant in many states of India (especially Rajasthan, Madhya Pradesh, Uttar Pradesh) and in rural population. It is estimated that about 70% girls are married off before the age of 18 years without their consent. Due to constant threat of sexual abuse, molestation, out of caste alliance and curse of dowry, parents often take the easy route of marrying off their daughters at an early age especially in families with poor socioeconomic status.

Early or teenage marriages are associated with several health hazards to the mothers and their babies. There is greater likelihood of more conceptions, abortions/stillbirths, pregnancy-induced hypertension, difficult deliveries, birth trauma and maternal malnutrition. There is increased risk of neonatal morbidity and mortality because of increased incidence of preterm and low birth weight or small-for-dates babies. Teenage mother is likely to have poor education and lack maturity to provide satisfactory parenting to look after the health and nutritional needs of her children. Due to increasing literacy, awareness, urbanization and improvement in the socioeconomic status, there has been a gradual increase in the age at marriage. The health care professionals (HCPs) and nurses should take initiative and responsibility to inform and educate the community about the health hazards of early marriages and motivate them to eliminate this social malady.

Sexual abuse and reproductive health According to WHO data, every year globally 150 million girls and 73 million boys under the age of 18 years are forced to have sexual intercourse or other forms of sexual and physical abuse. The problem has become worse due to breakdown of joint family system and because many mothers are working and are unable to guard them at home. It is unfortunate that in poor societies girls are exploited or forced into commercial sex work or sexual slavery. They are subjected to neglect, sexual and physical violence and psychological abuse. Due to unsafe sexual practices and poor concept of personal hygiene, there is high incidence of sexually transmitted diseases (STDs) and pelvic inflammatory disease (PID) with increased prevalence of tubal pregnancy and infertility.

Risk of HIV/AIDS Women are at a greater risk of contracting HIV than men and are often at the mercy of their sexual partners for use of condoms. In a global survey conducted in 2005, nearly half of the 39 million people infected with HIV were women. They pose a potential risk to transmit HIV to their innocent children during pregnancy, child birth and breastfeeding.

Maternal mortality It is estimated that globally every year nearly half a million women (one woman every minute) die as a result of complications of

46

46

pregnancy and child birth. In India, maternal mortality rate is extremely high with the current adjusted estimate of 178 maternal deaths per 100,000 child births accounting for 25% of all maternal deaths worldwide. Many of the maternal lives can be saved by providing basic health care services including universal antenatal care, availability of skilled birth attendants for all deliveries and emergency obstetric care for women who develop complications.

Women in old age Grandmothers are a great resource of knowledge and skills for mothercraft and child care. In many families, they are the mainstay of child care for working parents. But unfortunately, elderly women face double discrimination on the basis of both gender and old age. Women tend to live longer than men, they lack control of family resources and often face discrimination in our inheritance and property laws. They are at the mercy of the male members of the family and often live a life of neglect due to lack of any social support system in our country.

National Plan of Action for the Girl Child

During 1991–2000, Government of India launched a plan of action for improving the status of girl child by eliminating gender discrimination, prevention of female feticide and infanticide, provision of primary education and protection of girls against exploitation, assault and abuse. A sustained educational campaign by the Government of India and NGOs has been started to ensure that girls are accorded equal rights and opportunities without any discrimination. A happy and healthy girl child is indeed the harbinger of bright future and strong foundation of our society.

Beti Bachao Beti Padhao (BBBP) Yojana The Government of India launched the initiative, "Save Girl Child, Educate Girl Child" on 22 January, 2015 with an initial corpus of INR 100 crores (US $ 15 million). The scheme was launched to address the declining child sex ratio (CSR) which has dropped to 940 girls for every 1000 boys in 2011 because of antenatal sex determination by ultrasonography and selective female feticides. Moreover, there is neglect of health care, nutrition and education of girls in our patriarchial society. The discrimination against girl children occurs due to several socioeconomic factors. In Indian society, son is considered as the *waaris* or inheritor and protector of family assets, provides extra hands to look after the family business and for tilling the agricultural land and provides an assurance (often misplaced) that he would look after the parents in their old age. On the other hand, the girls are considered as a liability because of financial burden of dowry, greater responsibility on the part of parents for their supervision and protection, and they are "lost" to the family after their marriage because in-laws abode is considered as their "real home" in our culture.

The pilot project has been launched in 100 districts of the country with following aims and objectives: (i) prevention of female feticides, (ii) ensure survival and protection of girl child, (iii) ensure education of all girls, (iv) prevent child marriages and teenage pregnancies through compulsory registration of all marriages; (v) effective and stringent anti-dowry act; and (vi) providing financial incentives to parents of girl children. It is proposed to meet the objectives of the scheme by implementing following strategies throughout the country in a phased manner.

1. To launch a sustained social mobilization and communication campaign to create equal opportunities for upbringing and education of girl children.
2. Prevent female feticides and neglect of girl children to improve declining child sex ratio.
3. Identify and focus on gender critical districts for intensive and integrated implementation of BBBP strategies.
4. Mobilize and train the workers of Panchayati Raj institutions, urban local bodies and grassroot workers to serve as catalysts for social change in partnership with local community, women and youth groups.
5. Ensure that community welfare programs are responsive to gender bias and rights of children.

CHILD ABUSE AND NEGLECT

Children are most vulnerable section of our society and are at the mercy of their care takers to look after their basic needs of nutrition, health care, education, and protection. It is an unfortunate fact that a large number of children in less developed countries are living in poverty and are deprived of their rights of survival, optimal health, nutrition, education and protection from exploitation and discrimination. The World Health Organization has defined *Child Abuse* as a violation of basic human rights of a child. It includes all forms of physical and emotional maltreatment, neglect or negligent treatment, sexual harm, commercial or other exploitation, resulting in actual harm or potential harm to the child's health, survival, development and dignity in the context of a relationship of responsibility, trust or power. *Child Neglect* is defined as inattention or negligence by the care taker to provide for the health, education, nutrition, emotional development, shelter and safe living conditions to the child in the context of resources available to the family or care taker leading to harm to the child's health or physical, mental, moral, spiritual and social development. At times, the term *Child Maltreatment* is used, which includes all forms of physical and emotional ill treatment, sexual abuse, neglect and exploitation that results in actual or potential harm to the child's health, development or dignity. Over the years, the concept of Child Abuse and Neglect (CAN) has been widened to include a variety of exploitations like neglect (health care, nutrition, education, love), physical, emotional, social, political and sexual abuse **(Table 46.1)**.

Risk Factors

Child abuse can occur in any family, and at all levels of society. It is more common in families with poor socioeconomic status, poverty, lack of housing, lack of education, unemployment and alcohol abuse. There may be constant interparental conflicts or fights. It is more common when there are too many children in a family with predominence of female children. The child may be born of an unwanted pregnancy, may be odd looking and dark complexioned or have excessive crying, hyperactive and difficult child to rear. It is more common in children of single parents who are young or one of the parents may be a psychopath or suffered ill treatment from his or her own parents during their childhood. The child may run away from home if parents are authoritarian, rigid with military type or punitive style of discipline.

Sexual Abuse and Exploitation

Girls are more vulnerable to rape, trafficking and pornography but there is increasing incidence of sexual exploitation among boys. The perpetrators of most sexual crimes include relatives, acquantices, teachers, neighbours, employers and psychopaths. There is a need that parents, care takers and pediatricians should provide messages on personal space, and protection against sexually abusive experience. Children should be told to be wary if someone touches them inappropriately which makes them uncomfortable, titulates their erogenous body areas, or encourages the child to touch someone's private parts. Whenever someone is taking liberties with the child, he or she should inform the parents or care taker to prevent sexually abusive behavior.

The Ministry of Health and Family Welfare, Government of India has framed guidelines for doctors for handling victims of sexual assault or abuse, during the course of their duty. No hospital can deny evaluation and treatment of sexual assault victims, which has been made a cognizable criminal offence punishable with appropriate fine, imprisonment or both. Every physician working in the emergency department, should be aware of the Standard Operating Procedure (SOP) for assessment and management of sexual assault victims. All medicolegal examinations and procedures must respect the privacy of the victim and informed consent must be taken from the parents or care taker. The examination room should have adequate place, well-lighted examination table, equipment and supplies like sexual assault forensic evidence (SAFE) kit for collecting and preserving medicolegal evidence **(Figure 46.1)**.

Legislative Framework

The revised National Policy for Children (2013) has stipulated the upper age limit of children as 18 years and has affirmed the guidelines of the UN Convention on the Rights of the Child (UNCRC). The Government of India has assigned the responsibility to oversee the rights and protection of children to the Ministry of Women and Child Development. The National Commission for protection of Child Rights established in 2007,

---

Table 46.1 Common forms of child abuse and neglect

1. Physical violence, abuse and battered baby or shaken baby syndrome.
2. Parental neglect: Abandonment, desertion, lack of food, clothing, education, medical care, lack of love, emotional abuse, selling of children.
3. Sexual abuse: Fondling, inappropriate touching, rape or sodomy, prostitution, pornography.
4. Exploitation of children in various ways
   - Substance abuse
   - Sexual abuse and prostitution
   - Political abuse: Wars, party propaganda and electioneering
   - Entertainment abuse: Rope walking, fire jumping, bungee diving, street dancing, camel racing, dangerous stunts, circus, etc.
   - Child labor: Roadside-dhabas, tea stalls, domestic aides, cycle or auto repair shop, small scale industries like glass factory, cigarettes, fireworks, zari work, and carpet weaving; rag-picking, manual and agricultural worker, and shoe shiners.
   - Kidnapping children for begging, stealing, house breaking, thefts, gambling, smuggling and antisocial activities.
   - Trafficking of children for slavery, domestic and industrial labor, sexual abuse, prostitution.
5. Runaway children: Street children, substance abuse, antisocial activities like thefts, crimes, fights, *dada giri*, and delinquent children.

46

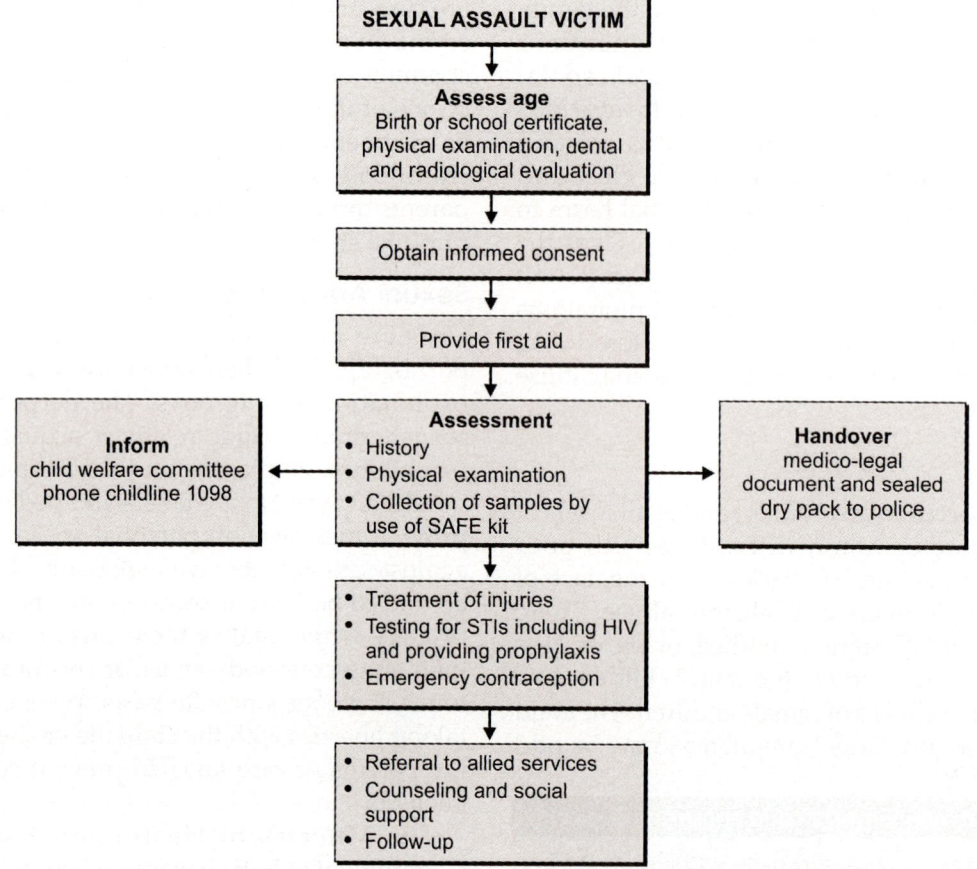

Figure 46.1 Algorithm for handling sexual assault victims
STIs: Sexually transmitted infections, HIV: Human immunodeficiency virus, SAFE kit: sexual assault forensic evidence kit
www.http://mohfw.nic.in.

is charged with the responsibility to look after the crimes against children and recommend punitive action against perpetrators of child abuse and neglect. The Government of India has launched an Integrated Child Protection Scheme in 2009. The guiding principle of the initiative is to recognize that child protection is a primary responsibility of the family, supported by community, government and civil society.

The legislative framework for children's rights is being strengthened and is currently governed by two legislations. The Juvenile Justice Act has been amended in 2006 and provides primary legal framework for both Children in Need of Care and Protection (CNCP) and Children in Conflict of Laws (CCL). The cases of children in need of protection and instances of child abuse are heard by Child Welfare Committee (CWC), which has a chairperson and four members, of whom atleast one is a woman and at last one is expert in children's issues. The legal and criminal matters pertaining to children are handled by Juvenile Justice Boards (JJBs), which have a Metropolitan or Judicial

Magistrate and two social workers, of whom one must be a woman. The protection of Children from Sexual Offences (POCSO) Act 2012 specifically addresses the issue of sexual offences committed against children, which until now was being tried under laws that did not differentiate between adult and child victims. The POCSO Act requires mandatory reporting of all cases of child sexual abuse by doctors and multidisciplinary professionals. The cases of child abuse can be referred to Child Welfare Committee (CWC) and Childline 1098 for necessary sociolegal action. The CLA 2013 and POCSO Act 2012 stipulates that any registered medical practitioner can carry out a medico legal examination of the victim of sexual assault and rape and the observations of the health care provider will stand in the court of law.

Prevention

Children are safe in a family when parents are well educated, emotionally stable without any ego problems or interparental conflicts. The government should provide adequate social services to promote universal education, provide employment skills and opportunities, family life education, development of mothercraft and fathercraft skills for child rearing. The life cycle approach for care of girl children should be promoted because it is the best investment for building a nation. The moral and spiritual values of the society need to be promoted by the teachers, religious leaders and politicians. It is nice to have disciplined children (who become disciplined and productive adults) but discipline should be inculcated with love and appreciation and not by criticism or corporal punishment. It is important to remember that children are inspired and motivated by a pat on their backs and are discouraged and humiliated by a kick on their ass.

BATTERED CHILD SYNDROME

Child neglect and "abuse" occurs when parents are maladjusted, there is financial stress, drug addiction or alcoholism. The pent up anger and frustration is vent out on children who serve as scapegoats. Both parents may indulge in battering but father is the usual villain especially when he is a step father or suspects infidelity on the part of his wife. Many parents who abuse their children were themselves victims of child abuse or may have a psychological disorder. Child abuse may also occur in institutions such as day care centers, schools, child care agencies like delinquent homes and orphanages. Children employed as domestic aides are being increasingly reported as victims of torture by their employers.

Clinical Features

Child abuse may occur at any age but is most common in toddlers and preschool children. In India, girl child is more often abused. There are features of neglect, emotional abuse, failure to thrive, undernutrition, and poor skin hygiene. Physical injuries are inflicted by pinching, pushing, beating with a stick or a belt or by twisting the extremities. There are evidences of multiple bruises, scratches, hematomas, fractures of long bones, ribs or skull *without giving any history of trauma*. There may be multiple fractures in various stages of healing. Chronic subdural hematoma with retinal hemorrhages are highly suggestive of battered child syndrome or shaken baby syndrome. There is evidence that one-third of severely shaken infants die and the majority of survivors develop long-term consequences such as mental retardation, cerebral palsy or blindness.

There may be tell tale marks of burns, scalds or burn marks inflicted by cigarette butts. Imaging studies are done to identify fractures and visceral injuries. There

may be evidences of sexual abuse. The child is frightened, lonely and aloof, and does not seek any comfort or solace from her parents. Children who are sexually abused exhibit symptoms of genital injury, pelvic inflammatory disease, sexually transmitted infections, abdominal pain, constipation, recurrent urinary tract infections and psychological problems.

Role of a Nurse

1. Injuries should be assessed and treated as per standard protocol and under the guidance of a pediatrician and orthopedic specialist. Nurse should provide tender loving care to the neglected child.
2. Family dynamics should be assessed for underlying factors leading to the child abuse.
3. The help of a social worker should be taken for home visiting and for taking history from neighbours and other family members.
4. The nurse should be non-critical and non-judgemental about the behavior of the parents who should be helped to mend their behavior with a warm and sensitive attitude without any anger or tone of punishment.
5. The support of child welfare agencies may be sought to provide necessary guidance to the family to prevent further abuse. Psychiatric consultation should be given to parents. De-addiction facilities should be provided if a parent is suffering from drug abuse or alcoholism. Punitive actions against parents or caretakers may be counterproductive.

STREET CHILDREN

It is a bounden duty of a nation to ensure that every child is adequately protected, housed, clothed, fed and educated and provided with opportunities to enjoy the freedom and pleasures of childhood. Street children are those children who loiter or live on the streets, pavements, wasteland and shanty dwellings. The contributing factors which force children to leave their homes include poverty, rapid urbanization, broken family, loss of parents, alcoholic or psychopathic father, natural or man made disasters, accidents, child abuse and neglect, population explosion and lack of housing facilities.

According to an estimate by UNICEF, there are about 100 million street children, out of which 70 million are in the developing countries. Majority of street children are boys. There are three groups of street children, (i) those who maintain a regular contact with their families and return back to home at night, (ii) children with occasional contact with their families and (iii) children without any contact with their families. Street children have no protection or supervision by adults. They have no source of secure livelihood and may do petty jobs like domestic work, cleaning job in a shop, tea stall and rag picking or indulge in unnatural sexual activities to earn money. These children may join organized child gangs which are controlled by the villains or *dadas* of the den.

Health Hazards

Street children live in most unhygienic and poor sanitary conditions and are vulnerable to a large number of water-borne diseases like recurrent diarrhea, dysentery, giardiasis, parasitic infestations, typhoid fever and viral hepatitis. They lack immunizations and are likely to suffer from vaccine-preventable diseases especially tuberculosis. They are likely to have frequent skin infections, scabies and lice. They are prone to develop psychosocial problems like juvenile delinquency and criminal activities, low self esteem, anger against society (due to big divide between rich and poor), sexual abuse with risk of sexually transmitted diseases, drug addictions and prostitution.

Prevention

There is a need for social and economic upliftment of all segments of society with the help of governmental schemes for social welfare, free and compulsory education, skill development schemes, employment opportunities with adequate wages, family life education and population control strategies, provision of homes and shelters for the homeless. Street children need protection, guidance, free education, health care, counseling and adoption opportunities for their rehabilitation. The non-government organizations like Child Relief and You (CRY) and the City Level Program of Action (CLPOA) have taken initiatives to launch welfare schemes for the benefit of abandoned and street children. These schemes provide a number of social services for the benefit of under-privileged children to look after their health, nutrition, education, recreation, vocational training and development of skills, and safe-guarding the fundamental rights of every child.

CHILD LABOR

Children belonging to poor socioeconomic segment of our society are forced to undertake gainful occupations to supplement the family income. It is more common in children belonging to rural areas and semiurban slums. According to International Labor Organization (ILO), child labor is defined as gainful employment of children below 15 years of age with the aim of earning livelihood for themselves and their families. Children may be made to work at home and away from home either in the unorganized or in the organized sectors. In unorganized sector, children are employed as agriculture labor, domestic servants, helpers and vendors in *dhabas* and tea stalls, shoe shine boys, rag pickers, etc. The child labor is most prevalent in the semiorganized sectors namely carpet weaving, zari embroidery, cigarette and *bidi* making, match and fireworks factories, glass industry, precious stone polishing, building construction, cycle and automobile workshops and garages. The common denominator of child labor is a large family with lack of financial resources for sustenance. Apart from poverty, other correlates include lack of education of parents, selfish and lazy parents, alcoholic or drug abuse father, single mother or separated parents, broken family and school dropouts. Children may be "sold" or kidnapped for exploitation as bonded labor.

Health Hazards

Children "lose their childhood" in pursuit of earning a livelihood at an age when they should be in school and enjoying life without any worries and responsibilities. Child labor adversely affects self esteem, social, emotional, psychological and moral development of children. The working children are at an increased risk of exposure to poor personal hygiene and environ-mental sanitation, lack of safe drinking water and inadequate food. They are prone to develop frequent respiratory infections, diarrheal diseases, tuberculosis, parasitic infestations, scabies, pyoderma and malnutrition. They are highly vulnerable to develop drug addictions, smoking, sexual abuse and risk of sexually transmitted diseases (STDs), pelvic inflammatory disease (PID), accidents and injuries. The child may suffer from work-related disorders (occupational health hazards) depending upon the nature of work in the factories.

Prevention of Child Labor

It is a national disgrace that millions of children in India "sacrifice their childhood" for the sake of earning livelihood for their parents and siblings. It is an unavoidable social malady which is pursued for the sake of survival. There is a need for social and political revolution to improve facilities for education, employment opportunities, better wages, family planning and avoidance of child marriages. There is a need not only for the availability of free compulsory education but schools should also provide other incentives like free mid-day meals, free books and stationery, basic health care, nutrition and family life education; and teaching of skills for earning. The concept of "earning while learning" needs to be promoted.

Indian constitution promotes the Rights of Children and protection against their exploitation. The Child Labor Protection and Regulation Act 1986, provides guidelines for restriction of child labor. The Supreme Court of India on 8th December, 1996, directed all state governments and union territories to take concrete steps to abolish child labor and instructed the government to establish child labor rehabilitation welfare fund. According to Child Labor (Protection and Regulation) Act 1986, no child below the age of 14 years can be employed for labor. The offending employers can be prosecuted and asked to pay a compensation of INR 20,000.00 against each child employee which is credited to the child labor rehabilitation welfare fund. In the current socioeconomic milieu of the country, it is difficult to abolish child labor but attempts should be made to restrict it and make it safer, dignified and more remunerative without any exploitation and bonding.

ADOPTION

Nature has queer ways of striking a balance in society. There are a large number of indigent couples who have plenty of children but no means or resources to provide them decent nurturing. And there are a number of couples from well-to-do families with unlimited resources who crave for children of their own. Almost 1–2% of couples are infertile and despite various therapeutic interventions and recourse to assisted reproductive technologies (in-vitro fertilization or IVF, gamete intrafallopian transfer or GIFT, zygote intrafallopian transfer or ZIFT and tubal ovum transfer or TOT) and surrogate motherhood, they are unable to beget children of their own. Adoption is a boon for them.

According to "Hindu Adoption and Maintenance Act 1956" there is a legal provision for needy parents to adopt children who are not biologically related to them. They can adopt a child from among children of their relatives who are willing to offer their child for adoption. More commonly the child is taken for adoption from an orphanage, foster home or from a hospital where children are abandoned by their unwed mothers or due to other social reasons. Adoption serves the felt needs and desires of both the needy couples as well as the children who get security and tender loving care from their adoptive parents.

Screening for Adoption

When children are adopted from an orphanage or a foster home, pediatrician is asked to examine the child for its suitability for adoption by assessing their physical growth, neuromotor development, nutritional status, presence of any contagious disease or developmental defect, and immunization record. Laboratory investigations are carried out for complete blood count, X-ray chest, Mantoux test and tests for sexually transmitted diseases like VDRL, HBsAg, HIV and if indicated TORCH profile.

Procedure for Adoption

Social worker or a public health nurse should provide guidance and support to the family for completing the formalities for adoption.

1. The eligibility for adoption can be checked on the Website of Central Adoption Resource Authority (CARA), Ministry of Women and Child Development or contact them at email: care_wcd@nic.in.
2. The adoptive parents should apply for adoption by filling the necessary form which should be signed by both the prospective parents.
3. The adoptive couple is required to produce a medical certificate regarding their inability to produce a child, marriage certificate, proof of age, income certificate or bank statement.
4. The social worker should provide information and data regarding the suitability of the adoptive parents. They should be psychologically and mentally sound, should have reasonable financial means, education, socioeconomic status and living conditions.
5. The child is handed over to the adoptive parents for foster care on a trial period. During this period, the social worker is asked to assess the suitability of adoptive parents and quality of care provided to the child by home visits. If a child is not able to adjust or when care provided by the adoptive parents is unsatisfactory, the agency has the right to take away the child and deny adoption.
6. When child is well adjusted and adoptive parents are found to be caring and considerate, legal adoption is confirmed. After legal adoption, the child gets all the rights and privileges which are granted to the biological child.

Role of a Public Health Nurse

The nurse should provide following guidance and support to the adoptive parents.

1. The adoptive parents and their family must have mutual agreement and acceptance for an adopted child.
2. The couple should be mentally and psychologically prepared and provided guidance for proper feeding, health care, immunizations, maintenance of personal hygiene, stimulation, and play activities.

46

3. Nurse should provide supportive care to reduce anxiety, tension and worry of the adoptive parents who feel incompetent and unprepared to undertake the unexpected parenting chores.

4. Every child who is adopted must be told, as early as the child can comprehend (usually around 5 years or school entry), that he or she is adopted and foster parents are now the real parents. When the adopted child comes to know about this fact from sources other than parents, it may cause severe psychological trauma due to betrayal and breach of trust and it may ruin relations between the foster parents and the child forever.

46

NATIONAL MATERNAL AND CHILD HEALTH PROGRAMS

India has a population of over one billion and 70 percent of the population lives in villages and almost one-third of the population is below the poverty line. Over 80 percent diseases occur due to non-availability of safe and potable drinking water. Maternal undernutrition, early and frequent pregnancies, lack of education and empowerment of women are adversely affecting the health of children by increased incidence of low birth weight babies, frequent occurrence of common day-to-day infections and high prevalence of mild to moderate protein-calorie malnutrition (stunting) and deficiency of micronutrients. There are issues pertaining to unreached children belonging to below poverty line (BPL) families, neglected and abused children, street children and exploited children (for sex and child labor). The state of environmental sanitation and personal hygiene is appalling. There is increasing pollution, contamination of vegetables, fruits and dairy products by toxins, adulterants and pesticides. Due to population boom, there is overcrowding and lack of basic amenities and facilities in the mushrooming slums and urban areas. The Government of India spends just 1.4% of gross domestic product (GDP) on public health, while people spend 3.3% of GDP by availing health care being provided in the private sector.

The main objective of national policy for children is to provide facilities and opportunities to the nation's children to grow up to become robust and sturdy citizens, physically fit, mentally alert, morally healthy, spiritually sound and endowed with skills, competence and social awareness for the society. In order to realize and achieve this goal, a number of national programs have been launched for the welfare of mothers and children. The National Commission for Children is charged to oversee the effective implementation of these programs.

1. *National nutrition programs and services* Applied Nutrition Program, Mid-day Meal Program, Special Nutrition Program, National Nutritional Anemia, Prophylaxis Program, National Goiter Control Program, Vitamin A Prophylaxis Program, Baby friendly Hospital Initiative (BFHI), etc.
2. *Child health services* School health services, integrated child development services (ICDS), under-fives and well baby clinics.
3. *Disease prevention services* Expanded Program of Immunization, Universal Immunization Program, and Pulse Polio Immunization Program.
4. *Integrated maternal and child health services* National Child Survival and Safe Motherhood Program (CSSM), Reproductive and Child Health Program (RCH).
5. *Integrated Management of Neonatal and Childhood Illnesses (IMNCI).*
6. *National School Health Program.*
7. *National Tuberculosis Control Program.*
8. *National Iodine Deficiency Disorders Control Program.*
9. *National Vector-Borne Disease Control Program.*
10. *National Rural Health Mission (NRHM).*
11. *National Urban Health Mission (NUHM).*

Some of the important national maternal and child health programs are discussed below.

Applied Nutrition Programs

This program was started in the year 1960 in a few states and then gradually implemented throughout the country. The program is assisted by International Agencies like WHO, UNICEF and FAO. The program was designed to meet the nutritional needs of vulnerable segments of our society like preschool children, pregnant and lactating mothers. The program aims at achieving self sufficiency by increasing food production by popularizing kitchen gardens, poultry units and development of fisheries. Nutrition education is being imparted for efficient utilization of locally produced foods and increased consumption of green leafy vegetables, seasonal fruits and protein-rich foods. The program has lost its initial enthusiasm and commitment.

Nutrition supplements are being provided as snacks and mid-day meals to preschool children in several government and public sector schools in the country. It is being done at the state level and there is no universal national policy.

Inview of wide spread prevalence of vitamin A deficiency leading to night blindness and keratomalacia, vitamin A prophylaxis program was piggy-backed with expanded program of immunization (EPI). Every infant is administered 1,00,000 units of vitamin A along with measles vaccine at 9 months followed by four more doses of 2,00,000 units each at 18, 24, 30 and 36 months (6 months intervals). The program is now restricted to certain endemic areas and high-risk populations. Due to the increasing awareness that isolated nutrient deficiencies are rare in clinical practice, the program is not pursued with its initial enthusiasm.

Baby Friendly Hospital Initiative (BFHI)

In order to encourage and promote exclusive breast-feeding to enhance child survival, BFHI was launched jointly by WHO and UNICEF in March, 1992. Bottle being the biggest killer of babies in developing countries, a mission approach has been launched globally to revive the dwindling practice of breast feeding. Efforts are being made to improve the knowledge, attitude and practices of health care workers by providing them with information, scientific facts and skills to promote exclusive breastfeeding during first 6 months of life. Mother–baby bonding at birth, avoidance of prelacteal feeds, early breast feeding and practice of keeping the baby and her mother in the rooming-in ward are encouraged. The representatives of infant food manufacturers are strictly forbidden to contact mothers or health care staff for distribution of low cost or free infant formula, feeding bottles or literature pertaining to formula feedings. The advertisements and promotion of breast milk substitutes in media and distribution of pamphlets, calendars and growth charts, etc. is against the Infant Milk Substitute (IMS) code of conduct and can attract penalty.

Ten steps for successful breastfeeding

The following ten steps are recognized as minimum global criteria for attaining the status of a Baby Friendly Hospital.

Step 1 Have a written breastfeeding policy that is routinely communicated to all health staff.

Step 2 Train health care staff in skills necessary to implement this policy.

Step 3 Inform all pregnant women about the benefits and management of breastfeeding.

Step 4 Help mothers to initiate breastfeeding within half-hour of birth.

Step 5 Show mothers how to breastfeed and how to maintain lactation, even if they are separated from their infants.

Step 6 Give newborn infants no food or drink other than breast milk, unless medically indicated.

Step 7 Practice rooming-in and allow mothers and infants to remain together round-the-clock.

Step 8 Encourage breastfeeding on demand.

Step 9 Give no artificial feeds or pacifiers (also called dummies and soothers) to breastfeeding babies.

Step 10 Foster the establishment of breastfeeding support groups and refer mothers to them on discharge from the hospital or clinic.

The procedure for recognition of a hospital as baby friendly

The BFHI movement is active in India under a National Task Force comprising of government of India, UNICEF, WHO and a large number of professional bodies and voluntary organizations. A number of regional workshops have been organized on lactation management and for training of BFHI assessors. The following three steps are followed for recognition of a hospital as baby-friendly.

1. A hospital that conducts a minimum of 250 deliveries per year can seek the recognition. After implementation of ten global steps for promotion of breast feeding, a duly completed self-assessment form and registration form are sent to the BFHI secretariat.

2. The hospital/nursing home meeting all the ten criteria is visited by an Assessor for on-the-spot checks and to interview the mothers and health care staff. The Assessor sends his report and observations to the BFHI secretariat which is reviewed by the Review Committee for final recommendation.

3. The hospital/s fulfilling the national BFHI requirements are recognized as "Baby-Friendly." The National Task Force organizes a public ceremony for presentation of BFHI recognition certificate and a logo-plaque. The hospitals who are unable to fulfill the required criteria for certification are informed regarding their short comings. They can reapply for certification at a later date after eliminating all the short comings.

Integrated Child Development Services Program (ICDS)

The Integrated Child Development Services (ICDS) Program was launched in the year 1975 on 2nd October on Gandhiji's birthday. It is world's largest outreach program for care and development of preschool children. In 2005, following a Supreme Court order, ICDS program was extended to cover the entire country. The program provides coverage to all pregnant and nursing mothers and their children below 6 years of age through a network of *Anganwadis* or "courtyard shelters". One anganwadi center (AWC) is provided

46

46

for 800 inhabitants covering on an average 30 under-6 children. During the financial year 2016–17, INR 17,408 crores were allocated to the program. The World Bank, UNICEF, World Food Program (WFP) and Christian Action Research and Education (CARE) are major partners to support this program. The specific objectives of ICDS program are listed below:

1. To improve the nutrition and health status of children in the age group 0–6 years.
2. To reduce the incidence, morbidity and mortality due to malnutrition and reduce school drop-out rate.
3. To impart health and applied nutrition education to mothers.
4. To promote optimal physical, psychological and social development of children.
5. To achieve effective coordination among different departments of government of India to improve health and welfare of children and mothers.

The *Anganwadi* worker is the key person in this program and she is recruited from amongst the local population. She should have basic qualification of matriculation and is given three months training to improve her knowledge and skills required to discharge her responsibilities. She provides supplementary nutrition, immunizations, health check-ups, nutrition and health education and non-formal education to preschool children. Due to various reasons the impact of the program has been limited. It is being felt that the image of the program needs to change from the food disturbursement program to a comprehensive development program for children, adolescent girls and women with the active involvement of the community and with the help of a streamlined management information system.

Expanded Program of Immunizations (EPI)

The EPI was launched by government of India in January 1978 to reduce the incidence of common vaccine-preventable diseases. The target population are under-five children and pregnant women. The services of EPI (BCG and OPV at birth, 3 primary doses of DPT and OPV with boosters at 1½ year and 4½ year, measles at 9 months and two doses of tetanus toxoid during pregnancy) are provided as part of the regular maternal and child health services at the subcenters, primay health centers, community hospitals, district hospitals and MCH centers in the urban areas. When EPI coverage was found to be low on evaluation, the Universal Immunization Program (UIP) was introduced in 1985, concentrating on target population of infants below one year of age.

Inorder to eradicate poliomyelitis, Pulse Polio Immunization (PPI) Program was launched by government of India in 1995. In this program, all children under the age of 5 years, are given additional doses of OPV on designated alternate sundays. These doses are in addition to the six doses of OPV given under EPI program. It is a matter of great satisfaction for public health authorities that after the global eradication of smallpox in December 1979, India has been declared as polio free on 13 January 2014 following the success of PPI program.

The Child Survival and Safe Motherhood (CSSM) Program

The National Population Policy of India has recognized the link between high infant mortality rate (IMR) and excessive population growth. According to latest World Population Prospects released by United Nations (Revised 2015), it is estimated that by 2022, India's projected population would be around 1419 million compared to China's population of 1409 million. The policy statement commits the nation to bring down IMR to less than 30 per 1000 live births by the year 2010. This would necessitate a rapid reduction in neonatal deaths which form a major component of infant mortality. The policy also aims to achieve 80 percent deliveries at health posts or institutions and 100 percent deliveries by trained health personnel by the year 2010. Unfortunately these targets have not been achieved. According to Sample Registration System (SRS) 2013, IMR is 40 per 1000 population while under-5 mortality rate (U5MR) is 52 per 1000 live births. In order to prevent maternal and under-5 morbidity and mortality, CSSM program was launched in 1992–93 and is jointly funded by World Bank and UNICEF. It is a comprehensive MCH program providing a package of services for the children (child survival component) and the mothers (safe motherhood component). Health education aimed at rapid recognition and appropriate management of diarrhea with ORS has been a major component of CSSM. The ARI control program was started in India in 1990. Early recognition and prompt treatment of ARI with cotrimoxazole has reduced mortality due to pneumonia. The program is being implemented through the existing network of subcenters, primary health centers, community health centers and district hospitals. In each district, 4–6 first referral units (FRUs) have been created by upgrading community health centers (CHCs).

Reproductive and Child Health (RCH) Program

From October 1997, National Family Welfare (NFW) Program and the National Child Survival and Safe Motherhood (CSSM) programs have been merged into Reproductive and Child Health (RCH) Program. In addition to the family planning and MCH services, the RCH program provides strategies for prevention, identification and management of reproductive tract infections (RTIs) and the sexually transmitted diseases (STDs). RCH program provides client-oriented and target-free approach and lays emphasis on the quality of services and satisfaction of the consumers. Instead of target-oriented centralized planning (top down approach), it is proposed to develop the services depending upon the felt needs of individuals and communities (bottom up approach) in each PHC area. There is a strong component of newborn care to improve newborn survival under the RCH program. The components of health services for children and mothers under RCH Program are shown in **Table 46.2**.

The current package of services being implemented by the Department of Family Welfare, Government of India for promotion of child health and survival is given below:

1. Implementation of exclusive breastfeeding up to the age of 6 months and promotion of appropriate practices related to complementary feeding.
2. Control of deaths due to respiratory infections.
3. Control of deaths due to diarrheal diseases.
4. Provision of essential newborn care.
5. Iron folic acid (IFA) supplements to children under five years of age.
6. Vitamin A supplements to children between 6 months and 3 years of age.
7. Integrated management of neonatal and childhood illnesses (IMNCI).

Breastfeeding

Objectives Exclusive breastfeeding for first 6 months of life should be promoted as (i) it is the ideal method of infant feeding, (ii) it is the single most effective intervention for reduction of infant mortality and (iii) it delays return of fertility in the mother because of its natural contraceptive effect (lactational amenorrhea).

Strategies The Government of India has established partnership with major professional bodies and various non-government organizations (NGOs). The Infant Milk Substitute (IMS) Act has been implemented to promote breastfeeding and ban advertisements and free distribution of milk formulae and feeding bottles. The various strategies for promotion of breastfeeding include (i) baby friendly hospital initiative (BFHI), (ii) lactation clinics and (iii) peer counseling.

Prevention of deaths due to respiratory infections

The strategies include promotion of immunization, increasing immunocompetence by adequate intake of diet and micronutrients, avoidance of exposure, early identification and prompt treatment of pneumonia by administration of cotrimoxazole.

Prevention of deaths due to diarrheal diseases

The occurrence of diarrheal disorders should be reduced by (i) promotion of breast feeding and avoidance of formula feeds with a bottle, (ii) ensuring intake of safe water, (iii) promoting practices of personal hygiene (hand washing, daily bath) for preparation and feeding of weaning food, and (iv) administration of rotavirus vaccine to those who can afford. Diarrheal deaths can be reduced by early identification of diarrhea and prompt administration of oral rehydration solution (ORS) and zinc supplements. There is a need to promote ORS as the "drug for diarrhea" and discourage unnecessary use of antibiotics and binding agents.

Provision of essential newborn care

The availability of essential newborn care should be promoted with the help of community health workers and accredited social health activists (ASHAs). The core components of essential newborn care are listed below:

1. Good quality antenatal care (at least 5 contacts).
2. Safe delivery at a health care facility by a trained midwife.

Table 46.2 Package of services under RCH Program	
Safe motherhood services	*Child survival services*
■ Two doses of tetanus toxoid during pregnancy	■ Essential newborn care
■ Prevention and treatment of anemia	■ Immunizations of under-5 children
■ Prevention and treatment of RTIs and STDs	■ Health education for promotion of breast feeding, nutrition and immunizations, etc.
■ Antenatal care and early identification of high-risk pregnancies	■ Appropriate case management of acute diarrhea
■ Deliveries by trained personnel	■ Appropriate case management of ARI
■ Management of obstetric emergencies	■ Vitamin A prophylaxis
■ Birth spacing	

RTI, reproductive tract infections; STD, sexually transmitted diseases; ARI, acute respiratory infection.

3. Optimal care of neonates at birth.
4. Prevention of hypothermia.
5. Promotion of exclusive breastfeeding.
6. Prevention, early recognition and prompt treatment of bacterial infections.

Iron and folic acid (IFA) supplementation

Objectives (i) Screening children for anemias and giving appropriate treatment when indicated (ii) Reducing overall prevalence of anemia by 25% and moderate-severe anemia by 50% in children.

Strategies (i) improve dietary intake to meet RDAs for all macro and micronutrients, (ii) dietary diversification by giving iron folate rich foods as well as those food items (like vitamin C) which promote iron absorption and (iii) health and nutrition education to promote intake of iron and folate-rich food stuffs.

Infants

   i. Promotion of exclusive breastfeeding for 6 months (iron in breast milk is highly bioavailable).
   ii. Promotion of iron-rich complementary feeding by intake of green leafy vegetables, iron-rich fruits (banana, apple, pomegranate), and egg yolk.
   iii. Identification of anemia in high-risk children and its prompt management.

Preschool children According to the survey carried out by National Nutrition Monitoring Bureau 2002, 67% of preschool children were anemic.

   i. Advocacy for dietary diversification.
   ii. Biweekly administration of 1 mL IFA syrup containing 20 mg elemental iron and 100 µg folic acid during 6–60 months of age.
   iii. Screening for high risk children and their prompt management.
   iv. In hookworm endemic areas, community education should be provided to avoid walking bare feet, screening for anemia and periodic deworming every 6 months.

Adolescent boys and girls (10–18 years)

There is high incidence of iron deficiency anemia in adolescents due to rapid growth, dietary inadequacy of iron, frequent infections and parasitic infestations.

   i. Information and counseling for improving dietary intake of iron rich foods and prevention of worm infestations.
   ii. Administration of supervised weekly supplements of iron-folic acid (IFA) tablets containing 100 mg elemental iron and 500 µg folic acid throughout the year (52 weekly doses).
   iii. Albendazole 400 mg every 6 months for deworming.

Women in reproductive age group (15–45 years)

Women of reproductive age group are at an increased risk of development of iron deficiency anemia due to blood loss through menstrual cycles, inadequate dietary intake and recurrent infections.

   i. Weekly supplements of iron-folic acid tablets (100 mg elemental iron plus 500 µg folic acid) throughout the calendar year, i.e. 52 weeks/year.
   ii. Bi-annual deworming with albendazole 400 mg.

Pregnant and lactating women

There are increased nutritional demands (to provide for the nutritional needs of fetus and young infant) and excessive blood loss during delivery. Iron-folic acid (IFA tablets containing 100 mg elemental iron and 500 µg folic acid) supplements are given daily for 100 days starting from mid-pregnancy. Medications are poorly tolerated during first trimester of pregnancy and in general should be avoided. Following delivery, IFA supplements are continued for another 100 days to replenish the nutritional losses that occur during pregnancy and delivery.

Vitamin A supplementation

Objectives To decrease prevalence of vitamin A deficiency from the current 0.7 to 0.3%.

Strategies

Infants (i) Health and nutrition education to encourage intake of colostrum, promote exclusive breast feeding for first 6 months, (ii) promote intake of vitamin A-rich complementary foods and (iii) provide a dose of vitamin A 1,00,000 i.u. at 9 months.

Children (i) Health and nutrition education to promote intake of vitamin A-rich foods, (ii) early detection and prompt treatment of infections and (iii) providing supplements of vitamin A in a dose of 2,00,000 i.u. at 18, 24, 30 and 36 months of age.

Sick children (i) all children with xerophthalmia should be treated at health care facilities, (ii) children suffering from measles should be given a dose of vitamin A and (iii) children with malnutrition should receive vitamin A supplements.

National Rural Health Mission (NRHM)

In view of the fact that 70% of 1.25 billion people of India live in one million villages and existing health services are both unsatisfactory and unavailed by the rural people, the government of India launched National Rural Health Mission (NRHM). The goal of NRHM is to improve the availability and accessibility of quality health care to people residing in rural areas with special focus to the most vulnerable segments of population, i.e. economically poor, women and children. The fiscal outlay of NRHM for 2016–2017 is in the range of INR 11,196 crores.

Core strategies

1. The National Rural Health Mission (2005–2012) seeks to provide quality health care to rural population throughout the country with special focus on 18 states which have weak public health indicators and poor infrastructure. It is envisaged to raise public spending on health from 0.9 to 2.3% of GDP.
2. The capacity and credibility of Panchayati Raj Institutions (PRIs) shall be enhanced to own, control and manage public health services. Village Health Committee of the Panchayat will over see the Health Plan of each village.
3. It is proposed to create a new cadre of community based female health functionaries, named as *accredited social health activists* (ASHAs) to provide health services at the doorstep of people.
4. The existent network of rural health services of subcenters, primary health centers (PHCs), community health centers (CHCs) and district hospitals shall be improved and energized to provide curative health services of a desired standard in accordance with the recommendations of Indian Public Health Standards for adequate personnel, equipment and management protocols.
5. Effective integration and implementation of core public health strategies like environmental sanitation and hygiene, availability of safe drinking water and promotion of optimal nutrition through a District Plan for Health. It is proposed to decentralize health programs and promote the concept of district management of health through the active participation of PRIs.
6. It is proposed to integrate all vertical health and family welfare programs at National, State, Block and District levels.
7. It seeks to promote local health traditions and indigenous medicines by providing ASHAs a kit of medicines containing AYUSH (ayurvedic, unani, siddha and homeopathy) and allopathic medicines to treat common day-to-day illnesses.
8. Efforts are being made to strengthen capacities for data collection, assessment and review for evidence-based planning, monitoring and supervision of health interventions.
9. Promotion and development of capacities for preventive health care strategies at all levels by promoting healthy lifestyle (controlling consumption of alcohol, tobacco, drug abuse), satisfactory environmental conditions, nutritious diet, and universal immunizations.
10. It seeks to improve access of rural people, especially poor women and children, to equitable, affordable, accountable and effective primary health care.

The goals or outcomes of NRHM are listed in **Table 46.3**.

Accredited Social Health Activists (ASHAs)

Accredited social health activists (ASHAs) shall be recruited by the panchayat in each village from among the married/widowed/divorced women with formal education up to 8th class and having effective communication, caring and leadership skills. She will be given 23 days induction training spread over 12 months along with on-the-job training and supervision.

1. ASHA is an honorary volunteer and shall receive performance-based compensation for promotion of

Table 46.3 Goals of National Rural Health Mission

- Infant mortality rate shall be reduced to 30/1000 live births.
- Maternal mortality ratio to be reduced to 100/100,000 live births.
- Total fertility rate shall be reduced to 2.1.
- Malaria mortality rate reduction by 50% up to 2010 and sustaining that level up to 2012.
- Kala azar mortality reduction rate: 100% by 2010 and sustaining elimination until 2012.
- Filaria/microfilaria reduction rate: 70% by 2010, 80% by 2012 and elimination by 2015.
- Dengue mortality reduction rate by 50% by 2010 and sustaining at that level until 2012.
- Japanese encephalitis mortality rate reduction by 50% by 2010 and sustaining at that level until 2012.
- Cataract operations: Increasing to 46 lakhs per year until 2012.
- Leprosy prevalence rate: Reduction from 1.8/10,000 in 2005 to less than 1/10,000 thereafter.
- Tuberculosis DOTS services: Maintain 85% cure rate through entire mission period.
- Upgrading community health centers to the level of Indian Public Health Standards.
- Increase utilization of first referral units (FRUs) from less than 20% to 75%.
- Engaging 250,000 female accredited social health activists (ASHAs) in 10 states.

46

universal immunizations, referral and escorting pregnant women for delivery at the PHC or CHC, construction of household toilets and participation in various ad hoc health care delivery programs.

2. She will serve as a bridge between the public health system and the community and shall be accountable to the panchayat.

3. She will facilitate implementation of the village health plan with the help of *anganwadi* worker, ANM, functionaries of other departments and self help groups, under the leadership of the village health committee of the panchayat.

4. She will be given a drug kit containing generic AYUSH and allopathic formulations for treatment of common day-to-day illnesses. She will provide directly observed treatment short-course (DOTs) of antitubercular drugs under Revised National Tuberculosis Control Program.

5. Under Janani Suraksha Yojana (JSY), ASHA would organize delivery care services at PHC or CHC for the registered expectant mothers, assist in providing immunizations to under-5 children and act as a propagator and motivator for family planning services.

Janani Suraksha Yojana (JSY)

Janani Suraksha Yojana (JSY) is a 100% centrally sponsored scheme under the overall umbrella of NRHM to promote institutional deliveries of below poverty line (BPL) families. JSY is launched in lieu of national maternity benefit scheme (NMBs) wherein better diet was provided to BPL families. The main philosophy of JSY is to provide universal antenatal care, ensure institutional deliveries and postpartum care of BPL families with an incentive of cash payment of INR 700.00. The salient strategic components of JSY are given below:

1. Early registration of all BPL pregnant women by ASHA or an equivalent village health worker.

2. Providing at least 3 antenatal evaluations by ANM and identification of high-risk or complicated cases.

3. Ensuring institutional delivery by organizing appropriate referral and providing transport to the pregnant BPL women. It is mandatory for ASHA to escort the woman in labor for delivery at the appropriate health care facility.

4. Providing immediate postpartum care and ensuring administration of BCG vaccination within 4–6 weeks.

5. Disbursement of cash assistance to the BPL beneficiary after the institutional delivery. ASHA also gets cash incentive of INR 600.00 to 1000.00 for doing her job well.

Janani-Shishu Suraksha Karyakram (JSSK)

The Ministry of Health and Family Welfare, Government of India launched *Janani-Shishu Suraksha Karyakram* (JSSK) in June 2011 as a national initiative under the ambit of *Janani Suraksha Yojana* (JSY) for the benefit of pregnant women and newborns. Under this program, every year one crore pregnant women and their newborns shall be provided completely free and cashless medical services in governmental health care facilities both in the rural and urban areas. *Janani-Shishu Suraksha Karyakram* will supplement the cash assistance given to pregnant women under JSY and is aimed at mitigating the burden of out of pocket expenses incurred by pregnant women (both normal deliveries and cesarean sections) and care of their newborns (up to 30 days after birth).

Rashtriya Kishor Swasthya Karyakram (RKSK)

India is home to 240 million adolescents (10 – 19 years) accounting for 21.4% of country's population. In order to enable adolescents to fulfil their optimal potential, significant investments must be made on several priority areas of their welfare, namely education, reproductive and sexual health, nutrition, mental health, injuries including domestic and gender based violence, substance abuse, communicable and non-communicable diseases.

Recognizing the special needs of adolescents, Ministry of Health and Family Welfare (MOHFW) has launched *Rashtriya Kishor Swasthya Karyakram* (National Adolescent Health Program) on 7th January, 2014. The key components of the program include achievement of their full genetic potential, gender equity, availability of strategic support and partnership with other stakeholders for making informed and responsible decisions related to their health and well being. MOHFW in collaboration with UNFPA has developed a National Adolescent Health Strategy for the benefit of adolescents. Instead of existing clinic-based curative approach, the program shall provide community-based holistic health promotive, preventive, curative and welfare services for the benefit of adolescents at their doorsteps, i.e. schools and community at large.

National Urban Health Mission (NUHM)

To improve the health status of community living in urban slums and vulnerable populations living in urban areas, such as homeless, rag-pickers, street children, construction site workers and temporary migrants, the Ministry of Health and Family Welfare, Government of India launched National Urban Health Mission on January 20, 2014. The aims of NUHM include, improvement of health status of indigent and disadvantaged urban population, (ii) strengthening of public health care system, (iii) involvement of the community and urban local bodies in health care delivery, and to (iv) complement the National Rural Health Mission under the umbrella of a unified National Health Mission.

Coverage and commitments

1. To provide health preventive, promotive and essential curative services to estimated 221.3 million urban population including around 77.5 million poor and vulnerable population living in the state capitals, district headquarters and all cities/towns with a population above 50,000.
2. To create 30–100 bedded urban community health centers for cities above 5 lakh population.
3. Creation of network of urban primary health centers for every 50,000 population located within or near slums and shanty settlements.
4. Strengthening of existing First Referral Units (FRUs), Urban Health Centers and Dispensaries in terms of adequate human resources, equipment, medicines and consumables.
5. To provide auxiliary nurse midwife (ANM) for every 10,000–12,000 population and accredited social health activist (ASHA) for every 200–500 slum and urban poor households.
6. Empowerment of communities through *Mahila Arogya Samiti* to look after the health needs of every 50–100 slum and/or urban poor dwellings.

India Newborn Action Plan (INAP)

Children are truly the foundation of a nation and Government of India has launched several programs for welfare of girls (future mothers), women and children. The country has witnessed dramatic reduction in maternal and child mortality rates over the past two decades. The child survival has increased in India by virtue of reduction of post-neonatal deaths by promotion of breastfeeding, immunizations, oral rehydration solution (ORS) for treatment of diarrhea and early administration of antibiotics for treatment of acute respiratory tract infections. However, neonatal mortality has reduced much less, thereby increasing the contribution of neonatal deaths to mortality of under-5 children from 41% in 1990 to 56% in 2012. Every year about 0.76 million newborns die in India mainly due to preventable causes and an equal number of pregnancies end as stillbirths which are often missed or ignored.

Newborn health has now captured the attention of policy makers at the highest level because further reduction in child deaths can be achieved by improving the survival of newborns. The Ministry of Health and Family Welfare, Government of India has recognised the importance of newborn health (and also their creators, the mothers) as a national priority and development necessity. Two important strategies and commitments in this direction include the National Rural Health Mission (NRHM) and the Reproductive, Maternal, Newborn, Child and Adolescent Health (RMNCH+A) Strategy. NRHM by virtue of its subsidiary programs has provided unprecedented attention by allocation of resources for newborn health. While RMNCH+A strategy has provided a paradigm shift to emphasize the need for continuum-of-care from girls-women-mothers-newborns-children and adolescents by strengthening the health care system from the grass roots to the tertiary care level.

The Ministry of Health and Family Welfare, Government of India launched India Newborn Action Plan (INAP) on 18th September 2014 as a national commitment towards global Every Newborn Action Plan (ENAP) launched at the 67th World Health Assembly in June 2014. The main focus of the program is to improve the health and welfare of women and launch interventions to reduce maternal deaths, neonatal deaths and stillbirths. The goal of the program is to achieve a target of "single digit neonatal mortality rate (NMR)" and a "single digit stillbirth rate (SBR)" by 2030. It is proposed to improve and scale-up the strategies for interventions and provide clear guidelines for their implementation, monitoring and evaluation. The INAP will be implemented within the existing framework of RMNCH+A and guided by the principles of integration, social and gender equity, quality of care, accountability and partnerships with all the stakeholders. The main focus of intervention packages would be to reduce stillbirths and improve newborn health and survival through a network of home-based newborn care (HBNC), newborn care corners (NBCC) and facility-based newborn care (FBNC) at community health centers or first referral units, special care newborn units (SCNUs) at sub-district and district hospitals, medical colleges and tertiary care centers. It is proposed to build a strategy of **"six pillars"** at all levels of health care to provide (i) preconception and antenatal care, (ii) care during labor and child birth (iii) care of the newborn at birth, (iv) care of healthy newborns, (v) care of small and sick newborns and (vi) care beyond newborn survival. Under the sixth pillar of "care beyond newborn survival", India has taken a vital step toward improving quality of life beyond newborn survival. It is proposed to take necessary steps towards improving the quality of life of survivors with birth

46

defects and those infants who develop neurodevelopmental delay and disabilities due to prematurity and sickness. The strong component of the program is a systematic approach with close monitoring and evaluation to meet pre-set well-defined indicators or targets. After the launch of India Newborn Action Plan (INAP), India envisions a health system that eliminates preventable deaths of newborns and stillbirths, and where every pregnancy is wanted, children survive, thrive and they reach there full genetic potential.

Innovative Training Programs

The Ministry of Health and Family Welfare, Government of India has launched several community based programs to improve the care and survival of newborn babies. No program can succeed unless the health care providers (HCPs), who are expected to oversee the program, are commited, motivated and adequately trained. Apart from formal training of various community based health workers (*Anganwadi* worker, community neonatal health worker, accredited social health activist, auxiliary nurse midwife), their knowledge and skills should be updated by organizing refresher courses and by harnessing innovative tele-education modules. Distance learning modules can be used for teaching and training of nursing and medical students, medical officers and pediatricians. E-learning training programs are available for various aspects of reproductive and child health, like essential care of the newborns, home care of newborns (HCNB), newborns care corners (NBCC), care of sick newborns, or facility based newborn care (FBNC), audio-visual webinars (http://www.newbornwhocc.org/wefinar-essential_newborn htm), "Adobe Connect", online continuous positive airway pressure (CPAP) course and IMCI computerized adaptation and training tool (ICATT) to promote integrated management of neonatal and childhood diseases. The online or digital training efforts can be further augmented by the mentors with the help of SMSs or e-mails and periodic questionnaires or MCQ interactions and evaluations. There is a need to create a pool of national and state level trainers to take forward the agenda of improving skills and managerial capabilities of HCPs in order to improve the health and wellbeing of mothers and their babies.

Strategies to Improve Newborn Health and Survival

The newborn care is the most urgent key health priority in our country and saving newborn babies should form a national agenda to achieve further reduction in infant mortality rate in order to achieve IMR of less than 10 per 1000 live births. The enhancement of neonatal and infant survival is truly the key to the success of family welfare program and stabilization of population dynamics which is a major public health issue in India. Neonates constitute the foundation of a nation and no sensible government can afford to neglect their needs and rights. The following strategies or Ten Commandments, with short-term and long-term goals, have been launched by the Government of India inorder to improve newborn health and survival and enhance the quality of life among those who survive.

1. A national movement "India Newborn Action Plan" (INAP) has been launched and is being pursued like a "Mission".
2. Efforts are being made to provide facilities to improve education, nutrition (life cycle approach), health and "status" of girls and women who indeed are the creators and sustainers of progeny.
3. Launch a nationwide socio-political movement to discourage early marriages, teenage and frequent pregnancies.
4. Introduce teaching of mothercraft and family life education to high school boys and girls.
5. Ensure antenatal care of good quality to all pregnant women.
6. High-risk pregnant women should be identified and referred to a higher level of care and confinement.
7. All deliveries should be conducted by trained and skilled health care attendants. And as a long-term policy, infrastructure and facilities are being created to ensure that every baby is born at a nearby health care facility.
8. The need for a greater focus on preventive rather than curative newborn services. Available health care professionals and a special cadre of community-based skilled birth attendants or village level newborn care workers (Accredited Social Health Activists or ASHAs) are being trained and effectively used to provide essential newborn care at the community level.
9. Supervised home care should be provided to moderately low birth weight babies (above 1800 g or >34 weeks gestation) and to all sick and stable babies through sustainable, doable and cost-effective community-based programs.
10. The available infrastructure, facilities and expertise for MCH services should be enhanced to provide good quality level II newborn care at the first referral units and district hospitals under the supervision of well-trained and dedicated health

care professionals. There is a need to harness the potential of information technology (IT) to promote innovative interventions, like e-learning, mHealth and introduce changes in health-seeking behavior.

BIBLIOGRAPHY

Aggarwal K, Dalwai S, Galagali P, Mishra D, Prasad C, et al. Recommendations on recognition and response to child abuse and neglect in Indian setting. *Indian Pediatr* 2010, 47: 493–504.

Integrated Management of Neonatal and Childhood Illness (IMNCI): Student's Handbook. *Ministry of Health and Family Welfare, Government of India*; 2007.

Ministry of Health and Family Welfare, Government of India. Guidelines and protocols. Medico-legal care of survivors/victims of sexual violence 2014. Available at www.http://mohfw.nic.in.

National Policy for Children, 2012. Available at http:pib.nic.in/newsite/erelease.aspx?relid = 94782.

Seth R. Child abuse and neglect in India. *Indian J Pediatr* 2015, 82(8): 707–714.

Srivastava RN. Child abuse and neglect: Asia Pacific Conference and the Delhi Declaration. *Indian Pediatr* 2011, 49:11–12.

Study on Child Abuse, India 2007. Ministry of Women and Child Development, Government of India. Available at www.wcd.nic.in/childabuse.pdf.

World Health Organization. Child maltreatment. Available at http://www.int/topics/child_abuse/en/.

46

Integrated Management of Neonatal and Childhood Illnesses (IMNCIs)

The WHO and UNICEF in collaboration with many other agencies, have adopted an integrated management of childhood illnesses (IMCI) approach in Child Health Programs in over 100 countries in mid-1990s. This strategy has been adopted and expanded in India to include neonatal care at home as well as in the health care facilities and renamed it as Integrated Management of Neonatal and Childhood Illnesses (IMNCIs). Health workers are trained with hands-on clinical practice for effective management of sick children aged between one week and five years. The new program is intended to integrate many well-known isolated interventions like universal immunization, exclusive breastfeeding during first 6 months of life, timely complementary feeding, essential newborn care, oral rehydration therapy for management of acute diarrhea and appropriate and timely use of antibiotics for treatment of neonatal sepsis and pneumonia in children. Algorithms have been developed to diagnose sepsis, measles, malaria, diarrhea, pneumonia and malnutrition. Apart from rational management of common diseases, health workers promote breastfeeding, provide immunizations, health and nutrition education. *The emphasis has shifted from purely curative services to a package of comprehensive health preventive and promotive services at each contact of the health worker with the consumers.* Therefore, IMNCI is not a new program but it is a new approach or a comprehensive health package to provide an holistic approach to harness greater benefits for the welfare and survival of children. The core strategy of the program is to provide integrated case management of the most common neonatal and childhood illnesses with a focus on most common causes of deaths in under-five children. The IMNCI strategy is being implemented in a phased manner for teaching of undergraduate medical and nursing students throughout the country.

Rationale

1. Improvement in child health and survival are not necessarily dependent on the use of sophisticated and expensive technologies.

2. An integrated approach is needed to manage sick children to achieve better outcomes.

3. A careful and systematic assessment of common symptoms and selected specific signs to provide rational and effective therapy.

4. Child health programs must go beyond tackling diseases of children and must address overall health and well-being of children by promotion of breastfeeding, provision of universal immunizations, and effective health and nutrition education.

Essential Components of the Program

The IMNCI guidelines for case management of common diseases have been divided into two age categories, that is, young infants from birth up to 2 months and children above 2 months up to 5 years of age. The salient guidelines of IMNCI are summarized below:

1. All sick infants up to 2 months of age must be assessed for "possible infection and jaundice" and they must be routinely evaluated for the major symptoms.

2. All sick children between 2 months and 5 years must be examined for "general danger signs" that indicate the need for immediate referral or admission to the hospital. They should be routinely assessed for major symptoms such as fever, cough, difficult or rapid breathing, diarrhea, and ear problems.

3. All under-5 children who are sick must be routinely assessed for nutritional and immunization status, feeding problems, and other common day-to-day problems.

4. A limited number of carefully selected clinical signs are used, based on their sensitivity and specificity, to diagnose common childhood diseases. These signs were selected considering the conditions and ground realities prevalent at the first-level health care facilities.

5. On the basis of a combination of various signs, the child is classified into various groups (instead of a diagnosis) and further divided into color-coded triage as *pink* which requires urgent referral or admission to a hospital, *yellow* when specific treatment

ment is required through the outpatient department and *green* which calls for home management.

6. The IMNCI guidelines address most but not all the major reasons for which a sick infant or child is brought to the clinic. The guidelines, for example, do not describe the management of trauma or other acute emergencies because of various accidents or injuries and also do not cover care of the baby at birth.

7. The management procedures outlined in the IMNCI protocols use a limited number of essential drugs and encourage active participation by caretakers in the treatment of sick infants and children.

8. An essential component of IMNCI guidelines lays emphasis on providing counseling and guidance to care takers about home care, optional feeding, administration of oral rehydration fluids, immunizations and healthy family lifestyle and the need for further management and follow-up.

In order to launch integrated management of childhood illnesses (IMCI) in the country, Government of India established a core group with representatives from Indian Academy of Pediatrics (IAP), National Neonatology Forum (NNF) of India, National Antimalaria Program (NAMP), Department of Women and Child Development (DWCD), Child-in-Need Institute (CINI), WHO, UNICEF, eminent pediatricians and neonatologists and the representatives from Ministry of Health and Family Welfare, Government of India. The Core Group developed Indian version of IMCI and renamed it as Integrated Management of Neonatal and Childhood Illnesses (IMNCI). The major components of this strategy are listed below:

1. Strengthening the skills of health care workers.
2. Strengthening of health care infrastructure.
3. Involvement of the community.

The first two components are facility-based IMNCI and the third is community-based IMNCI.

The salient features of the Indian adaptation are listed below:

i. Incorporation of neonatal care because neonatal deaths account for two-thirds of infant mortality.
ii. Inclusion of neonates between 0 and 7 days.
iii. Incorporating national guidelines on malaria, anemia, vitamin A prophylaxis and immunization schedule.
iv. Training program of health workers reduced from 11 days to 8 days.
v. Training protocols includes sick young infants up to 2 months of age.
vi. Proportion of training time devoted to sick young infant and sick child is almost identical.

IMNCI Case Management Process

Steps of case management process are shown in **Figure 47.1**:

Step 1: Assess the young infant/child
Step 2: Classify the illness
Step 3: Identify treatment
Step 4: Treat the young infant/child
Step 5: Counsel the mother
Step 6: Follow-up care

Classification of Patients

IMNCI classification charts describe the steps of case management process: Assess, classify and identify treatment **(Chart 47.1)**. There are separate classification boxes for main symptoms, nutritional status and anemia. Classification tables are used starting with the pink rows. If the young infant or child does not have the severe classifications, look at the yellow rows. If the young infant or child does not have any of the signs in the pink or yellow rows, select the classification in the green row. If the young infant or child has signs from more than one row, the more severe classification is selected. However, if the classification chart has more than one arm (e.g. possible bacterial infection/jaundice, diarrhea in a sick child), one may use more than one classification from that box.

IMNCI classifications are not necessarily specific diagnoses, but they indicate what action needs to be taken. All classifications are color-coded: pink calls for hospital referral or admission, yellow for initiation of treatment, and green means that the child can be sent home with necessary medicines and careful advice on when to return.

Effective Communication with the Care Provider

It is critical to communicate effectively with the infant's mother or caretaker. Proper communication helps to reassure the mother or caretaker that the infant will receive appropriate care. In addition, the success of home treatment depends on how well the mother or caretaker knows about giving the treatment and understands its importance.

ASSESS AND CLASSIFY THE SICK YOUNG INFANT UP TO 2 MONTHS AGE

Young infants (infants age <2 months) have special characteristics that must be considered when classifying their illness. They can become sick and die very quickly from serious bacterial infections. They frequently have only general nonspecific signs such as inactivity or lethargy, fever or low body temperature. Mild chest

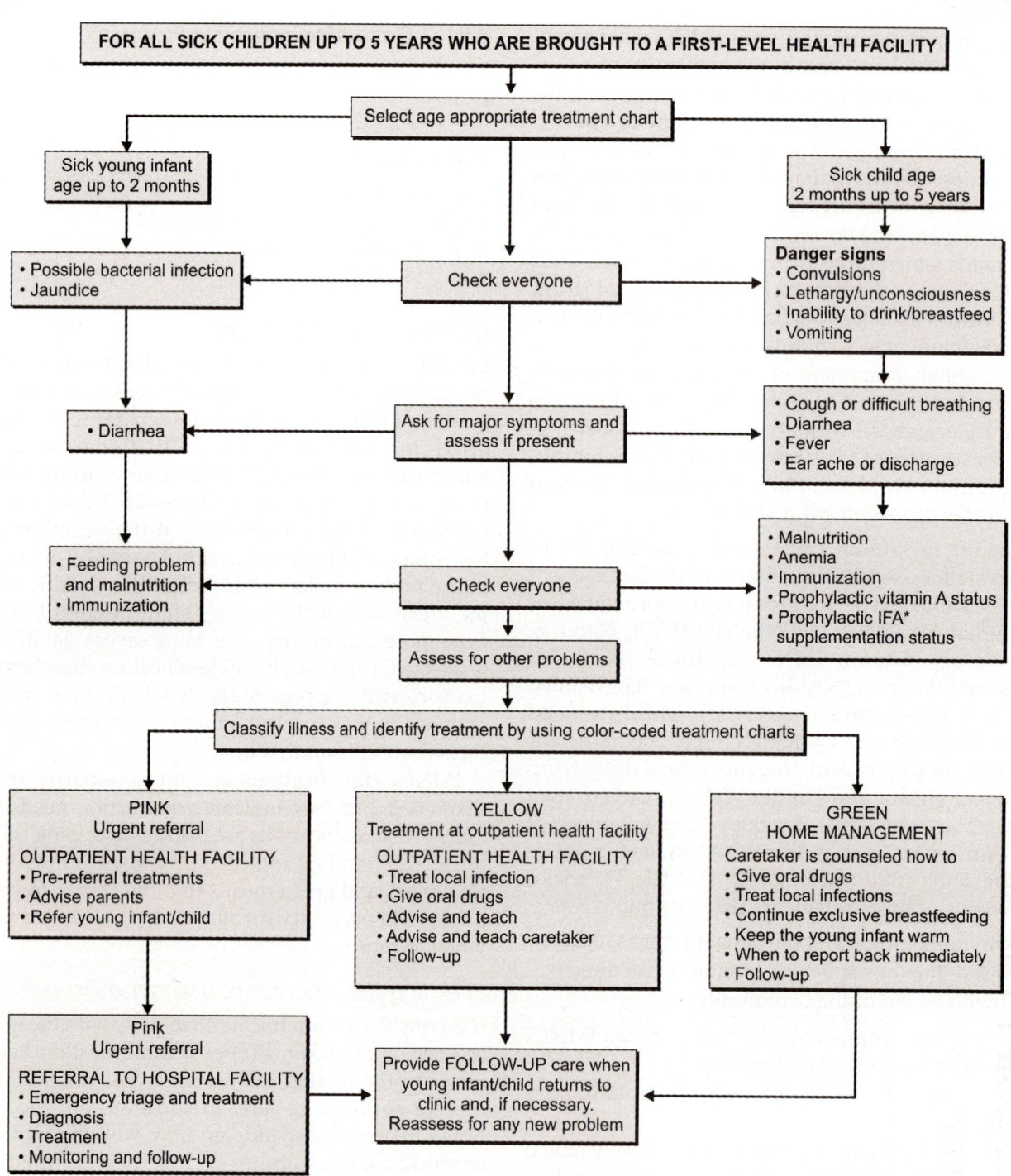

FOR ALL SICK CHILDREN UP TO 5 YEARS WHO ARE BROUGHT TO A FIRST-LEVEL HEALTH FACILITY

Select age appropriate treatment chart

Sick young infant age up to 2 months

Sick child age 2 months up to 5 years

Check everyone

• Possible bacterial infection
• Jaundice

Danger signs
• Convulsions
• Lethargy/unconsciousness
• Inability to drink/breastfeed
• Vomiting

Ask for major symptoms and assess if present

• Diarrhea

• Cough or difficult breathing
• Diarrhea
• Fever
• Ear ache or discharge

Check everyone

• Feeding problem and malnutrition
• Immunization

• Malnutrition
• Anemia
• Immunization
• Prophylactic vitamin A status
• Prophylactic IFA* supplementation status

Assess for other problems

Classify illness and identify treatment by using color-coded treatment charts

PINK
Urgent referral

OUTPATIENT HEALTH FACILITY
• Pre-referral treatments
• Advise parents
• Refer young infant/child

YELLOW
Treatment at outpatient health facility

OUTPATIENT HEALTH FACILITY
• Treat local infection
• Give oral drugs
• Advise and teach
• Advise and teach caretaker
• Follow-up

GREEN
HOME MANAGEMENT

Caretaker is counseled how to
• Give oral drugs
• Treat local infections
• Continue exclusive breastfeeding
• Keep the young infant warm
• When to report back immediately
• Follow-up

Pink
Urgent referral

REFERRAL TO HOSPITAL FACILITY
• Emergency triage and treatment
• Diagnosis
• Treatment
• Monitoring and follow-up

Provide FOLLOW-UP care when young infant/child returns to clinic and, if necessary. Reassess for any new problem

Figure 47.1 IMNCI case management process

indrawing is normal in young infants because their chest wall is soft. For these reasons, assessment, classification and treatment of young infant is somewhat different from an older infant or young child. The assessment procedure for this age group includes a number of important steps that must be followed by the health care provider, including: (i) history taking and communicating with the caretaker about the young infant's problem; (ii) checking for possible bacterial infection/jaundice; (iii) assessing for diarrhea if present; (iv) checking for feeding problem or malnutrition; (v) checking immunization status; and (vi) assessing other problems.

Checking for Possible Bacterial Infection/Jaundice

In the first step, all sick young infants are examined to assess for signs of possible bacterial infection and jaundice.

Chart 47.1

ASSESS AND CLASSIFY THE SICK YOUNG INFANT UP TO 2 MONTHS AGE

ASSESS   CLASSIFY   IDENTIFY   TREATMENT

USE ALL BOXES THAT MATCH INFANT'S SYMPTOMS AND PROBLEMS TO CLASSIFY THE ILLNESS

ASK THE MOTHER WHAT THE YOUNG INFANT'S PROBLEMS ARE
- Determine if this is an initial or followup visit for this problem
  - if followup visit, use the followup instructions on the bottom of this chart
  - if initial visit, assess the young infant as follows:

A child with a pink classification needs URGENT attention. Complete the assessment and pre-referral treatment immediately so referral is not delayed

CHECK FOR POSSIBLE BACTERIAL INFECTION/JAUNDICE

ASK:

Has the infant had convulsions?

LOOK, LISTEN, FEEL:

- Count the breaths in one minute

  Repeat the count if elevated

- Look for severe chest indrawing
- Look for nasal flaring

  } YOUNG INFANT MUST BE CALM

- Look and listen for grunting
- Look and feel for bulging fontanel
- Look for pus draining from the ear
- Look at the umbilicus. Is it red or draining pus?
- Look for skin pustules. Are there 10 or more skin pustules or a big boil?
- Measure axillary temperature (if not possible, feel for fever or low body temperature)
- See if the young infant is lethargic or unconscious
- Look at the young infant's movements. Are they less than normal?
- Look for jaundice. Are the palms and soles yellow?

	SIGNS	CLASSIFY AS	IDENTIFY TREATMENT (Urgent prereferral treatments are in bold print)
Classify ALL YOUNG INFANTS	• Convulsions or • Fast breathing ≥60 breaths per minute or more) or • Severe chest indrawing or • Nasal flaring or • Grunting or • Bulging fontanel or • ≥10 or more skin pustules or a big boil or • Axillary temperature 37.5°C or above (or feels hot to touch) or temperature less than 35.5°C (or feels cold to touch) or • Lethargic or unconscious or • Less than normal movements	**POSSIBLE SERIOUS BACTERIAL INFECTION**	➤ *Give first dose of intramuscular ampicillin and gentamicin* ➤ *Treat to prevent low blood sugar* ➤ *Warm the young infant by skin to skin contact if temperature less than 36.5°C (or feels cold to touch) while arranging referral* ➤ *Advise mother how to keep the young infant warm on the way to the hospital* ➤ *Refer URGENTLY to hospital*
	• Umbilicus red or draining pus or • Pus discharge from ear or • <10 skin pustules	**LOCAL BACTERIAL INFECTION**	➤ *Give oral amoxicillin for 5 days* ➤ Teach mother to treat local infections at home ➤ Followup in 2 days
And if the infant has jaundice	• Palms and soles yellow or • Age < 24 hr or • Age 14 days or more	**SEVERE JAUNDICE**	➤ *Treat to prevent low blood sugar* ➤ *Warm the young infant by skin to skin contact if temperature less than 36.5°C (or feels cold to touch) while arranging referral* ➤ *Advise mother how to keep the young infant warm on the way to the hospital* ➤ *Refer URGENTLY to hospital*
	• Palms and soles not yellow	**JAUNDICE**	➤ Advise mother to give home care for the young infant ➤ Advise mother when to return immediately ➤ Followup in 2 days
And if the temperature is between 35.5 and 36.4°C	• Temperature between 35.5 and 36.4°C	**LOW BODY TEMPERATURE**	➤ Warm the young infant using skin-to-skin contact for one hour and REASSESS If no improvement, refer ➤ Treat to prevent low blood sugar

*If referral is not possible, see the section **Where Referral Is Not Possible** in the module **Treat the Young Infant and Counsel the Mother***

47

(Contd.)

47

Chart 47.1 (Contd.)

(Contd.)

THEN ASK:
Does the young infant have diarrhea?*

IF YES, ASK: **LOOK AND FEEL:**

- For how long?
- Is there blood in the stool?

- Look at the young infant's general condition. Is the infant:
  - Lethargic or unconscious?
  - Restless and irritable?
- Look for sunken eyes
- Pinch the skin of the abdomen Does it go back:
  - Very slowly (longer than 2 seconds)?
  - Slowly?

Classify DIARRHEA

for DEHYDRATION

	Classification	Signs	Treatment

	SEVERE DEHYDRATION	**Two of the following signs:**
		• Lethargic or unconscious
		• Sunken eyes
		• Skin pinch goes back very slowly
			➤ *Give first dose of intramuscular ampicillin and gentamicin*
			➤ *If infant also has low weight or another severe classification:*
			  – *Refer URGENTLY to hospital with mother giving frequent sips of ORS on the way*
			  – *Advise mother to continue breastfeeding*
			  – *Advise mother how to keep the young infant warm on the way to the hospital*
			OR
			➤ If infant does not have low weight or any other severe classification:
			  – Give fluid for severe dehydration (Plan C) and then refer to hospital after rehydration

	SOME DEHYDRATION	**Two of the following signs:**
		• Restless, irritable
		• Sunken eyes
		• Skin pinch goes back slowly
			➤ *If infant also has low weight or another severe classification*
			  – *Give first dose of intramuscular ampicillin and gentamicin*
			  – *Refer URGENTLY to hospital with mother giving frequent sips of ORS on the way*
			  – *Advise mother to continue breastfeeding*
			  – *Advise mother how to keep the young infant warm on the way to the hospital*
			➤ *If infant does not have low weight or another severe classification:*
			  – Give fluids for some dehydration (Plan B)
			  – Advise mother when to return immediately
			  – Followup in 2 days

	NO DEHYDRATION	Not enough signs to classify as some or severe dehydration	➤ Give fluids to treat diarrhea at home (Plan A) ➤ Advise mother when to return immediately ➤ Followup in 5 days if not improving
and if diarrhea 14 days or more	**SEVERE PERSISTENT DIARRHEA**	Diarrhoea lasting 14 days or more	➤ Give first dose of intramuscular ampicillin and gentamicin if the young infant has low weight, dehydration or another severe classification ➤ Treat to prevent low blood sugar ➤ Advise how to keep infant warm on the way to the hospital
and if blood in stool	**SEVERE DYSENTERY**	Blood in the stool	➤ Give first dose of intramuscular ampicillin and gentamicin if the young infant has low weight, dehydration or another severe classification ➤ Treat to prevent low blood sugar ➤ Advise how to keep infant warm on the way to the hospital

* What is diarrhea in a young infant?

If the stools have changed from usual pattern and are many and watery (more water than fecal matter). The normally frequent or loose stools of a breastfed baby are not diarrhea

*#If referral is not possible, see the section **Where Referral Is Not Possible** in the module **Treat the Young Infant and Counsel the Mother***

Chart 47.1 (Contd.)

THEN CHECK FOR FEEDING PROBLEM & MALNUTRITION:

ASK:

- Is there any difficulty feeding?
- Is the infant breastfed? If yes, how many times in 24 hr?
- Does the infant usually receive any other foods or drinks? If yes, how often?
- What do you use to feed the infant?

IF AN INFANT: Has any difficulty feeding, or
Is breastfeeding less than 8 times in 24 hr, or
Is taking any other foods or drinks, or
Is low weight for age,

AND

Has no indications to refer urgently to hospital:

ASSESS BREASTFEEDING:

Has the infant breastfed in the previous hour?

If the infant has not fed in the previous hour, ask the mother to put her infant to the breast. Observe the breastfeed for 4 minutes

(If the infant was fed during the last hour, ask the mother if she can wait and tell you when the infant is willing to feed again)

- Is the infant able to attach?
  no attachment at all   not well attached   good attachment

  TO CHECK ATTACHMENT, LOOK FOR:
  - Chin touching breast
  - Mouth wide open
  - Lower lip turned outward
  - More areola visible above than below the mouth

  (All of these signs should be present if the attachment is good)

- Is the infant suckling effectively (that is, slow deep sucks, sometimes pausing)?
  not suckling at all   not suckling effectively   suckling effectively

  Clear a blocked nose if it interferes with breastfeeding

- Look for ulcers or white patches in the mouth (thrush)

Does the mother have pain while breastfeeding?

If yes, look and feel for:
- Flat or inverted nipples, or sore nipples
- Engorged breasts or breast abscess

LOOK, FEEL:

Determine weight for age

Classify FEEDING

Signs	Classify as	Treatment
• Not able to feed, or • No attachment at all, or • Not suckling at all, or • Severely underweight (<–3 SD)	**NOT ABLE TO FEED: POSSIBLE SERIOUS BACTERIAL INFECTION OR SEVERE MALNUTRITION**	➤ *Give first dose of intramuscular ampicillin and gentamicin* ➤ *Treat to prevent low blood sugar* ➤ *Warm the young infant by skin-to-skin contact if temperature less than 36.5°C (or feels cold to touch) while arranging referral* ➤ *Advise mother how to keep the young infant warm on the way to the hospital* ➤ *Refer URGENTLY to hospital#*
• Not well attached to breast, or • Not suckling effectively, or • Less than 8 breastfeeds in 24 hr, or • Receives other foods or drinks, or • Thrush (ulcers or white patches in mouth), or • Moderately underweight (<–2 to –3 SD), or • Breast or nipple problems	**FEEDING PROBLEM OR LOW WEIGHT FOR AGE**	➤ If not well attached or not suckling effectively, teach correct positioning and attachment ➤ If breastfeeding less than 8 times in 24 hr, advise to increase frequency of feeding ➤ If receiving other foods or drinks, counsel mother about breastfeeding more, reducing other foods or drinks, and using a cup and spoon ➤ If not breastfeeding at all, advise mother about giving locally appropriate animal milk and teach the mother to feed with a cup and spoon ➤ If thrush, teach the mother to treat thrush at home ➤ If low weight for age, teach the mother how to keep the young infant with low weight warm at home ➤ If breast or nipple problem, teach the mother to treat breast or nipple problems ➤ Advise mother to give home care for the young infant ➤ Advise mother when to return immediately ➤ Followup any feeding problem or thrush in 2 days ➤ Followup low weight for age in 14 days
• Not low weight for age (≥–2SD) and no other signs of inadequate feeding	**NO FEEDING PROBLEM**	➤ Advise mother to give home care for the young infant ➤ Advise mother when to return immediately ➤ Praise the mother for feeding the infant well

*#If referral is not possible, see the section **Where Referral Is Not Possible** in the module **Treat the Young Infant and Counsel the Mother***

47

47

The bacterial infection can be serious blood-borne bacterial infection or a localized infection such as skin infection or ear infection.

The clinical signs which point to possible serious bacterial infection are: Convulsions (as part of the current illness); and fast breathing (the cut-off rate to identify fast breathing in young infants is 60 breaths per minute or more). If the breathing rate is 60 breaths or more, the count should be repeated, because the breathing rate of a young infant is often irregular; if the second count is also 60 breaths or more, the young infant has fast breathing); severe chest indrawing; nasal flaring; grunting; bulging anterior fontanel; >10 skin pustules; axillary temperature >37.5°C or <35.5°C; lethargy or unconsciousness; and less than normal body movements. Presence of any of these signs indicates possible serious bacterial infection which may be a part of sepsis or pneumonia. A young infant with possible serious bacterial infection is referred urgently to hospital after giving first dose of antibiotics. The mother is advised to continue breastfeeding and to keep the baby warm on the way to hospital.

Pus or redness around the umbilicus, presence of <10 skin pustules or pus draining from ear is classified as local bacterial infection and treated with oral antibiotics.

Jaundice is the visible manifestation of elevated serum bilirubin. Occurrence of jaundice within first 24 hr of birth or after 14 days of age, or deep jaundice visible as yellow palms and soles suggests pathological jaundice and is classified as a severe illness necessitating urgent referral to a hospital for evaluation **(Chart 47.1)**. An infant aged 1–13 days who has jaundice but palms and soles are not yellow, is advised home care but should be advised to come for follow-up after 2 days and told when to return back immediately.

In addition to possible bacterial infection and jaundice, sick young infants with temperature between 35.5 and 36.5°C are classified to have low body temperature. This may be due to environmental factors or because of infection. Such infants are warmed using skin-to-skin contact and reassessed after one hour. If the temperature becomes normal and the infant has no other features for pink classification, he can be sent home after advising the mother on how to keep the baby warm. If the temperature is still below 36.5°C the infant should be referred to the hospital.

Assessment of an Infant with Diarrhea

Diarrhea is a main symptom, which is assessed if the mother says it is present. Exclusively breastfed infants normally pass frequent soft stools immediately after each feed. This should not be confused with diarrhea.

A young infant is said to have diarrhea if the stools have changed from usual pattern and the child is passing many watery stools (more water than fecal matter). A sudden change in the established frequency and consistency of stools is labelled as diarrhea.

All infants with diarrhea should be assessed for presence of dehydration. A number of clinical signs are used to determine the level of dehydration: infant's general condition (lethargic or unconscious or restless/irritable); sunken eyes and elasticity of skin (skin pinch goes back very slowly, slowly or immediately). In addition the infant is assessed for persistent diarrhea and dysentery.

Persistent diarrhea is an episode of diarrhea, with or without blood, which begins acutely and lasts at least 14 days. Persistent diarrhea is usually associated with weight loss and often with serious nonintestinal infections. Persistent diarrhea in a young infant is considered as a severe illness and requires urgent referral. Similarly, visible blood in stool in a young infant is classified as dysentery and the infant should be referred to the hospital.

All young infants with diarrhea are classified for degree of dehydration and in addition may be classified if they have persistent diarrhea and/or dysentery. Young infants with severe dehydration will need IV fluids while those with some dehydration are treated as plan B with oral rehydration. Young infants with no dehydration will require more fluids to prevent dehydration.

Checking for Feeding Problems or Malnutrition

All sick young infants seen in outpatient health facilities should be routinely evaluated for adequate feeding and weight gain. Weight-for-age compares the young infant's weight with the infants of the same age in the reference population (WHO-NCHS reference). The very low weight-for-age or severely underweight identifies children whose weight is –3 standard deviations below the mean weight of infants in the reference population (Z score <–3). The low weight-for-age or moderately underweight identifies children whose weight is –2 standard deviations below the mean weight of infants in the reference population (Z score <–2). Infants who are very low weight-for-age are given pink classification and should be referred to a hospital. Infants who are low weight-for-age need special attention to feed them and for keeping them warm.

To assess the young infant for feeding problems, the mother is asked specific questions about infant feeding to determine if the feeding practices are optimal. The weight of the child and feeding history is taken into consideration to determine if breastfeeding technique needs to be checked. An exclusively breastfed infant who is not low weight-for-age does not require any intervention and therefore is not observed for breastfeeding. If the mother gives history of feeding problem or the infant is low-weight-for-age and has no indication for referral, the mother is observed for breastfeeding. Breastfeeding is observed to see the signs of attachment and whether the infant is suckling effectively. Mothers of infants with problems in feeding are counseled appropriately. Infants who are not low-weight-for-age and have no feeding problem are classified as 'no feeding problem' and counseled about home care of young infant.

Checking Immunization Status

Immunization status should be checked in all sick young infants. A young infant who is not sick enough to be referred to a hospital should be given the necessary immunizations before he is sent home.

Assessing Other Problems

All sick young infants need to be assessed for other potential problems mentioned by the mother or observed during the examination. If a potentially serious problem is found or there are no means in the clinic to help the infant, he should be referred to the hospital.

Identify Treatment Options

The next step is to identify treatment required for the young infant according to the classification. All the treatments required are listed in the 'Identify Treatment' column of the ASSESS and CLASSIFY THE SICK YOUNG INFANT, **Chart 47.1**. If a sick young infant has more than one classification, treatment required for all the classifications must be identified. The first step is to determine if there is a need to refer the child to the hospital.

All infants and children with a severe classification (pink) are referred to a hospital as soon as assessment is completed and necessary pre-referral treatment is administered. Successful referral of severely ill infants to the hospital depends on effective counseling of the caretaker. The first step is to give urgent pre-referral treatment (written in bold font in the treatment section of chart). The options include:

- Administering first dose of antibiotic.
- Treatment of severe dehydration.
- Warming the young infant using skin-to-skin contact (kangaroo-mother-care) and keeping the infant warm on the way to the hospital.

- Prevention of hypoglycemia with breastmilk; if young infant is not able to swallow give expressed breast milk/appropriate animal milk with added sugar by nasogastric tube.
- In young infants with diarrhea, give frequent sips of ORS solution on the way to the hospital.

Treatment in the Outpatient Clinic and at Home

Young infants who have localized infection, feeding problem or low weight, or diarrhea with some dehydration, should have treatment initiated in clinic which should be continued at home **(Table 47.1)**. Counseling a mother/caretaker is critical for home care. The health professional should use good communication skills while counseling the mother/caretaker for treatment **(Box 47.1)**.

Table 47.1 Treatment guidelines for managing sick young infant in the outpatient department or at home

Treatment of local infections

- Local bacterial infection: Give oral amoxicillin or co-trimoxazole for 5 days (avoid co-trimoxazole in infants < 1 month of age, who are premature or jaundiced)
- Skin pustules or umbilical infection: Teach to apply gentian violet paint twice daily at home.
- Discharge from ear: Teach to dry the ear with a cotton wick.

Some and no dehydration

Treat dehydration as per WHO guidelines for treatment of dehydration.

Feeding problem or low weight

- Skin pustules or umbilical infection: Teach to apply gentian violet
- Teach correct positioning and attachment for breastfeeding
- Teach the mother to manage breast and nipple problems
- Treat thrush: Tell the mother to paint the mouth of the young infant with gentian violet 0.25% twice daily
- Feeding with a cup and spoon: Wherever indicated, teach the mother correct technique of feeding
- Counsel the mother/caretaker about other feeding problems.

Keep the young infant warm

Teach the mother how to keep the young infant with low weight or low body temperature warm (do not bathe the young infant but sponge with lukewarm water to clean, provide skin-to-skin contact; keep the room warm): clothe the baby in 3–4 layers properly covering the head with a cap and hands and feet with mittens and socks respectively, cover the baby and the mother with additional quilt or shawl, especially in cold weather).

47

Box 47.1 | **Effective communication and counseling (APAC)**

- *Ask and listen:* Ask the mother/caretaker and listen carefully to find out the young infant/child's problems and what the mother/caretaker is already doing for the young infant/child
- *Praise:* Praise the mother/caretaker for what she has done well
- *Advise and teach:* Advise the mother/caretaker how to take care of young infant/child at home (for tasks which require mother/caretaker to carry out treatment at home: Give information, show an example, and let her practice)
- *Check:* Before the mother/caretaker leaves, always check her understanding by asking questions to find out what she understands and what needs further explanation

ASSESS AND CLASSIFY THE SICK CHILD BETWEEN 2 MONTHS UP TO 5 YEARS AGE

The assessment procedure is similar to that of young infant including: (i) history taking and communicating with the caretaker about the child's problem; (ii) checking for general danger signs; (iii) checking main symptoms; (iv) checking for malnutrition; (v) checking for anemia; (vi) assessing the child's feeding; (vii) checking immunization status; and (viii) assessing other problems (Chart 47.2).

Identification of Danger Signs

A sick child brought to an outpatient facility may have signs that clearly indicate a specific problem. For example, a child may present with cough and chest indrawing which indicate severe pneumonia. However, some children may present with serious, nonspecific signs called General Danger Signs that do not point to a particular diagnosis. For example, a child who is lethargic or unconscious or excessively irritable or crying inconsolably may have meningitis, severe pneumonia, cerebral malaria or any other severe disease. Great care should be taken to ensure that these general danger signs are not overlooked because they suggest that a child is severely ill and needs urgent attention. The following general danger signs should be routinely checked in all children: (i) history of convulsions during the present illness, (ii) unconsciousness or lethargy, (iii) inability to drink or breastfeed when mother tries to breastfeed or to give the child something to drink, and (iv) child vomits everything.

If a child has one or more of these signs, he must be considered seriously ill and will almost always need referral. In order to start treatment for severe illnesses

without delay, the child should be quickly assessed for the main symptoms and malnutrition and referred urgently to a hospital.

Assessment of Main Symptoms

After checking for general danger signs, the health care provider must enquire about the following main symptoms: (i) cough or difficult breathing; (ii) diarrhea; (iii) fever; and (iv) ear problems. If the symptom is present the child is evaluated for that symptom (Chart 47.2).

Cough or difficult breathing A child with cough or difficult breathing may have pneumonia or severe respiratory infection. In developing countries, pneumonia is often due to bacteria. The most common pathogens are *Streptococcus pneumoniae* and *Haemophilus influenzae*. Many children are brought to the clinic with less serious respiratory infections. Most children with cough or difficult breathing have only a mild infection. They do not need treatment with antibiotics. Their families can manage them at home. Very sick children with cough or difficult breathing need to be identified as they require antibiotic therapy. Fortunately, one can identify almost all cases of pneumonia by checking for two clinical signs, i.e. fast breathing and chest indrawing. Chest indrawing is a sign of severe pneumonia.

Clinical Assessment and classification A child presenting with cough or difficult breathing should first be assessed for general danger signs. This child may have pneumonia or severe respiratory infection. Three key clinical signs are used to assess a sick child with cough or difficult breathing: *fast breathing* (cut-off respiratory rate for fast breathing is 50 breaths per minute or more for a child 2 months up to 12 months, and 40 breaths per minute or more for 12 months up to 5 yr); *lower chest wall indrawing and stridor in a calm child.* Based on a combination of the above clinical signs, children presenting with cough or difficult breathing can be classified into one of the three categories. A child with general danger sign or chest indrawing or stridor is classified as severe pneumonia or very severe disease and merits urgent referral to the hospital. A sick child with cough who has fast breathing is classified as pneumonia and his treatment initiated in clinic with oral antimicrobials. A child with cough with none of these signs is classified as cough and cold and given home remedies to soothe throat and mother is counseled for home care.

A child with cough or cold normally improves in one week. However, a child with chronic cough (more than 30 days) needs to be further assessed (and, if needed, referred) to exclude tuberculosis, asthma, whooping cough or any other problem.

Chart 47.2

ASSESS AND CLASSIFY THE SICK CHILD AGE 2 MONTHS UP TO 5 YEARS

ASSESS   CLASSIFY   IDENTIFY TREATMENT

ASK THE MOTHER WHAT ARE THE CHILD'S PROBLEMS?

- Determine if this is an initial or follow-up visit for this problem
  If follow-up visit, use the follow-up instructions on *TREAT THE CHILD* chart
  If initial visit, assess the child as follows:

CHECK FOR GENERAL DANGER SIGNS

ASK:
- Is the child able to drink or breastfeed?
- Does the child vomit everything?
- Is the child having convulsions?

LOOK:
See if the child is lethargic or unconscious

A child with any general danger sign needs URGENT attention; complete the assessment and give the pre-referral treatment immediately so that referral is not delayed

USE ALL BOXES THAT MATCH THE CHILD'S SYMPTOMS AND PROBLEMS TO CLASSIFY THE ILLNESS

THEN ASK ABOUT MAIN SYMPTOMS:
Does the child have cough or difficult breathing?

IF YES, ASK: *LOOK, LISTEN:*
For how long?
- Count the breaths in one minute
- Look for chest indrawing
- Look and listen for stridor

CHILD MUST BE CALM

Classify COUGH or DIFFICULT BREATHING

Age:	Fast breathing is:
2 months to 12 months	50 breaths per minute or more
12 months to 5 years	40 breaths per minute or more

SIGNS	CLASSIFY AS	IDENTIFY TREATMENT (Urgent pre-referral treatments are in bold print)
• Any general danger sign, or • Chest indrawing, or • Stridor in a calm child	SEVERE PNEUMONIA OR VERY SEVERE DISEASE	➤ *Give first dose of injectable chloramphenicol (If not possible give oral amoxycillin)* ➤ *Refer URGENTLY to hospital #*
Fast breathing	PNEUMONIA	➤ *Give Amoxycillin for 5 days* ➤ Soothe the throat and relieve the cough with a safe remedy if child is 6 mo or older ➤ Advise mother when to return back immediately ➤ Follow-up in 2 days
No signs of pneumonia	NO PNEUMONIA: COUGH OR COLD	➤ If coughing for more than 30 days, refer for assessment ➤ Soothe the throat and relieve the cough with a safe home remedy if child 6 mo or older ➤ Advise mother when to return back ➤ Follow-up in 5 days if not improving

#If referral is not possible, see the section *Where Referral is Not Possible in the module. Treat the Child*

(Contd.)

47

Chart 47.2 (*Contd.*)

Does the child have diarrhea?

IF YES, ASK: **LOOK AND FEEL:**

- For how long?
- Is there blood in the stool?

- Look at the child's general condition
  Is the child:
  Lethargic or unconscious?
  Restless and irritable?
- Look for sunken eyes
- Offer the child fluid
  Is the child:
  Not able to drink or drinking poorly?
  Drinking eagerly, thirsty?
- Pinch the skin of the abdomen
  Does it go back:
  Very slowly (longer than 2 seconds)?
  Slowly?

Classify DIARRHEA

	Signs	Classify as	Treatment
for DEHYDRATION	Two of the following signs: • Lethargic or unconscious • Sunken eyes • Not able to drink or drinking poorly • Skin pinch goes back very slowly	**SEVERE DEHYDRATION**	➢ If child has no other severe classification: – Give fluids for severe dehydration (Plan C) ➢ *If child also has another severe classification:* *Refer URGENTLY to hospital# with mother giving frequent sips of ORS on the way. Advise the mother to continue breastfeeding* ➢ *If child is 2 years or older and there is cholera in your area, give doxycycline for cholera*
	Two of the following signs: • Restless, irritable • Sunken eyes • Drinks eagerly, thirsty • Skin pinch goes back slowly	**SOME DEHYDRATION**	➢ Give fluids and food for some dehydration (Plan B) ➢ *If child also has a severe classification:* *Refer URGENTLY to hospital# with mother giving frequent sips of ORS on the way. Advise the mother to continue breastfeeding* ➢ Advise mother when to return back ➢ Follow-up in 5 days if not improving
	Not enough signs to classify as some or severe dehydration	**NO DEHYDRATION**	➢ Give fluids, zinc supplements and food to treat diarrhea at home (Plan A) ➢ Advise mother when to return back ➢ Follow-up in 5 days if not improving
and if diarrhea 14 days or more	Dehydration present	**SEVERE PERSISTENT DIARRHEA**	➢ Treat dehydration before referral unless the child has another severe classification ➢ **Refer to hospital#**
	No dehydration	**PERSISTENT DIARRHEA**	➢ Advise the mother on feeding a child who has PERSISTENT DIARRHEA ➢ **Give single dose of vitamin A** ➢ Give zinc supplements daily for 14 days ➢ Follow-up in 5 days
and if blood in stool	Blood in the stool	**DYSENTERY**	➢ *Treat for 3 days with ciprofloxacin* ➢ *Treat dehydration* ➢ Give zinc supplements daily for 14 days ➢ Follow-up in 2 days

#If referral is not possible, see the section *Where Referral Is Not Possible* in the module. *Treat the Child*

(*Contd.*)

Chart 47.2 (Contd.)

Does the child have fever?
(by history or feels hot or temperature 37.5°C* or above)

IF YES:
Decide Malaria Risk: High or Low

THEN ASK:
- Fever for how long?
- If more than 7 days, has fever been present everyday?
- Did the child suffer from measles within the last 3 months?

LOOK AND FEEL:
- Look or feel for stiff neck
- Look and feel for bulging fontanel
- Look for runny nose

Look for signs of MEASLES
- Generalized rash and
- One of these: cough, runny nose, or red eyes

If the child has measles now or within the last 3 months:
- Look for mouth ulcers
  Are they deep and extensive?
- Look for pus draining from the eye
- Look for clouding of the cornea

Classify FEVER

HIGH MALARIA RISK
High Malaria Risk

Signs	Classify as	Treatment
• Any general danger sign, or • Stiff neck, or • Bulging fontanel	VERY SEVERE FEBRILE DISEASE	➤ *Give first dose of IM quinine after making a blood smear / RDT* ➤ *Give first dose of IV or IM chloramphenicol (If not possible, give oral amoxicillin)* ➤ *Treat the child to prevent low blood sugar* ➤ Give one dose of paracetamol in clinic for high fever (38.5°C or above) ➤ *Refer URGENTLY to hospital#*
Fever (by history, or feels hot, or temperature 37.5°C or above)	MALARIA	➤ *Give oral antimalarials for HIGH malaria risk area after making a blood smear* ➤ Give one dose of paracetamol in clinic for high fever (38.5°C or above) ➤ Advise mother when to return back immediately ➤ Follow-up in 2 days if fever persists ➤ If fever is present everyday for more than 7 days, refer for assessment

LOW MALARIA RISK
Low Malaria Risk

Signs	Classify as	Treatment
• Any general danger sign, or • Stiff neck, or • Bulging fontanel	VERY SEVERE FEBRILE DISEASE	➤ *Give first dose of IM quinine after making a blood smear* ➤ *Give first dose of IV or IM chloramphenicol (If not possible, give oral amoxicillin)* ➤ *Treat the child to prevent low blood sugar* ➤ Give one dose of paracetamol in clinic for high fever (38.5°C or above) ➤ *Refer URGENTLY to hospital#*
• NO runny nose, and • NO measles, and • NO other cause of fever	MALARIA	➤ *Give oral antimalarials for LOW malaria risk area after making a blood smear / RDT* ➤ Give one dose of paracetamol in clinic for high fever (38.5°C or above) ➤ Advise mother when to return back ➤ Follow-up in 2 days ➤ If fever is present everyday for more than 7 days, refer for assessment
• Runny nose PRESENT or • Measles PRESENT or • Other cause of fever PRESENT**	FEVER: MALARIA UNLIKELY	➤ Give one dose of paracetamol in clinic for high fever (38.5°C or above) ➤ Advise mother when to return back ➤ Follow-up in 2 days ➤ If fever is present everyday for more than 7 days, refer for assessment

If MEASLES Now or within last 3 months, Classify

Signs	Classify as	Treatment
• Any general danger sign, or • Clouding of cornea, or • Deep or extensive mouth ulcers	SEVERE COMPLICATED MEASLES	➤ *Give first dose of vitamin A* ➤ *Give first dose of injectable chloramphenicol (if not possible give oral amoxycillin)* ➤ *If clouding of the cornea or pus draining from the eye, apply tetracycline eye ointment* ➤ *Refer URGENTLY to hospital*
• Pus draining from the eye, or • Mouth ulcers	MEASLES WITH EYE OR MOUTH COMPLICATIONS	➤ Give first dose of vitamin A ➤ If pus draining from the eye, treat eye infection with tetracycline eye ointment ➤ If mouth ulcers, treat with gentian violet ➤ Follow-up in 2 days
Measles now or within the last 3 months	MEASLES	Give first dose of vitamin A

---

* This cut off is for axillary temperatures; rectal temperature cutoff is approximately 0.5°C higher
** Other causes of fever include cough or cold, pneumonia, diarrhea, dysentery and skin infections
*** Other important complications of measles include pneumonia, stridor, diarrhea, ear infection, and malnutrition and are classified in other tables

If referral is not possible, see the section **Where Referral Is Not Possible in the module **Treat the Child**

47

(Contd.)

Chart 47.2 (Contd.)

Does the child have an ear problem?

IF YES, ASK:

LOOK AND FEEL:

- Is there ear pain?
- Is there ear discharge? If yes, for how long?
- Look for pus draining from the ear
- Feel for tender swelling behind the ear

> **Classify EAR PROBLEM**

Signs	Classify	Treatment
Tender swelling behind the ear	**MASTOIDITIS**	➤ *Give first dose of injectable chloramphenicol (if not possible give oral amoxycillin)* ➤ *Give first dose of paracetamol for pain* ➤ **Refer URGENTLY to hospital**#
• Pus is seen draining from the ear and discharge is reported for less than 14 days, or • Ear pain in present	**ACUTE EAR INFECTION**	➤ **Give Amoxycillin for 5 days** ➤ Give paracetamol for pain ➤ Dry the ear with a cotton wick ➤ Follow-up in 5 days
Pus is seen draining from the ear and discharge is reported for 14 days or more	**CHRONIC EAR INFECTION**	➤ Dry the ear with a cotton wick ➤ Topical ciprofloxacin ear drops for 2 weeks ➤ Follow-up in 5 days
• No ear pain • No pus seen draining from the ear	**NO EAR INFECTION**	No additional treatment

#If referral is not possible, see the section *Where Referral Is Not Possible in the* module. **Treat the Child**

47

(Contd.)

Chart 47.2 (*Contd.*)

THEN CHECK FOR MALNUTRITION

LOOK AND FEEL:

- Look for visible severe wasting
- Look for edema of both feet
- Determine weight-for-age

Classify NUTRITIONAL STATUS

Signs	Classification	Treatment
• Visible severe wasting, or • Edema of both feet	SEVERE MALNUTRITION	➤ Give single dose of vitamin A ➤ Prevent low blood sugar ➤ *Refer URGENTLY to hospital#* ➤ *While referral is being organized, warm the child* ➤ *Keep the child warm on the way to hospital*
Very low weight-for-age	VERY LOW WEIGHT	➤ Assess and counsel for feeding If feeding problem, follow-up in 5 days ➤ Advise mother when to return immediately ➤ Follow-up in 30 days
Not very low weight-for-age and no other sign of malnutrition	NOT VERY LOW WEIGHT	➤ If child is less than 2 yr old, assess the child's feeding and counsel the mother on feeding according to the FOOD box on the *COUNSEL THE MOTHER* chart – If there is a feeding problem, follow-up in 5 days ➤ Advise mother when to return immediately

THEN CHECK FOR ANEMIA

LOOK:

- Look for palmar pallor. Is it:
  – Severe palmar pallor?
  – Some palmar pallor?

Classify ANEMIA

Signs	Classification	Treatment
Severe palmar pallor	SEVERE ANEMIA	➤ *Refer URGENTLY to hospital#*
Some palmar pallor	ANEMIA	➤ Give iron folic acid therapy for 14 days ➤ Assess the child's feeding and counsel the mother on feeding according to the FOOD box on the *COUNSEL THE MOTHER* chart – If there is a feeding problem, follow-up in 5 days ➤ Advise mother when to return immediately ➤ Follow-up in 14 days
No palmar pallor	NO ANEMIA	➤ Give prophylactic iron folic acid if child 6 mo or older

THEN CHECK THE CHILD'S IMMUNIZATION *, PROPHYLACTIC VITAMIN A & IRON-FOLIC ACID SUPPLEMENTATION STATUS

IMMUNIZATION SCHEDULE:

AGE	VACCINE
Birth	BCG + OPV-0
6 weeks	DPT-1 + OPV-1 (+ HepB-1**)
10 weeks	DPT-2 + OPV-2 (+ HepB-2**)
14 weeks	DPT-3 + OPV-3 (+ HepB-3**)
9 mo	Measles
16–18 mo	DPT Booster + OPV
60 mo	DT

PROPHYLACTIC VITAMIN A
Give a single dose of vitamin A:
100,000 IU at 9 mo with measles immunization
200,000 IU at 16–18 mo with DPT Booster
200,000 IU at 24 mo and then every 6 mo till 60 mo of age

PROPHYLACTIC IFA
Give 20 mg elemental iron +100 mcg folic acid (one tablet of Pediatric IFA or 5 ml of IFA syrup or 1 ml of IFA drops) for a total of 100 days in a year after the child has recovered from acute illness if:
➤ The child is 6 mo of age or older, and
➤ Has not received Pediatric IFA tablet/syrup/drops for 100 days in last one year

* A child who needs to be immunized should be advised to go for immunization the day vaccines are available at AW/SC/PHC
** Hepatitis B to be given wherever included in the immunization schedule

ASSESS OTHER PROBLEMS

MAKE SURE CHILD WITH ANY GENERAL DANGER SIGN IS REFERRED after first dose of an appropriate antibiotic and other urgent treatments
Exception: Rehydration of the child according to Plan C may resolve danger signs so that referral is no longer needed

#If referral is not possible, see the section *Where Referral Is Not Possible* in the module. *Treat the Child*

(Contd.)

47

Diarrhea

A child with diarrhea passes stools with more water than normal. A child with diarrhea may have (i) acute watery diarrhea (including cholera); (ii) dysentery (bloody diarrhea); or (iii) persistent diarrhea (diarrhea that lasts 14 days or more).

Most diarrheal episodes are caused by agents for which antimicrobials are not effective and therefore antibiotics should not be used routinely for treatment of diarrhea. Antidiarrheal drugs do not provide practical benefits for children with acute diarrhea, and some may have dangerous side effects.

Clinical assessment and classification All children with diarrhea should be assessed for dehydration based on the following clinical signs: *child's general condition* (lethargic or unconscious or restless/irritable); *sunken eyes; child's reaction when offered to drink* (not able to drink or drinking poorly or drinking eagerly/thirsty or drinking normally) and *elasticity of skin* (skin pinch goes back very slowly, slowly or immediately). In addition, a child with diarrhea should be asked how long the child has had diarrhea and if there is blood in the stool. This will allow identification of children with persistent diarrhea and dysentery.

Children with severe dehydration require immediate IV infusion according to WHO treatment guidelines described in plan C. Children with some dehydration require active oral treatment with ORS as per plan B. Patients with diarrhea and no dehydration are advised to give more fluids than usual to prevent dehydration according to WHO treatment plan A.

All children with persistent diarrhea are classified based on presence or absence of dehydration. Children with persistent diarrhea and dehydration are classified as severe persistent diarrhea and need to be referred to hospital after treatment of dehydration. Children with persistent diarrhea and no dehydration can be safely managed on outpatient basis with appropriate feeding. Children with dysentery are given effective antibiotics for shigellosis.

Fever

Fever is a very common condition and is often the main reason for bringing children to the health center. It may be caused by minor viral infections, but may also be the most obvious sign of a life-threatening illness, e.g. *P. falciparum* malaria or meningitis. When diagnostic capacity is limited, it is important to identify those children who need urgent referral with appropriate pre-referral treatment (antimalarial or antibacterial). All sick children should be assessed for fever if it is reported by mother or fever is present on examination.

Clinical assessment and classification In endemic areas, the risk of malaria transmission is defined by areas of high and low malaria risk in the country. National Anti-Malaria Program (NAMP) has defined areas depending on risk of malaria. History of duration of fever is important in evaluating fever. If fever has persisted daily for more than seven days, the child needs to be referred to hospital for assessment and diagnostic tests. The other signs looked for in a child with fever include general danger signs (assessed earlier) and signs of meningitis, e.g. *bulging fontanel and stiff neck*. Besides these, signs of measles and runny nose are also looked for.

If the child has measles currently or within the last three months, he should be assessed for possible complications. Some complications of measles are assessed as main symptoms, e.g. cough/difficult breathing, diarrhea and ear infection. Clouding of cornea and mouth ulcers are assessed along with measles. Clouding of cornea is a dangerous eye complication. If not treated, cornea can ulcerate and cause blindness. An infant with corneal clouding needs urgent treatment with vitamin A.

Before classifying fever, one should check for other obvious causes of fever. Children with fever are classified based on the presence of any of the general danger signs, stiff neck, level of malaria risk in the area and presence/absence of symptoms like runny nose, measles or clinical signs of other possible infection. In high malaria risk area, all children with fever need to get antimalarial treatment as per NAMP guidelines. In areas with low malaria risk, children with fever with no other obvious cause are classified as malaria and should be evaluated with blood smear and treated with oral antimalarial drugs (chloroquine). In low malaria risk area, children with fever due to another cause (e.g. cough and cold or ear infection or diarrhea) are classified as fever, malaria unlikely and given symptomatic treatment for fever.

Ear Problems

A child with an ear problem may have acute otitis, media. If the infection is not treated, the ear drum may perforate. Ear infections are the main cause of deafness in low-income areas, which leads to learning problems. The middle ear infection can also spread from the ear and cause mastoiditis and/or meningitis. The sick child is assessed for ear infection if any ear problem is reported.

Clinical assessment and classification The mother is asked about history of ear pain and ear discharge or pus. The child is examined for tender swelling behind the ear. Based on these clinical findings, a child can be classified as mastoiditis, acute ear infection, chronic ear infection or no ear infection. Children with mastoiditis are classified as severe illness and referred urgently to hospital. Children with acute ear infection are given oral antibiotics and those with chronic ear infection are advised to keep the ear dry by wicking.

Assessment of Malnutrition

After assessing for general danger signs and the four main symptoms, *all children should be assessed for malnutrition*. There are two main reasons for routine assessment of nutritional status in sick children: (i) to identify children with severe malnutrition who are at increased risk of mortality and need urgent referral to provide active treatment; and (ii) to identify children with suboptimal nutritional status resulting from ongoing deficits in dietary intake plus repeated episodes of infection and who may benefit from nutritional counseling.

Classification of Malnutrition

Visible severe wasting This is defined as severe wasting of the shoulders, arms, buttocks, and legs, with ribs easily seen, and indicates presence of marasmus. When wasting is extreme, there are many folds of skin on the buttocks and thighs. It looks as if the child is wearing baggy pants. The face of a child with visible severe wasting may still look normal. The child's abdomen may be large or distended.

Edema of both feet The presence of edema in both feet may signal kwashiorkor.

Weight-for-age Plotting weight for age in the growth chart, based on reference population, helps to identify children with low (Z score less than –2) or very low (Z score less than –3) weight-for-age, these children are at increased risk of infection and poor growth and development.

Checking for Anemia

All children should be assessed for anemia. The most common cause of anemia in young children in developing countries is nutritional or because of parasitic or helminthic infestations.

Clinical assessment and classification Palmar pallor can help to identify sick children with severe anemia. Whenever feasible, diagnosis of anemia can be supported by using a simple laboratory test for hemoglobin estimation. For clinical assessment of anemia, the color of the child's palm is compared with examiner's own palm. If the skin of the child's palm is pale, the child has *some palmar pallor*. If the skin of the palm is very pale or so pale that it looks white, the child has *severe palmar pallor*. Based on severity of palmar pallor it is classified as severe anemia, anemia or no anemia.

Feeding History and Problems

All children less than 2-yr-old and all children classified as anemic or very low weight need to be assessed for feeding even if they have a normal Z score. Feeding assessment includes questioning the mother or caretaker about feeding history. The mother or caretaker should be given appropriate advice to help overcome any feeding problems.

To assess feeding, ask the mother, whether she breastfeeds her child (how many times during the day and night), does the child take any other food or fluids (what food or fluids, how many times a day, how the child is fed, how large are the servings, who feeds the child) and during the illness, has the child's feeding changed (if yes, how?).

Identify feeding problems When counseling a mother about feeding, one should use good communication skills. It is important to complete the assessment of feeding by referring to age appropriate feeding recommendations and identify all the feeding problems before giving advice. In addition to differences from the feeding recommendations, some other problems may become apparent from the mother's answers. Other common feeding problems are: *Difficulty in breastfeeding, use of feeding bottle, lack of vigorous sucking and not feeding well during illness.* IMNCI guidelines recommend locally acceptable, available and affordable foods for feeding a child during sickness and health.

Checking for Immunization, Vitamin A and Folic Acid Supplementation Status

The immunization status of every sick child brought to a health facility should be checked. Children who are well enough to be sent home can be immunized. After checking immunization status, determine if the child needs vitamin A supplementation and/or prophylactic iron folic acid supplementation.

Assessment for other Problems

The IMNCI clinical guidelines focus on five main symptoms. In addition, the assessment steps within each main symptom take into account several other common problems. For example, conditions such as meningitis, sepsis, tuberculosis, conjunctivitis, and different causes of fever such as ear infection and sore

47

throat are routinely assessed within the IMNCI case management protocol. If the guidelines are correctly applied, children with these conditions will receive presumptive treatment or urgent referral. Nevertheless, health care providers still need to consider other causes of severe or acute illness.

Treatment

All therapeutic options are listed in the Identify Treatment column of the *Assess and Classify the Sick Child Age 2 Months up to 5 Years* **(Chart 47.2)**. All sick children with a severe classification (pink) are referred to a hospital as soon as assessment is completed and necessary pre-referral treatment is administered. If a child has severe dehydration and no other severe classification, and IV infusion is available in the outpatient clinic, an attempt should be made to rehydrate the sick child. The principles of referral of a sick child are similar to those described for a sick young infant.

Referral of Children 2 Months up to 5 Years of Age

Possible pre-referral treatment(s) options includes:

- For convulsions diazepam IV or rectally. If convulsions continue after 10 min give a second dose.
- First dose of appropriate intramuscular antibiotic—chloramphenicol or ampicillin + gentamicin or ceftriaxone (for severe pneumonia or severe disease; very severe febrile disease; severe complicated measles; mastoiditis). Give oral antibiotic if injectable antibiotics are not available.
- First dose of quinine (for severe malaria) as per national guidelines.
- Vitamin A (persistent diarrhea, measles, severe malnutrition).
- Prevention of hypoglycemia with breast milk or sugar water.
- Oral antimalarials as per guidelines.
- Paracetamol for high fever (38.5°C or above) or pain.
- Tetracycline eye ointment (if clouding of the cornea or pus draining from eye).
- Frequent sips of ORS solution on the way to the hospital in sick children with diarrhea.

If a child does not need urgent referral, check to see if the child needs nonurgent referral for further assessment; for example, for a cough that has lasted more than 30 days, or for fever that has lasted seven days or more. These referrals are not as urgent, and other necessary treatments may be done before transporting for referral.

Treatment in the Outpatient Clinic and at Home

Identify the treatment options with each non-referral classification (*yellow* and *green*) in the IMNCI chart. Treatment uses a minimum of affordable essential drugs. Following guidelines for treatment need to be followed:

- Counseling a mother/caretaker for looking after the child at home is very important. Good communication skills based on principles of APAC are helpful for effective counseling.
- Give appropriate treatment and advice for 'yellow' and 'green' classifications as detailed in **Table 47.2**.

Counseling the Mother or Caretaker

A child who is seen at the clinic needs to continue treatment, optional feeding and fluids at home. The child's mother or caretaker also needs to recognize when the child is not improving, or is becoming sicker. The success of home treatment depends on how well the mother or caretaker knows to give treatment, understands its importance and knows when to return

Table 47.2 Treatment guidelines for managing a sick child in the OPD and at home

- *Pneumonia, acute ear infection* Give the first dose of the antibiotics in the clinic and teach the mother how to give oral drugs, cotrimoxazole or amoxicillin.
- *Dysentery* Give the first dose of the antibiotic in the clinic and teach the mother how to give oral drug, like ciprofloxicin for 3 days.
- *Cholera* In areas where cholera can not be excluded, children more than 2-year-old with severe dehydration should be given a single dose of doxycycline.
- *Dehydration and persistent diarrhea* Treat 'some' and 'no' dehydration and persistent diarrhea as per standard WHO guidelines.
- *Persistent diarrhea and severe malnutrition*, give single dose of vitamin A in the clinic.
- *Measles* Give two doses of vitamin A (first dose in clinic and give mother one dose to be given at home the next day).
- *Malaria* Treat as per recommendations
- *Anemia* Give iron folic acid for 3 months
- *Cough and cold* If the child is 6 months or older, use safe home remedies (continue breastfeeding, use honey, tulsi, ginger and other safe home remedies).
- *Local infection* Teach the mother or caretaker how to treat the infection at home. Instructions may be given about how to treat eye infection with tetracycline eye ointment; dry the ear by wicking to treat ear infection; and treat mouth ulcers or thrush with gentian violet.
- For acute diarrhea, persistent diarrhea and dysentery, give zinc (10–20 mg) supplements for 14 days.

Table 47.3 Mother should report immediately if she notices following symptoms

Young infant (age 0–2 mo)	*Sick child (2 mo–5 yrs)*
■ Refusing breastfeeding or drinking poorly	■ Not able to drink or breastfeed
■ Becomes sicker	■ Becomes sicker
■ Develops fever or cold to touch	■ Develops fever
■ Fast/difficult breathing	■ Child with cough and cold develops fast/difficult breathing
■ Blood in stools (if infant has diarrhea)	■ Child with diarrhea passes blood in stool or drinking poorly
■ Yellow palms and soles (if jaundiced)	

to a health care provider. Some advice is simple; sometimes advice requires teaching the mother or caretaker how to do a task. When you teach a mother how to treat a child, use three basic teaching steps: *give information; show an example; let her practice.*

- Advise to continue feeding and increase intake of fluids during illness
- Teach how to give oral drugs or to treat local infection
- Counsel to solve feeding problems (if any)
- Advise when to return **(Table 47.3)**. Every mother or caretaker who is taking a sick child home, needs to be advised about when to return back to a health facility. The health care provider should (i) teach signs that signify need for immediate return back to

health care provider, (ii) advise when to return for a follow-up visit, and (iii) schedule the next well-child or immunization visit.

BIBLIOGRAPHY

Integrated Management of Neonatal and Childhood Illness. Training Modules for Physicians. *Ministry of Health and Family Welfare, Govt. of India,* 2003.

World Health Organization. Integrated Management of Childhood Illness. WHO/CHD/97.3.A –3.G, *WHO, Geneva,* 1997.

World Health Organization. Integrated Management of the Sick Child. *Bull WHO* 1995; 73:735–40.

World Health Organization. Management of the Child with a Serious Infection or Severe Malnutrition: Guidelines for care at the first-referral level in developing countries. *WHO, Geneva,* 2000.

47

Medications and Supportive Nursing Care

Administration of drugs is one of the most important responsibilities of a nurse working in the pediatric ward. She should discharge this responsibility with utmost care, commitment and caution. World Health Organization is promoting the safety of medicines for children because they are more prone to develop adverse drug reactions. It is estimated that 1 in 10 children admitted in the hospital experience an adverse drug reaction, which must be documented and reported to the pharmacovigilance authorities. Before administration of any medication, the nurse must ask for any history of adverse drug reaction in the child or family members. In order to avoid errors and accidents in administration of medicines to children, the following seven "Rights" should be followed:

i. Right patient (check with hospital identification tag and from the mother or attendant).
ii. Right medicine with valid expiry date (check twice).
iii. Right dose and dilution (in case of IV medicines).
iv. Right route of administration.
v. Right timing
vi. Right documentation
vii. Right of the parents and child to know about the benefits and adverse effects of the drug.

Calculation of Drug Dosage

Children are not mini-adults and there is no reliable formula to calculate dose of drugs in children on the basis of adult dose. The dose of drugs in children is expressed per unit body weight or surface area (SA). The calculations based on surface area are more accurate because SA is proportional to the metabolic rate. But in clinical practice the dosages are calculated on the basis of body weight due to convenience and ease. A handbook or manual of drug dosages should be available in the ward for easy reference. Whenever in doubt, the manufacturer's instructions regarding dosage, dilution, mode of administration and side effects should be consulted when giving medicines to newborn babies and infants due to their small doses and greater risk of over dosing and toxicity. The dose of drugs need to be appropriately modified in children suffering from hepatic dysfunction and renal failure. In malnourished children, due to associated hypoproteinemia, the level of free or active drug is likely to be higher. Moreover, there is reduced biotransformation or detoxification of drugs in the liver with a greater risk of toxicity. When doses of drugs are calculated on the basis of actual body weight, malnourished children are likely to get a lower dose of drug for their age which can provide the desired therapeutic benefits. In obese children, dose should be calculated on the basis of ideal body weight instead of actual body weight. The nurse should be familiar with the dosages of commonly used life-saving drugs and their side effects.

Oral Medications

Most children hate medicines and it needs lot of patience and tact on the part of nurse to given them medicines. The nurse should establish a good rapport and develop a knack to get the cooperation of the child under her care. It may be easier and more convenient for the mother to administer oral medicine but nurse must ensure that the medicine is administered to the child in her presence. Medicines are absorbed better on empty stomach (especially penicillin, erythromycin, eltroxin, antiemetics and antitubercular drugs) but most drugs are preferably administered after or in-between meals to reduce gastric side effects and improve their tolerance.

Drop formulations are preferred in young infants due to small volume of the medicine to be administered. In preschool children, syrup or suspension formulation is usually given. Dispersible tablets or mouth dissolving tablets can be given to children above 2–3 years of age. Most school-going children should be able to swallow tablets or capsules but at times even an adolescent child may refuse to take a tablet. Rarely, a child is more keen to swallow a tablet instead of taking a liquid formulation. Some children are extremely prone to vomit when a medicine is given to them.

Mother should hold the infant in her lap in a semi-upright position while giving medicine to him. Medicine can be given with a spoon or preferably with a plastic syringe or dropper. The exact amount to be administered should be measured with a syringe or by the graduated dispenser provided by the manufacturer. Medicine should not be poured on the dorsum of tongue but instead between the side of the tongue and the cheeks. No medicine should be mixed in the milk or food because the child may stop taking milk or food after this procedure. Medicine can be mixed in fruit juice or any other sugar-based drink. The medicine or crushed tablet can be mixed in honey or fruit juice.

The toddlers create the greatest fuss in taking medicines and need to be handled with understanding and firmness. The attention is diverted and child is held firmly while giving the medicine. In a struggling child, due care should be exercised to prevent choking and aspiration. If the medicine is vomited out immediately (within 15 minutes) after the administration, doctor should be notified and medicine is readministered. The older child should be dealt with understanding and explanation that the medicine will make him feel better and he will be able to go home sooner.

Some medicines are given sublingual (midazolam, nifedipine) and as a nasal spray (Insed, DDAVP). It is hoped that nasal spray of insulin will be available in the near future for control of diabetes mellitus. Some vaccines are administered through nasal route.

Rectal Medications

Rectal medications are not popular or well accepted in our culture except glycerine suppositories for relief of constipation. Rectal route of medication is used in children with persistent vomiting and ambulatory or home treatment of seizures or when medication cannot be given orally due to irritant nature of drug. Certain medications are available in liquid form in a prefilled syringe with a nozzle (diazepam) or a medicated suppository (paracetamol). The suppository is a medicated solid formulation in a tapered or bullet shape, which can be introduced through the anus into the rectum. The medication is placed beyond the anal sphincter. After insertion of the medicine in rectum, the mother is asked to hold the buttocks firmly for a few minutes or buttocks are taped so that medicine stays in the rectum.

Parenteral Medications

In critically sick children admitted to the hospital, drugs are administered through intramuscular or intravenous route. In life-saving situations, IV route is preferred especially in newborn babies because absorption through IM route is slow and unsatisfactory. Intramuscular medication is avoided in children with bleeding disorder or when volume of the drug is more than 2 mL or drug is likely to cause local irritation and severe pain. Most vaccines are administered through subcutaneous or intramuscular route in the antero-lateral part of mid-thigh or deltoid region. Vaccines should not be given in the gluteal region due to slow and unsatisfactory absorption.

Intravenous medications should preferably be given with due aseptic precautions through an indwelling catheter to reduce the risk of leakage in the extravascular region. Drugs should not be mixed before administration. They should be appropriately diluted as per instructions of the manufacturer before administration. They can be injected as a slow bolus directly through the indwelling cannula or by puncturing the access port of the infusion set or through 3-way stopcock by wearing gloves and observing strict aseptic precautions. At times drugs are administered slowly over a period of 15–30 minutes through a micro-burette set or infusion pump. In case of certain drugs, they can be added to the infusion fluid in the bottle (like sodium bicarbonate, potassium chloride, calcium gluconate, inotropic agents, etc.). Drugs should not be added to the blood or blood products and TPN solution. They should be properly diluted in the diluent recommended by the manufacturer. It is preferable to avoid adding drugs to the infusate containing sodium bicarbonate.

In newborn babies, formulations with the lowest strength should be used, e.g. use 10 mg/mL concentration of gentamicin injection rather than 40 mg/mL. In view of small volumes and low dosages, it is preferable to use 1.0 mL or tuberculin syringe for giving medications to newborn babies. The drug should be properly and accurately diluted to administer the correct dose to young infants. When injectable form of the drug contains sodium, the amount of sodium being administered should be monitored. *The amount of diluent and flush fluid administered through IV medications should be recorded and subtracted from total daily fluids as a safeguard against over infusion.* When a new or infrequently used drug is being given, it is advised to read the manufacturer's instructions.

48

Topical Medications

For instillation of *eye drops*, child is restrained by the mother in a supine position. The nurse washes her hands and stands at the head-end or right side of the child. The eye dropper is held in the right hand resting over the child's forehead. With the index finger of the left hand, the lower fornix of the conjunctival sac is exposed by applying gentle downward and backward pressure. Two drops of the medicine are released into the eye by lowering the nozzle of the dropper to a few millimeters of the exposed conjunctival sac. The medication should not be dropped directly over the cornea. The procedure is repeated on the other side. The same procedure is followed for instillation of eye ointment which is applied to the exposed lower fornix of the conjunctival sac at night for sustained effect. It is preferable to use single use ointment applicaps to reduce the risk of cross infection. Even when only one eye is infected, the drops are instilled in both the eyes by putting the drops first in the normal eye and then into the infected one.

For instillation of *nose drops*, child lies on his back, a blanket roll or pillow is placed under the shoulders to hyperextend the neck. Child's face is held with the left hand encircling the chin and cheeks while drops are instilled with the right hand. The nozzle of the dropper is directed just inside the nostril and 2–3 drops of the medicine are instilled. While instilling the drops, the head is turned slightly to the other side so that the drops stay in the nostril instead of rushing directly into the pharynx. Medicated decongestant nose drops should preferably be avoided (because of rebound nasal congestion) and instead 0.6% saline solution should be used. In young infants, nose drops should be instilled 15 minutes before the feed so that by the time feed is offered to the baby, the nose block is relieved. *Oily solutions should never be instilled into the nose due to potential risk of aspiration and development of lipoid pneumonia.*

For instillation of *ear drops*, child is restrained in the lateral position. The medicine dropper is held by the nurse in her right hand which is placed over the check of the baby. The tragus of the ear is pulled directly backwards in infants and backwards and upwards in case of children to straighten the ear canal. The nozzle of the dropper is brought near the opening of the ear and 2–3 drops are instilled. The ear is gently massaged and child is kept in the same position for 1–2 minutes for effective distribution of the medicine in the ear canal. The procedure is repeated in the other ear by turning the child over to the other side. A cotton pledget can be inserted into the ear canal to prevent leakage of medication.

Medications Directly Administered into the Lungs (Aerosol Therapy)

Easy access of the airways through mouth and nose provides an opportunity to administer bronchodilators, mucolytic agents and corticosteroids directly to the upper and lower airways. The advantages include prompt therapeutic response, need for a lower dosage and reduced risk of side effects. *Acute attack of bronchial asthma is best managed by administration of aerosolized bronchodilators with the help of an inhaler or by nebulization.*

Nebulization In acute attack of bronchial asthma, a heavy duty nebulizer is used to administer aerosole of bronchodilators and steroids. It is an electrical devise and drug is administered with the help of a air compressor. Oxygen at a flow rate of 6–8 liters/min can be used to deliver the drug when hypoxia is present in a severe case. Drug is dissolved in normal saline and taken in a volume of 3 mL. In young children, it is best given through a mask by enclosing his mouth and nose **(Figure 48.1)**. Child is asked to breathe slowly and deeply. The drug is nebulized over a period of 10–15 minutes. It is recommended to give 3 doses at an interval of 20 minutes to abort an attack. It is preferable to use a disposable mask for each patient to prevent risk of cross infection.

Metered-dose inhaler (MDI) with a spacer This method of drug delivery is as effective as nebulization but more doses are required. A spacer device must be used in children because of poor hand-lung coordination while using MDI in children **(Figure 48.2)**.

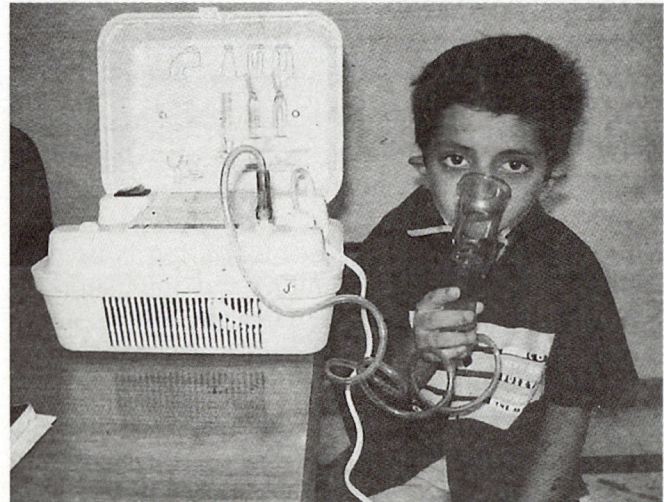

Figure 48.1 Nebulization with the help of an electrically operated nebulizer which can be used at home. It is preferable to use a mask enclosing nose and mouth in a pre-school child. In a life-threatening situation, oxygen should be used at a flow rate of 6–7 liters/min in a hospital setting

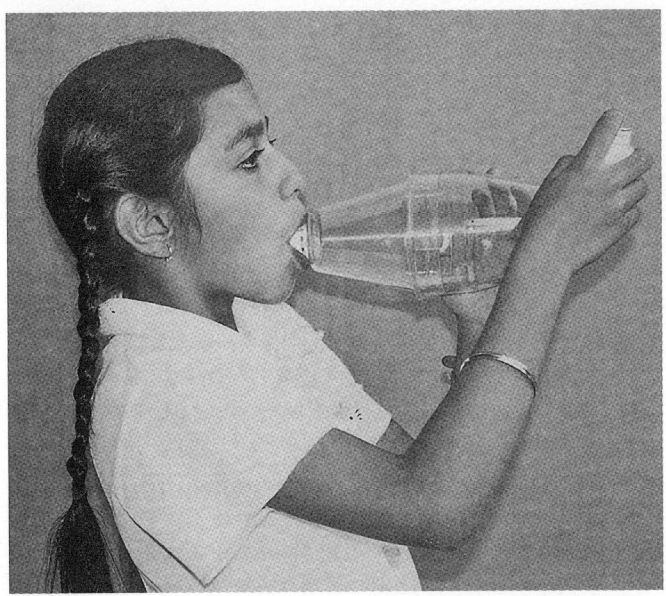

Figure 48.2 In a pre-school child, metered-dose inhaler is used with a spacer device. Children above 3 years can grasp the oral piece of the spacer with their lips while in younger children a mask is attached to the outlet of the spacer

It can be used both with a mask or with the help of a mouth piece through which child breathes. The canister is shaken thoroughly and two puffs are delivered into the spacer or holding device and child is asked to breathe through the mouth slowly and deeply for alteast 15 seconds. During an acute attack two puffs should be taken after every 5 minutes till the attack subsides. MDI with a spacer is as effective as a nebulizer but 4–6 doses of MDI are equivalent to one dose administered through the nebulizer. The spacer should be washed with a detergent every week and air dried.

Rotahaler A rotahaler delivers medication in a powdered form and is more convenient to use in children because it needs less coordination for effective delivery of drug. The capsule is inserted in the "capsule hold" and the rotahaler is rotated to break the capsule and powdered medicine is released in the delivery chamber. The child breathes out and then holds snugly the mouthpiece and takes a deep breath and holds the breath for a few seconds. The child breathes out through the nose and takes a deep breath through the mouth again to inhale the medicine into the lungs a couple of times (**Figure 48.3**). The rotahaler chamber should be kept clean and dry.

Humidification

Humidification has a soothing effect an respiratory passages, relieves congestion and loosens thick secretions to facilitate expectoration. Humidification is

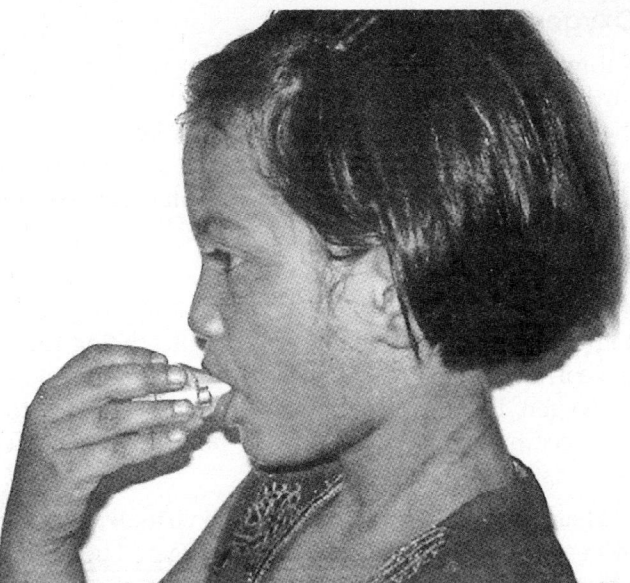

Figure 48.3 Rotahaler is a useful device for use by school-going children because it can be easily carried to school. The capsule containing the powdered medication is inserted in the "capsule hold" and rotahaler is rotated to break the capsule to deliver the powdered medicine in the delivery chamber. The child is asked to breathe out, hold the mouthpiece of the rotahaler snugly with her lips and take a deep breath to inhale the medicine into the lungs. The child may need to take a couple of breaths to inhale all the powdered medicine into the lungs

48

useful to relieve nasal congestion and treat inflammatory conditions of lungs like bronchitis or bronchiolitis, bronchopneumonia and cystic fibrosis.

The compressed air or oxygen is passed through water contained in a nebulizer which converts liquid into a fine spray of mist. The mist can be delivered to the child through a mask, head box or a small tent. This provides cool mist for humidification. The box or canopy of the tent should be kept clean and dry to ensure clear view of the child. The position of the child should be frequently changed and chest physiotherapy should be done to loosen the secretions and facilitate their expectoration. Young children are likely to swallow the phlegm and pass it in the stool or vomit it out.

Humidification can also be provided through a facial steamer or an electric kettle. Nasal decongestion can be enhanced by adding some carom or thymol seeds (*ajwain*) in the water of facial steamer. Infant in the mother's lap or child can be kept at a distance of about one foot from the steamer. Adolescent children can breathe-in the steam through their mouth from the snout of a porcelein kettle containing boiling water. *When providing humidification through steam, utmost care should be taken to prevent the risk of scalds.*

Oxygen Therapy

Room air provides only 21% oxygen while in many cardiorespiratory disorders causing hypoxia, oxygen therapy is life saving. Oxygen should be warmed to room temperature and humidified by passing it through a bottle containing sterile water. Dry oxygen should not be given due to risk of causing irritation of air passages and cough.

Incubator Oxygen can be given to a newborn baby being nursed in the incubator. Incubator being rather large in size, there is considerable wastage and leakage of oxygen. Even when a baby is lying in the incubator, it is recommended to use a head box or oxyhood for administration of oxygen.

Head box Oxygen tents have been virtually replaced by head boxes for administration of oxygen. The square-shaped box is moulded as a single piece from transparent plastic or perspex material. The box is provided with an adjustable neck port or a flexible occluding collar to create an effective seal to prevent free entry of environmental air into the box. The oxygen tube is attached to the nozzle located on the head end side of the box so that high concentration of oxygen are achieved around the face of the baby. Depending upon the flow rate of the oxygen and size of the head box, different concentrations of oxygen in the box can be achieved to meet the needs of the baby **(Figure 48.4)**. The concentration of the oxygen in the head box can be raised by increasing flow rate of the oxygen till cyanosis disappears and arterial oxygen saturation (SaO$_2$) of the baby is kept between 90 and 95%. In newborn babies arterial oxygen tension (PaO$_2$) should also be monitored and maintained between 50 and 80 mm Hg to prevent the risk of development of retinopathy of prematurity (ROP). Oxygen is life saving but both expensive as well as toxic. It should be used in the lowest concentration to relieve cyanosis or maintain normal arterial oxygen saturation and it must be discontinued when oxygen therapy is no longer required.

Mask In an older cooperative child, a disposable polythene bag can be used for administration of oxygen. Mask is snugly affixed on the face enclosing mouth and nose of the child. Oxygen is turned on and flow rate is adjusted and maintained on the basis of arterial oxygen saturation of the child who is attached to a pulse oximeter.

Nasal catheter The catheter with multiple side holes is passed through the nose till its tip reaches the nasopharynx just behind the uvula. It is securely taped to the upper lip and cheek. Oxygen is delivered at a rate of 2 liters/min to avoid excessive irritation of the nasopharynx. The skin should be kept clean and nostril kept lubricated with an antibiotic cream and kept free of any crusts.

Nasal prongs A twin-holed nasal prongs can be used for administration of oxygen at a low flow rate of 1–2 liters/min. The nasal prongs are inserted into the nostrils of the infant and catheter is affixed with the help of a micropore tape or an elastic band **(Figure 48.5)**. Catheter is attached to the humidified oxygen source and oxygen delivered at a rate of 2 liters per minute. This modality is better accepted because it does not cause local irritation due to the catheter.

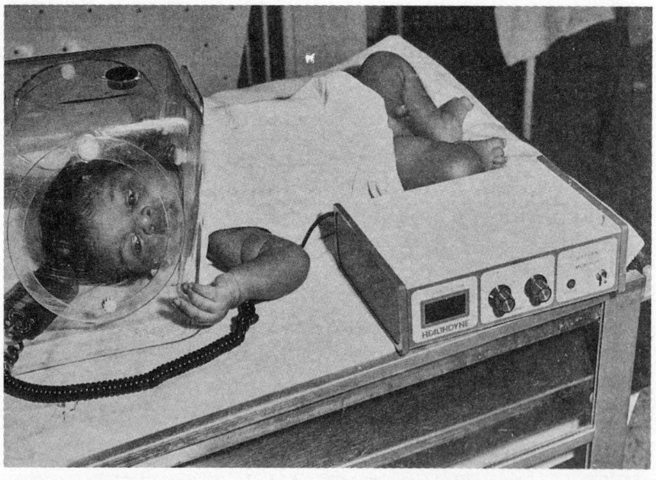

Figure 48.4 Oxygen head box. It is useful to achieve high ambient oxygen concentration around the face and minimize the wastage of oxygen. The concentration of oxygen in the box should be periodically checked with an oxygen analyzer

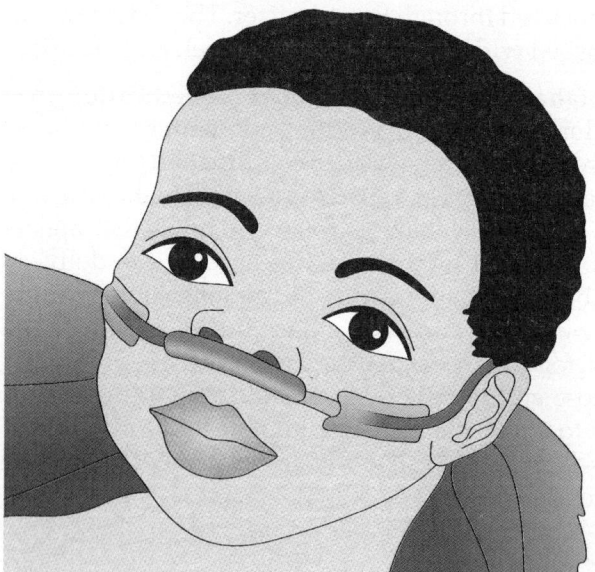

Figure 48.5 Administration of oxygen with the help of nasal prongs. The method is convenient and there is no wastage of oxygen

Phototherapy

Hyperbilirubinemia due to elevation of indirect bilirubin may cause damage to the basal ganglia of the brain in newborn babies. Phototherapy is a non-invasive method to bring down the bilirubin level by exposing the skin of the baby to blue or cool white light between 450 and 460 nm wave length. Light converts the bilirubin to non-toxic water soluble compounds which are excreted in the urine and stool. The flux of the light should be checked with the help of a fluxmeter and kept between 8 and 12 uw/cm^2/nm for effective phototherapy. The light source (tubes/halogen bulbs) need to be changed every 3 months or after 1000 hours of use or when ends of the tubes turn black. Other more effective phototherapy modalities incude blue light emitting diodes, fiberoptic cool BiliBlanket, and double surface phototherapy.

Procedure Baby is undressed completely but diaper is kept on to protect the gonads. Eyes are covered with eye patches to prevent damage to the retina. Nude baby is kept under the light source at a distance of 45 cm **(Figure 48.6)**. The efficacy of phototherapy is enhanced by using blue light emitting diodes (LEDs), reducing the distance between the light source and baby, and by exposing the skin of the baby to the light source both from above and below. The baby is turned every 2 hours or after each feed to expose maximum area of skin to light. Baby should be given frequent breast feedings but no supplements of extra water or milk is required. Phototherapy is stopped when serum bilirubin returns to a safe value as per the NICU protocol. Nurse should monitor the following parameters during phototherapy:

1. Temperature every 2 hours.
2. Ensure adequate breast feeding so that baby passes urine 6 and 8 times/day.
3. Daily weight record.
4. Serum bilirubin as per unit protocol.
5. Side effects of phototherapy like skin rash, loose greenish stools, hypo- or hyperthermia, dehydration (excessive weight loss), and bronze baby syndrome. Skin of the baby becomes bronze colored when a baby with conjugated hyperbilirubinemia is placed under light.

Blood Transfusion

The indications for blood transfusion include severe anemia (hemoglobin <5 g/dL), acute hemorrhage, hematological malignancy, following surgery and certain life-threatening conditions. Blood must be collected from voluntary donors and screened for malaria, VDRL, HIV, HBsAg, and HBcAg. Washed red blood cells (packed cell transfusion) without plasma

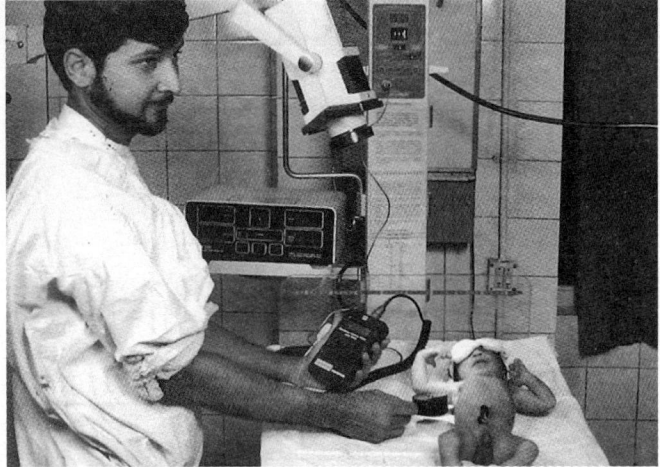

Figure 48.6 Baby under phototherapy unit. Note the effective shielding of eyes to protect against retinal damage. The flux of the phototherapy unit is being checked with a flux meter

proteins, leukocytes and platelets are preferred for correction of chronic anemia because of low risk of transfusion reactions and volume overload. When transfusion is given to replenish blood volume, whole blood should be transfused.

Procedure Intravenous line should be established with physiological saline. The blood transfusion should be started within 30 minutes following the arrival of blood from the blood bank. Check the bag of blood for patient's name, age, hospital registration number and expiry date. Verify the blood group and Rh type of blood in the bag and that of the patient. Inspect the blood against light for any abnormal color, gas bubbles, clumping or extraneous material. Ask the parents whether the child has had a previous reaction to transfusion of blood or blood products. The bag of blood must have a filter and some centers use an additional filter in the infusion set. Replace the 0.9% saline infusion drip with the blood bag and start infusion slowly for treatment of chronic anemia and rapidly for replacement of acute blood loss. The blood should be transfused over a period of maximum of 4 hours to reduce the risk of contamination by bacteria.

Monitoring Monitor the rate of infusion and record the infusion as per intravenous infusion guidelines. Monitor child's temperature, pulse and respiration rates every 15 minutes during the first hour and then every 30 minutes until blood transfusion is complete. *No medications should be administered through the blood transfusion set.* If any reaction occurs, stop the transfusion immediately and inform the doctor. **Table 48.1** outlines various reactions to blood transfusion and their management.

48

Table 48.1 Common reactions during blood transfusion

Reaction	Manifestations	Management
Hemolytic reaction	Chills, rigors, fever, breathlessness, hematuria, shock and renal failure	Stop transfusion, retain the sample of donor's and patient's blood. Inform doctor and treat shock due to hemolysis.
Febrile reactions	Fever or chills	Stop transfusion and give paracetamol
Allergic reactions*	Urticarial rash, wheezing, breathlessness, and stridor due to laryngeal edema	Stop transfusion. Give adrenaline IM and hydrocortisone IV
Circulatory** overload	Chest pain, breathlessness, distended neck veins, enlarging liver size, and crackles at the base of lungs	Place the child in an upright position and give IV furosemide

*Prophylactic antihistaminic may be given if child had a reaction to a previous blood transfusion.
**In children with chronic or long standing anemia, furosemide should be given before starting transfusion with packed red blood cells.

Platelet Transfusion

Platelet concentrate is given to children with bleeding manifestations due to thrombocytopenia. The risk of bleeding appears when platelet count drops below $5000/mm^3$. Platelets are also matched according to ABO and Rhesus blood group as in case of blood transfusion but in an emergency situation unmatched platelet concentrate can be given. The life span of transfused platelets is around 4 days and repeated platelet transfusions may be needed till underlying disease process is controlled.

The procedure is similar to blood transfusion. The bag containing platelets should be agitated during the procedure to prevent clumping of platelets. Platelets are transfused rapidly during 20–40 minutes. The child should be watched for fluid over load and allergic reaction. Adverse reactions to administration of platelets are best treated by administration of an antihistamine drug.

Emergency Trolley

The crash cart should be kept ready at all times in the Pediatric Intensive Care Unit to provide CPR facilities and life-sustaining medications as and when required **(Table 48.2)**. The trolley should be checked in each duty shift to ensure that all equipment and supplies are available and are functional and emergency drugs have valid expiry dates.

DOSAGES OF COMMONLY USED DRUGS

1. **Analgesic-antipyretic agents**

   Acetyl salicylic acid 10–15 mg/kg/dose PO every 4–6 hr

   Caution Avoid in children with viral fever due to risk of development of Reye syndrome

   Paracetamol (acetaminophen) 15 mg/kg/dose PO q 4–6 hr up to maximum of 60 mg/kg in 24 hr, 10 mg/kg/dose IM.

   Ibuprofen 10 mg/kg/dose PO q 6–8 hr.

   Mefenamic acid 7.5 mg/kg/dose PO q 6–8 hr.

2. **Narcotic analgesics (opioids)**

   Fentanyl 1.0–5.0 μg/kg/dose q 1–4 hr IV as a continuous infusion @ 1–5 μg/kg/hr.

   Pethidine hydrochloride 1–2 mg/kg/dose IM or IV

   Morphine sulfate 0.1–0.2 mg/kg/dose SC or IV q 4 hr.

   Caution Keep naloxone (0.01 mg/kg IV) ready as an antidote in case of respiratory depression.

3. **Sedatives**

   Chloral hydrate 7.5–15 mg/kg/dose PO q 6–8 hr.

   Triclofos sodium 20 mg/kg/dose PO

   Diazepam 0.1–0.2 mg/kg/dose oral, IM or IV

   Ketamine 0.5–2.0 mg/kg/dose IV slowly and 2.5–5.0 mg/kg/dose IM

   Midazolam 0.5–0.75 mg/kg/dose oral and 0.05–0.15 mg/kg/dose IM or IV

   Caution Avoid combining it with fentanyl but it is complementary to ketamine.

4. **Anticonvulsants**

   Carbamazepine 10–30 mg/kg/day q 8–12 hr PO

   Clobazam 0.3–1.0 mg/kg/day q 12 hr

   Lorazepam 0.05–0.1 mg/kg/dose IV or IM, may repeat after 10–15 min

   Diazepam 0.25–0.5 mg/kg/dose per rectum. 0.25–0.5 mg/kg/dose IV every 5 minutes for control of status epilepticus.

   Phenobarbitone sodium 15–20 mg/kg IV loading dose followed by 5–8 mg/kg/day q 12–24 hr PO for maintenance.

Table 48.2 Basic contents of pediatric emergency trolley

Airway maintenance

- Oropharyngeal airways of different sizes
- Endotracheal tubes 2.5–3.5 mm for newborn babies and 4.0 mm for infants. In older children ET tube size in mm = Age in years/4 + 4
- Laryngoscopes with straight handles for infants and older children
- Laryngeal mask airways and disposable face masks of different sizes
- Self-inflating Ambu bags and masks of different sizes
- T-piece or anesthetic circuit
- Ambient oxygen monitor
- Oxygen saturation monitor (pulse oximeter)
- Mechanical ventilators

Cardiac monitoring

- Cardiac monitor
- Non-invasive blood pressure monitor, sphygmomanometers and blood pressure cuffs of different sizes
- Portable ECG machine
- Defibrillator with pediatric paddles (4.5 cm) for infants and adult paddles (8.0 cm) for older children

Drugs and intravenous fluids

- Infusion pumps
- Saline/dextrose 500 mL bags in various concentrations, Ringers' lactate solution
- Dextran and plasma expander solution
- Emergency drug box containing adrenaline, sodium bicarbonate, naloxone, inotropes, cardiotonics, lignocaine, atropine sulfate, anticonvulsants, hydrocortisone, antihypertensives, antiemetics, antibiotics, diphenhydramine hydrochloride, chloral hydrate, specific antiodotes, etc.
- Heavy duty nebulizer with various bronchodilator solutions for nebulization.

Miscellaneous equipment

- Stethoscope
- Intravenous infusion set
- Intravenous cannulae, scalp-vein needles and CVP cannulae
- Intravenous cut-down set
- Surgical gloves, disposable syringes and needles of different sizes and gauges
- Intraosseous and spinal needles
- Suction tubes, feeding tubes, rectal tubes, catheters, thoracostomy tubes and disposables, etc.
- Mediswabs
- Scissors
- Water-based lubricant gel
- Surgical tape, leucoplast and micropore
- Splints of different sizes
- Blood specimen bottles, labels, etc.
- Surgical procedure trays: Vascular cut down, tracheostomy, cricothyroidotomy, thoracostomy, pericardiocentesis, paracentesis sets, peritoneal dialysis kit, and exchange blood transfusion set.

48

Phenytoin sodium 15–20 mg/kg/dose IV loading dose slowly and adequately diluted with normal saline. Maintenance dose 5–8 mg/kg/day single dose oral. Avoid IM administration due to erratic absorption.

Paraldehyde 0.1–0.2 mg/kg/dose deep IM or 0.3 mL/kg/dose per rectum mixed with coconut oil.

Valproate sodium 10–15 mg/kg/day q 8–12 hr PO with weekly increments to reach up to maximum dose of 60 mg/kg/day.

5. **Antibiotics**

Amikacin 15–20 mg/kg/day IM or IV q 8–12 hr

Cefixime 8 mg/kg/day q 12 hr or 24 hr PO, IM, IV

Cefotaxime sodium 100–150 mg/kg/day q 6–8 hr IM or IV

Ceftriaxone sodium 50–75 mg/kg/day q 12–24 hr IV

Gentamicin sulfate 5.0-7.5 mg/kg/day IM or IV q 8–12 hr

Cephalexin 25–50 mg/kg/day oral q 6–8 hr

Erythromycin 30–50 mg/kg/day oral q 6–8 hr

Azithromycin 10 mg/kg/day q 12–24 hr

Amoxycillin 25–50 mg/kg/day oral q 8 hr. High doses can be used IV for treatment of septicemia

Penicillin G benzathine 6,00,000 units IM below 6 years and 12,00,000 units IM above 6 years of age every 3 weekly for prophylaxis against rheumatic fever.

Caution Keep epinephrine handy to treat anaphylaxis

Ciprofloxacin 20–30 mg/kg/day oral q 12 hr

Ofloxacin 15 mg/kg/day oral q 12 hr

Norfloxacin 10–15 mg/kg/day oral q 12 hr

6. **Antiemetics**

Metoclopramide hydrochloride 0.2 mg/kg/dose q 6–8 hr oral, IM or IV

Domperidone 0.2–0.4 mg/kg/dose q 6-8 hr oral

Ondansetron hydrochloride dihydrate <4 yr: 2 mg q 4 hr; 4–11 yr: 4 mg q 4 hr; >12 yr: 8 mg q 4 hr PO Intravenous dose is 0.15–0.45 mg/kg

7. **Antimalarials**

Chloroquine phosphate 10 mg of base/kg oral stat followed by 5 mg/kg at 6 hr, 24 hr and of the doctor 48 hr. Give IM or IV under direct supervision of the doctor.

Quinine dihydrochloride For cerebral malaria, 20 mg/kg is given in a concentration of 1 mg/mL of normal saline or 5% dextrose over a period of 4 hr as a loading dose followed by 10 mg/kg every 8 hours as an infusion over 4 hours. Shift to oral therapy as soon as possible.

P. falciparum **resistant malaria**

Artesunate 4 mg/kg once daily for 3 days plus single dose of sulfadoxine-pyremethamine (25 mg/1.25 mg/kg) single dose on day 1 or mefloquine 25 mg/kg in 2 divided doses (15 mg/kg in the morning and 10 mg/kg evening) on day 2 and day 3.

OR

Fixed-dose combination of artemether (20 mg) and lumefantrine (120 mg) can be used as a 6 dose regimen given twice a day for 3 days. The dose is based on body weight:

5–14 kg 1 tablet, 15–24 kg 2 tablets, 25–35 kg 3 tablets and >35 kg 4 tablets. First dose is given at the time of diagnosis followed by another dose after 8 hours and then twice daily on day 2 and day 3.

8. **Antitubercular drugs**

Pyrazinamide 25–35 mg/kg/day (max 200 mg) single dose oral on empty stomach for 2 months

Isoniazid 10 mg/kg/day (max 300 mg) single dose oral up to 6–9 months

Rifampicin 10 mg/kg/day (max 600 mg) single dose oral on empty stomach for 6–9 months

Streptomycin sulfate 15 mg/kg/day (max 1.0 g) IM single dose for 2 months

Ethambutol 20–25 mg/kg/day single (max 1500 mg) dose oral for 4 weeks followed by 15 mg/kg/day for 6–9 months

9. **Anthelmintics**

Albendazole 200 mg single dose in children below 2 years and 400 mg single dose in children above 2 years of age.

Mebendazole 100 mg twice a day for 3 days

Levamisole 2 mg/kg/day single dose for ascariasis, 50 mg every 6 hourly for 4 doses for treatment of hookworm infestation.

10. **Bronchodilators**

Adrenaline (epinephrine) 0.01 mL/kg per dose (maximum 0.5 mL per dose) of 1: 1000 solution IM. Intravenously it is given 10 fold diluted, 0.1 mL/kg per dose of 1:10,000 solution for cardiac arrest. For laryngeal edema and acute bronchiolitis 0.3–0.5 mL/kg of 1:10,000 solution is diluted in 3 mL of normal saline and given through a nebulizer.

Aminophylline 5–7 mg/kg loading dose diluted in 25–30 mL normal saline IV followed by 0.5–0.9 mg/kg/hr constant infusion.

Salbutamol 0.1–0.4 mg/kg/dose q 8 hr oral

Theophylline 15–25 mg/kg/day q 8 hr oral

11. **Cardiotonics**

Digoxin Digitalizing dose for neonates and infants is 0.06 mg/kg/day, children >2 yr 0.04 mg/kg/day oral (parenteral dose is 2/3 rd of oral). One-half of the digitalizing dose is given stat, followed by 1/4th after 8 hr and remaining 1/4th after 16 hr. The daily maintenance dose is about 1/4th of the initial digitalizing dose.

Dopamine Dopamine infusion is started at a rate of 5 µg/kg/min which is slowly increased to 20 µg/kg/min. One mL of dopamine dissolved in 100 mL of 5% dextrose gives a concentration of 400 µg/mL.

Dobutamine 5–20 µg/kg/min IV constant infusion

12. Diuretics

Furosemide 1–2 mg/kg/dose oral q 12 hr. The IV dose is one-half of the oral dose.

Hydrochlorthiazide 1–2 mg/kg/dose q 12 hr oral.

13. Corticosteroids

Betamethasone 0.1–0.2 mg/kg/day q 8 hr oral. It is 7–10 times more potent than prednisolone.

Cortisone acetate 0.7–1.0 mg/kg/day q 8 hr oral for physiological requirements.

Dexamethasone 0.5 mg/kg/dose q 6 hr IV for shock and cerebral edema.

Hydrocortisone sodium succinate 25–50 mg/kg/dose q 4–6 hr IV for status asthmaticus and shock.

Prednisolone 1–2 mg/kg/day q 6–8 hr oral after meals.

Deflazacort 1–2 mg/kg q 6–8 hr oral.

Methyl prednisolone 30 mg/kg/dose IV bolus over 10–15 min daily for 3–5 days.

14. Miscellaneous agents

Atropine sulfate 0.02 mg/kg/dose IV or SC (minimum dose 0.2 mg).

Naloxone hydrochloride 0.1–0.2 mg/kg IV every 2–3 min for 3 doses (maximum total dose 2 mg).

Calcium gluconate 1–2 mL/kg/dose of 10% solution diluted with equal volume of distilled water or double volume of 5% dextrose, given slowly IV over 10 minutes. Stop the infusion if heart rate drops below 100/min. Calcium gluconate should not be added to the infusate containing sodium bicarbonate because of risk of precipitation.

Sodium bicarbonate 1–2 mEq/kg/dose or 0.3 × body weight in kg × base deficit. The available 7.5% solution of sodium bicarbonate provides 0.9 mEq/mL of bicarbonate.

Potassium chloride 1–2 mEq/kg/day q 8 hr oral. Intravenous concentration should not exceed 40 mEq/L. 1.0 mL of 15% solution of potassium chloride provides 2.0 mEq of potassium.

Caution Administer only when urine flow is established.

Lignocaine 1.0 mg/kg/dose IV bolus every 5 minutes up to a maximum total dose of 5 mg/kg followed by constant IV infusion @ 10–15 mg/kg/min.

Flunarizine 5 mg single daily oral dose in children above 5 years for prophylaxis against migraine.

Lansoprazol 1.0 mg/kg/day q 12–24 hr.

Methotrexate 5–10 mg/m^2 oral on empty stomach once a week.

Prostaglandin E$_1$ 0.05–0.4 µg/kg/min by continuous intravenous infusion through a large vein or umbilical artery catheter. The maintenance dose to keep the ductus open is only 0.01 µg/kg/min.

Source: Singh M, Deorari AK. *Drug Dosages in Children.* New Delhi, CBS Publishers and Distributors Pvt. Ltd. 9th Edition, 2015.

48

BIBLIOGRAPHY

Blair W, Smith B. Nursing documentation: Framework and barriers. *Contemporary Nurse* 2012, 41(2): 160–168.

Cates CC, Bara A, Crilly JA. Holding chambers versus nebulizers for beta-agonist treatment of acute asthma. *Cochrane Database Syst Rev* 2003, (3): 000052.

Collins SA, Cato K, Albers D, et al. Relationship between nursing documentation and patients mortality. *Am J Crit Care* 2013, 22(4): 306–313.

Ferguson SL. To err is human: strategies for ensuring patient safety and quality when caring for children. *J Pediatr Nurs* 2001, 16(6): 438–440.

Hughes RG, Edgerton EA. Reducing pediatric medication errors: children are specially at risk for medication errors. *Am J Nurs* 2005, 105(5): 79–84.

Maisels MJ, McDonagh AF. Phototherapy for neonatal jaundice. *N Engl J Med* 2008, 358(9): 920–928.

Singh M. Phototherapy. In: Care of the Newborn. New Delhi, CBS Publishers and Distributors Pvt. Ltd, Revised 8th Edition 2016, p 338–341.

Woods D, Thomas R, Holl J, et al. Adverse events and preventable adverse events in children. *Pediatrics* 2005, 115(1): 155–160.

49

Nursing Procedures

A nurse is expected to perform or assist the doctor to perform a large number of procedures to examine and monitor sick children, undertake diagnostic investigations and provide therapeutic interventions. *She is the most important member of the health team to seek cooperation of sick children and provide emotional support to the family.*

Role of a Nurse

1. The nurse should have the necessary knowledge and skills to assist the physician to undertake various procedures.
2. She should record vital signs and various anthropometric indices.
3. She should explain the nature of procedure, drugs to be used for analgesia and sedation and likely complications to the family and allay their concern and anxiety. *It is essential to take written informed consent prior to any procedure from the parent or legal guardian of the child.*
4. The child should be prepared and told about the nature of procedure in a simple language to allay his fear and anxiety. Apart from verbal guidance, nurse can take the help of visual aids like simple line drawings or a doll to explain the nature of the procedure.
5. She should ensure strict asepsis protocol to reduce the risk of infection and complications.
6. The child must be provided with adequate analgesia and sedation to reduce anxiety and pain to the bare minimum.
7. Nurse can explain to the family to exploit the concept of role-playing at home before the actual procedure or surgery. The diabetic child who needs insulin injections can role-play by giving an injection to a doll.
8. The safety of a diagnostic and therapeutic procedure is of utmost importance. The nurse should know the likely complications of the procedure so that relevant monitoring can be done after the procedure to identify them early and manage promptly.

VITAL SIGNS

In critically sick children, vital signs are monitored continuously with the help of a multi-channel vital sign monitor to ensure accuracy and save the time of nurses. But it must be remembered that machines are as good as the women or men handling and maintaining them. *Even when a sick child is hooked on to a vital sign monitor, it is important for the nurse to record the observations in the case file and check the vital signs manually to ascertain the accuracy of vital sign monitor from time to time.* The vital signs include temperature, pulse, respiration (TPR) and blood pressure.

Temperature Oral temperature is considered as the reference temperature and is taken by placing the clinical thermometer under the tongue. In children below 5 years, skin or rectal or eardrum temperature can be taken. For details of methods to record body temperature refer to **Chapter 31**.

Pulse The pulse should be recorded when child is at rest or during sleep because crying, activity, anxiety and restlessness may increase the pulse rate. Radial pulse is usually recorded by placing middle and index fingers gently over the outer side of supine or anterior surface of the wrist. It should be recorded for full one minute by watch. Pulse can also be recorded from the femoral (groin), carotid (neck), brachial (elbow) and anterior tibial (ankle) arteries. In infants and newborn babies, radial pulse is difficult to feel and instead apical impulse or heart beat may be recorded by palpation or with the help of a stethoscope. Rate, volume, rhythm and character of the pulse are noted.

Respiration Respirations should be recorded in a quiet resting child because crying and activity also increase the breathing rate. Rate, regularity, depth (whether deep or shallow), normal or labored, suprasternal and intercostal retractions and movements of the alae nasi should be noticed.

Blood pressure It is conventionally recorded in the upper arm at the site of brachial artery. The child should be quiet and lying supine in bed. The appropriate size of cuff, which should cover two-thirds of the upper arm should be used. The recommended cuff size in infants under one year of age is 2.5 cm, 1–4 years 5 cm, 5–9 years 9 cm and over 10 years is 13 cm. *When cuff width is too narrow for the upper arm it gives erroneously high blood pressure and when cuff is too wide the blood pressure recording is likely to be low.* Cuff is wrapped snugly over the upper arm with its lower margin about 2–3 cm above the elbow.

Palpatory method Cuff is inflated to above the anticipated blood pressure of the patient inorder to obliterate the radial or brachial pulse. The cuff is gradually and slowly deflated till the radial or brachial pulse can be felt again. This gives only systolic pressure of the patient.

Auscultatory method Cuff is inflated to obliterate the arterial pulse. Brachial artery in the cubital fossa (medial or inner side of elbow) is auscultated while gradually and slowly deflating the cuff. The point at which the sound is first heard gives the systolic blood pressure. The cuff is further deflated slowly while listening to the sound. When the sound becomes muffled, it is taken as diastolic blood pressure. The difference between the systolic and diastolic blood pressure provides the pulse pressure (strength or volume of the pulse).

Flush method This method is used in small infants and instead of pulse, flushing or blanching of the hand is used to record systolic blood pressure. This method is time consuming and unreliable and has been replaced by technology-based recording of blood pressure.

Blood pressure monitor Doppler system based on the principle of oscillometry and sound waves provides an accurate and non-invasive means for recording blood pressure in newborn babies and critically sick children. The ultrasonic waves are picked up by the transducer located in the cuff. The instrument provides continuous digital display of heart rate, systolic, diastolic and mean blood pressure. There is a provision for an alarm or warning signal when blood pressure falls or rises beyond certain preset limits.

Intra-arterial blood pressure Direct arterial blood pressure can be recorded by introducing a transducer into the umbilical artery or a peripheral artery in critically sick newborn babies and infants. The method is accurate but rather invasive and fraught with several complications. The normal range of vital signs at different ages is given in **Chapter 1**.

INTAKE-OUTPUT CHARTING

Accurate charting of 24-hour fluid intake and output is of great importance in management of critically sick children **(Box 49.1)**. It provides guidelines for administration of fluids and allows assessment of renal function.

Fluid intake All fluids (oral and parenteral), their nature and volume taken over a period of 24 hours should be recorded in a chart. Apart from intravenous fluids, accurate record of infused blood and blood products, flush fluids and drug diluents and vehicles, etc. should be maintained. The patients's attendants should be instructed to assist in keeping an accurate record of oral intake.

Fluid output The total output of fluids in the form of urine, stools, vomitings, nasogastric aspirate, enterostomy leakage, etc. should be recorded. In boys urine can be collected by attaching a condom or test tube while urine collection bag is more suitable for urine collection in girls. Catheterization should be avoided as far as possible due to risk of causing urinary tract infection. Catheterization is done in children with renal shut down or when accurate urine collection is not possible by any other means in a critically sick child. The total urine output of 24 hours is divided by the body weight and 24 to calculate urine output in mL/kg/hr, which is an important index of renal function.

In children with acute gastroenteritis, the ongoing fluid losses from intestines (vomiting and diarrheal stools) should be calculated and replenished through intravenous fluids. It is not possible to make an accurate assessment of fluid losses through vomitings and stools but a rough estimate is made by assuming 5 mL/kg

Box 49.1 Conditions demanding accurate intake-output charting*

- Persistent vomiting, diarrhea and dehydration due to any cause
- Hypovolemia, circulatory collapse or shock
- Congestive heart failure
- Renal dysfunction or renal shut down
- Severe thermal burns
- Drowning
- Diabetes mellitus and insipidus
- Pre- and post-surgical patients
- Failure of any major organ or multiorgan dysfunction
- CNS conditions like head injury, meningitis, encephalitis and raised intracranial tension

*All children admitted to NICU and PICU need accurate monitoring of fluid intake and output.

for each vomiting and 10 mL/kg for each watery stool. Accurate estimate of fluid losses through gastric aspirate or from enterostomy stoma should be maintained. Gastric aspirate is replaced by physiological saline while intestinal fluid losses are replenished with N/2 dextrose-saline.

ANTHROPOMETRY

Anthropometric measurements of children should be taken during their routine visits for vaccinations, whenever they report to the out patient department or get admitted to the hospital.

Weight Weight is taken nude or with identical clothes each time. The weight may be recorded on a beam type mechanical weighing scale (Detecto scale with an accuracy of ±20 g). The scale should be frequently checked with standard weights and zero error must be adjusted before weighing. Electronic weighing scales are available for infants and children with a of resolution ±1 g, 5 g and 10 g) and should be preferred for their accuracy and convenience **(Figures 49.1 and 49.2)**.

In field conditions, salter spring machine is quite satisfactory because it is cheap and convenient to carry. The machine is hung from the hook or held by an attendant and baby is placed on the sling attached to the bottom hook. The weight should be recorded on the Road-to-Health cards especially in under-5 children.

Length and height In infants below 2 years of age, recumbent length is measured with the help of an infantometer while in older children standing height is taken. Accurate recording of length or height is difficult and often unreliable but it is a better index of physical

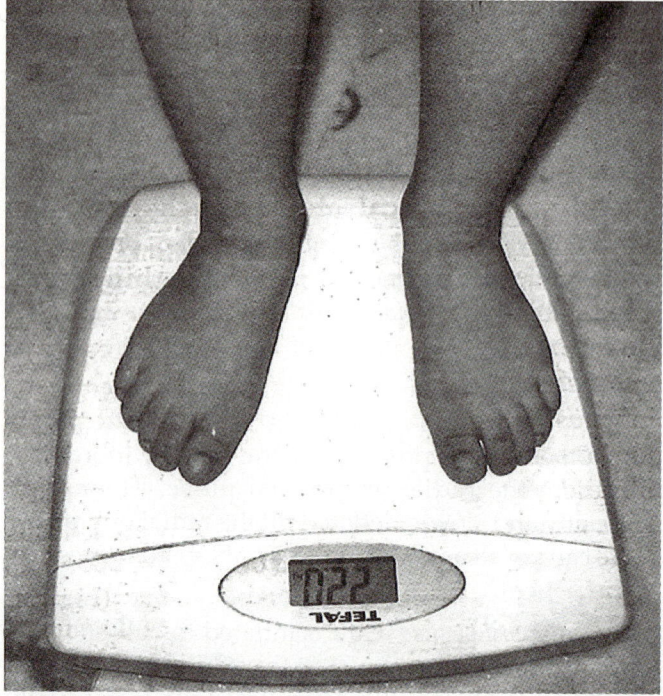

Figure 49.2 Electronic weighing scale for taking weight of children above 2 years of age with a resolution of ±100 g. Electronic scales are convenient, time saving and accurate compared to mechanical weighing scales

growth. The infant is placed supine on the infantometer. Assistant or mother is asked to hold the head snugly against the fixed vertical plank. The legs are fully extended by pressing at the knees and the movable foot plank of the infantometer is firmly opposed against the soles and length is read from the scale **(Figure 49.3)**. In practice, it is difficult to extend both the legs of an infant while it is convenient and satisfactory to extend only one leg and record the length.

In older children who can stand, height can be measured by the rod attached to the lever type weighing machine or by an in-built stadiometer affixed on the wall or simply by making the child stand against a wall on which a measuring scale is inscribed. The head of the child should be held erect with eyes aligned horizontally and ears vertically without any tilt **(Figure 49.4)**.

Head circumference The occipitofrontal head circumference (OFC) should be measured with a nonstretchable fiber-glass tape. The tape should encircle over the most prominent parts of the occiput and supraorbital frontal areas **(Figure 49.5)**. Head circumference is recorded in preschool children because adult head size is achieved by 5–6 years of age.

Chest circumference The chest circumference is measured at the level of nipples **(Figure 49.6)**. The chest circumference equals head circumference around

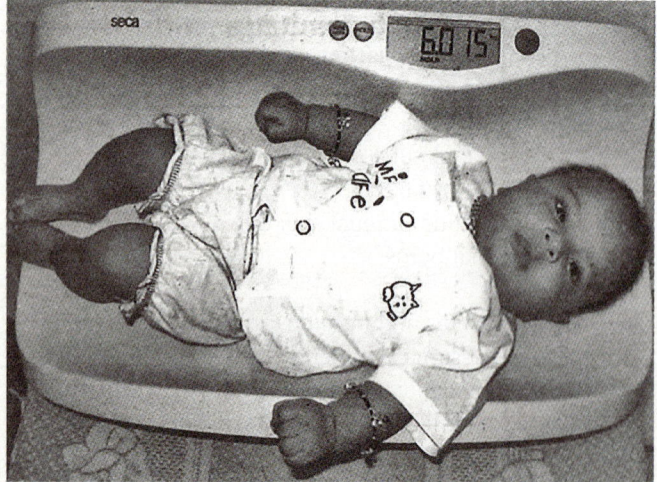

Figure 49.1 Electronic baby weighing scale with a resolution of ±5 g

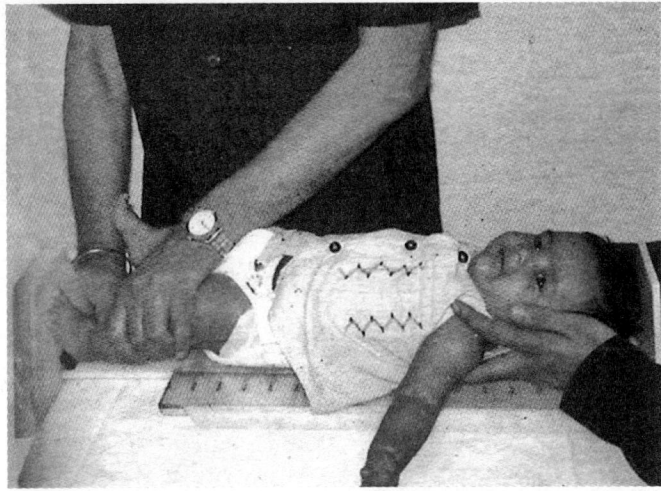

Figure 49.3 Method for recording length on an infantometer. Infant is placed supine on the infantometer with vertex of head touching the fixed plank while one leg is straightened and aligned with the movable plank of the infantometer. Mother or attendant is asked to hold the head firmly against the fixed plank while nurse or physician restrains and straightens one leg firmly to snugly align the sole of the foot with the movable plank of the infantometer

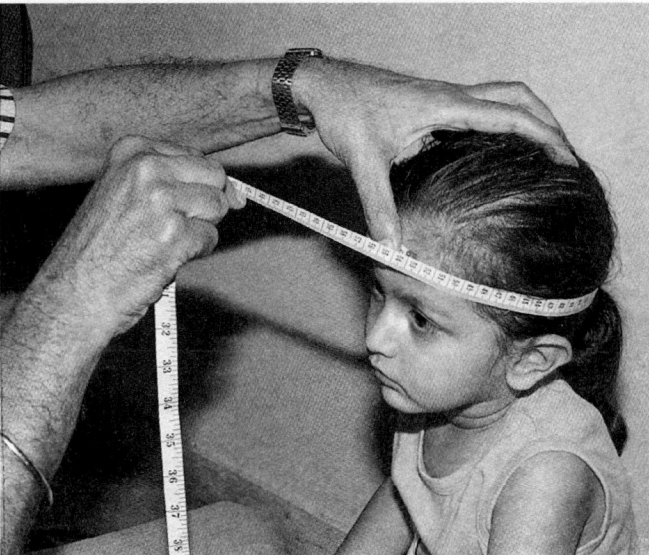

Figure 49.5 Method for recording head circumference. Use a non-stretchable fiber-glass tape and encircle the most prominent parts of occiput and supraorbital ridges

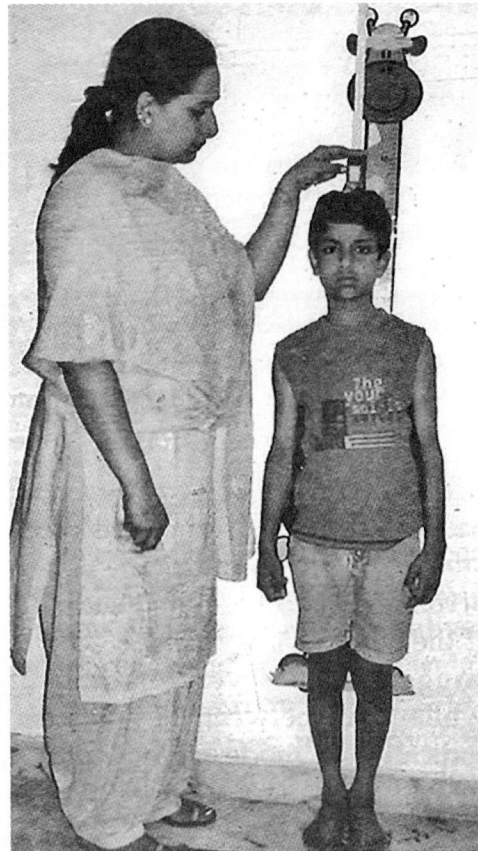

Figure 49.4 Method of recording height with the help of a stadiometer. Note the correct posture with perfect alignment of eyes and ears of the child

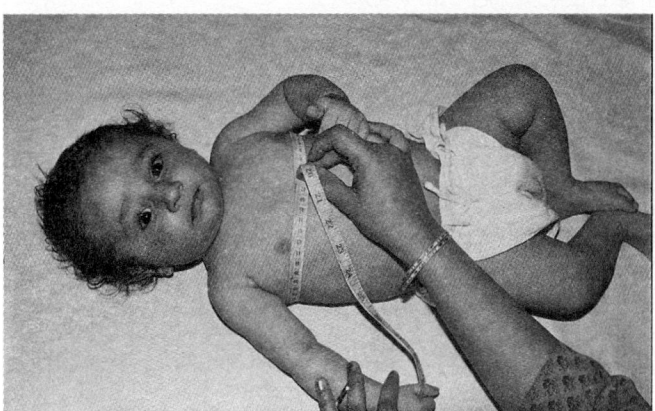

Figure 49.6 Measurement of chest circumference at the level of nipples

months to one year of age but thereafter chest grows more rapidly as compared to the brain. In malnourished children, chest size may be significantly smaller than the head circumference because growth of the brain is less affected by undernutrition.

Mid-upper arm circumference During 1–5 years of age, mid-upper arm circumference (MUAC) remains reasonably static between 15 and 17 cm among healthy children because fat of early infancy is gradually replaced by muscles. Mid-upper arm circumference is measured with a fiber-glass tape or steel tape at the midpoint between acromion and olecranon (**Figure 49.7**). If the MUAC is less than 12.5 cm, it is suggestive of severe malnutrition while MUAC between 12.5 and 13.5 cm is indicative of moderate malnutrition.

49

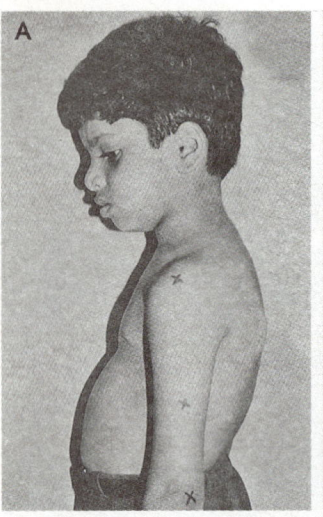
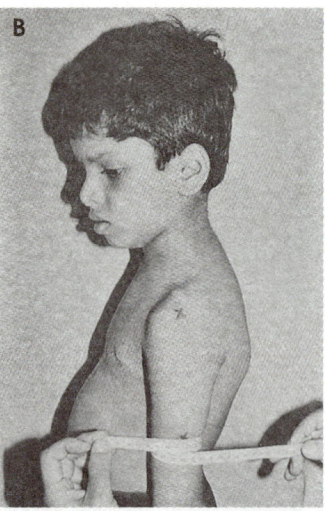

Figure 49.7 Method for recording mid-upper arm circumference. (A) Midpoint between acromion and olecranon is identified. (B) The circumference is measured with the help of a fiber-glass tape. The measurement should be taken only in children between the ages of 1 and 5 years

| Table 49.1 Mid-upper arm circumference for different heights | |
Mid-upper arm circumference (cm)	Height (cm)
12.50	70.00
12.75	80.00
13.00	90.00
13.25	97.50
13.50	103.50
13.75	106.50
14.00	110.00
14.25	113.50
14.50	116.00
14.75	118.00
15.00	121.00
15.50	125.00
16.00	129.00
16.50	133.00

Bangle test can be used for quick assessment of arm circumference. A fiber-glass bangle of internal diameter of 4 cm is slipped above the forearm. If the bangle passes above the elbow, it suggests that upper arm circumference is less than 12.5 cm and child is malnourished.

Shakir tape is a fiber-glass tape with red (less than 12.5 cm), yellow (12.5–13.5 cm) and green shading (> 13.5 cm) so that paramedical workers can assess the nutritional status without having to remember the normal limits of mid-arm circumference.

Quack stick is developed on the principle that acute starvation severely affects MUAC while height is unaffected. The child appears tall, thin and wasted. The Quack stick is a meter rod with two set of markings. The expected height of the child against various sizes of mid-upper arm circumference is inscribed on the rod. **Table 49.1** shows mid-upper arm circumference for different heights. The malnourished child would be taller than the anticipated height derived from the MUAC.

Weight-for-age The child is considered as *underweight* when his weight is less than 2 SD of the median weight-for-age of NCHS or WHO reference standards.

Height-for-age *Stunting* is diagnosed when height-for-age of the child is below 2 SD of the expected median height-for-age of NCHS or WHO reference standards.

Weight-for-height Weight-for-height is expressed as a percentage of the reference median weight expected on the basis of the height. When weight-for-height is less than 2 SD of the expected median weight-for-height of NCHS or WHO reference standards it is indicative of *acute malnutrition* or *wasting*. A weight-for-height of greater than 2SD of NCHS standards or above 95th percentile is suggestive of obesity.

Body mass index Body mass index (BMI) is calculated as weight in kg as a ratio of (height in meters)^2. BMI-for-age charts are available for the diagnosis of obesity. A BMI-for-age of >90th percentile is suggestive of overweight and when it is more than 95th percentile or it is associated with triceps or subscapular skinfold thickness-for-age of >90th percentile it is diagnostic of adolescent obesity.

BODY HOLDS AND RESTRAINTS

A nurse is often required to hold the child while assisting the pediatrician to examine and do various procedures on the child. Sometimes it may be necessary to use certain restraints to restrict the movements of the sick baby in the bed. However, the use of restraints should be restricted to the minimum. These should never be used as a punishment. *Efforts should be made to seek cooperation of the child by handling him in a playful manner and indiscriminate use of restraints should be avoided.* School-going children should be taken into confidence by explaining the nature of procedure to reduce their fear and anxiety. The restraints should be well padded and should not be too tight to cause constrictions or undue pressure on the underlying part. The restraints should be removed 2–3 times in a day to inspect and clean the underlying area.

ENT examination Throat is examined by focusing torch light over the back of throat. In a struggling infant, mother or nurse should hold the child in her lap. She holds and immobilizes the head with one hand and restrains both the arms of the child with the other hand **(Figure 49.8)**. Alternatively, before holding the child in the lap, he may be securely wrapped in a sheet to restrain his arms. The neck should be slightly extended and physician examines the throat with the help of torch light and a wooden spatula to depress the tongue. The child often cries which provides a good view of the throat.

Throat can also be examined in a supine position. The arms are extended over the head and both head and the arms are restrained by the mother or nurse **(Figure 49.9)**. The legs can be restrained by wrapping them in a blanket. In most children above 2 years of age throat can be examined without any restraint and without using a wooden spatula. Child is simply asked to open his mouth widely and say Ah…Ah….

For otscopic examination of the ears, child sits in a side posture in the lap of the mother or nurse. Arms are restrained with one hand while head is firmly steadied by the other hand **(Figure 49.10)**. After introducing otoscope in the ear canal, pinna is pulled directly backwards in infants and upwards and backwards in older children to get a clear view of the tympanic membrane.

Arm-leg hold The child lies supine on the examination table and nurse stands at the head-end of the table. She bends over the child to firmly hold the child's knees while keeping the legs apart and encircles her elbows around the arms and trunk to restrain the upper part of body. This hold allows examination of the groin and perineal region and is useful for getting femoral blood sample.

Head-leg hold Nurse stands on the side of the table and child lies on his side with face towards the nurse. She places one hand and arm over and around the head and neck area and the other over and around the thighs. She then firmly pulls both her arms towards her body to obtain a desired spinal curve to perform lumbar puncture.

Mummifying The child's arms can be restrained with the help of a bed sheet. Child's right arm is folded in a sheet and both ends of the sheet are pulled under his back and left arm is wrapped with the doubled sheet which is again pulled under his back. This leaves head, neck, trunk and legs uncovered for examination. Inorder to restrain the child more securely, to undertake a procedure, the doubled sheet under the back is again brought infront around the right arm, taken around the left arm and finally tucked under his back.

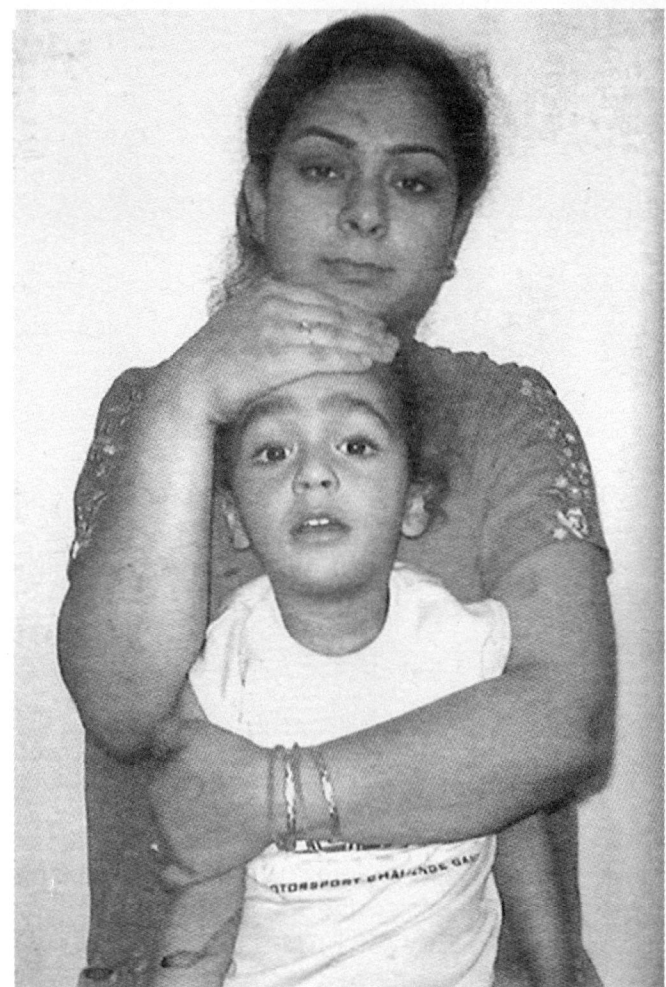

Figure 49.8 Restraining an infant and pre-school child for examination of throat. Mother is asked to restrain the child by immobilizing his head with one hand and encircling the limbs with the other hand

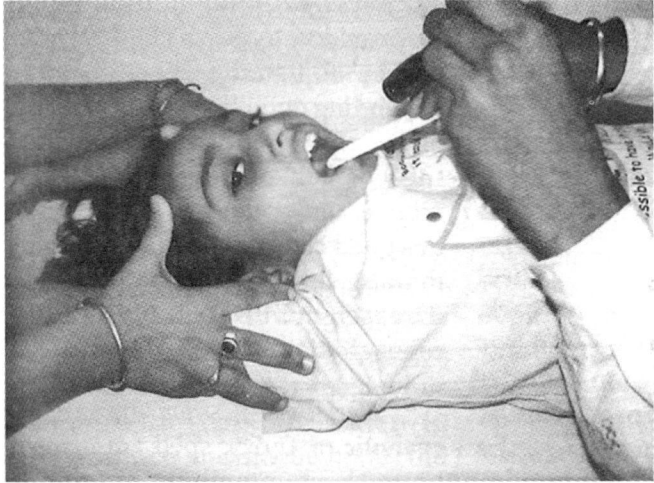

Figure 49.9 Throat can also be examined in a supine position by slightly extending the head and restraining the arms and head of the child by the mother as shown in the photograph

49

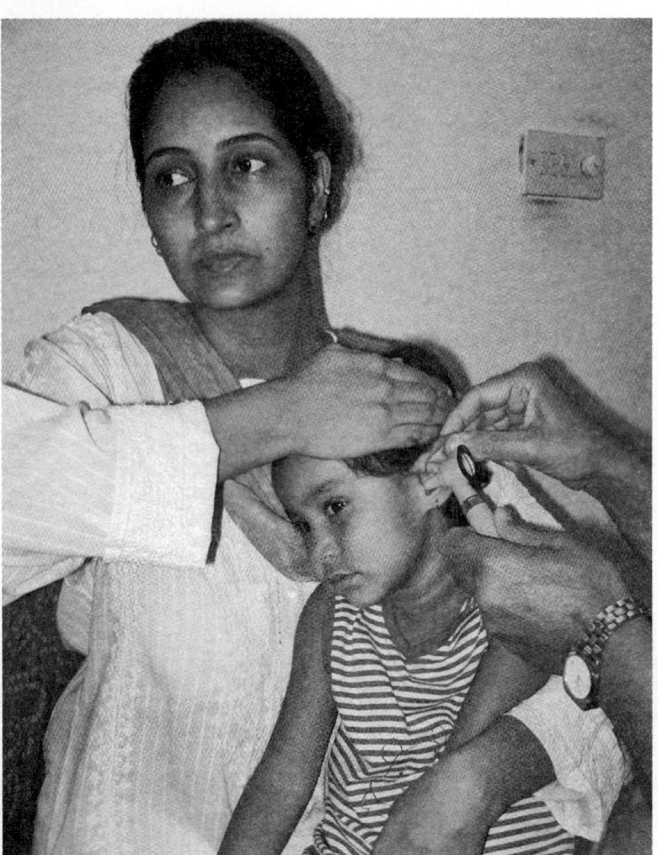

Figure 49.10 Position and restraining the child for otoscopic examination of the ear. The attendant should be asked to hold the child firmly to avoid any damage to the ear canal

Body restraint Restless and delerious child can be restrained in a bed having side railings. The child can be worn a jacket having strings on the back, by encircling his arms and legs, which are then secured to the frame of the cot. Tying the arms and legs of the child with the help of ropes or bandages with a clove-hitch knot appear rather crude and inhuman.

Elbow restraint Elbow restraint is used to prevent the infant from flexing his elbow so that he is unable to remove the nasogastric tube or scalp vein, reach to his face (operated cleft lip, cleft palate), and infant having eczema. Elbow is extended, padded and bandaged with a wooden spatula placed on the anterior or flexor aspect.

NURSING POSITIONS

During certain clinical situations and disease states, children are placed in various special positions to provide them comfort and speedy recovery.

Upright position Patients with congestive heart failure and bronchial asthma feel comfortable in upright or semi-upright position. Back rest can be provided to older children which can be adjusted at various angles depending upon the need and comfort of the child. In infants, head-end of the cot can be raised by placing pillows under the mattress. Specially designed chairs are available to nurse infants with gastroesophageal reflux disease (GERD) to prevent regurgitation.

Knee-chest position Infants with cyanotic or anoxic spell are placed in knee-chest position to provide comfort and abort the attack.

Lateral or side position The child is placed in a semiprone or side position to maintain an open airway following a surgical procedure in the throat and in children with seizures and unconsciousness. This position is also used for inserting a thermometer, suppository, doing a rectal examination and for giving an enema.

Prone position The child is nursed in a prone or face down position (on his abdomen) when there is meningomyelocele, teratoma, injury or burns on the back. Soft pillows or water mattress can be used to make the child comfortable. Infants with respiratory distress feel comfortable in a prone position. *When an infant is placed in a prone position, he should be constantly observed due to increased risk of sudden infant death syndrome (SIDS).*

Total body splint The baby is placed over a well-padded crucifix splint and limbs are restrained with the help of lightly tied bandages. This splint is ideal for newborn babies to perform exchange blood transfusion.

COLLECTION OF LABORATORY SAMPLES

The samples for investigations must be properly collected, stored and transported to the laboratory. The specimens and samples should be properly labelled with name, age, sex, ward, bed number and central registration number of the patient to avoid any mix-up.

Urine Collection

When urine specimen is required for culture, perineum and genitals should be washed thoroughly with soap and water. In girls, labia majora and minora should be separated while washing with soap and water. In boys, prepuce should be retracted back (after 2 years age) and glans penis cleaned with soap and water. *Antiseptic soap or solution should not be used for cleaning while collecting urine sample for culture.*

Mid-stream or clean-catch specimen This method is suitable to collect urine specimen in an older and cooperative child. The child is asked to pass urine in the bedpan or commode. After the small amount of urine has been voided, urinary stream is directed towards a wide-mouth sterile bottle. After the desired amount of urine has been collected, the child voids the remaining urine into the bedpan or commode.

Some intelligent mothers can collect mid-stream urine sample even in infants with some skill and patience. When infant is expected to pass urine after a feed, he is held from both the thighs over a wash basin. Mother produces a hissing sound or tap of the wash basin is opened to simulate the sound of passage of urine. When baby voids, an assistant or nurse collects the mid-stream sample of urine in a sterile bottle. The urine sample is first processed for plating and culture studies while the remaining urine can be subjected to routine and microscopic examination.

A collecting-bag or a test tube sample In male infants, urine sample can be collected either by using a collection bag or a condom, or by simply affixing a test tube over the penis **(Figure 49.11)**. In female infants, it is very difficult to prevent contamination of urine from feces. The child lies supine with hips flexed and thighs widely separated. Protective covering is removed from the adhesive of the collecting bag. The bag is then firmly applied to the perineum by enclosing vulvar area in the bag. The child should be constantly watched for passage of urine. As soon as the urine is voided, bag is gently removed and urine sample is transferred to the specimen bottle. *The sample collected with the help of a urine collection bag is not suitable for culture studies.*

Catheterization Despite using aseptic precautions, this method of urine collection is associated with potential risk of introducing infection. Its use is restricted for conducting certain diagnostic procedures (micturating cystourethrogram) or for collection of 24-hour urine in critically sick children or patients with renal shut down. In boys, use of a condom is suitable for collection of urine over several days. A rubber tube is attached, after making a hole in the bottom of the condom, to periodically drain and collect the urine after each voiding.

The child lies in a recumbent position and area is prepared aseptically by using sterile towels and drapes to cover legs, perineum and abdomen. The nurse should wear sterile gloves and stand on right side of the child. Labia majora are cleaned with moistened sterile swabs 2–3 times, working from front to backwards (from vulva towards anus), using a swab once only. Then labia majora are separated to expose labia minora which are cleaned similarly. Finally labia minora are separated and vestibule is cleaned. External urethral opening is located as a small dimple lying above or anterior to the opening of vagina. With the left hand, labia minora are held apart and with the right hand a catheter lubricated with sterile saline solution, held about 2–3 cm from the tip, is gently introduced into the urethra till urine flows. The urine should be directly collected into a sterile container. After the bladder has been emptied, catheter is pinched and withdrawn gently. When urinary output needs to be monitored for several days, an indwelling catheter (size 8–10 Foley catheter) is inserted and is taped to the groin.

Suprapubic bladder aspiration Suprabubic aspiration of urinary bladder is done in newborn babies and young infants for sterile collection of urine sample for culture studies because urinary bladder is an abdominal organ in infants. Strict aseptic precautions are taken by use of sterile drapes and gloves. Procedures is done one hour after the feed when bladder is likely to be full. Suprapubic skin is cleaned with povidone-iodine and alcohol. Needle (21 gauge) with a 10 mL syringe is inserted 1.0 cm above the symphysis pubis in the midline **(Figure 49.12)**. Needle is advanced directly backwards. Syringe is tilted towards abdomen and gradually withdrawn while applying gentle negative pressure. Procedure is safe but transient hematuria is common.

49

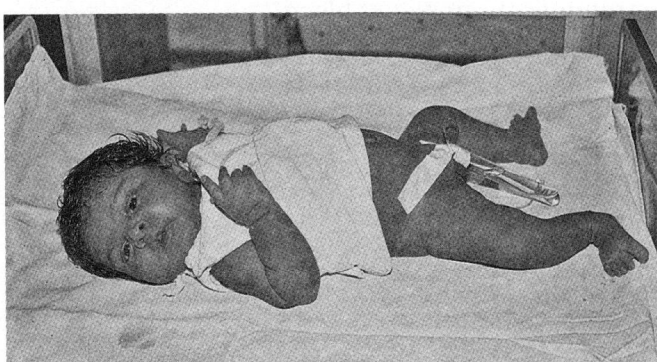

Figure 49.11 Urine being collected with a test tube in a male infant

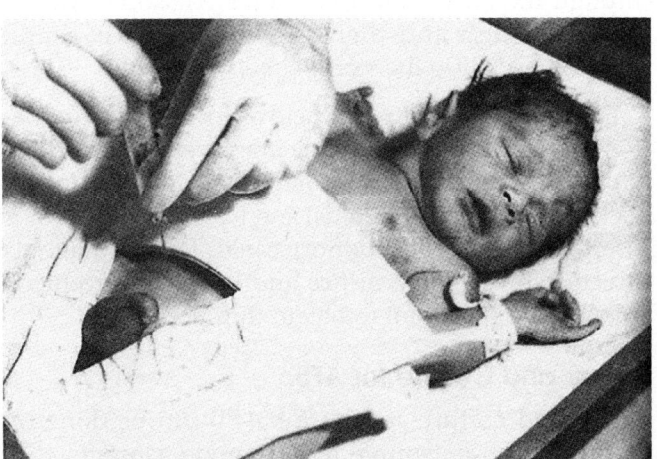

Figure 49.12 Suprapubic bladder aspiration

Stool Sample

Stool sample can be collected directly from the napkin or potty into a wide-mouthed bottle with the help of a wooden spatula. When stool contains mucus or blood, the sample should include those abnormal components.

For purposes of culture studies, rectal swab is more appropriate. The rectal swab is available as a sterile applicator dressed in a lubricated glass sheath. It is introduced for 1–2 cm beyond the anal sphincter, swab applicator is then pushed beyond the end of the sheath. The swab is then inserted back into the sheath and taken out and replaced into the tube.

Swabs

Swabs are obtained from inside the body orifices or from the skin surface for Gram staining and bacteriological or viral studies. Sterile dressed cotton applicators contained in sterile plugged tubes are supplied by the department of microbiology. As far as possible swab should be taken before any antiseptic or antibiotic is used. The swab should be immediately returned back to the container and sent to the laboratory before it dries up.

Throat swab Child is held as for ENT examination. Mouth is opened, tongue is depressed with a spatula and swab is introduced deep into the throat to touch tonsillar areas. The swab is quickly withdrawn, placed in the sterile test tube and sent to the laboratory. Care should be taken that the swab should not touch the lips or tongue on entering or while being removed from the mouth.

Nasopharyngeal or cough swab Cough swab may be used in cases of whooping cough and bronchopneumonia. Child sits or is held as for ENT examination. The swab supported on a flexible wire is introduced through the nostril till it reaches the nasopharynx. It induces cough and then swab is withdrawn and replaced back into the sterile tube.

Ear swab Child sits or is held as for an ear examination with ear to be swabbed facing the examiner. Pinna of the ear is pulled upwards and backwards (or directly backwards in case of infants) and a sterile speculum is inserted into external auditory canal. The head light is directed towards the orifice and swab is introduced through the speculum to obtain the specimen.

Smear and Culture for AFB

Smear and culture studies for AFB can be done on sputum, gastric aspirate, lymph node aspirate, cold abscess, pleural or peritoneal aspirate.

Sputum examination All efforts should be made to demonstrate bacteriological evidence of tuberculosis before starting antitubercular therapy. Young children do not expectorate, they either swallow or vomit out the bronchial exudates. Adolescent children with fibrocaseous tuberculosis should be evaluated by examining two samples of early morning sputum for AFB smear, culture and antibiotic sensitivity studies. In young children with radiological changes suggestive of pulmonary tuberculosis, induced sputum (following nebulization with hypertonic or 3% saline) or bronchoalveolar lavage (BAL) after endotracheal intubation can be collected and processed for smear, culture (BACTEC) and PCR (Gene Xpert®) studies for acid fast bacilli (AFB) or *Mycobacterium tuberculosis*.

Gastric aspirate for AFB Children with pulmonary tuberculosis are unable to expectorate sputum, which is usually swallowed into the stomach. A nasogastric tube is inserted into the stomach after the dinner and left in-situ whole night. Early morning, before awakening the child, gastric contents are aspirated and sent to the laboratory for identification of acid fast bacilli on smear examination after centrifugation. The centrifuged aspirate is also processed for culture of AFB by BACTEC system which provides a much faster report compared to the conventional system.

Blood Samples

Due aseptic precautions should be taken to collect blood samples. *Gloves should be worn as part of universal precautions against risk of HIV infection.* Skin should be prepared by application of povidone-iodine which should be allowed to dry for one minute followed by cleaning with 70% isopropyle alcohol. The amount of blood taken for various investigations must be recorded in the case file. *It is important to remember that 10 mL of blood from a 2 kg infant represents about 6% of his blood volume.* It is desirable to have micromethods technology so that biochemical parameters are checked with micro or ultramicro samples of blood.

Capillary blood Heal (newborn babies and infants) and finger tip can be used to collect capillary blood sample. To reduce pain and discomfort, infant can be offered breastfeeding or glucose or sucrose water. The baby should be cuddled and caressed during and after the procedure. The site can be warmed with a warm sterile towel or warm moist cotton pledget to produce hyperemia. For heel prick, most lateral or medial sites (avoid centre of the sole) are chosen for puncture **(Figure 49.13)**. Foot is grasped in left hand, it is dorsiflexed so that the engorged heel pulp stands out. The lancet is pushed to a depth of 2 mm, it is rotated

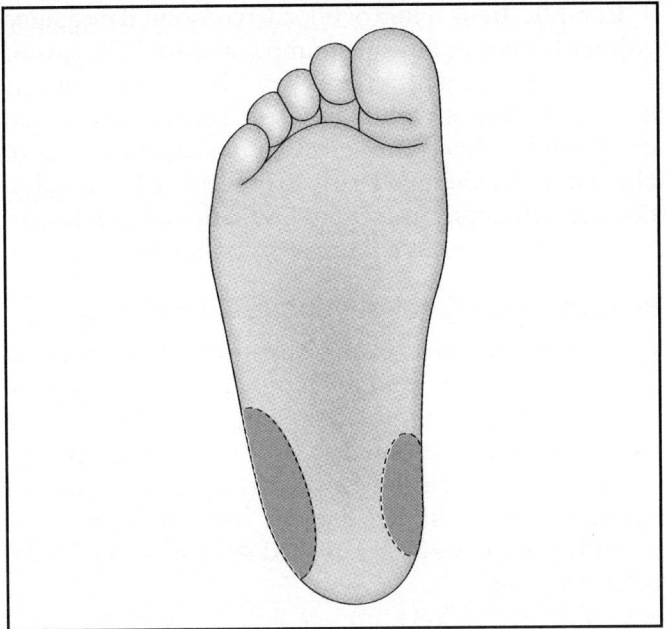

Figure 49.13 Appropriate and safe sites for obtaining capillary blood sample from the heel

and pulled out. The limb is kept in a dependent position. The first drop is wiped away with a sterile cotton. The subsequent drops are directly collected into a container or sucked into a heparinized capillary tube. Bleeding is stopped by holding a gauze pad against the puncture site. Healex spray or 2% mercurochrome or betadine and a Band-Aid is applied to disinfect and seal the puncture site.

Venous blood With due aseptic precautions, blood is collected from superficial veins on the scalp or limbs (avoid central veins like femoral and jugular). Assistant can hold the limb proximal to venipuncture site or a tourniquet may be used to make the veins engorged or prominent. Cold light or illuminator can be used to visualize the vein during the procedure. In newborn babies, 23 gauge needle with broken hub can be used. It is often difficult to obtain the blood by suction because of thin veins. The blood is collected directly into the specimen container as it flows dropwise from the needle. After removing the needle, bleeding is stopped by local pressure with a swab or gauze. Healex spray or 2% mercurochrome is applied to disinfect and seal the site of puncture.

Blood culture sample Use of sterile gloves and strict asepsis of skin with application of povidone-iodine for one minute are mandatory. The blood should be directly transferred to the culture bottle after sterilizing its stopper on a flame. The ratio of blood to the volume of culture medium should be 1:10, i.e. 1.0 mL blood should be poured in a culture bottle containing 10 mL

of the medium. The culture bottle should be kept in the incubator or immediately sent to the laboratory. *It should never be kept in the refrigerator as it will suppress the growth of bacteria.*

INTRAVENOUS ACCESS

The infusion can be set up in a peripheral vein by percutaneous venipuncture with a small-vein or scalp-vein infusion set. **Figure 49.14** shows various body sites having superficial veins to establish intravenous access. It is, however, preferable to use a percutaneous venous catheter (medicath or angiocath) because of reduced risk of dislodegment and leakage.

Small-vein set Any peripheral vein can be used for infusion though scalp veins are easy to puncture due to relative immobility and ease of splintage. The set is attached to a syringe containing normal saline and flushed. Grasp the rubber finger grip (butterfly) of the needle and pierce the skin gently. The bevel of needle should face upwards and it should be inserted along the direction of flow of blood. The needle course is directed just under, and almost parallel to the skin. Coming over the vein, pierce it while applying gentle negative pressure by the syringe. The blood would appear in the tube immediately upon entry of the vein. Sometimes with 24 to 26 gauge needle and when the patient is in shock, the blood may not show in the tubing. Slowly flush the needle with saline and look

49

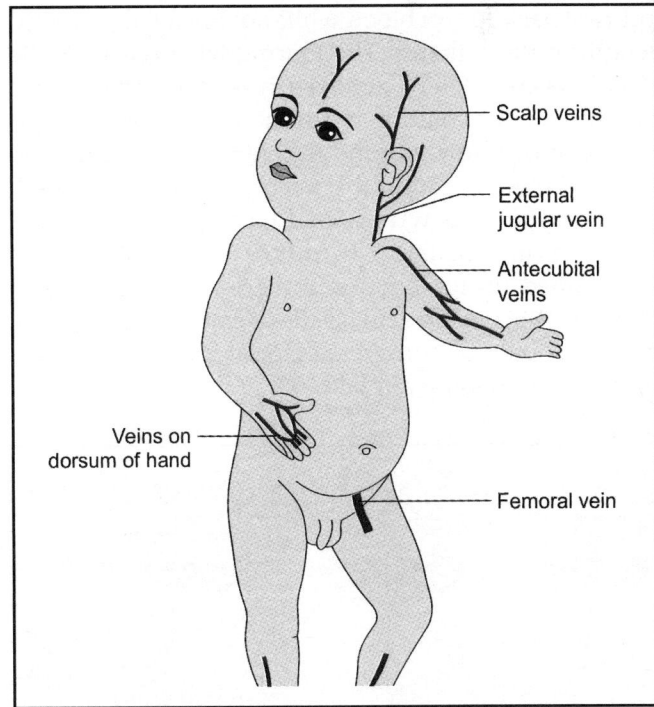

Scalp veins

External jugular vein

Antecubital veins

Veins on dorsum of hand

Femoral vein

Figure 49.14 Sites for intravenous access

for swelling proximal to the needle tip. Secure the needle and tubing to the site with adhesive tape as shown in **Figure 49.15** and adjust the flow rate. Check flow rate regularly to prevent under or overinfusion. Measured volume infusion sets (burette set) and infusion pumps are ideal to regulate the rate of infusion in young children.

Catheter needle Small-vein sets have been replaced by use of needle-catheter sets because of ease of fixation and feasibility of prolonged use. Vein is made prominent by applying a tourniquet proximal to the site of vein puncture. Rubbing alcohol makes superficial veins more prominent and they can also be visualized with the help of a cold light illuminator. The catheter with 24 gauge needle (neoflon or venflon) is grasped between the thumb and forefinger with its attached syringe resting against the palm of the operator's hand. The vein may be approached from above, at a venous junction or from the side. The skin adjacent to the vein is briskly punctured with the needle-catheter held approximately 10–15 degrees to the skin or axis of the arm. Once beneath the dermis, the angle is narrowed so that the catheter is nearly flush with the axis of the vein. When blood is seen in the needle hub, the catheter and needle are advanced along the course of the vein for additional 2 to 3 mm. If a syringe is attached to the catheter, it is aspirated to observe the free return of blood. The plastic catheter is then advanced gently into the vein while the needle is held stationary. Slight pressure may be applied at the tip of the catheter to prevent backflow of blood while advancing the desired length of the catheter. The tourniquet is released, the needle is completely removed from the catheter and an intravenous solution is attached. Sterile dressing is placed at puncture site and the entry point of catheter. The catheter is secured by micropore tape. The limb may be splinted with a padded wooden spatula. Intravenous infusion through a cannula can be maintained up to 72 hours if there is no blockage or leakage. When scalp vein needle or catheter is removed, the site should be compressed for at least two minutes and sterile dressing applied.

Complications Fluid overload may occur if measured volume burette or infusion pump is not used. Prolonged restraint is frequently necessary unless veins on the dorsum of hand or scalp are used. Local swelling and thrombophlebitis can occur. Extravasation of fluid or blood must be identified early to prevent local complications. In neonates, intravenous lines constitute an important portal and source for nososcomial infections.

Percutaneous Central Venous Catheterization

Central venous line is established for a long-term access for administration of intravenous fluids or parenteral nutrition. They are useful for monitoring central venous pressure **(Figure 49.16)**. The procedure is technically difficult and should be conducted by an experienced operator with strict aseptic precautions. The cannulation can be accomplished through a peripheral or central vein.

Subclavian vein catheterization The infant is sedated and placed supine with a towel roll between the scapulae. The head is turned away from the side of needle insertion and shoulders are dropped down. The skin is prepared with spirit-betadine-spirit and infiltrated with 1% xylocaine. The introducer needle of 3 Fr. silastic or silicone catheter is inserted through the skin, at a point joining outer one-third with the inner two-thirds of the clavicle. The needle is kept almost parallel to the chest wall and directed towards the sternal notch. When blood flow is established, the guide wire is inserted and catheter is advanced to lie at the junction of the superior vena cava with right atrium. The position of the catheter tip should be confirmed radiographically. The insertion site is covered with a transparent surgical dressing. The procedure is blind and associated with risk of development of pneumothorax, hemothorax and inadvertent puncture of subclavian artery.

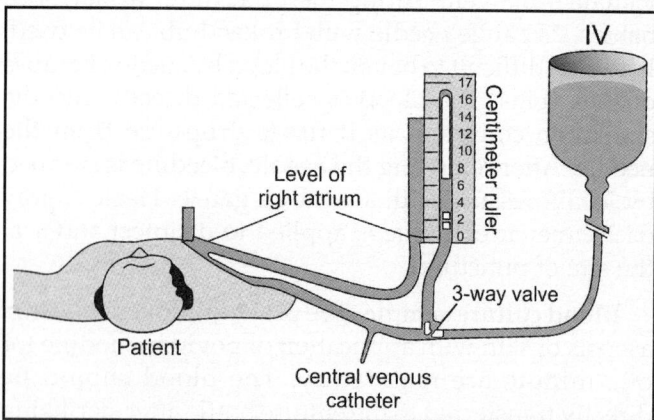

Figure 49.16 Technique for recording central venous pressure. The zero mark of the centimeter ruler is placed opposite the level of right atrium

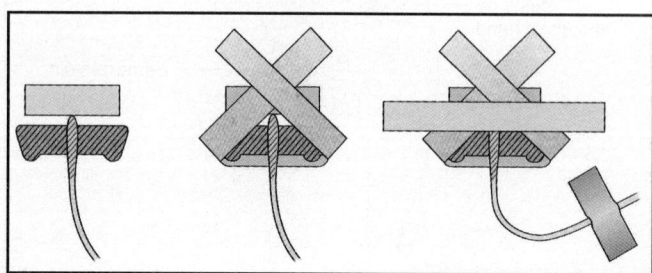

Figure 49.15 Method to securely affix the scalp vein set

Peripheral or external jugular vein catheterization

The cannulation is done through external jugular, basilica or greater saphenous vein. Silicone or silastic 2 Fr. catheter with an introducer needle is used. The site is prepared with spirit-betadine-spirit. The vein is identified with cold light and needle with catheter is inserted. The catheter is advanced after removing the needle so that its tip is positioned at the junction of superior vena cava with right atrium. The position of the catheter tip is confirmed radiographically. The procedure is safe and common complications include infection, thrombosis and thrombophlebitis.

Intraosseous Access

When veins are collapsed in critically sick children with dehydration or shock, intraosseous access can be used for administration of fluids, blood and even drugs . The major merits of intraosseous (IO) technique are its rapidity, high success and low complication rates. Intraosseous access can be reliably achieved in 30 to 60 seconds in most cases, even by health care providers with minimal experience. This route delivers the drug or fluids into the noncollapsible marrow venous plexus from where the emissary veins carry them to the general circulation. It being a large vascular bed, rapid infusions required for volume resuscitation in cases of shock can also be administered through this route. Blood transfusion, irritant infusions, catecholamine infusions and even viscous drugs have been successfully administered through this route. In addition to infusion, the procedure allows bone marrow aspiration which can be analysed for pH, pCO_2, blood culture and blood typing and crossmatching.

Procedure The technique of IO line placement is simple. A bone marrow needle with stylet or the specially designed intraosseous needles are recommended. However, in a desperate situation any wide bored strong needle, especially if it has a stylet can be used. The needle is inserted into the medial surface of tibia 1–3 cm below the tibial tuberosity. This point is generally one finger breadth below and just medial to the tibial tuberosity. The needle should be kept approximately perpendicular to the surface of the bone. The advancing force over the needle head is released as soon as a sudden decrease in resistance to forward motion of the needle is felt **(Figure 49.17)**. A test injection of 10 mL normal saline can be used to ascertain the position of the needle. The insertion is successful and the needle is clearly in the marrow cavity if the following conditions are fulfilled:

i. A sudden decrease in resistance occurs as the needle passes through the bony cortex into the marrow.

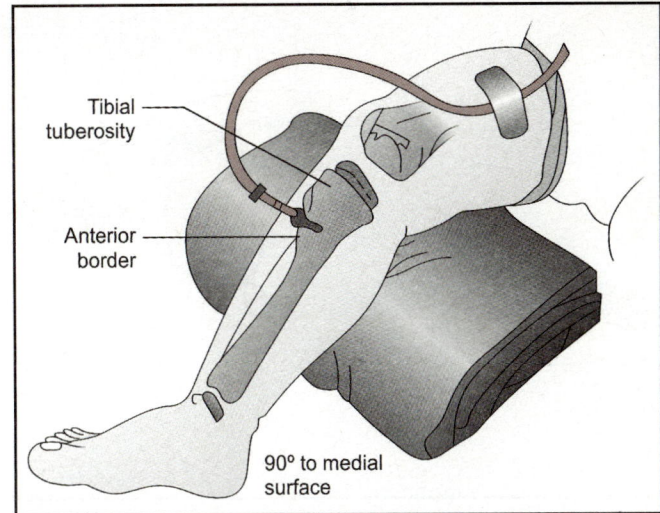

Figure 49.17 Procedure for setting up an intraosseous infusion

ii. The needle can remain upright without any support.

iii. Fluids flow through the needle freely without any evidence of subcutaneous infiltration. If there is any evidence of infiltration or if test injection fails, a second attempt at intraosseous cannulation should be performed on the contralateral tibia.

Distal femur, medial malleolus and anterior superior iliac spine are the alternative recommended sites for IO infusion in children. IO access can be used in all age groups, including preterm babies. In older children and adults, distal tibia, anterior superior iliac spine, distal radius or distal ulna can be used. Sternal IO cannulas for adults are now available.

Umbilical Vein Catheterization

Umbilical vein catheterization is done to establish access for short-term administration of fluids and drugs, conducting exchange blood transfusion and for monitoring central venous pressure.

Procedure

1. Use strict aseptic measures by wearing gloves, mask and gown and using a surgical drape with a central hole. Prepare the cord and surrounding skin upto radius of 5 cm with alcohol-povidone-alcohol.

2. Grasp cord stump with toothed forceps and cut the cord with a scalpel 2 cm from the base. Identify the umbilical vein which is large in size and thin walled and usually located at 6 o'clock **(Figure 49.18)**.

3. Gently insert tips of iris forceps into lumen of the vein and remove any blood clots.

49

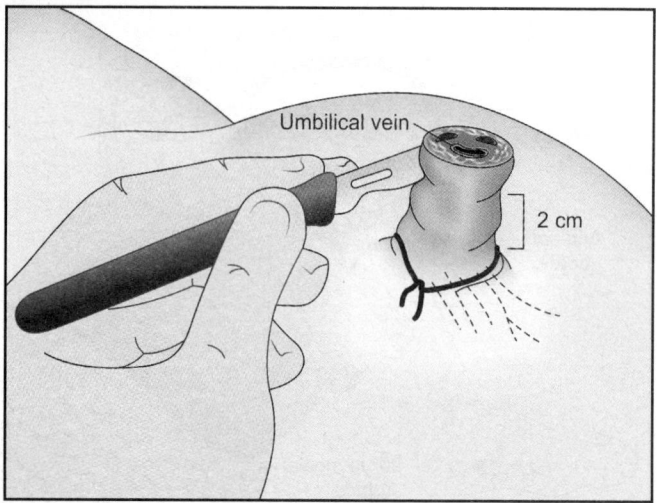

Figure 49.18 Cutting the umbilical stump about 2 cm from skin for placement of umbilical venous catheter

4. Select an appropriate-sized catheter (5 Fr for <3.5 kg and 8 Fr for >3.5 kg), fill it with normal saline, and attach a syringe and stopcock.

5. Introduce the catheter for 2–3 cm into the vein and apply gentle suction. If no blood comes out, withdraw the catheter, remove the clot again and reinsert.

6. When free flow of the blood is obtained, the catheter is inserted to the desired length (see the graph) to ensure that catheter tip lies in ductus venosus or inferior vena cava. If catheter meets any obstruction during insertion to the desired length, withdraw the catheter by 2 cm, rotate it and reinsert.

7. The position of the tip of the catheter can be checked on X-ray of abdomen. The catheter tip should lie opposite D9–D10 vertebrae just above the dome of right diaphragm.

8. Secure the catheter in place with a purse-string suture. Never leave the catheter open to atmosphere due to risk of air embolism. Tape the catheter away from the perineum to prevent soiling with urine and feces. Routine cord care should be continued without covering the stump with any dressing.

Umbilical Arterial Line

Umbilical arterial line allows for frequent arterial blood sampling for monitoring of arterial blood gases (ABGs) of babies on assisted ventilation and for direct and continuous measurement of systemic blood pressure with a transducer.

Procedure

1. Use strict aseptic precautions by wearing gloves, mask, gown and using sterile drape with a central hole. Prepare the cord and surrounding skin up to radius of 5 cm with alcohol-providone-alcohol.

2. Grasp the cord stump with toothed forceps and cut the cord with a scalpel 1 cm from skin.

3. Squeeze the cord between thumb and index finger for 2 minutes. This will cause dilatation of umbilical arteries due to hypoxia and would facilitate cannulation. Two umbilical arteries can be identified as thick-walled white structures that protrude slightly from the cut surface.

4. To further dilate the artery, grasp the cord stump with a toothed forceps holding it at a point close to the artery to be catheterized. Introduce one of the limbs of curved iris forceps into the lumen of the artery upto a depth of 0.5 cm. After some dilatation, introduce the closed tip of the iris forceps and gently dilate the artery upto the depth of 1 cm by opening the forceps and maintaining pressure for 15–30 seconds. Keep the umbilical artery stretched and dilated with curved iris forceps while inserting the catheter (Figure 49.19).

5. Select the appropriate sized catheter (3.5 Fr <1250 g, 5.0 Fr >1250 g), fill it with heparinised saline and attach a syringe and stopcock.

6. Insert the catheter for at least 2 cm into the umbilical artery and remove the iris forceps. Grasp the cord again with toothed forceps and gently pull the cord towards head of the infant while catheter is pushed caudally. The mild traction of the cord will facilitate passage of the catheter at an angle between the cord and skin.

7. After inserting catheter to a depth of 5 cm, verify the correct intraluminal position of the catheter by

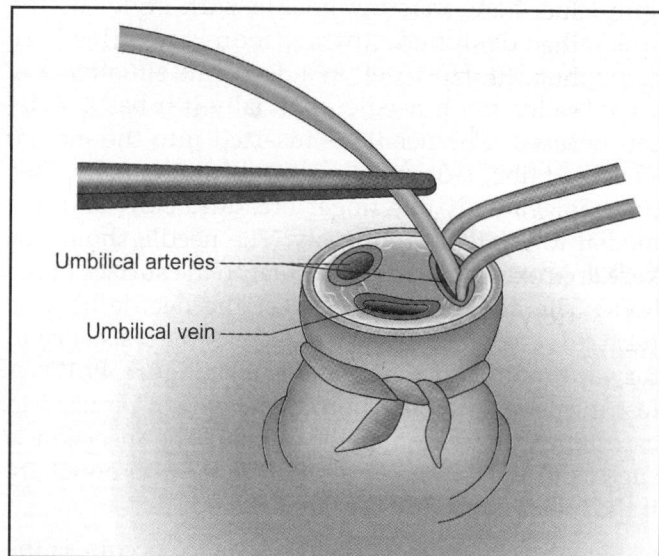

Figure 49.19 Dilatation of umbilical artery and insertion of catheter

aspirating blood. When blood is aspirated the catheter should be cleared by injecting flush solution.

8. Insert the catheter to the desired length (refer to the graph) either to be placed at a low position (L3–L4) or high position (T6–T9) which is confirmed by taking an X-ray of abdomen. If there is development of sudden cyanosis or blanching and discoloration of the buttock or leg on one side, catheter should be removed.

9. Apply purse-string suture and affix the catheter away from the perineum. If desired, catheter can be secured with a tape bridge. Routine cord care is continued without applying any local dressing. The patency of arterial line is maintained by continuous infusion of physiological saline @ 0.5–1.0 mL per hour by using an infusion pump.

10. Arterial blood sample for ABGs is obtained as follows:
    i. Use strict aseptic precautions and clean the side port of 3-way stopcock with alcohol.
    ii. Place gauze piece under the stopcock and unscrew the cap of the hub.
    iii. Attach 5 mL syringe to the hub and turn 3-way stopcock to connect syringe to the catheter. Withdraw 2–3 mL blood, close the luer-lock and remove the syringe.
    iv. Attach 2 mL empty syringe and collect the blood sample by opening the luer-lock.
    v. After collection of blood sample, re-attach 5 mL syringe (containing blood and heparinized saline which was initially withdrawn) and push the blood back into the baby after opening the luer-lock. Flush 1 mL heparinized saline and then close the luer-lock. Put the cap over the hub. Restart the slow infusion of heparinized saline to maintain the patency of the catheter. Maintain an accurate record of all infusions whether for flushing, administration of drugs or for maintenance of catheter patency.

Radial Artery Cannulation

Radial artery cannulation is done for obtaining frequent arterial blood samples for monitoring ABGs and for direct measuring of arterial blood pressure.

Procedure

1. *Modified Allen's* test is done to assess adequacy of collateral circulation through ulnar artery. Compress infants's hand with firm pressure (to blanch it) and simultaneously occlude the ipsilateral radial and ulnar arteries with index finger and thumb of other hand. After a few seconds, release the baby's hand and it should appear pale. Now release the pressure over the ulnar artery while maintaining firm pressure over the radial artery. Reperfusion of the entire palm should occur within few seconds if there is collateral circulation from ulnar artery. Radial artery cannulation should be done only if ulnar collateral circulation is satisfactory.

2. Strict aseptic precautions should be taken by wearing gloves, gown and mask. Restrain infant's forearm and hand with wrist in extension. Apply alcohol-providone-alcohol over the front of wrist at the proposed site of puncture.

3. Locate the radial artery by palpation or transillumination.

4. Insert neoflon at 30°–40° angle to skin **(Figure 49.20)**. Remove the stylet and withdraw cannula slowly until arterial blood flow is seen.

5. Advance cannula into the artery for 5–6 cm, attach three-way stopcock and infuse heparinised saline @ 1.0 mL/hr through an infusion pump **(Figure 49.21)**.

6. Secure venflon with a skin stitch and transparent tape or micropore to allow constant visualization of skin entry site and fingers of the baby.

7. Change IV tubing and flushing solution every 24 hours.

8. The following procedure should be followed by the nurse to collect the arterial blood sample:
    i. Wash hands and put on gloves.
    ii. Clean side port of 3-way stopcock.
    iii. Place sterile gauze piece underneath the hub.
    iv. Unscrew the cap of hub and attach 5 mL syringe.
    v. Open 3-way stopcock and withdraw 2–3 mL blood. Close the luer-lock and remove the syringe.

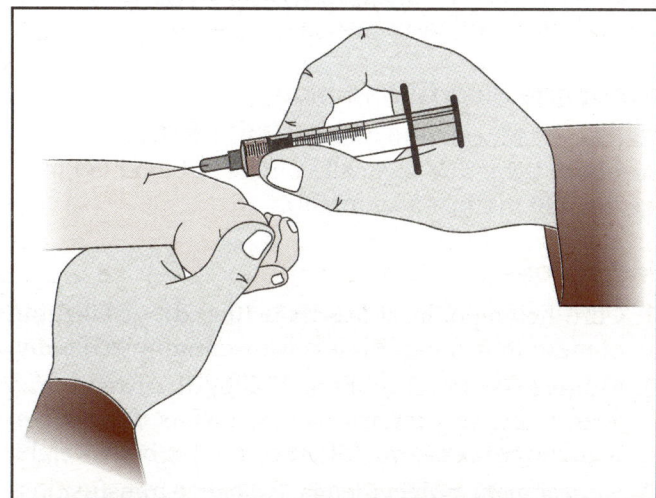

Figure 49.20 Direct puncturing of radial artery for collection of sample of arterial blood for gases

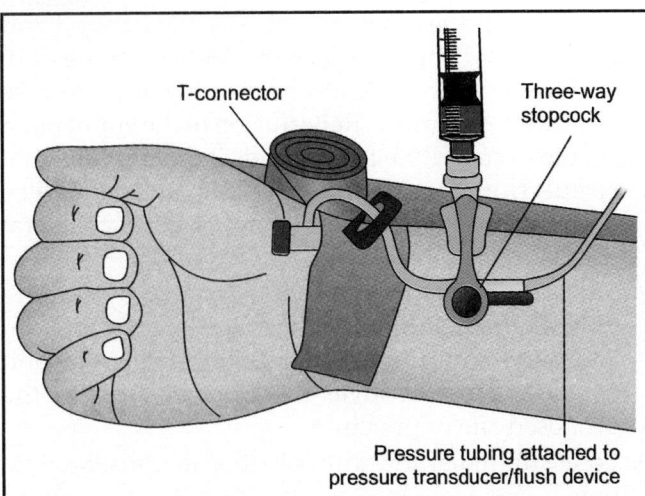

T-connector

Three-way stopcock

Pressure tubing attached to pressure transducer/flush device

Figure 49.21 Radial artery indwelling catheter set up for continuous monitoring of arterial blood pressure and frequent blood sampling

vi. Attach 2 mL syringe and collect blood sample for ABG study. Close the luer-lock and remove the syringe and send it to the laboratory. Maintain accurate record of total amount of blood sample taken and saline infusion given to the baby.

vii. Attach 5 mL syringe (containing initially withdrawn blood), open luer-lock and push the blood back into the baby. Flush the catheter with 1.0 mL heparinised saline and then close the luer-lock. Put the cap over the hub, and restart continuous heparinised saline infusion at the desired rate.

Caution Observe closely for any bleeding and signs of vasospasm, i.e. hand and fingers becoming cold, pale or blotchy. Notify the physician immediately if there is any suspicion of vasospasm.

Exchange Blood Transfusion

Exchange blood transfusion (EBT) is feasible in a newborn baby due to small volume of blood (80 mL/kg, i.e. 240 mL in a 3 kg infant).

Indications

1. Cord hemoglobin of less than 10 g/dL or bilirubin of more than 5 mg/dL in a Rh-isoimmunized baby.
2. Indirect serum bilirubin of 20 mg/dL or more in a term baby. In preterm babies, EBT is done when bilirubin crosses 10 mg/dL for each 1.0 kg body weight.
3. Symptomatic polycythemia. Exchange transfusion is done with normal saline.
4. Disseminated intravascular hemolysis

5. Life-threatening metabolic disorders
6. Acute renal and hepatic failure
7. Septicemia with sclerema
8. Drug toxicity
9. Partial exchange blood transfusion for chronic anemia

Choice of blood Fresh acid-citrate-dextrose (ACD) or citrate-phosphate-dextrose (CPD) blood (not more than 72 hours old) is used for EBT. In emergency situations, O Rh-negative blood can be used without cross matching. Subsequently, ABO-type specific Rh-negative blood cross matched with maternal serum is used in babies with Rh-isoimmunization. In ABO hemolytic disease of the newborn, O Rh-specific blood with low titer of anti-A and anti-B antibodies is preferred or O Rh-specific RBCs are suspended in AB plasma. Effective exchange is achieved by performing the procedure with double the blood volume of the baby, i.e. 160 mL/kg.

Procedure

1. Strict aseptic precautions should be observed by wearing gown, mask and gloves and use of surgical drapes with a central hole.
2. Baby is affixed to a well padded crucifix splint, placed under a radiant warmer and attached to a vital sign monitor for a continuous display of temperature, heart rate, breathing rate, blood pressure and arterial oxygen saturation (SpO_2 or SaO_2).
3. Under full aseptic conditions, umbilical vein is cannulated as described on page 475. The catheter is attached to two 3-way taps so that its leads are connected to the umbilical catheter, syringe, donor blood and a sterile container for waste. The blood should be pre-warmed by using a blood warmer or immersing the blood bag in a water bath at 37°C.
4. The blood is withdrawn with gentle suction and donor's blood is injected slowly in aliquots of 10–20 mL depending upon the size of the baby. During the procedure, the bottle of donor's blood is gently agitated from time to time to keep the RBCs and plasma mixed. The jammed syringes and blocked 3-way connectors are rinsed with heparinized saline (10 units of heparin/mL).
5. Accurate record of IN/OUT of blood and condition of the baby is maintained by the nurse. Whenever untoward signs appear (restlessness, grunting, rapid breathing, tachycardia, fall in oxygen saturation, etc.), the procedure is withheld till condition of the baby improves.

6. After every 100 mL of exchange, venous pressure should be checked and 1.0 mL calcium gluconate is administered slowly if ACD or CPD blood is used for exchange.

7. After completion of the procedure, the catheter is filled with heparinized normal saline and umbilical stump is sprayed with an antibiotic powder. There is no need to administer prophylactic antibiotics when procedure is conducted under strict aseptic conditions.

Complications In experienced hands, EBT is a safe procedure without any complications or mortality. The common complications include transmission of blood-borne pathogens (malarial parasites, CMV, HIV, HBV, HCV), over-loading of circulation or shock, electrolyte disturbances (hyperkalemia, hypocalcemia, metabolic acidosis) and hypoglycemia following exchange transfusion with heparinized blood.

INJECTIONS

Children are scared of injections and they cry more due to fear and anxiety rather than pain of injection. *The common practice of giving threats of injections and doctors to children to modify their behavior is condemned.* In ambulatory pediatric practice, there is no need to give injections except for administration of vaccines, treatment of anaphylaxis, long-acting penicillin prophylaxis for rheumatic fever and doing intradermal skin tests. There is a wrong belief that medicines work better or faster when given parenterally. If a child is really sick to need parenteral medications, he usually needs admission to the hospital. Disposable syringes and needles should be used to reduce the risk of infection and transmission of hepatitis B and C virus and HIV. Injection site should be cleaned with isopropyl alcohol. Rubber diaphragm of the vial should also be cleaned with an alcohol swab. Small children should be held by the mother in the lap or restrained on the table by the mother or attendant. The child should be cuddled and caressed after the injection. The older children should be assured that injection will merely hurt like the bite of an insect to allay their fear and anxiety.

Intradermal injection Intracutaneous injection is given for administration of certain vaccines (BCG, antirabies) and for doing intradermal tests like Mantoux test and Schick test, to test drug sensitivity and for desensitization. Injection is given with 26 gauge short-bevelled needle attached to a tuberculin syringe. Skin is cleaned with soap and water or sterile saline, it is stretched with left hand. Syringe is held in the right hand with bevel of the needle facing upwards. Needle is inserted into the skin (not under the skin). When complete bevel gets inserted into the skin, 0.1 mL of medicine is injected which produces a wheal of 5 mm at the site of injection. BCG vaccine is given intradermally over the lateral side of top of the left shoulder while in Mantoux test 0.1 mL 2 TU PPD is injected intradermally on the middle of the flexor or volar surface of the left forearm. The injected site is examined after 48–72 hours to look for any swelling or induration. When largest diameter of induration is more than 10 mm, it indicates that child has had exposure to tubercle bacilli (natural infection or BCG vaccination) or is currently suffering from tuberculosis. In an immuno-compromised child (HIV infection, chemotherapy, steroids, following measles), induration of more than 5 mm is considered as positive. *Erythema or redness alone is of no significance.*

Subcutaneous (hypodermic) injection The common sites for giving subcutaneous injection are outer aspect of upper arm (deltoid muscle), anterior or lateral aspect of thigh (vastus lateralis) and under the skin of abdomen (insulin and antirabies injection). Skin is pinched between the thumb and forefinger of left hand and needle is inserted at 45° with the right hand. The left hand then supports the needle and syringe and drug is injected slowly. After withdrawal of needle, the swab is kept over the injection site and it is gently massaged to disperse the medicine and kept pressed till bleeding stops. In subcutaneous injection, the absorption of medicine is slow because of poor blood supply in the subcutaneous region.

Intramuscular injection The sites with good muscle mass and lack of any underlying blood vessels or nerve are chosen for intramuscular injections. In infants and preschool children, anterolateral aspect of mid-thigh (rectus femoris or vastus lateralis muscle) is the preferred site for intramuscular injection **(Figures 49.22 and 49.23)**. In children above 5 years of age, intramuscular injection can be given over the outer aspect of upper arm just below the shoulder (deltoid muscle) **(Figure 49.24)**. The upper and outer quadrant of buttocks (gluteal muscle) is avoided due to potential risk of causing damage to the sciatic nerve and reserved for giving an oily injection or when the volume of drug is large. The volume of fluid or medicine to be injected should be limited to 0.5 mL in an infant, 1.0 mL in a toddler and 1.5–3.0 mL for an older child or adolescent. The skin at injection site is cleaned with alcohol and stretched by thumb and forefinger of left hand. The needle is inserted quickly at right angle, the drug is injected slowly and needle withdrawn quickly. Before injecting the drug, gentle negative pressure is applied to make sure that needle has not inadvertently entered

49

49

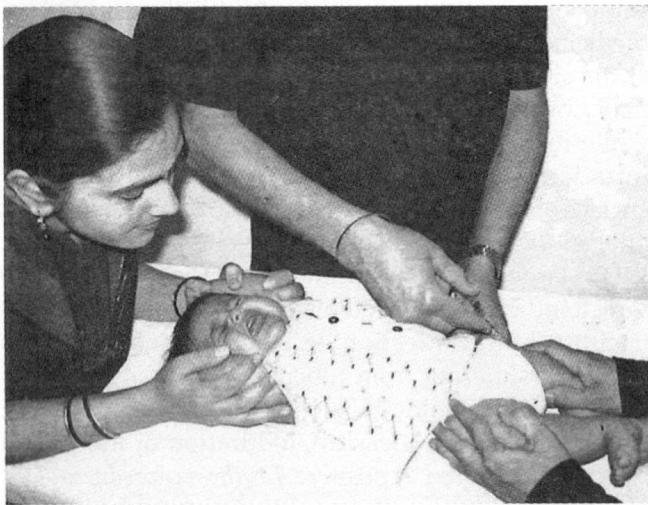

Figure 49.22 Mother is asked to restrain the arms of the baby and talk with her to provide comfort. Father or attendant is asked to firmly immobilize the thigh and injection is given at the anterolateral site over the midthigh region

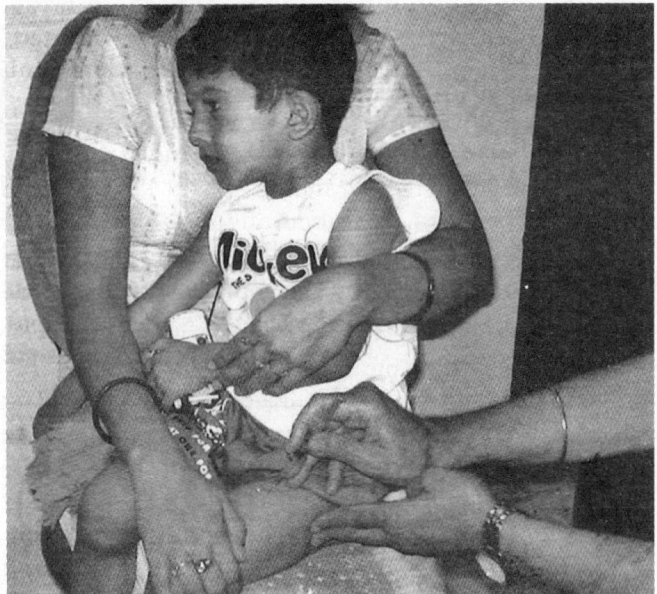

Figure 49.23 Toddler is best injected while being held by the mother in the comfort of her lap. She is asked to restrain his arms with one hand and thigh to be injected with the other hand

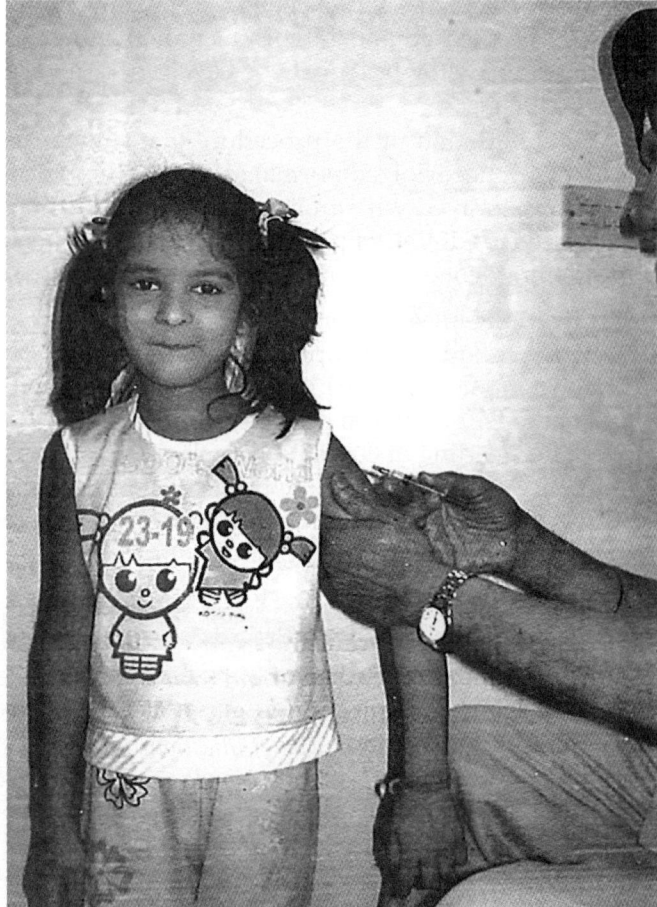

Figure 49.24 Most school-going children cooperate for receiving vaccine shot over the deltoid region. The attention of the child is distracted while giving the injection

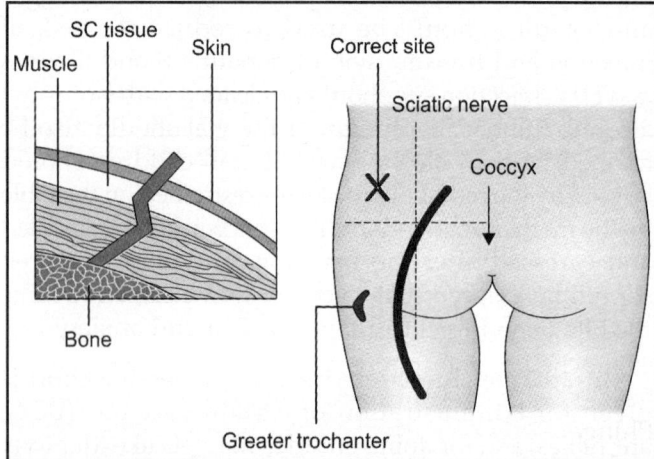

Figure 49.25 The landmarks to identify the correct site for injection into the buttock to prevent damage to the sciatic nerve

into a blood vessel. If blood is withdrawn, needle should be pushed further before injecting the medicine. After the withdrawal of the needle, puncture site should be gently massaged and kept pressed with a medicated swab till bleeding stops. The safe site for giving injection at the gluteal site is shown in **Figure 49.25**. The child lies in prone position (on his tummy) or semiprone or lateral position and buttock is divided into four quadrants. *The injection is given into the upper and outer* *quadrant to prevent damage to the sciatic nerve.* Intramuscular injection should not be given to a child with a bleeding or coagulation disorder and subcutaneous injection is associated with lower risk of bleeding. In order to reduce the risk of needlestick injury, the disposable needle should not be recapped, bent or broken.

ENTERAL FEEDING AND PROCEDURES

Gastric intubation Tube is inserted into the stomach for feeding, gastric aspiration and stomach wash or lavage. The tube may be inserted through the mouth for doing a lavage but nasogastric intubation is preferred for feeding or prolonged gastric aspiration because of ease of fixing a nasogastric tube. Non-irritating PVP and plastic tubes can be safely kept in-situ for several days. Tip of the patient's little finger provides a useful guide regarding the maximum diameter of the tube that can be passed through the nose. In newborn babies and infants, 3, 5, 6, or 9 Fr and for older children 9–15 Fr size tubes are used for nasogastric intubation. For orogastric intubation, a larger sized tube (9–18 Fr) is used.

Tube length is measured and ear marked. For orogastric intubation, tube length is measured from bridge of the nose to the xiphisternum. For nasogastric intubation, tube is measured from bridge of the nose to the tragus of the ear and then to the xiphisternum **(Figure 49.26)**. The child lies supine and may need to be restrained or mummified if uncooperative. Tube is lubricated with glycerine or sterile saline (never with an oil). The tube is inserted through the nose (or the mouth) into the esophagus and down to stomach upto the marked length keeping the neck slightly flexed. Inadvertent passage into the trachea provokes sudden choking and coughing. The position of the tube in the stomach is checked and confirmed as follows:

i. Auscultation over the epigastrium for gurgling sounds on injection of air.

ii. Aspiration of acidic stomach contents.

iii. Instillation of 1–2 mL of sterile distilled water should not provoke any coughing and choking.

A 20 mL syringe containing the milk or special feed is attached to the tube and raised above the level of head. Feed is allowed to flow into stomach by gravity. Plunger should not be used to push the feed. After giving the feed, tube is flushed with sterile water to avoid clogging or blockage of the tube. After feeding, the child is kept supine and turned to the right. The tube is securely affixed on the face with a milipore tape **(Figure 49.27)**.

Gastric lavage A large-bored tube is passed through the mouth. The child is effectively restrained in left

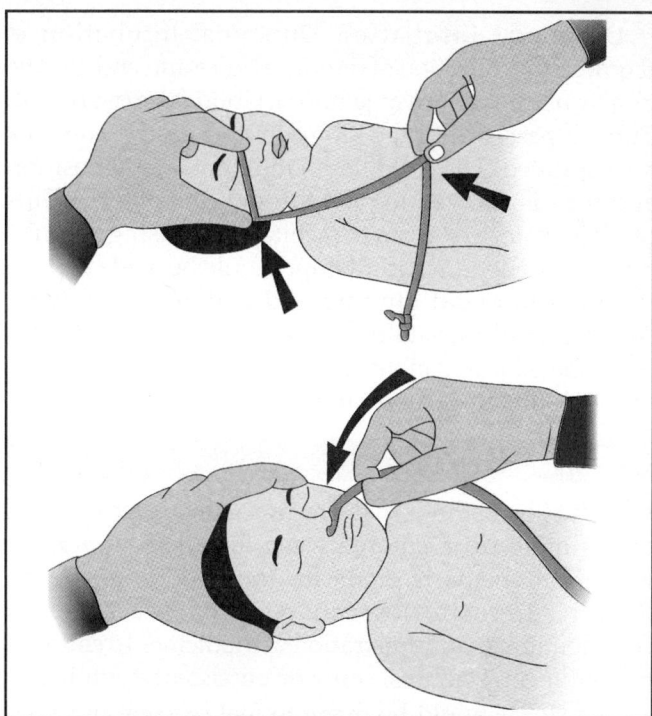

Figure 49.26 Measuring the length of the nasogastric tube and technique of insertion of nasogastric tube

49

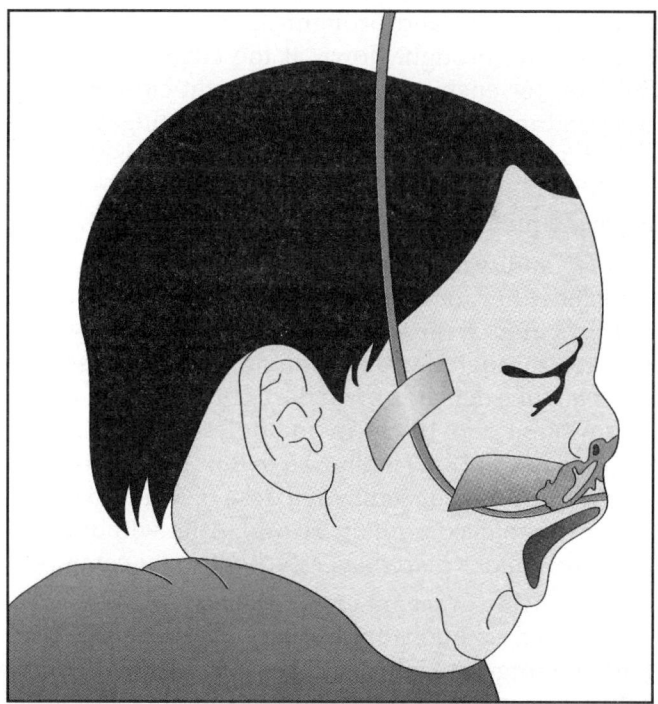

Figure 49.27 Effective fixation of nasogastric tube on the face with a milipore tape

lateral position. 30–60 mL of lavage fluid (usually normal saline) is introduced and withdrawn alternately. The position of the child is varied during the procedure to ensure effective lavage of the stomach.

Duodenal intubation Duodenal intubation is required for collection of duodenal juice and endoscopic biopsy of duodenum or jejunum. Child fasts overnight. Tube is passed into the stomach and gastric contents are aspirated. The child lies in the right lateral position and tube is allowed to pass through the pylorus. Sips of plain water are given to facilitate the passage of tube into the duodenum. No attempt should be made to push the tube to avoid kinking and coiling of the tube. Aspiration of bile-stained alkaline contents indicates that tube is located in the duodenum. The exact position of the radiopaque tube can be checked radiologically.

ENEMAS

Introduction of fluids in the rectum to evacuate the hard stools or to do a colonic wash is called an enema. Retention enema is given for therapeutic purposes. Rectal suppositories can be used for relief of constipation or administration of medicines to children having fever, seizures, coma or persistent vomiting.

The child should be made to feel relaxed and void urine before the procedure. Strict privacy should be ensured for adolescent children. The child lies in the left lateral position with a macintosh underneath. Lower limbs are flexed and brought up to the chest while buttocks are brought down at the edge of the table. Solution for enema should be brought close to body temperature. Enema catheter and connecting tubes are filled with enema solution to displace the air. Traditional soap and water enemas have been replaced by ready made or disposable enemas.

Soap and water enema Terminal 5–10 cm of rectal catheter (12 Fr for infant and 14–18 Fr for older child) is lubricated with liquid paraffin or vaseline and inserted through the anal opening. Depth of insertion of rectal tube depends upon the age of child, i.e. 2.5 cm in an infant and 10 cm in an adolescent child. Soap solution (5% at 38°C) is allowed to flow by gravity from the funnel into the rectum in a dose of 50 mL per year of age (up to maximum of 750 mL). After withdrawl of catheter, child is placed over the bed pan or commode.

Disposable evacuant enema Ready-made hypertonic evacuant solutions are available in disposable plastic bags having insertion or injection nozzles. Enema solution is warmed by placing it in basin of water at 40°C. Lubricated enema nozzle is passed beyond the anal sphincter after removing the cap. The enema solution is slowly injected by gradually rolling up the plastic bag. The child's buttocks are kept strapped for sometime to soften the stools before evacuation. The desired amount of enema fluid should be injected depending upon the manufacturer's instructions.

Olive oil (or liquid paraffin, glycerin) enema It is used to soften the hard and impacted fecoliths in children with intractable constipation. Warm olive oil is slowly injected through the anus. The amount of olive oil to be administered depends upon the age of the child (10 mL per year of age). Enema is administered slowly over a period of 10–15 minutes and catheter withdrawn gently. Foot-end of the bed is raised and buttocks are strapped to delay evacuation.

Saline bowel wash Bowel or colonic wash is done with 0.9% sodium chloride solution (physiological saline or normal saline) at a rate of 30 mL per year of age. Plain water should not be used for bowel wash as it may lead to water intoxication. Bowel wash is done prior to proctoscopy, colonoscopy and barium enema studies.

Retention enema This is a therapeutic enema and child is encouraged to retain the injected medicine in the enema fluid as long as possible. Medicated enema fluid is injected very slowly, foot-end of the bed is raised and buttocks are strapped after the procedure. The commonly used retention enemas include use of prednisolone solution in ulcerative colitis and hypertonic magnesium sulfate (25%) to reduce intracranial pressure and paraldehyde for control of seizures. Medicated suppositories or rectal solutions are available for administration of certain drugs (diazepam, paracetamol) to children who are unable to take them orally.

Manual evacuation of feces At times, when fecoliths are impacted, they may be removed manually. The child lies in the same position as recommended for the procedure of enema. Gloved well-lubricated index finger is inserted into the rectum and fecal masses are broken into several pieces and extracted gently into a receiver till all the fecoliths are removed. Application of a local anesthetic at the perianal area may facilitate the procedure by reducing pain.

SUCTIONING

In critically sick children, when airway is compromised due to excessive secretions in the nose or oral cavity, suction is required to improve oxygenation. Suction is often required in babies with upper GI anomalies, seizures, bulbar palsy, coma, surgical procedure, assisted ventilation and tracheostomy.

Oro- and nasopharyngeal suction Strict aseptic precautions should be used by wearing gloves. The suction catheter and gloves should be changed everytime suction is performed. Suction pressure (suction machine or piped suction source) should be maintained between 60 and 80 mm Hg (60–80 cm H_2O) to prevent damage to the mucosa. Measure the length of catheter from mouth or nose up to suprasternal notch. The wide-bored suction catheter is passed upwards and backwards either from the nose or mouth. Intermittent negative suction is applied while gently withdrawing the catheter. The procedure is repeated couple of times to suck out all secretions. In a community setting or when mechanical suction source is not available, the nurse can use a manual mucus extractor to suck the secretions.

Oral airway In a comatosed child, an oral airway is inserted to prevent the tongue falling backwards in order to maintain the patency of the air passages. It is important to select an appropriate sized airway for insertion because a small airway may push the tongue into posterior pharynx while a large airway may itself block the oropharynx. Airway is measured by placing it over the cheek. When its outer flange is aligned at the level of central incisors, the distal end of the airway should reach up to the angle of the jaw.

Ask an assistant to open the jaws ith both hands. Airway is slowly and gently pushed inside the oral cavity by keeping the distal opening facing upwards towards the palate. When airway reaches the back of the tongue, it is rotated 180° so that its bite block is aligned with central incisors and its flange is snugly positioned along the lips. Keep the oral cavity free of secretions by regular suctioning around the airway.

Endotracheal suction Infants and children on assisted ventilation need periodic suctioning through endotracheal tube to remove mucus and secretions. Chest physiotherapy should precede suctioning to loosen the secretions. The procedure should be conducted under proper sterile conditions by wearing surgical gloves and using disposable sterile packs containing suction catheters and a bowl. The size of the suction catheter should be such that it should not completely block the ET tube. Before the procedure, the infant should be ventilated with a bag using 100 percent oxygen. The suction is carried out in three positions of the head namely straight, right rotation and left rotation. The suction catheter is introduced through the in-built port so that ET tube does not need to be disconnected. The suction catheter is inserted 0.5 cm beyond the end of the ET tube. After introduction of catheter, suction is applied continuously while gradually withdrawing the catheter. The suctioning should be limited to periods of 10 seconds followed by hyperventilation with oxygen. When secretions are thick and viscid their suctioning may be facilitated by instillation of 1–2 mL of normal saline or acetylcystein.

The patient is hand ventilated for 60 seconds after instillation of saline or acetyl cystein before suctioning is done. The tracheal secretions should be periodically sent for culture and antibiotic sensitivity pattern. During the procedure, the patient should be closely watched and should be attached to a pulse oximeter and cardiac monitor.

Tracheostomy suction With due aseptic precautions, insert a wide-bored suction catheter through the tracheostomy tube up to 0.5 cm beyond the end of the tube. Gentle negative suction (60–80 mm Hg) is applied and suction catheter is gradually removed while rotating the catheter. The suction should not be applied for more that 10–15 seconds at a time. When secretions are thick and viscid, 1–2 mL of normal saline or acetylcysteine should be instilled before suctioning.

Complications Suctioning should be done only when indicated because it is associated with discomfort, irritation and several other complications, which are listed below:
  i. Gagging, coughing and hypoxia
  ii. Laryngospasm
  iii. Tachycardia and bradycardia
  iv. Increase in intracranial pressure and blood pressure
  v. Damage to the mucosa
  vi. Risk of infection

Steam Inhalation

Steam inhalation is useful to loosen thick secretions in the respiratory tract, promote expectoration and relieve inflammatory congestion in the upper airways. It is dangerous to give steam inhalation by boiling water in a household kitchen utensil. It is preferable and safer to use a facial steamer. Switch off the fan or air conditioner. Steamer should be filled with water upto the desired level. You can put some carom seeds (*ajwain*) in the water to facilitate relief of nasal congestion. Steamer should be placed on a table and child should sit at a distance of about one foot with his face aligned at the level of steamer's nozzle. The nostrils should be cleaned off any secretions before the start of procedure. School going child can sit comfortably on a chair while a younger child must be held in mother's lap. *Never leave the child alone during steam inhalation due to risk of scalds.* There is no need to cover the child and steamer with a blanket or sheet because it is uncomfortable and scary to the child. Steam should be given for atleast 10 minutes 2 to 3 times in a day. During the procedure, face and nostrils should be cleaned off sweat and secretions with a face towel. Encourage the child to blow the nose and expectorate airway secretions during

49

and after steam inhalation. In infants, the nose can be cleared by aspirating with a nasal aspirator. The nurse or mother should be asked to provide chest physiotherapy after steam inhalation. In a child with croup or stridor, steam inhalation can be given in the bathroom by opening the shower after putting the geyser on. Steam inhalation is contraindicated in a child with respiratory difficulty and bronchospasm.

Chest Physiotherapy

In children with chronic suppurative lung disease like persistent pneumonia, bronchiectasis, cystic fibrosis and lung abscess, chest physiotherapy is done to facilitate drainage of bronchial secretions and exudates. Steam inhalation and use of bronchodilators enhance the efficacy of chest physiotherapy. Depending upon the bronchopulmonary segment to be drained, the child is positioned appropriately with head end kept low. The hand is cupped and by keeping the wrist loose, the chest wall is clapped with the cup of the hand so that a hollow sound is heard. The procedure is continued for 10–15 minutes by keeping the child in various positions to drain specific areas or bronchopulmonary segments of the affected lung/s. The procedure should be abandoned if child develops any respiratory distress or tachycardia.

Oxygen Saturation Monitoring

Pulse oximetry provides non-invasive technology for rational and safe administration of oxygen to sick babies. Arterial oxygen saturation (SpO$_2$ or SaO$_2$) is monitored with a pulse oximeter in infants and children with tachypnea, respiratory distress, apneic attacks and cyanosis. Children on assisted ventilation and during resuscitation and CPR, should be hooked to a pulse oximeter **(Figure 49.28)**. The instrument provides direct read-out of SpO$_2$ or SaO$_2$ and heart rate.

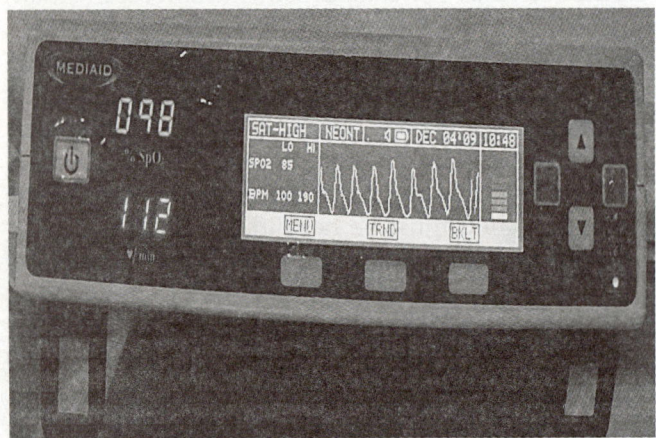

Figure 49.28 Pulse oximeter for monitoring arterial oxygen saturation and heart rate

Procedure

1. Assemble all the necessary equipment including simultaneous monitoring of ambient oxygen analyzer.
2. Affix sensor probe of pulse oximeter over the foot or hand of the baby. In older children, sensor can be affixed over the thumb or big toe.
3. Ensure that two sides of the sensor probe are directly opposite to each other and it is snugly affixed with the help of a tape or a wrap. One side of the probe emits light while the photodiode on the other side picks up the transmitted light. The reusable sensor probes should be cleaned with alcohol in-between patients to reduce the risk of nosocomial infection.
4. Set high and low alarm limits for oxygen saturation and heart rate (2% above and below desired limits). Periodically check displayed heart rate with actual heart rate as obtained on auscultation of the heart. If there is disparity between the two values, the oxygen saturation readings may not be reliable.
5. Record heart rate, respiratory rate, SpO$_2$ and ambient oxygen concentration (FiO$_2$) hourly. Maintain SpO$_2$ between 90 and 95% in newborn babies and above 85% in infants and older children.
6. Keep a close watch over the skin site where sensor is affixed for any skin damage and change the site atleast once per shift.

Precautions

1. Pulse oximetry is unreliable if there is poor tissue perfusion or cold extremities due to hypothermia and shock.
2. Excessive movements of limb and exposure of sensor to strong light gives false readings.
3. Do not apply cuff of blood pressure monitor on the limb where oxygen sensor is affixed.
4. Oxygen saturation monitors are unreliable for detection of hyperoxia. In preterm babies, monitoring of arterial oxygen tension (PaO$_2$) by frequent ABGs is mandatory to safeguard against development of retinopathy of prematurity (ROP).
5. The heart rate display provided by the pulse oximeter must tally with the heart rate obtained manually by auscultation or taken by another vital sign monitor, otherwise oxygen saturation values may not be reliable.

Radiant Warmer (open care system)

Radiant warmers are extremely useful to provide radiation heat source to maintain warm microenvironment for newborn babies and infants. They may be manually-controlled or servo-controlled, i.e. heat out put from the warmer is automatically modified (raised or lowered) by the thermostat to maintain the desired skin temperature of the baby. The manual mode is used initially to prewarm the cot or for rapid warming of a hypothermic baby. When a radiant warmer is attached to a baby cot, it is called open care system (as opposed to an incubator which is a closed system.).

1. The radiant warmer and open care system is better than an incubator because it provides easy access to the baby for nursing care and various procedures. The risk of nosocomial infection is also lower compared to an incubator **(Figure 49.29)**.

2. The major drawbacks of open care system include unnecessary or excessive handling of the baby and excessive evaporative heat losses. A cap and cotton frock can be worn to reduce water loss from the skin.

3. Radiant warmer should not be exposed to strong draught or air currents and room temperature should be kept above 26°C.

4. Open care system is used in the initial care of sick and preterm babies needing assisted ventilation and other life support interventions. Once baby is stable, he is shifted to the incubator.

5. When using the manual mode of open care system, baby's temperature should be checked continuously with a telethermometer or recorded manually on a regular basis.

6. In servo-controlled system, the skin sensor is affixed midway between xiphisternum and umbilicus. Skin temperature is set at 36.5°C. *It is important to ensure that the skin probe should never come off the skin because of danger of hyperthermia or excessive warming of the baby.* When sensor gets dislodged, thermostat perceives the temperature of the nursery (which is around 26°C) and radiant warmer continues to generate heat (in trying to raise the nursery temperature to the set skin sensor temperature of 36.5°C), thus raising the baby's temperature to a dangerous level.

7. Open care system should be kept clean and disinfected by mopping with 2% bacillocid during each shift.

Incubator Care

Incubators or isolettes are useful to keep the baby warm, provide isolation, reduce handling, administer oxygen and increase humidity to reduce evaporative skin losses. When a preterm baby is hemodynamically stable, he is best nursed in an incubator **(Figure 49.30)**.

1. Incubator can be used on air mode or manual mode and servo-controlled or skin-temperature control mode. In air mode, the desired ambient temperature around the baby is set and the heater output adjusts itself to maintain it. The appropriate set temperature is decided by using the thermoneutral temperature charts based on gestation and postnatal age of the

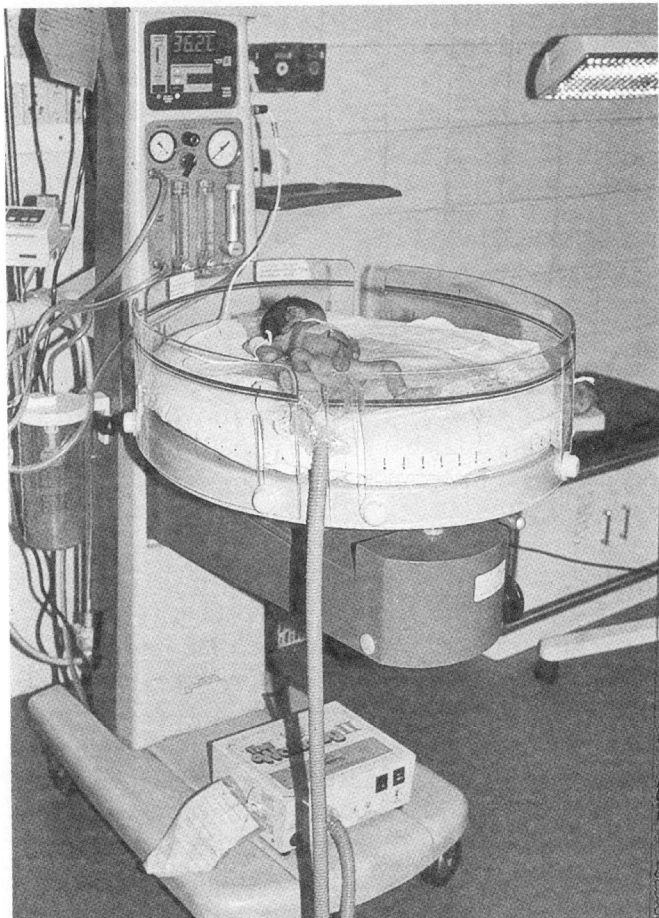

Figure 49.29 Open care system. It is equipped with overhead heat and light source along with servocontrol facility

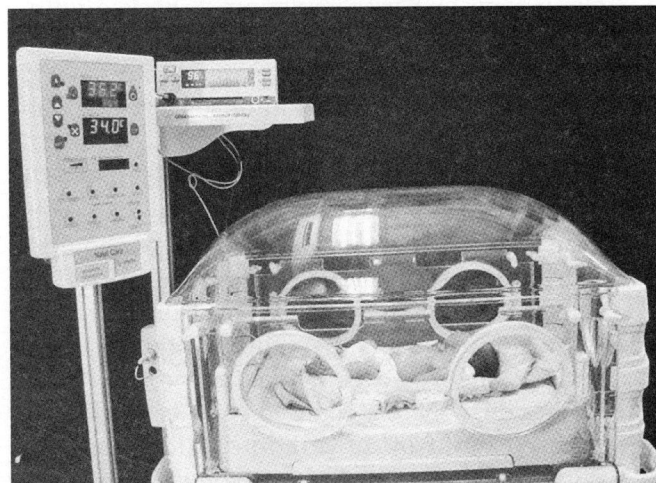

Figure 49.30 Intensive care double-walled incubator. It is provided with portholes and circulation of filtered air with a provision to increase humidity

49

baby. When ambient temperature is maintained in the thermoneutral range, the oxygen and caloric consumption of the baby is lowest with enhanced survival. The air temperature sensing probe is placed near the baby and care is taken to ensure that it is not displaced or covered.

2. In servo-controlled mode or skin temperature control, skin sensor is attached firmly over the anterior abdominal wall midway between epigastrium and umbilicus and set at 36.5°C. The feedback mechanism modifies heater output to keep the body temperature of the baby close to the set temperature. *When using servo-controlled mode, care should be taken to ensure that the skin probe does not get dislodged which may lead to dangerous over heating of the baby.*

3. The baby in the incubator should preferably be nursed clothed and with a cap, mittens, socks and a frock.

4. Incubator should not be placed close to the wall as it will hamper air circulation. Double-walled incubators (or baby can be enclosed in a perspex dome shield) are preferred due to less radiation and convective heat losses.

5. Humidification reduces insensible water losses but is associated with increased risk of nosocomial infection with *Pseudomonas* and *Klebsiella*. Humidification is mandatory in babies weighing less than 1.0 kg. Humidification chamber is filled with sterile water and 1–2 mL of glacial acetic acid or vinegar is added to reduce colonization with bacteria. Humidification water must be changed daily.

6. Baby in the incubator should be nursed through portholes without opening the front panel. Babies on warmers or in incubators with skin probes, need to have their axillary temperatures checked with a clinical thermometer every 2–4 hours to ensure that it is maintained between 36.5°C and 37.2°C. Wide fluctuations in skin temperature suggest that baby is unstable or ill.

7. Incubators and warmers should be maintained in working condition and calibrated every 4–6 months by the biomedical engineer. Strict asepsis should be ensured by proper house keeping routines and cleaning schedule followed by the nurses (refer to **Chapter 6** for details). Air filter of the incubator should be changed every 3 months because when it becomes dirty there is reduced entry of oxygen and increased build up of carbon dioxide inside the incubator. The sleeves of access windows should be changed daily and washed. Incubator canopy should not be cleaned with alcohol due to risk of making it foggy and disfigured.

LUMBAR PUNCTURE (Spinal tap)

Lumbar puncture is done to obtain cerebrospinal fluid (CSF) for cytology, biochemical analysis, PCR and culture studies. The procedure is also done to monitor CSF pressure, intrathecal drug administration and for decompression in children with pseudotumor cerebri and hydrocephalus. It is a safe procedure when performed with due asepsis and when there are no contraindications.

Contraindications

1. Raised intracranial pressure with papilledema (when sutures are closed) because of risk of uncal herniation and sudden death.
2. Persistent seizures with worsening level of consciousness.
3. Local infection of skin over the lumbar area.
4. Bleeding diathesis.
5. In a critically sick child with shock, the procedure is postponed till child is stable.

Procedure The nurse prepares the family and child for a lumbar puncture by briefly explaining the need, steps involved and safety of the procedure. The consent form should be duly signed by the family member or attendant. The nurse has an important responsibility to restrain the child for the procedure. The operator wears the surgical gown, mask and gloves to ensure strict asepsis. The child is placed on its side (lateral recumbent position) near the edge of a table or trolley. The nurse flexes the back of the child (to increase distance between the intervertebral spaces) by placing one hand or arm around the child's neck and other arm over the buttocks and back of thighs. The neck is flexed toward the chest and knees are drawn toward the abdomen so that back is maximally rounded. In neonates and infants, the procedure can be done in a sitting position.

Skin over the dorsum of back is prepared with surgical alcohol-povidone-alcohol and draped with a sterile sheet. Intervertebral space between L_4 and L_5 is identified by using iliac crest as a landmark, which correspond to it. The site of puncture is infiltrated with local anesthetic. The lumbar puncture needle is inserted above L_5 spine and advanced to reach ligamentum flavum, which is pierced with a gentle pressure. When needle pierces the dura, the pressure gives way. The stylet of lumbar puncture needle is removed and CSF allowed to flow into a sterile collection bottle. A manometer may be attached to the needle to determine the CSF pressure. In children younger than 2 years, a disposable 18–20 FG needle can be used without any local anesthetic.

During the procedure, the nurse should keep a watch on the color and breathing of the child. When CSF is blood stained, it should be collected in three collection bottles to see whether it remains uniformly blood tinged (subarachnoid hemorrhage) or CSF is initially red colored and becomes clear as it flows (traumatic puncture). Collect 0.5 mL CSF in ethylene diamine tetra-acetic acid (EDTA) bottle for cell count and 1–2 mL in plain vial for culture and biochemistry. After withdrawing the needle, the puncture site is sealed with tincture benzoin or micropore seal to prevent oozing of CSF. The CSF for cytology should be examined without any delay and preferably within 30 minutes. After lumbar puncture, the child is kept supine in bed for a couple of hours to reduce the risk of headache.

BIBLIOGRAPHY

Bowden VR, Greenberg CS. Pediatric Nursing Procedures. *Lippincott Williams and Wilkins*. 3rd Edition, 2011.

Harrison D, Beggs S, Stevens B. Sucrose for procedural pain management in infants. *Pediatrics* 2012, 130(5): 918–925.

Kalia K. Pediatric Nursing Procedures. *New Delhi, Jaypee Bros*, 2012.

Lodha R, Kabra SK, Sinha A, Thukral A (Eds). Pediatric Procedures. *New Delhi, CBS Publishers and Distributors Pvt. Ltd*. First edition, 2014.

Metheny NA, Meert KL. Monitoring feeding tube placement. *Nutr Clin Pract* 2004, 19(5): 487–495.

Shah PS, Herbozo C, Aliwalas L, el al. Breastfeeding or breast milk for procedural pain in neonates. *Cochrane Database Syst. Rev* 2012, 12: CD004950. doi:10.1002 14651858.CD004950. pub3.

49

Glossary of Common Medical Conditions

A

Abortion The loss of an embryo or fetus before 20 weeks of gestation or of a fetus weighing less than 500 g is called abortion or miscarriage. Almost 20% of pregnancies end in miscarriage.

Abscess A collection of pus due to pyogenic infection at any site of the body is called abscess. It is usually associated with fever, swelling, pain, redness and warmth. The abscess must be incised and drained for prompt relief. Tuberculous lymphadenitis may produce a cold abscess.

Acne Appearance of black heads (comedones) with palpable small nodules on the face are suggestive of acne vulgaris. The skin lesions may become infected and pustular by unnecessary handling. They may occur in children of both sexes during adolescence. The skin lesions may also occur over the upper back and shoulders. They occur due to hormonal changes and herald the onset of puberty.

Acquired immunodeficiency syndrome (AIDS) It is a life-threatening viral infection due to HIV that can be transmitted to the child from his mother during late pregnancy or delivery, through breast milk or transfusion of infected blood, blood products or needles. In adolescents (and adults), it commonly occurs by indulging in unsafe sexual encounters with multiple partners and anal sex. The child suffers from frequent respiratory and GI infections and fails to grow properly. The disease can be prevented but there is no satisfactory cure.

Adenoids Adenoids are small pads of lymphatic tissue at the back of the nose. In some allergic children, they get enlarged causing blockage of nose. The child has to keep his mouth open for breathing. The mouth remains open during sleep, snoring is common and jaw hangs down giving a dull appearance to the face which is called as "adenoid facies".

Adolescence The period (10–16 years in girls and 12 to 18 years in boys) during which the child goes through the process of sexual maturation is called adolescence. There are profound physical, emotional and psychological changes during this period.

Adoption Adoption of a child refers to the legal process of becoming a non biological parent. The child may be adopted from among children of a relative or more commonly from an orphanage, foster home or from a hospital when a child is abandoned by her unwed mother or because of other social reasons.

Aerophagy Swallowing of air (aero: air, phagy: swallowing) while feeding is common in bottle fed babies. The eructation of air bubble may lead to regurgitation of some curdled milk which is called possetting or simply regurgitation of feeds.

Allergic conjunctivitis There is inflammation of one or both eyes because of allergic reaction to pollen or mold spores. It is characterized by watering of eyes, irritation or itching and redness of conjunctiva.

Allergic rhinitis It is an immunoglobulin E-mediated inflammation of the nasal mucosa in response to airborne allergens, such as pollen, dust mites, animal dander and mold. There is sudden onset of nasal itching, sneezing, and profuse watery discharge from nose and eyes without any fever.

Allergy It is an unusual response or reaction to substances which are otherwise harmless. The allergic tendency is usually hereditary or familial when it is called atopy. The allergic response may occur to practically any item which is inhaled (dust, pollen, molds, fungus, animal hair, smoke, cockroaches, mosquito repellants, etc.), eaten (drugs or medicines, milk, nuts, eggs, fish, chocolates, food color and preservatives, etc.) or applied on the skin (soap, talcum powder, cosmetics, hair dyes, synthetic fabric, and leather).

Alopecia Baldness or absence of hair over the head due to any cause.

Amblyopia There is defective vision or 'lazy eye' in a child with wandering, non-fixing but normal looking eyes. The eyes may have a variable concomitant squint and are malaligned.

Amebiasis It is characterized by intestinal infection due to *Entameba histolytica* (producing acute dysentery) and rarely trophozoites may involve liver to produce amebic abscess or disseminate to distant organs through bloodstream.

Amenorrhea Cessation of menstrual periods is called amenorrhea and usually signify either onset of pregnancy or menopause. It may also occur due to chronic systemic, endocrinal and psychological disorder.

Amniocentesis The technique of collecting amniotic fluid during pregnancy for diagnostic purposes is called amniocentesis. It is best performed during 15–16 weeks of pregnancy.

Anaphylaxis It is a dramatic onset of immediate IgE-mediated life-threatening reaction to a drug, food or insect bite. There is sudden onset of intense pruritus, sinking sensation like syncope and angioedema involving upper airways (difficulty in breathing, stridor), eyelids, lips and tongue. Administration of adrenaline 0.01 mL/kg of 1: 1000 solution IM is life saving. The maximum dose is 0.5 mL which can be repeated every 15–30 minutes for 2 to 3 doses.

Anemia In healthy children, the skin looks pink due to hemoglobin content in the red blood cells. Anemia is a condition when the hemoglobin content of the blood is below normal. The child looks pale, listless and tires easily.

Anorexia nervosa A rare psychological eating disorder among adolescent girls who have an abnormal fear of obesity, distorted body image and they practically starve themselves by refusing to eat.

Antibiotic (anti: against, bio: life) A chemical substance that inhibits the growth or kills bacteria. They have no effect on viruses. It is preferable to use the terms like antibacterial, antiviral, antifungal, antiparasitic agents which are more appropriate and explanatory.

Aphthous ulcers These are painful white ulcers with red margins over the gums and inner lining of mouth cavity (buccal mucosa). Due to pain, there is excessive salivation and child refuses to eat. They are caused by recurrent infections by herpes simplex or adenovirus.

Appendicitis Appendix is a finger-like appendage on the intestine at the junction between small and large intestine (cecum). Appendicitis is inflammation of the appendix due to infection. It is associated with fever, vomiting, pain and tenderness over the right lower abdomen (iliac region).

Arthralgias They are characterized by non-specific pain or discomfort in one or several joints without any localized inflammatory signs. The common causes of arthralgias in children include growing pains, trauma, transient synovitis, osteochondrosis and acute leukemia.

Arthritis Inflammation of the joints resulting in pain and swelling due to infection or autoimmune disorder.

Ascariasis Infestation with round worms is called ascariasis. It may be associated with increased appetite and abdominal pain. At times there may be no symptoms.

Asthma Wheezing and difficulty in breathing due to allergic condition of air passages is called bronchial asthma. There is constitutional or hereditary predisposition. The symptoms occur due to bronchospasm, i.e. reversible narrowing of air passages.

Atopy There is genetic or familial tendency for development of allergic or hypersensitivity disorders such as eczema, atopic dermatitis, hay fever and bronchial asthma. It is an immediate hypersensitivity disorder that is mediated through IgE antibodies.

Attention deficit hyperactivity disorder (ADHD) These children may have learning disability due to hyperactivity and poor attention span. They are unable to sit still and are perpetually moving, fidgeting, squirming and poking their fingers into everything. They have an impulsive behavior, blurting out answers before completion of questions and have trouble waiting for their turn.

Autism The mental development may be normal up to certain age and then these children regress especially in their social interactions and speech. They lack emotional warmth and do not like to be held or cuddled. They have no or brief eye contact. They may have intense liking for some inanimate object or toy and react violently to any change in their environment and daily routines. They can be mistaken with children having mental retardation.

B

Bacteria Disease causing germs which produce pus and are not visible to the naked eye. They can be seen under the light microscope.

Balanitis Inflammation of the tip of penis, often associated with a bead of pus and redness. There may be associated urinary tract infection and difficulty in passing urine.

Bed wetting (nocturnal enuresis) Most children are dry at night by the age of 4 to 5 years. However, there is no definite age by which a child learns to remain dry at night. In general, when a school-going (not play school!) child continues to wet his bed regularly (not occasionally) it is called nocturnal enuresis or bed-wetting.

Bell's palsy There is sudden onset of unilateral lower motor neuron facial nerve palsy like a bolt from the blue. There may be history of exposure to cold or preceding viral infection. Prognosis is usually good.

Birth asphyxia When baby fails to get enough oxygen before and during the process of delivery, it is called birth asphyxia. The cry may be delayed and there may be no breathing efforts for several minutes after birth. The baby may develop convulsions during first day of life and may be sluggish or inactive to suck feeds effectively.

Birth marks The presence of areas of skin discoloration of any shape, size and color are called birth marks. They are usually present at birth but may appear anytime during early infancy. The color of the birth mark may be milky white, pale, dark brown, black, blue or pink-red.

Blinking Involuntary opening and closing of eyelids is called blinking. It is a protective mechanism against dust and bright light and helps to keep the eyes uniformly moist. Excessive or repetitive blinking may be a habit disorder, tics, attention seeking behavior, suggestive of dandruff or an allergic disorder.

Body mass index (BMI) It is calculated by the formula $\frac{\text{Weight (kg)}}{\text{Height (meters)}^2}$. A BMI-for-age of higher than 85th percentile is suggestive of overweight and when it is more than 95th percentile, it is diagnostic of obesity.

Boils A painful pus-filled bump under the skin is called a boil or impetigo. The infection starts in the root of hair follicle or sebaceous glands and is most commonly caused by *Staphylococcus aureus*.

Bowed legs In normal newborns when legs are extended, they form a concavity toward inner side due to genu varus. Bowing of legs is normal during first year of life. It is gradually replaced by physiological knock knees.

Breast milk jaundice Breastfed babies have a greater incidence and severity of jaundice. Jaundice may last for 6–10 weeks. The infant remains active, feeds well and passes yellow-colored stools and water-like urine. It is a benign condition and does not need any treatment.

Breath holding spells These are extreme forms of temper tantrums which usually occur in sensitive and stubborn children of over indulgent parents or grandparents. The baby cries either due to temper tantrum or injury, cries loudly, holds his breath during a prolonged uninterrupted spell of crying and becomes blue and limp or stiff. These spells may occur at any age but are most common between 6 months and 3 years.

Bronchiolitis It is an acute viral infection (usually due to respiratory syncitial virus or RSV) of lungs commonly occurring during 6 months to 2 years of age. There is fever, symptoms of common cold and increasing respiratory difficulty with wheezing. The condition may be confused with pneumonia or bronchospasm due to asthmatic bronchitis.

Bruxism The grinding of teeth during sleep is called bruxism. Some children may grind their teeth during waking hours. It is not a sign of worm infestation. It may be a symptom of release of tension or stress at night due to unexpressed anger and resentment during the day. It is a benign condition and disappears spontaneously.

C

Cancer Abnormal, excessive and disordered growth of cells that are malignant and invade the surrounding tissues and may disseminate and invade tissues and organs at distant sites (metastases).

Candida albicans A yeast-like fungus that may cause a diaper rash and infection in the mouth (thrush). Fungal infections are common in immunocompromised children and patients receiving broad-spectrum antibiotics.

Caput succedaneum There is a boggy, diffuse edematous swelling of soft tissues of scalp over the presenting part in a baby born by vaginal delivery. The swelling is present at birth, it is pitting, non-fluctuant and not limited by sutures unlike, cephalhematoma.

Cardiopulmonary resuscitation (CPR) An emergency procedure to maintain airways, breathing and circulation by using artificial breathing and chest compressions in children who develop respiratory failure, cardiac arrest or combined cardiorespiratory arrest.

Caries teeth Caries occur due to excessive intake of sweets (chocolates, candies, soft drinks, etc.) which promote the growth of bacteria in the mouth leading to erosion of hard covering of teeth which is called enamel. The destruction of teeth may lead to formation of cavities which is usually associated with toothache. Caries may involve both primary (milk teeth) as well as permanent teeth.

Celiac disease It is a T cell immune-mediated enteropathy to gluten, which is found in wheat, rye and barley. It is characterized by chronic or recurrent diarrhea (after weaning), severe growth retardation, anemia and a variety of other intestinal and extraintestinal manifestations. Elevation of antibodies against human recombinant tissue transglutaminase (tTG IgA) enzyme and global villus atrophy on duodenal biopsy are diagnostic.

Cephalhematoma There is subperiosteal collection of blood secondary to difficult or vacuum assisted vaginal delivery. The fluctuant swelling appears after 2–3 days and does not cross the suture lines. Depending upon its size, the swelling resolves spontaneously over a period of few days or weeks.

Cerebral palsy Delayed motor milestones (delay in head control, sitting, standing, walking, holding objects, etc.) with stiffness or spasticity of limbs is called cerebral palsy. It occurs due to brain damage before, during or soon after birth. It may be associated with convulsions and mental retardation. The condition is non-hereditary and nonprogressive.

Chickenpox (chhotti mata) It is a viral infection due to varicella. There are "crops" of skin rashes (red patches, red pimples, blisters like "dew drops", etc.) mostly on the trunk with fever and itching. Following recovery, some individuals may manifest with herpes zoster or shingles (painful streak of blisters on one side of the trunk) during adulthood.

Chikungunya It is a viral disease which is transmitted to human by the bites of female species of *Aedes aegypti*. There is acute onset of fever, nausea, headache, redness of eyes, skin rash, severe back pain and widespread arthralgias involving both large and small joints. The disease is self-limiting but joint disability may last for several months or years in some patients.

Choking The mechanical obstruction of the flow of air from the environment to the lungs is called choking. It may be partial or complete, and may occur due to inhalation of a foreign body or compression of upper airway because of angioneurotic edema or external compression.

Chorionic villus sampling It is a prenatal test in which a sample of chorionic villi is removed from the placenta for antenatal diagnosis of a genetic disorder in the fetus. The procedure can be performed from the cervix (transcervical) or the abdominal wall (trans-abdominal).

Circumcision A surgical procedure to remove the foreskin of penis. It may be undertaken for religious or medical reasons.

Cleft palate There is an opening or cleft in the roof of the mouth due to failure of the palatal shelves to come fully together and fuse. It can occur alone or in combination with cleft lip.

Club foot (talipes equinovarus) It is a congenital deformity where one or both the feet are stretched downwards (plantar flexed) and turned inwards (adducted) towards each other.

Color blindness There is reduced ability to differentiate between different colors especially red and green. It is an X-linked disorder that affects 8% men. The disability is life long and there is no specific treatment.

Colostrum The yellowish-thick milk produced during first 2 to 3 days after delivery is called colostrum. It is rich in protein and is replete with protective antibodies. It should never be discarded or denied to the baby.

Coma A deep state of unconsciousness from which a person cannot be aroused by any painful stimulus.

Common cold It is viral infection causing symptoms of fever, runny nose, cough and sneezing due to upper respiratory catarrh. It is a self-limiting disease caused by over 200 antigenically distinct viral agents.

Congenital disorder When a condition exists before, at or soon after birth due to a fetal or developmental cause, it is called congenital. It may be hereditary (genetic) or it may occur due to adverse environmental factors. The disorder may be seen at birth or manifestations may appear later in life.

Congenital malformations (anomalies) These are developmental defects which occur during the phase of embryogenesis, i.e. first 3 months of fetal life. The anomalies may be minor and merely cosmetic or they may be life-threatening by involving vital organ of the body. They are usually present at birth but may be detected any time later in life.

Conjunctivitis It is characterized by redness of one or both the eyes with thin or thick pus discharge. It may occur due to infection (bacterial or viral) or chemical irritation by lamp black soot (*kajal*) or collyrium (*surma*) or as an allergic reaction.

Constipation When a child lacks regular bowel habit and does not pass the stools at least once in a day it is called constipation. Passage of hard stools may produce a small tear (fissure) in the anal orifice leading to pain and bleeding during attempts at defecation, thus further aggravating constipation.

Contraception The methods or devices used to prevent pregnancy are called contraception or birth control. The most common method used is the barrier method with the help of a condom. The condom used by the male partner, not only provides contraception but also protects against development of sexually transmitted diseases.

Convalescence It is a period of recovery and recuperation following an illness. The duration of convalescence depends upon the type and severity of illness. During convalescence, child needs nutritious diet (for catch-up growth) and extra attention.

Convulsion (seizure) Sudden stiffening or twitching movements of a limb or whole body with or without loss of consciousness is called a convulsion, seizure or fit. It may be associated with staring look or uprolling of eyeballs.

Cradle cap Greasy, yellowish crust on the scalp due to excessive production of sebum in newborn babies. It is a form of seborrhea (*roosi*) or dandruff and may cause skin rash with irritation and itching on the face or skin creases.

Cretinism The clinical syndrome due to congenital deficiency of thyroid hormone in children is called cretinism. It is an important cause of preventable and readily treatable cause of mental deficiency.

Croup It is characterized by a harsh, vibratory, high-pitched inspiratory sound with labored breathing. The croupy sound is heard during each breath that the baby takes in (inspiratory sound). The condition may be caused by swelling of larynx because of viral infection or allergic reaction (anaphylaxis) and laryngospasm due to tetany.

Cyanosis When hemoglobin is not properly oxygenated because of serious diseases of the heart or lungs, the blood becomes blue due to formation of carboxy-hemoglobin. Nails, lips and tongue would look blue. Isolated blueness of fingers or toe nails (peripheral cyanosis) may occur because of exposure to cold.

D

Dandruff (*Roosi*) There are whitish-brown flakes on the scalp hair, due to excessive production of sebum and it may even affect the eyebrows and eyelashes. A cradle cap (scaly crust over the top of head) in young infants is a form of dandruff.

Dehydration Deficiency of water in the body (commonly due to vomiting and diarrhea) is called dehydration. The child is irritable because of excessive thirst, eyes are sunken, oral mucosa becomes dry and skin is dry, shrivelled and inelastic. When urine output is reduced or no urine is passed over 6 hours in an infant and 12 hours in an older child, and the child becomes drowsy, it indicates that dehydration is severe.

Dengue fever It is a viral infection due to one of the three dengue viruses transmitted by the bite of infected mosquitoes called *Aedes aegyptiae*. It is characterized by fever, severe backache or bodyaches, skin rash (pin point bleeding spots) and pain in the eyes. Bleeding manifestations, exudation of plasma in subcutaneous tissues and circulatory collapse occurs in serious form of the disease.

Diabetes mellitus Children develop early-onset type-1 or insulin-dependent diabetes mellitus due to lack of insulin because of damage to the pancreas. There is marked elevation of blood glucose with leakage of glucose in the urine. Disease is characterized by excessive appetite (polyphagia), marked urination (polyuria), excessive thirst (polydypsia) and progressive weight loss. In some children, disease may manifest as a life-threatening emergency with sudden onset of vomitings, abdominal pain, fever, drowsiness or coma due to diabetic ketoacidosis.

Diarrhea There is increased frequency of stools which may be semiloose or watery. There is sudden change in the established frequency of bowel motions. Crying may be due to abdominal colic but more often it is due to thirst because of dehydration. The frequency of stooling may vary from 4–5 per day to more than 50 times in a day.

Down syndrome See mongolism.

Drooling The constant dribbling of saliva or watering of mouth is called drooling. It may occur due to excessive production of saliva or because of inability to swallow it. The common causes include mouth ulcers, teething, mouth breathing, cerebral palsy, autism, and bulbar palsy.

Duchenne muscular dystrophy It is a sex-linked or X-linked muscular dystrophy which is limited to boys. There is a progressive loss of muscular activity with difficulty to go upstairs. The child finds great difficulty to stand up from sitting position (Gower sign). The calf muscles are abnormally bulky and prominent.

Dysentery When diarrheal stools contain blood and mucus, it is called dysentery.

Dyslexia It is characterized by difficulty in reading and writing with poor spellings, handwriting and drawing skills in a child with an average or above average intelligence. The child is competent in other skills such as oral class work, puzzles and games. The disorder may run in families.

Dysmenorrhea The occurrence of pain and discomfort or cramps immediately before and during menstruations is called dysmenorrhea. Dysmenorrhea is common during onset of menstrual periods, may be primary or idiopathic, or it may be associated with some pathology in the reproductive organs.

E

Ectopic pregnancy The pregnancy that gets lodged at a site other than the uterus, most commonly in one of the fallopian tubes.

Eczema The allergic condition of the skin is called eczema. In infants, it usually appears as red patches with papules and vesicles on both cheeks and later may spread to the whole body especially creases and flexural surfaces of joints. There is severe itching which makes the child irritable with disturbed sleep pattern. The condition is called atopic dermatitis when there is a family history of allergy.

Edema Accumulation of fluids in the tissues leading to puffiness of face, swelling of feet and boggyness over lower back (in infants).

Encephalitis Acute inflammation of the brain or encephalon is called encephalitis. There is sudden onset of fever, headache, confusion, drowsiness and seizures. It may be associated with meningitis, when it is called meningoencephalitis.

Encopresis Soiling of under pants with feces, because of overflow of feces due to persistent constipation as a consequence of psychological refusal to evacuate bowels.

Enuresis See bed-wetting.

Epilepsy When there are repeated convulsions due to a brain disorder it is called epilepsy. Most epileptic children have normal intelligence and in a significant proportion of cases no cause is found even on detailed investigations. Family history may be positive.

Epistaxis There is bleeding from one or both nostrils. The swallowed blood may be vomited or passed in stools (black stools called melena).

Evening colic It is characterized by sudden onset of bouts of unexplained, inconsolable crying spells in the evening after a few days or weeks of birth. The crying episodes occur due to intestinal colic because of "blocked wind" and are associated with excessive gurgling sounds on palpation of abdomen. The condition resolves spontaneously after 4–6 weeks of nightmare!

Exanthematous illness The infective illnesses which are associated with characteristic skin eruption (exanthemata) are called exanthematous illness. Most commonly they occur due to viral infections (measles, rubella, chickenpox, roseola infantum, herpes zoster,

hand-foot-mouth disease) but can also occur in associated with bacterial infections ilke scarlet fever, meningococcemia, typhus and typhoid fever. They may be associated with internal eruptions over the mucosal surfaces which is called as enanthem. Koplik spots are the characteristic enanthem of measles.

F

Failure to thrive A syndrome in which a young child fails to have satisfactory weight gain and linear growth (poor gain in height) due to a chronic illness or psycho-social reasons.

Family life education It pertains to knowledge and skills for healthy functioning of family unit by virtue of good communication skills, knowledge of human psychology, decision making skills, positive self-esteem and healthy interpersonal relationships. It also indudes knowledge and skills about creative expression of love and safe sexual activity between a man and a woman. It is desirable to impart knowledge and skills pertaining to family life and reproductive health to boys and girls of middle school (5th grade onwards).

Febrile convulsions Seizures occurring in association with fever in children between 6 months to 3 years age. The condition is benign and does not lead to epilepsy.

Fetus Baby in the mother's womb is called fetus. During first 9 weeks it is called an embryo.

Fever Elevation of oral body temperature to above 100°F (37.8°C) is called fever.

Fluorosis It is a chronic condition caused by excessive intake fluorine contaminated water. In human dwellings where fluorine content of water exceeds 2 ppm (>2 mg/L), the population is at risk to develop fluorosis. The usual features including mottling and discoloration of teeth, crippling deformities of long bones and spine.

Fomites Any inanimate object or article capable of transferring an infectious agent from one individual to the other is called a fomite. Infact, the diseases that spread by droplet or fecal-oral transmission often do so through fomites.

Fontanels The gaps or soft spots between the skull bones at birth are called fontanels. These gaps are present to allow the brain to grow during infancy and early childhood. The largest fontanel (anterior fontanel) is located on the top of the head or crown. It feels soft to touch because it is not covered by any skull bone and may show pulsations with each heart beat. It usually closes by the age of 12 to 18 months.

Food poisoning Intake of contaminated food (Road-side *Dhabha* or food prepared for social functions or stale food) is followed by sudden occurrence of severe vomitings, abdominal cramps and diarrhea. When food is contaminated with toxins, the symptoms appear within few hours, while in case of infected food, the onset of symptoms is delayed depending upon the incubation period of pathogens. Foods eaten raw or without cooking are more likely to cause infection or infestation. Water, meat, eggs, milk, and dairy products are commonly contaminated.

G

Galactogogues The substances that promote lactation are called galactogogues. A large number of kitchen items are credited to improve lactation but none is satisfactory. The list includes *shatavari*, fenugreek, fennel, anise, milk thistle, alfa alfa, vervain, oatmeal, etc. Pharmaceutical agents like domperidone and metoclopramide may improve lactation by interacting with dopamine D_2 receptors to increase the production of prolactin.

Gastroenteritis See diarrhea.

Gastroesophageal reflux Regurgitation of stomach contents into the esophagus because of laxity of gastroesophageal junction which may lead to heart burn, vomiting and aspiration into the lungs. It may cause wheezing in young infants.

Genetic disorders A genetic disorder is caused by an abnormality in an individual's DNA. It may be a single gene disorder (inborn error of metabolism) or may occur due to presence of an additional (trisomy 21 or Down syndrome) or absence (XO or Turner syndrome) of an entire chromosome.

Geographic tongue The presence of bizarre shapes and patterns of grey-white areas on the upper surface of tongue with advancing slightly elevated margins resembling like a map is called geographic tongue. The shape and pattern of the map may change from time to time. The condition is of no significance and does not require any treatment.

Ghutti *Janam ghutti* is an ayurvedic concoction of several ingredients which is used for treatment of a variety of disorders in infants like constipation, diarrhea, colic, wind, teething, etc. It has no proven utility and should preferably be avoided.

Goiter Enlargement or swelling of thyroid gland (which is located on the front of middle of the neck) is called goiter.

Growing pains Children between 2 and 10 years of age often complain of pains in the legs especially during the evening. Pain is usually due to fatigue because of excessive physical activity throughout the day. The condition is often called as "growing pains" because children are actively growing during this period. The pain can be relieved by hot water bath, massage and use of paracetamol.

H

Habit spasms See tics.

Halitosis It is defined as bad breath or unpleasant odor in the exhaled breath. The common causes include blocked nose or mouth breathing; poor orodental hygiene, chronic infection in the nose or sinuses, liver dysfunction and chronic lung disease or bronchiectasis.

Hay fever See allergic rhinitis

Health Health is not merely freedom from disease but it is a state of physical, mental, emotional, social and spiritual wellbeing. There should be feeling of vigour, happiness, poise, peace and confidence in all day-to-day activities.

Heat exhaustion When children play outdoors during hot dry summer months they may develop heat exhaustion due to loss of body fluids and salts because of profuse sweating. The child may complain of headache, weakness and dizziness. Skin is cool and wet due to sweating.

Heat stroke Excessive exposure to extremely hot and dry weather may lead to failure of the body cooling mechanisms when sweat glands are over whelmed. There is sudden rise in body temperature above 105°F (hyperpyrexia). Skin may be dry due to lack of sweating. The child may develop convulsions and becomes delirious, drowsy and even unconscious. Liver dysfunction is invariable.

Hematemesis When vomiting is tinged or mixed with blood it is called hematemesis. It may occur due to bleeding in stomach or due to swallowed blood (epistaxis or bleeding in mouth).

Hematoma A localized collection of blood externally or internally, either spontaneously or following an injury (trauma) is called hematoma.

Hematuria Passage of blood in the urine is called hematuria. It may be microscopic or gross.

Hemophilia It is a sex-linked disorder causing excessive bleeding on minor injury in boys. It is a metabolic disorder due to deficiency of antihemophiliac globulin or factor VIII which is required to stop bleeding.

Hemoptysis Spitting of blood-tinged sputum is called hemoptysis. The common causes include re-infection tuberculosis, pneumonia, swine flu, bronchiectasis, mitral stenosis and pulmonary edema.

Hepatitis Inflammation of liver due to a variety of causes (mostly due to viruses and toxins) is called hepatitis. There is loss of appetite, vomiting, jaundice (yellowness of eyes), high colored urine, pain and tenderness over the liver area (right upper abdomen).

Hernia The protrusion of intestines through the body orifices (like umbilicus, inguinal canal) due to straining and crying is called hernia. It is a boggy, soft swelling which disappears on lying down or by gentle pressure.

Hiccups Sudden, spasmodic contractions of diaphragm with audible sounds are called hiccups. They are common in healthy newborn babies due to distension of stomach after a feed.

Hydrocele It occurs due to collection of fluid in the sac around the testes (scrotum). Unlike hernia, the swelling cannot be reduced by pressure or on lying down. It is usually seen in newborn babies and young infants and disappears spontaneously by 6 months of age.

Hydrocephalus There is excessive accumulation of fluid in the ventricles of brain leading to excessive increase in the size of head, prominent veins over the forehead, bulging of anterior fontanel and downward rolling of eyes (setting-sun sign).

Hyperhidrosis Excessive sweating due to any cause is called as hyperhidrosis. In some children, excessive sweating is physiological or familial, and does not need any treatment. The common causes of hyperhidrosis include over clothing, exercise, humid and warm environment, acute infection, use of antipyretic and hyperthyroidism.

I

Immunization It is a process of producing protective antibodies against serious life-threatening diseases by injecting killed or tamed microbes or by giving toxins of the microbes. Antigen-based vaccines are being increasingly prepared by modern genetic engineering or recombinant technology. Some vaccines provide life-long protection after a single injection while in others booster doses are required to enhance and sustain the level of protective antibodies.

Impetigo Boils over the skin are called impetigo. They are more common in summer and occur due to sweating and poor personal hygiene.

Inflammation A combination of signs and symptoms due to a localized infection are called inflammation. There is fever, swelling, pain, tenderness (pain on touching), redness and warmth at the site of infection.

Inflammatory bowel disease (IBD) It occurs due to an altered immune response of the host to bacterial flora of the gut because of environmental and genetic factors. There are episodes of diarrhea, abdominal pain, passage of blood and mucus in stools (ulcerative colitis, Crohn's disease).

Intelligence quotient It is an estimate of intelligence of person which includes comprehension, analytical ability, reasoning, memory and attention span. The mental capabilities or cognition can be assessed by a number of intelligence tests to calculate mental age of the child. Intelligence quotient is calculated by expressing the mental age of the child as a percentage of his chronological or actual age. The child with an average intelligence has an IQ between 85 and 115.

In-toeing The toes are turned inward like a pigeon (pigeon-toes) due to internal rotation of tibia. It is a common condition in toddlers and usually resolves spontaneously in due cause of time.

Intrauterine growth retardation The fetal growth does not keep pace with duration of gestation either due to adverse uterine conditions or because of fetal abnormalities. When birth weight of a baby is less than 10th percentile for the period of gestation, he is called small-for-dates or labelled to have intrauterine growth retardation.

Intrauterine infection The occurrence of fetal infection in-utero is designated as intrauterine infection. They are rare but may occur due to a variety of pathogens like viruses, bacteria, spirochetes and protozoa. They are popularly described with an acronym of TORCH wherein T stand for toxoplasma, O for others (syphilis, gonococcal ophthalmia, tuberculosis, malaria, varicella, hepatitis B, Coxsackie B, Echo, Parvovirus B19 and HIV), R for rubella, C for cytomegalovirus and H for herpes simplex hominis. Due to relatively a large basket of "others", TORCH acronym has become obsolete and not commonly used.

Irritable bowel syndrome (IBS) It is characterized by vague symptoms of crampy upper abdominal discomfort, altered bowel movements (diarrhea or passage of motion after every meal, constipation), sense of incomplete evacuation, bloating and belching. It is a psychosomatic disorder of unknown etiology affecting school-going children and adolescents.

J

Jaundice Yellowness of eyes (due to elevation of serum bilirubin) and passage of dark turmeric-colored urine is called jaundice.

Junk food The pre-prepared 'fast food' or packaged food that has low nutritional content or contains high concentration of ingredients which can adversely affect the health of the consumer, are labelled as junk food. These pre-cooked foods are deficient in protein, vitamins, minerals and fiber. They are loaded with sugar, saturated fats, trans fats, salt and calories. The examples of western junk food include hamburgers, hot dogs, pizzas, noodles, tacos, processed food, carbonated beverages, snack food and desserts. The commonly consumed Indian junk food include *pakoras, mathis, aloo tikkie, samosa, bathooras, poories, namkeen, paranthas,* etc.

K

Kangaroo-mother care Kangaroo-mother care (KMC) or skin-to-skin contact is based on marsupial care-giving concept of kangaroos to keep their babies in a maternal pouch. Kangaroo-mother care may be continuous or intermittent and can be provided by mother or any other care giver including father. It is a cost-effective and useful strategy to enhance the survival of LBW babies in developing countries having constraints of financial resources and technology.

Kegel exercises The exercises that are done to improve the tone of perineal muscles are called kegel exercises. They are useful to improve the strength of perineal muscles during pregnancy. Mother is asked to contract or tense the perineal muscles, the way it is done to stop passage of urine and stool. She is asked to hold the muscles tight as long as she can do and then slowly release and relax the muscles for several seconds. She is advised to do at least 20–25 repetitions of kegels at various times of the day while sitting, standing, attending phone, watching TV, lying down or doing household chores.

Kernicterus It is a bilirubin encephalopathy due to elevated unconjugated bilirubin level during first week of life. The neonatal features include lethargy, shrill cry, "setting sun sign", seizures, backward arching of neck and trunk (opisthotonos). During follow-up, these infants manifest neuromotor retardation, rigidity of limbs, yellow staining of teeth and deafness.

Knock knees A deformity of the legs wherein when knees touch each other, the ankles are wide apart. Most healthy preschool children have mild knock knees with a distance of <5 cm between two ankles when child stands with knees touching together.

L

Laryngomalacia There is flaccidity or easy collapsibility of aryepiglottic folds of wind pipe or larynx, which produces a stridor or crowing sound after one or two weeks of birth. The stridor is inspiratory, low-pitched, vibratory or fluttering in character like undulating flutter of curtains exposed to a blast of wind. The condition is benign and intermittent and resolves spontaneously in a few months.

Leprosy It is a chronic infectious disease caused by *Mycobacterium leprae* which predominantly affect the skin and nerves and may cause severe disfigurement and disability. Infection is transmitted after a long and close contact with an infectious patient of leprosy.

Leukemia The cancer of blood (usually white blood cells) is called leukemia and it can occur at any age.

Lockjaw Inability to open the mouth is called lockjaw or trismus. In association with muscle spasms on touch, it is a classical sign of tetanus. Other causes of lockjaw include arthritis of temporomandibular joint, injury to the jaw, syndrome of brainstem dysfunction, tumor, encephalitis, phenothiazine toxicity and strychnine poisoning.

Low birth weight baby A baby with a birth weight of less than 2500 g (<5.5 lbs) is called a low birth weight baby. The baby may be born early (premature) or born at term but suffered from intrauterine growth restriction (IUGR).

M

Malaria It occurs due to infection with blood parasites, which are transmitted by the bites of infected female anopheles mosquitoes. The two common parasites are *P. vivax* and *P. falciparum*. It is usually characterized by sudden onset of high grade fever with feeling of chills and rigors (shivering). In *P. vivax* infection, fever typically occurs on alternate days.

Mantoux test It is a test to assess the delayed hyper-sensitivity skin response to *Mycobacterium tuberculosis*. It is also called tuberculin test, PPD test and Pirquet test. 0.1 mL of 2 Tu PPD RT23 is injected intradermally over anterior surface of left forearm. The test site is examined after 48–72 hours for development of swelling or induration (not erythema or redness). When induration is 10 mm or more, the test is reported as positive. The positive test indicates that either the patient is suffering from tuberculosis or he had exposure to tuberculosis in the past.

Measles (*Khasra*) It is a common viral infection which starts with fever, cough and cold. After 4 days, fever shoots up and child develops a pink rash starting on the face and then spreading to the whole body.

Meningitis Infection of the brain with inflammation of its membranes or meninges covering the brain and spinal cord is called meningitis. It may be caused by pyogenic bacteria, tubercular bacilli, viruses and fungi. It is characterized by fever, headache, vomiting, photophobia and neck rigidity.

Mental retardation Mental retardation or mental subnormality is a generalized neurodevelopmental disorder characterized by significantly impaired intellectual and adaptive functioning. It may be isolated or associated with motor disability, seizures and abnormalities in special senses.

Metabolic syndrome X It is a metabolic disorder which is associated with five risk factors like obesity (BMI >30 kg/m^2), high blood pressure (>130/85 mm Hg), elevated blood sugar (insulin resistance), high serum triglycerides (>150 mg/dL) reduced level of high-density lipoproteins (HDL < 40 mg/dL). The syndrome X is a recognized risk factor for development of cardiovascular disease and type 2 diabetes mellitus in adult life.

Microcephaly When head size is abnormally small, it is called microcephaly. It may occur due to early fusion of sutures and skull bones (craniosynostosis) or poor growth of brain. The latter is usually associated with mental deficiency.

Micronutrients The chemical elements or nutrients required in trace amounts for the normal growth, development, physiological and metabolic wellbeing of living organism. They include vitamins and trace minerals.

Migraine A specific type of periodic headache which is often one sided and usually associated or preceded by nausea, vomiting and visual disturbances. Migraines are more common in girls and often run in families.

Milestones of development The important stages in the development of children are called milestones. The components of development include motor (gross and fine), social, adaptive and speech. The key milestones in infancy include social smile (6–8 weeks), head control (4 months), sitting (6 months), crawling (8–10 months), standing (10–12 months), and walking (12–18 months).

Mongolian blue spots These are flat blue-gray skin marks with irregular shapes over lower back and buttocks which are present at birth. They are benign and disappear spontaneously after a few months or years. They have nothing to do with mongolism or Down syndrome.

Mongolism (Down syndrome) It is a chromosomal disorder, where instead of normal pair of 21 chromosomes, there is one additional 21 chromosome (trisomy-21). The child has typical soft round face, small head, widely spaced upward slanted eyes, single transverse crease (simian crease) in the palms, flabby muscles and mental subnormality.

Motion sickness (travelling sickness) During travel by road or sea, some individuals develop nausea, vertigo (spinning of head) and vomiting. It usually occurs travelling in a car or bus through a hilly track having curves and culverts up and down the hill.

Mumps (*Kanpedey*) In this viral infection, there is painful swelling of one or both the parotid glands which are located infront of the angles of the jaw and below the lobules of ears.

N

Newborn baby Infant during first 28 days of life is called a newborn baby or neonate.

O

Obesity When body mass index (BMI) is above 85th percentile, it is suggestive of overweight while obesity is diagnosed when BMI is equal to or more than 95th percentile. BMI (kg/m^2) is calculated by the formula: $\dfrac{\text{Weight (kg)}}{\text{Height (meters)}^2}$. The commonly accepted BMI ranges are underweight: <18.5, normal weight: 18.5 to 25, overweight: 25 to 30, obese: >30.

Oral rehydration solution Oral rehydration solution (ORS) is a specially formulated electrolyte solution which is given to prevent and treat dehydration due to acute gastrointestinal disorders and reduces the need for intravenous rehydration therapy. The currently recommended WHO-ORS contains sodium chloride 2.6 g (140 mOsm/L), potassium chloride 1.5 g (20 mOsm/L), trisodium citrate 2.9 g (10 mOsm/L), glucose 13.5 g (75 mOsm/L) in one liter of water. It is one of the greatest advances of 20th century to reduce the risk of diarrhea-related mortality in children.

Osteomyelitis Bacterial infection of the bone associated with signs of inflammation is called osteomyelitis. Drainage of pus and antibiotic treatment may be required for several weeks due to poor penetration of antibiotics because of poor blood supply to the bone.

Otitis media Infection of middle ear usually following an episode of common cold. If diagnosis is delayed, the ear drum perforates with discharge of pus through the ear.

P

Pacifier The use of a pacifier or dummy (binky, soother or teether) nipple is a common practice in the West to keep the infant pacified while mother is busy with her household chores. It is a rubber, plastic or silicone nipple which is given to the cranky infant to suck and remain quiet. It should be avoided in Indian setting because of risk of colic, diarrhea, ear infection and malnutrition.

Pelvic inflammatory disease (PID) Ascending infection of the genital tract, uterus and fallopian tubes in adolescent girls due to poor hygienic conditions or unsafe sex. It is caused by bacteria (usually chlamydia, gonococci and a variety of other pathogens) and may cause infertility (inability to conceive) due to blockage of fallopian tubes if not treated promptly with antibiotics.

Phimosis When foreskin (prepuce) of the penis cannot be retracted it is called phimosis. Foreskin is normally not retractable during first 2 years of life.

Pica Eating of mud or other non-edible objects is called pica. It may lead to frequent episodes of diarrhea and worm infestation or lead poisoning. It may be a symptom of iron deficiency and often resolves after administration of iron supplements.

Placenta previa Placenta is located in the lower segment of the uterus leading to antepartum hemorrhage (APH) at the onset of labor.

Pneumonia Infection of lungs (due to bacteria, viruses, fungi) is called pneumonia. It may affect one (lobar pneumonia) or both the lungs (bronchopneumonia or double pneumonia). It is often preceded by common cold. The child has fever, cough, rapid and distressed breathing.

Poliomyelitis It is a water-borne viral infection which affects the spinal cord. The initial symptoms are like common cold with body aches and stiffness of back and neck. It may be followed by sudden development of flaccid (limp) asymmetric paralysis of one or several limbs. There may be breathing difficulty when chest muscles are affected.

Post-term infant Baby born after 42 weeks of pregnancy is called post-term or post mature.

Prebiotics The non-digestible food ingredients or dietary fiber and substrates (such as fructo-oligosaccharide, galacto-oligosaccharide, oligofructose and inulin) that promote the growth of probiotics are called prebiotics.

Preterm baby Any baby born before 37 weeks of pregnancy is called premature or preterm baby.

Prickly heat (miliria rubra) During hot and humid weather, development of fine pinhead-sized pinkish itchy rash on the neck and trunk is called prickly heat.

Probiotics The health-friendly bacteria in the gut are called probiotics (promote life). They are present in plenty in human milk (*Lactobacillus acidophilus*, *Bifidobacterium*) and yoghurt or curd. They prevent the entry of harmful bacteria and food allergens through gut, promote digestion and absorption of food and stimulate gut immunity.

Puberty When a child has achieved complete sexual maturation to become an adult, he or she has attained puberty. It is a state of sexual development when an adolescent becomes an adult and is capable to beget or bear children. The girl starts menstruating (12–14 years) and the boy would have achieved adult size of the genitals (14–16 years).

Q

Q fever It is a zoonotic disease caused by *Coxiella burnetii* through contact with an aborting or parturient cattle, sheep and goats. The common symptoms include fever, chills, night sweats, headache and chest pain. Abortion and premature delivery may occur if infection occurs during pregnancy.

Quinsy The development of peritonsillar abscess between one of the tonsils and pharyngeal wall is called quinsy. It is a serious complication of untreated tonsillitis which is characterized by high grade fever, hoarseness of voice, toxemia, dysphagia, and obvious unilateral bulge of one of the tonsils. It is a definitive indication for tonsillectomy.

R

Rabies It is a life-threatening viral infection which is usually caused by the bite of a rabid dog. It can also occur due to the bite by infected monkeys, mongoose, bats, cats, foxes and jackals. There are acute neurological manifestations with severe agitation and spasms of muscles of swallowing at the sight of water (hydrophobia). It can be prevented by vaccination and administration of human rabies immunoglobulins (RIG) but once disease occurs it is invariably fatal.

Retinopathy of prematurity Retinopathy of prematurity (ROP) is a dreaded complication of unmonitored oxygen therapy in preterm babies with a gestation of less than 34 weeks. It is characterized by abnormal proliferation of small retinal blood vessels as a consequence of high oxygen tension in arterial blood and is a leading cause of preventable blindness in developed countries.

Rhesus isoimmunization Rhesus incompatibility between the mother and her baby (Rh-negative mother and Rh-positive fetus) is an important cause of rhesus isoimmunization which can lead to development of severe jaundice in a newborn baby. It is preventable by timely administration of anti-D antibodies intramuscularly during pregnancy (28–32 weeks) and within 72 hours of delivery.

Rheumatic fever When a sore throat due to streptococcal infection is not adequately treated, it may be followed 2 weeks later by development of fever, migratory joint pains and damage to the heart.

Rheumatoid arthritis It is an autoimmune disorder causing intractable and recurrent inflammatory involvement of multiple joints with special predilection for the small joints.

Rickets Rickets is a disease of growing bones in children due to deficiency of vitamin D. In adults, vitamim D deficiency causes osteomalacia.

Rubella (German measles) It is a viral infection which produces a mild disease with skin rash. There may be symptoms of common cold for 1–2 days followed by diffuse maculo-papular reddish skin rash over the trunk. There may be painful enlargement of lymphnodes located on the back of the neck. When German measles occurs in early pregnancy there is a risk of development of serious congenital malformations in the fetus (congenital rubella syndrome). It is characterized by triad of cataract, sensorineural deafness and congenital heart disease (patent ductus arteriosus and pulmonary artery stenosis).

S

Scabies This is an infection due to a tiny female mite (*Sarcoptes scabiei*) because of poor personal hygiene and use of infected bed sheets. There are pinhead sized pimples between the webs of fingers, wrists, body creases and genital area. Itching is marked and worse at night.

Sexually transmitted diseases (STDs) Diseases contracted by indulging in unsafe sexual practices with multiple sex partners. The list includes candida albicans, gonorrhea, syphilis, chlamydiae, mycoplasma, genital herpes, venereal warts, chancroid, lymphogranuloma venereum, HIV, human papillomavirus, and pelvic inflammatory disease.

Sinusitis Infections and inflammation of sinuses is called sinusitis. The sinuses are air-filled spaces which are located in the bones around the nose, forehead, cheeks and eyes. The usual symptoms include persistent fever, discomfort and local tenderness, blocked nose with purulent discharge, non-resonant voice, sogginess and black circles under the eyes.

Spina bifida A congenital defect characterized by incomplete closure of spinal vertebrae that encase the spinal cord. The defect may be silent or associated with a boggy swelling due to protrusion of spinal membranes or part of the neural tissue through the defect (meningocele or meningomyelocele). The latter may be associated with hydrocephalus and neurological deficits in the lower limbs.

Squint The eyes are not properly aligned and they look in different directions (crossed eyes). Squint is common during early life but usually disappears spontaneously by the age of 6 months. It may be paralytic or concomitant (due to amblyopia or lazy eye).

Stillbirths Intermediate and late fetal deaths after the gestation of 20 weeks or fetal weight of more than 500 g or lenght of more than 25 cm are designated still births.

Stridor It is a harsh, high-pitched vibratory respiratory sound, usually inspiratory but may be biphasic in character. It is produced by turbulence of airflow through partially blocked upper airway (larynx and trachea). It is usually associated with brassy or barking cough and hoarseness of voice. The term is interchangeably used with croup.

Stunting It is a measure of chronic malnutrition when height-for-age is below minus 2 standard deviations (severe stunting) of the median WHO child growth standards. In India, almost one-half (48%) of under-5 children are stunted.

Stye Inflammation of the eyelid due to infection of the follicle of the eye lashes is called stye. It may occur due to rubbing of eyes with dirty fingers, use of lamp black soot (*kajal*) or general run down condition of health.

Swaddling Swaddling is a cultural practice in temperate countries where infants are tightly wrapped in a sheet or blanket to restrain and restrict movements of their limbs. Infant is disturbed less and is able to sleep better and maintain body temperature in winter. The practice is gradually waning off due to increased risk of sudden infant death syndrome (SIDS) and developmental dysplasia of the hip (DDH).

Syncope Syncope or fainting or swooning is a temporary loss of consciousness and muscle strength due to sudden drop in blood pressure. It may be preceded or associated with lightheadedness, dizziness, sweating, pallor, and blurred vision. It is common in adolescent girls. The common causes include anxiety, pain, orthostatic hypotension, abnormal heart rhythm, cardiac valvular dysfunction, hypoxia and hypoglycemia.

T

Teeth grinding See bruxism.

Tetany The neuromuscular irritability and spasm of skeletal muscles due to hypocalcemia is called tetany. Rarely, it may be associated with spasm of larynx (laryngospasm) leading to breathing difficulty and stridor.

Thalassemia major It is a genetic disorder, which is characterized by formation of defective hemoglobin. Instead of mature or adult hemoglobin, there is excessive amount of fetal hemoglobin. The child manifests with progressive anemia from early life requiring repeated blood transfusions. Both parents carry the abnormal gene and have minor thalassemia. Bone marrow or stem cell transplant, a complex and expensive technology, may provide cure. Thalassemia minor is associated with mild anemia with elevated levels of HbA_2 hemoglobin.

Thrush This is an infection of the oral cavity caused by a fungus (*Candida albicans*). There are white patches with red margins distributed over the tongue and the inner surface of lips and cheeks. The child may have difficulty in feeding due to pain and discomfort.

Tics Habit spasms or tics are stereotyped, involuntary non-rhythmic and repetitive movements of a particular part of the body. The common tics include shrugging of shoulders, blinking of eyes, twisting of neck and throat clearing noises or dry coughing.

Toe-walking Most infants walk on their toes unlike adults who walk heel-to-toes. The habit of toe-walking gradually disappears but may persist in patients with cerebral palsy, Duchenne muscular dystrophy, and autism spectrum disorder.

Tonsillitis Infection and inflammation of tonsils may occur due to a bacterial or viral infection. There is fever, sore throat and tonsils are markedly enlarged and intensely red in color.

Tonsils Tonsils are pads of lymphoid tissue, one on either side of the throat. These can be seen as rounded projections in the throat on asking the child to widely open his mouth.

Torticollis It is a condition of sudden onset with dystonic turning or twisting of head towards one side with painful spasm of neck muscles. The condition is also called wry neck. The top of head is tilted to one side while chin points to the other side. The condition may be congenital or acquired due to sudden exposure to cold, inflammatory condition of neck muscles, trauma and intake of certain drugs.

Typhoid fever It is a water-borne infection due to *Salmonella typhi*. There is a history of prolonged fever with toxemia but without any specific diagnostic symptoms. When a fever does not resolve by 5–7 days time, the possibility of typhoid fever should be seriously considered.

U

Undescended testis Cryptorchidism or undescended testis is diagnosed when one or both testes fail to descend into scrotal sac. Almost 30% of preterm infants have undescended testis but overall incidence of cryptorchidism is about 1% at one year of age. The condition should not be confused with retractable testis.

Urticaria (*Hives, chhapaaki*) It is an allergic disorder with sudden appearance of red blotchy patches over the skin with raised irregular margins. The central areas are relatively pale. There is intense itching. The patches may be very large in size when it is called giant urticaria. It may occur due to allergic response to an infection, drugs, certain eatables or internal diseases.

V

Varicella See chickenpox.

Viruses They are extremely tiny (15–300 nm size which is about one-hundredth the size of an average bacterium) disease producing germs which are not visible under the ordinary microscope. They can even pass through fine filters which usually retain bacteria. They can be seen under an electron microscope.

Vitamins Vitamins are micronutrients which are essential for the nutritional and metabolic needs of the body. They are classified into two broad groups; water soluble (vitamin B complex, vitamin C) and fat soluble (vitamin A, vitamin D, vitamin E and vitamin K).

W

Warts They are thick, rough papules or elevations with irregular surface mostly distributed on the dorsum of hands and fingers. They are caused by a viral infection.

Wheezing It is a rasping or audible whistling sound produced as a result of obstruction or spasm of the bronchial tubes.

Weaning It is a process of gradually introducing semisolid foods and reducing the intake of mother's milk. After 6 months of age, breastfeeding alone is not able to sustain the growth of the infant unless home-made nutritious weaning foods are introduced to meet the increasing nutritional demands.

Whooping cough (pertussis) It is caused by an infection with a bacterium called *Bardotella pertussis*. There are initial symptoms of common cold which are followed by intractable spasmodic bouts of coughing. During the bout of coughing face becomes red and child may vomit. The prolonged bout of cough is followed by a loud croaky sound or a "whoop" when child takes in a deep breath.

X

Xerophthalmia There is dryness of eyes because of failure to produce tears, mostly as a consequence of vitamin A deficiency. There is dryness of cornea and conjunctiva which becomes lusterless, dry and wrinkled and if untreated may progress to corneal ulceration and blindness.

Y

Yaws It is a rare chronic disfiguring and debilitating disease most commonly affecting children and caused by pertenue subspecies of *Treponema pallidum*. There is development of nodules on the skin which ulcerate and become intractable. There is thickening of the skin of palms and soles with involvement of small bones and disfigurement of nose. The disease is nonsexual in nature and is spread by direct contact.

Z

Zoonosis The diseases transmitted from animals and vertebrates to human beings are called zoonosis. Animals may serve as a principal or intermediate host or reservoir of infection. The infection may be transmitted directly from the animal to the human being or with the help of another vector such as mosquitoes, fleas and ticks.

Appendices

Appendix I Weight and measurement conversion tables			
Weight equivalents		**Height and weight conversion factors**	
Apothecary	*Metric*	*To convert*	*Multiply by*
1 grain	60 mg or 0.05 g	Inches to centimeters	2.54
15 grain	1000 mg or 1.0 g	Inches to meters	0.0254
60 grain (1 dram)	4 g	Feet to meters	0.3048
8 dram (1 oz)	30 g	Pounds to kilograms	0.4535
1 pound (16 oz)	480 g	Kilograms to pounds	2.2
2.2 pounds	1 kg		

Liquid measures				
Apothecary		*Metric (approximately)*	*Household measures*	
1 minim (drop)		0.06 mL	Teaspoon	5 mL
15 minims		1.0 mL	Tablespoon	15 mL
60 minims (1 fl dram)		3.7 mL	Cup or *katori*	150 mL
8 fl dram (1 fl oz)	29.6 mL	30.0 mL	Glass	250 mL
16 fl oz (1 pint)	473.2 mL	500.0 mL		
32 fl oz (1 quart)	946.4 mL	1000.0 mL		
1 gallon		4 quarts		

Appendix II Temperature equivalents			
Celsius	*Fahrenheit*	*Celsius*	*Fahrenheit*
35.0	95.0	38.6	101.4
35.4	95.7	39.0	102.2
35.8	96.4	39.4	102.9
36.0	96.8	39.8	103.6
36.4	97.5	40.2	104.3
36.8	98.2	40.6	105.1
37.0	98.6	41.0	105.8
37.4	99.3	41.4	106.5
37.8	100.0	41.8	107.2
38.2	100.7	42.0	107.6

The normal body temperature of 98.4 F° corresponds to 36.9 C°. To convert Fahrenheit to Celsius subtract 32 and divide by 1.8. To convert Celsius to Fahrenheit multiply by 1.8 and add 32.

Appendix III Approximate caloric and protein content of common Indian food stuffs (per 100 g)

Food stuff	Calories (kcal)	Protein (g)
Wheat	350	11.0
Rice	345	6.5
Pulses/legumes	350	20–25
Leafy vegetables	25–50	2.0–5.0
Other vegetables, roots and tubers	50–100	1.0–2.5
Groundnuts	550	25.0
Apple	60	0.2
Banana	120	1.2
Flesh foods	150–200	20
Egg	180	13.0
Cow's milk	70	3.5
Ghee and oil	900	–
Sugar	400	–

Adapted from Food and Health, Eds. VR. Murthy, BR. Rama Sastri, K. Srilakshmi. National Institute of Nutrition, Hyderabad, 1979.

1. Standard hen's egg weighs 50–60 g and provides 300 mg cholesterol.

2. *Khichdi* gruel and cooked pulses contain one part of dry food stuff and 4 parts of water. Cooked rice contains one part of rice and one part of water.

3. Average sized *chapati* has 50 g wheat flour.

Appendix IV Recommended daily requirements of balanced diet for Indian children (grams)

Food stuffs	1–3 years	4–6 years	7–9 years	10–12 years	13–18 years**
Cereals	150	200	250	320	400–450
Pulses	40–50*	50–60*	60–70*	60–70*	60–70*
Green leafy vegetables	50	75	75	100	100
Other vegetables, roots and tubers	30	50	50	75	150
Fruits	50	50	50	50	50
Milk	200–250*	200–250*	200–250*	200–250*	200–250*
Fats and oil	20	25	30	35	35–50
Meat, fish or eggs	30	30	30	30	60
Sugar and jaggery	30	40	50	50	50

Adapted from Nutritive Values of Indian Foods, Gopalan C, Rama Sastri BR, Balasubramanian SC (Eds.) Nutritive Values of Indian Foods. ICMR, Hyderabad, India 1980.

* Higher values refer to vegetarian subjects.

** Requirements are higher in adolescent boys than girls.

Appendix V Chronology of human dentition

	Primary or deciduous teeth*			
	Eruption		Shedding	
Teeth	Mandibular	Maxillary	Mandibular	Maxillary
Central incisors	5–7 months	6–8 months	6–7 years	7–8 years
Lateral incisors	7–10 months	8–11 months	7–8 years	8–9 years
Canines	16–20 months	16–20 months	9–11 years	11–12 years
First molars	10–16 months	10–16 months	10–12 years	10–11 years
Second molars	20–30 months	20–30 months	11–13 years	10–12 years

(Contd.)

Appendix V Chronology of human dentition (Contd.)

Secondary or permanent teeth*

Teeth	Begins at	Complete at	Mandibular	Maxillary
Central incisors	3–4 mo	9–10 y	6–7 y	7–8 y
Lateral incisors	Mand. 3–4 mo	10–11 y	7–8 y	8–9 y
	Max. 10–12 mo			
Canines	4–5 mo	12–15 y	9–11 y	11–12 y
First premolars	18–21 mo	12–13 y	10–12 y	10–11 y
Second premolars	24–30 mo	12–14 y	11–13 y	10–12 y
First molars	Birth	9–10 y	6–7 y	6–7 y
Second molars	30–36 mo	14–16 y	12–13 y	12–13 y
Third molars	Mand. 8–10 y	18–25 y	17–22 y	17–22 y
	Max. 7–9 y			

mand, mandible; max, maxilla; mo, months; y, year (s).

There is a wide variation in the eruption of the teeth which is genetically determined. Delayed or advanced dentition is poorly correlated both to the nutritional status and development of the child.

*Milk teeth or primary teeth are white in color and have a smooth edge in contrast to permanent teeth, which have an ivory-white or off-white color and have a finely serrated edge.

Appendix VI Normal blood pressure values at various ages

Age	Mean systolic ±2 SD		Mean diastolic ±2 SD	
	(kPa)	(mm Hg)	(kPa)	(mm Hg)
Newborn	10.6 ± 2.1	80 ± 16	6.1 ± 2.1	46 ± 16
6–12 mo	11.8 ± 3.9	89 ± 29	8 ± 1.3	60 ± 16
1 y	12.8 ± 4	96 ± 30	8.8 ± 3.3	66 ± 25
2 y	13.2 ± 3.3	99 ± 25	8.5 ± 3.3	64 ± 25
3 y	13.3 ± 3.3	100 ± 25	8.9 ± 3.1	67 ± 23
4 y	13.2 ± 2.7	99 ± 20	8.6 ± 2.7	65 ± 20
5–6 y	12.5 ± 1.9	94 ± 14	7.3 ± 1.2	55 ± 9
6–7 y	13.3 ± 2	100 ± 15	7.5 ± 1.2	56 ± 9
7–8 y	13.6 ± 2	102 ± 15	7.5 ± 1.1	56 ± 8
8–9 y	14.0 ± 2.1	105 ± 16	7.6 ± 1.2	57 ± 9
9–10 y	14.2 ± 2.1	107 ± 16	7.6 ± 1.2	57 ± 9
10–11 y	14.8 ± 2.3	111 ± 17	7.7 ± 1.3	58 ± 10
11–12 y	15.0 ± 2.4	113 ± 18	7.8 ± 1.3	59 ± 10
12–13 y	15.3 ± 2.5	115 ± 19	7.8 ± 1.3	59 ± 10
13–14 y	15.7 ± 2.5	118 ± 19	8 ± 1.3	60 ± 10

Source: Forfar JO, Arneil GC. In: Textbook of Pediatrics. 3rd ed. London: Churchill Livingstone; 1984, p 1977–1991.

mo, months(s); SD, standard deviation; y, year(s).

Note: Blood pressure measurement should be made using a cuff covering two-thirds of the upper arm. (1 mm Hg is approximately equal to 133 Pascals (pa) or 1 kilo Pascal = 7.5 mm Hg).

Appendix VII Oxygen therapy and delivery devices

Device	Flow rate	Oxygen concentration
Low flow systems		
Nasal cannula	1–6 Lit/min	Maximum 45%
Nasal catheter	1–6 Lit/min	Maximum 45%
Face mask	5–10 Lit/min	35–60%
Venturi type mask	5–10 Lit/min	25–60%
High flow systems		
Oxygen hood	10–15 Lit/min	80–90%
Partial rebreathing mask	10–12 Lit/min	50–60%
Non-rebreathing mask	10–12 Lit/min	Up to 90%
Anesthesia bag with a non-rebreathing mask	10–12 Lit/min	Up to 95%

lit, liters; min, minutes

Appendix VIII Weight-for-age and length-for-age boys

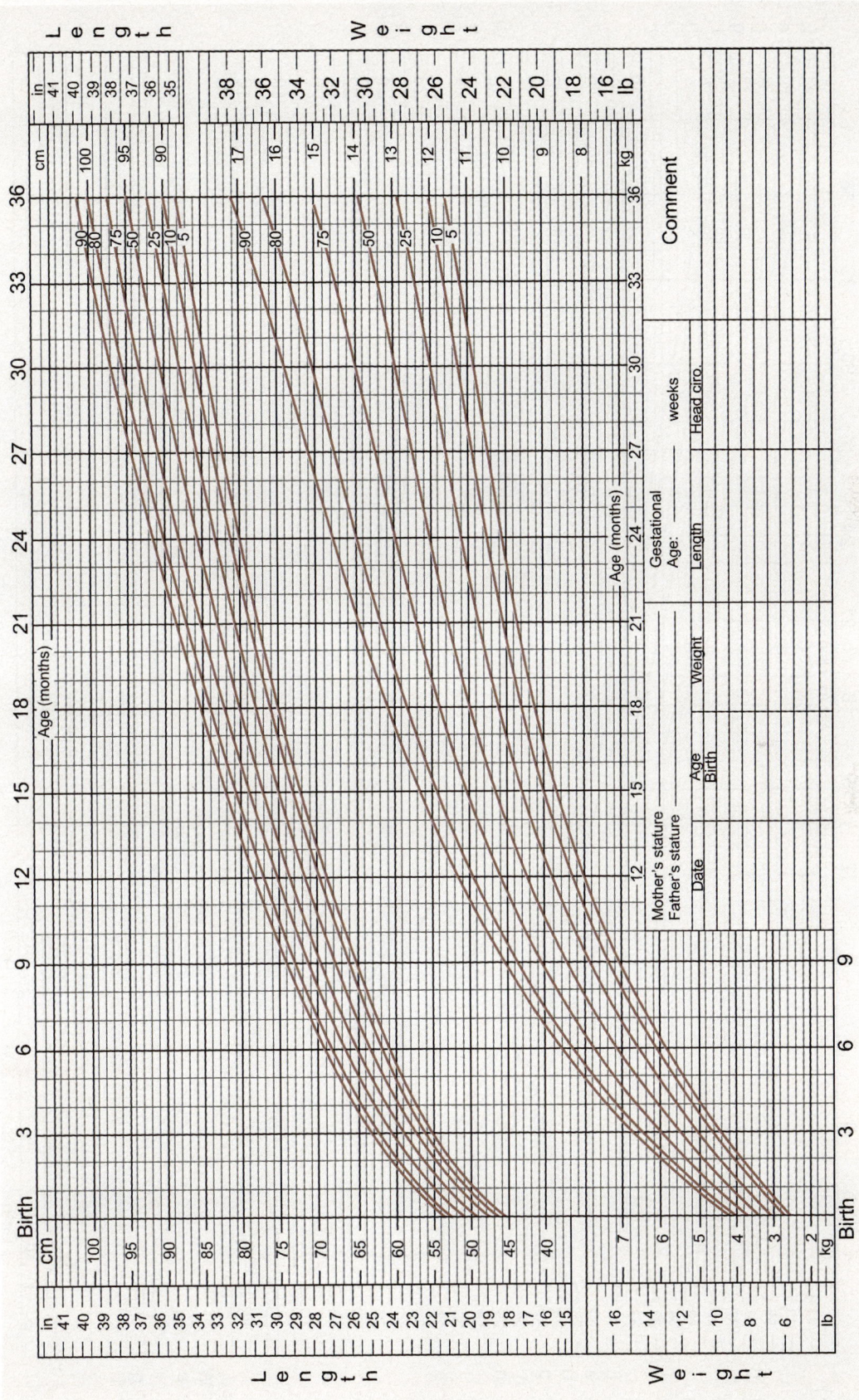

Appendix IX Weight-for-age and length-for-age girls

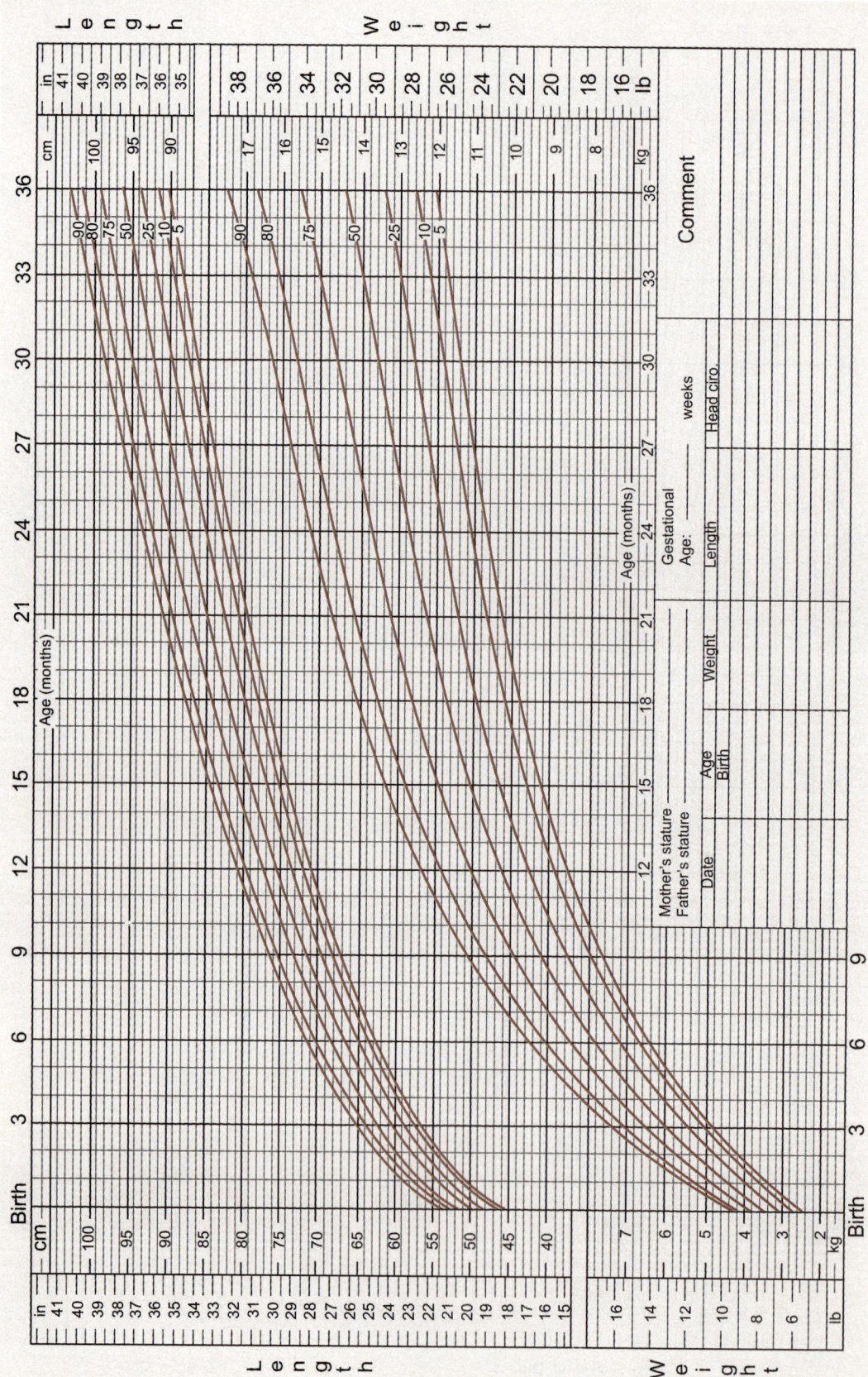

Appendix X Weight-for-age for boys birth to 5 years (percentiles)

Year : Month	Months	3rd	15th	Median	85th	97th
0 : 0	0	2.5	2.9	3.3	3.9	4.3
0 : 1	1	3.4	3.9	4.5	5.1	5.7
0 : 2	2	4.4	4.9	5.6	6.3	7.0
0 : 3	3	5.1	5.6	6.4	7.2	7.9
0 : 4	4	5.6	6.2	7.0	7.9	8.6
0 : 5	5	6.1	6.7	7.5	8.4	9.2
0 : 6	6	6.4	7.1	7.9	8.9	9.7
0 : 7	7	6.7	7.4	8.3	9.3	10.2
0 : 8	8	7.0	7.7	8.6	9.6	10.5
0 : 9	9	7.2	7.9	8.9	10.0	10.9
0 : 10	10	7.5	8.2	9.2	10.3	11.2
0 : 11	11	7.7	8.4	9.4	10.5	11.5
1 : 0	12	7.8	8.6	9.6	10.8	11.8
1 : 1	13	8.0	8.8	9.9	11.1	12.1
1 : 2	14	8.2	9.0	10.1	11.3	12.4
1 : 3	15	8.4	9.2	10.3	11.6	12.7
1 : 4	16	8.5	9.4	10.5	11.8	12.9
1 : 5	17	8.7	9.6	10.7	12.0	13.2
1 : 6	18	8.9	9.7	10.9	12.3	13.5
1 : 7	19	9.0	9.9	11.1	12.5	13.7
1 : 8	20	9.2	10.1	11.3	12.7	14.0
1 : 9	21	9.3	10.3	11.5	13.0	14.3
1 : 10	22	9.5	10.5	11.8	13.2	14.5
1 : 11	23	9.7	10.6	12.0	13.4	14.8
2 : 0	24	9.8	10.8	12.2	13.7	15.1
2 : 1	25	10.0	11.0	12.4	13.9	15.3
2 : 2	26	10.1	11.1	12.5	14.1	15.6
2 : 3	27	10.2	11.3	12.7	14.4	15.9
2 : 4	28	10.4	11.5	12.9	14.6	16.1
2 : 5	29	10.5	11.6	13.1	14.8	16.4
2 : 6	30	10.7	11.8	13.3	15.0	16.6
2 : 7	31	10.8	11.9	13.5	15.2	16.9
2 : 8	32	10.9	12.1	13.7	15.5	17.1
2 : 9	33	11.1	12.2	13.8	15.7	17.3
2 : 10	34	11.2	12.4	14.0	15.9	17.6
2 : 11	35	11.3	12.5	14.2	16.1	17.8
3 : 0	36	11.4	12.7	14.3	16.3	18.0
3 : 1	37	11.6	12.8	14.5	16.5	18.3
3 : 2	38	11.7	12.9	14.7	16.7	18.5
3 : 3	39	11.8	13.1	14.8	16.9	18.7
3 : 4	40	11.9	13.2	15.0	17.1	19.0
3 : 5	41	12.1	13.4	15.2	17.3	19.2
3 : 6	42	12.2	13.5	15.3	17.5	19.4
3 : 7	43	12.3	13.6	15.5	17.7	19.7
3 : 8	44	12.4	13.8	15.7	17.9	19.9
3 : 9	45	12.5	13.9	15.8	18.1	20.1
3 : 10	46	12.7	14.1	16.0	18.3	20.4
3 : 11	47	12.8	14.2	16.2	18.5	20.6
4 : 0	48	12.9	14.3	16.3	18.7	20.9
4 : 1	49	13.0	14.5	16.5	18.9	21.1

(Contd.)

Appendix X Weight-for-age for boys birth to 5 years (percentiles) *(Contd.)*						
Year : Month	*Months*	*3rd*	*15th*	*Median*	*85th*	*97th*
4 : 2	50	13.1	14.6	16.7	19.1	21.3
4 : 3	51	13.3	14.7	16.8	19.3	21.6
4 : 4	52	13.4	14.9	17.0	19.5	21.8
4 : 5	53	13.5	15.0	17.2	19.7	22.1
4 : 6	54	13.6	15.2	17.3	19.9	22.3
4 : 7	55	13.7	15.3	17.5	20.1	22.5
4 : 8	56	13.8	15.4	17.7	20.3	22.8
4 : 9	57	13.9	15.6	17.8	20.5	23.0
4 : 10	58	14.1	15.7	18.0	20.7	23.3
4 : 11	59	14.2	15.8	18.2	20.9	23.5
5 : 0	60	14.3	16.0	18.3	21.1	23.8

Source: de Onis M, Garza C Onyango AW, Martorell R. WHO child growth standards. *Acta Paediatrica (Suppl)* 2006, 450:1–110 and www.who.int/childgrowth/standards/en/.

Appendix X Weight-for-age for girls birth to 5 years (percentiles)						
Year : Month	*Months*	*3rd*	*15th*	*Median*	*85th*	*97th*
0 : 0	0	2.4	2.8	3.2	3.7	4.2
0 : 1	1	3.2	3.6	4.2	4.8	5.4
0 : 2	2	4.0	4.5	5.1	5.9	6.5
0 : 3	3	4.6	5.1	5.8	6.7	7.4
0 : 4	4	5.1	5.6	6.4	7.3	8.1
0 : 5	5	5.5	6.1	6.9	7.8	8.7
0 : 6	6	5.8	6.4	7.3	8.3	9.2
0 : 7	7	6.1	6.7	7.6	8.7	9.6
0 : 8	8	6.3	7.0	7.9	9.0	10.0
0 : 9	9	6.6	7.3	8.2	9.3	10.4
0 : 10	10	6.8	7.5	8.5	9.6	10.7
0 : 11	11	7.0	7.7	8.7	9.9	11.0
1 : 0	12	7.1	7.9	8.9	10.2	11.3
1 : 1	13	7.3	8.1	9.2	10.4	11.6
1 : 2	14	7.5	8.3	9.4	10.7	11.9
1 : 3	15	7.7	8.5	9.6	10.9	12.2
1 : 4	16	7.8	8.7	9.8	11.2	12.5
1 : 5	17	8.0	8.8	10.0	11.4	12.7
1 : 6	18	8.2	9.0	10.2	11.6	13.0
1 : 7	19	8.3	9.2	10.4	11.9	13.3
1 : 8	20	8.5	9.4	10.6	12.1	13.5
1 : 9	21	8.7	9.6	10.9	12.4	13.8
1 : 10	22	8.8	9.8	11.1	12.6	14.1
1 : 11	23	9.0	9.9	11.3	12.8	14.3
2 : 0	24	9.2	10.1	11.5	13.1	14.6
2 : 1	25	9.3	10.3	11.7	13.3	14.9
2 : 2	26	9.5	10.5	11.9	13.6	15.2
2 : 3	27	9.6	10.7	12.1	13.8	15.4
2 : 4	28	9.8	10.8	12.3	14.0	15.7
2 : 5	29	10.0	11.0	12.5	14.3	16.0
2 : 6	30	10.1	11.2	12.7	14.5	16.2
2 : 7	31	10.3	11.3	12.9	14.7	16.5
2 : 8	32	10.4	11.5	13.1	15.0	16.8

(Contd.)

Appendix X Weight-for-age for girls birth to 5 years (percentiles) (Contd.)						
Year : Month	Months	3rd	15th	Median	85th	97th
2 : 9	33	10.5	11.7	13.3	15.2	17.0
2 : 10	34	10.7	11.8	13.5	15.4	17.3
2 : 11	35	10.8	12.0	13.7	15.7	17.6
3 : 0	36	11.0	12.1	13.9	15.9	17.8
3 : 1	37	11.1	12.3	14.0	16.1	18.1
3 : 2	38	11.2	12.5	14.2	16.3	18.4
3 : 3	39	11.4	12.6	14.4	16.6	18.6
3 : 4	40	11.5	12.8	14.6	16.8	18.9
3 : 5	41	11.6	12.9	14.8	17.0	19.2
3 : 6	42	11.8	13.1	15.0	17.3	19.5
3 : 7	43	11.9	13.2	15.2	17.5	19.7
3 : 8	44	12.0	13.4	15.3	17.7	20.0
3 : 9	45	12.1	13.5	15.5	17.9	20.3
3 : 10	46	12.3	13.7	15.7	18.2	20.6
3 : 11	47	12.4	13.8	15.9	18.4	20.8
4 : 0	48	12.5	14.0	16.1	18.6	21.1
4 : 1	49	12.6	14.1	16.3	18.9	21.4
4 : 2	50	12.8	14.3	16.4	19.1	21.7
4 : 3	51	12.9	14.4	16.6	19.3	22.0
4 : 4	52	13.0	14.5	16.8	19.5	22.2
4 : 5	53	13.1	14.7	17.0	19.8	22.5
4 : 6	54	13.2	14.8	17.2	20.0	22.8
4 : 7	55	13.4	15.0	17.3	20.2	23.1
4 : 8	56	13.5	15.1	17.5	20.4	23.3
4 : 9	57	13.6	15.3	17.7	20.7	23.6
4 : 10	58	13.7	15.4	17.9	20.9	23.9
4 : 11	59	13.8	15.5	18.0	21.1	24.2
5 : 0	60	14.0	15.7	18.2	21.3	24.4

Appendix XI Length-for-age for boys birth to 2 years (percentiles)						
Year : Month	Months	3rd	15th	Median	85th	97th
0 : 0	0	46.3	47.9	49.9	51.8	53.4
0 : 1	1	51.1	52.7	54.7	56.7	58.4
0 : 2	2	54.7	56.4	58.4	60.5	62.2
0 : 3	3	57.6	59.3	61.4	63.5	65.3
0 : 4	4	60.0	61.7	63.9	66.0	67.8
0 : 5	5	61.9	63.7	65.9	68.1	69.9
0 : 6	6	63.6	65.4	67.6	69.8	71.6
0 : 7	7	65.1	66.9	69.2	71.4	73.2
0 : 8	8	66.5	68.3	70.6	72.9	74.7
0 : 9	9	67.7	69.6	72.0	74.3	76.2
0 : 10	10	69.0	70.9	73.3	75.6	77.6
0 : 11	11	70.2	72.1	74.5	77.0	78.9
1 : 0	12	71.3	73.3	75.7	78.2	80.2
1 : 1	13	72.4	74.4	76.9	79.4	81.5
1 : 2	14	73.4	75.5	78.0	80.6	82.7
1 : 3	15	74.4	76.5	79.1	81.8	83.9
1 : 4	16	75.4	77.5	80.2	82.9	85.1
1 : 5	17	76.3	78.5	81.2	84.0	86.2

(Contd.)

Appendix XI Length-for-age for boys birth to 2 years (percentiles) (*Contd.*)

Year : Month	Months	3rd	15th	Median	85th	97th
1 : 6	18	77.2	79.5	82.3	85.1	87.3
1 : 7	19	78.1	80.4	83.2	86.1	88.4
1 : 8	20	78.9	81.3	84.2	87.1	89.5
1 : 9	21	79.7	82.2	85.1	88.1	90.5
1 : 10	22	80.5	83.0	86.0	89.1	91.6
1 : 11	23	81.3	83.8	86.9	90.0	92.6
2 : 0	24	82.1	84.6	87.8	91.0	93.6

Appendix XI Height-for-age for boys 2 to 5 years (percentiles)

Year : Month	Months	3rd	15th	Median	85th	97th
2 : 1	25	82.1	84.7	88.0	91.2	93.8
2 : 2	26	82.8	85.5	88.8	92.1	94.8
2 : 3	27	83.5	86.3	89.6	93.0	95.7
2 : 4	28	84.2	87.0	90.4	93.8	96.6
2 : 5	29	84.9	87.7	91.2	94.7	97.5
2 : 6	30	85.5	88.4	91.9	95.5	98.3
2 : 7	31	86.2	89.1	92.7	96.2	99.2
2 : 8	32	86.8	89.7	93.4	97.0	100.0
2 : 9	33	87.4	90.4	94.1	97.8	100.8
2 : 10	34	88.0	91.0	94.8	98.5	101.5
2 : 11	35	88.5	91.6	95.4	99.2	102.3
3 : 0	36	89.1	92.2	96.1	99.9	103.1
3 : 1	37	89.7	92.8	96.7	100.6	103.8
3 : 2	38	90.2	93.4	97.4	101.3	104.5
3 : 3	39	90.8	94.0	98.0	102.0	105.2
3 : 4	40	91.3	94.6	98.6	102.7	105.9
3 : 5	41	91.9	95.2	99.2	103.3	106.6
3 : 6	42	92.4	95.7	99.9	104.0	107.3
3 : 7	43	92.9	96.3	100.4	104.6	108.0
3 : 8	44	93.4	96.8	101.0	105.2	108.6
3 : 9	45	93.9	97.4	101.6	105.8	109.3
3 : 10	46	94.4	97.9	102.2	106.5	109.9
3 : 11	47	94.9	98.5	102.8	107.1	110.6
4 : 0	48	95.4	99.0	103.3	107.7	111.2
4 : 1	49	95.9	99.5	103.9	108.3	111.8
4 : 2	50	96.4	100.0	104.4	108.9	112.5
4 : 3	51	96.9	100.5	105.0	109.5	113.1
4 : 4	52	97.4	101.1	105.6	110.1	113.7
4 : 5	53	97.9	101.6	106.1	110.7	114.3
4 : 6	54	98.4	102.1	106.7	111.2	115.0
4 : 7	55	98.8	102.6	107.2	111.8	115.6
4 : 8	56	99.3	103.1	107.8	112.4	116.2
4 : 9	57	99.8	103.6	108.3	113.0	116.8
4 : 10	58	100.3	104.1	108.9	113.6	117.4
4 : 11	59	100.8	104.7	109.4	114.2	118.1
5 : 0	60	101.2	105.2	110.0	114.8	118.7

Appendix XI Length-for-age for girls birth to 2 years (percentiles)

Year : Month	Months	3rd	15th	Median	85th	97th
0 : 0	0	45.6	47.2	49.1	51.1	52.7
0 : 1	1	50.0	51.7	53.7	55.7	57.4
0 : 2	2	53.2	55.0	57.1	59.2	60.9
0 : 3	3	55.8	57.6	59.8	62.0	63.8
0 : 4	4	58.0	59.8	62.1	64.3	66.2
0 : 5	5	59.9	61.7	64.0	66.3	68.2
0 : 6	6	61.5	63.4	65.7	68.1	70.0
0 : 7	7	62.9	64.9	67.3	69.7	71.6
0 : 8	8	64.3	66.3	68.7	71.2	73.2
0 : 9	9	65.6	67.6	70.1	72.6	74.7
0 : 10	10	66.8	68.9	71.5	74.0	76.1
0 : 11	11	68.0	70.2	72.8	75.4	77.5
1 : 0	12	69.2	71.3	74.0	76.7	78.9
1 : 1	13	70.3	72.5	75.2	77.9	80.2
1 : 2	14	71.3	73.6	76.4	79.2	81.4
1 : 3	15	72.4	74.7	77.5	80.3	82.7
1 : 4	16	73.3	75.7	78.6	81.5	83.9
1 : 5	17	74.3	76.7	79.7	82.6	85.0
1 : 6	18	75.2	77.7	80.7	83.7	86.2
1 : 7	19	76.2	78.7	81.7	84.8	87.3
1 : 8	20	77.0	79.6	82.7	85.8	88.4
1 : 9	21	77.9	80.5	83.7	86.8	89.4
1 : 10	22	78.7	81.4	84.6	87.8	90.5
1 : 11	23	79.6	82.2	85.5	88.8	91.5
2 : 0	24	80.3	83.1	86.4	89.8	92.5

Appendix XI Height-for-age for girls 2 to 5 years (percentiles)

Year : Month	Months	3rd	15th	Median	85th	97th
2 : 1	25	80.4	83.2	86.6	90.0	92.8
2 : 2	26	81.2	84.0	87.4	90.9	93.7
2 : 3	27	81.9	84.8	88.3	91.8	94.6
2 : 4	28	82.6	85.5	89.1	92.7	95.6
2 : 5	29	83.4	86.3	89.9	93.5	96.4
2 : 6	30	84.0	87.0	90.7	94.3	97.3
2 : 7	31	84.7	87.7	91.4	95.2	98.2
2 : 8	32	85.4	88.4	92.2	95.9	99.0
2 : 9	33	86.0	89.1	92.9	96.7	99.8
2 : 10	34	86.7	89.8	93.6	97.5	100.6
2 : 11	35	87.3	90.5	94.4	98.3	101.4
3 : 0	36	87.9	91.1	95.1	99.0	102.2
3 : 1	37	88.5	91.7	95.7	99.7	103.0
3 : 2	38	89.1	92.4	96.4	100.5	103.7
3 : 3	39	89.7	93.0	97.1	101.2	104.5
3 : 4	40	90.3	93.6	97.7	101.9	105.2
3 : 5	41	90.8	94.2	98.4	102.6	106.0
3 : 6	42	91.4	94.8	99.0	103.3	106.7
3 : 7	43	92.0	95.4	99.7	103.9	107.4
3 : 8	44	92.5	96.0	100.3	104.6	108.1
3 : 9	45	93.0	96.6	100.9	105.3	108.8

(Contd.)

Appendix XI Height-for-age for girls 2 to 5 years (percentiles) *(Contd.)*

Year : Month	Months	3rd	15th	Median	85th	97th
3 : 10	46	93.6	97.2	101.5	105.9	109.5
3 : 11	47	94.1	97.7	102.1	106.6	110.2
4 : 0	48	94.6	98.3	102.7	107.2	110.8
4 : 1	49	95.1	98.8	103.3	107.8	111.5
4 : 2	50	95.7	99.4	103.9	108.4	112.1
4 : 3	51	96.2	99.9	104.5	109.1	112.8
4 : 4	52	96.7	100.4	105.0	109.7	113.4
4 : 5	53	97.2	101.0	105.6	110.3	114.1
4 : 6	54	97.6	101.5	106.2	110.9	114.7
4 : 7	55	98.1	102.0	106.7	111.5	115.3
4 : 8	56	98.6	102.5	107.3	112.1	116.0
4 : 9	57	99.1	103.0	107.8	112.6	116.6
4 : 10	58	99.6	103.5	108.4	113.2	117.2
4 : 11	59	100.0	104.0	108.9	113.8	117.8
5 : 0	60	100.5	104.5	109.4	114.4	118.4

Appendix XII Head circumference-for-age for boys birth to 5 years (percentiles)

Year : Month	Months	3rd	15th	Median	85th	97th
0 : 0	0	32.1	33.1	34.5	35.8	36.9
0 : 1	1	35.1	36.1	37.3	38.5	39.5
0 : 2	2	36.9	37.9	39.1	40.3	41.3
0 : 3	3	38.3	39.3	40.5	41.7	42.7
0 : 4	4	39.4	40.4	41.6	42.9	43.9
0 : 5	5	40.3	41.3	42.6	43.8	44.8
0 : 6	6	41.0	42.1	43.3	44.6	45.6
0 : 7	7	41.7	42.7	44.0	45.3	46.3
0 : 8	8	42.2	43.2	44.5	45.8	46.9
0 : 9	9	42.6	43.7	45.0	46.3	47.4
0 : 10	10	43.0	44.1	45.4	46.7	47.8
0 : 11	11	43.4	44.4	45.8	47.1	48.2
1 : 0	12	43.6	44.7	46.1	47.4	48.5
1 : 1	13	43.9	45.0	46.3	47.7	48.8
1 : 2	14	44.1	45.2	46.6	47.9	49.0
1 : 3	15	44.3	45.5	46.8	48.2	49.3
1 : 4	16	44.5	45.6	47.0	48.4	49.5
1 : 5	17	44.7	45.8	47.2	48.6	49.7
1 : 6	18	44.9	46.0	47.4	48.7	49.9
1 : 7	19	45.0	46.2	47.5	48.9	50.0
1 : 8	20	45.2	46.3	47.7	49.1	50.2
1 : 9	21	45.3	46.4	47.8	49.2	50.4
1 : 10	22	45.4	46.6	48.0	49.4	50.5
1 : 11	23	45.6	46.7	48.1	49.5	50.7
2 : 0	24	45.7	46.8	48.3	49.7	50.8
2 : 1	25	45.8	47.0	48.4	49.8	50.9
2 : 2	26	45.9	47.1	48.5	49.9	51.1
2 : 3	27	46.0	47.2	48.6	50.0	51.2
2 : 4	28	46.1	47.3	48.7	50.2	51.3
2 : 5	29	46.2	47.4	48.8	50.3	51.4
2 : 6	30	46.3	47.5	48.9	50.4	51.6

(Contd.)

Appendix XII Head circumference-for-age for boys birth to 5 years (percentiles) *(Contd.)*

Year : Month	Months	3rd	15th	Median	85th	97th
2 : 7	31	46.4	47.6	49.0	50.5	51.7
2 : 8	32	46.5	47.7	49.1	50.6	51.8
2 : 9	33	46.6	47.8	49.2	50.7	51.9
2 : 10	34	46.6	47.8	49.3	50.8	52.0
2 : 11	35	46.7	47.9	49.4	50.8	52.0
3 : 0	36	46.8	48.0	49.5	50.9	52.1
3 : 1	37	47.9	48.1	49.5	51.0	52.2
3 : 2	38	46.9	48.1	49.6	51.1	52.3
3 : 3	39	47.0	48.2	49.7	51.2	52.4
3 : 4	40	47.0	48.3	49.7	51.2	52.4
3 : 5	41	47.1	48.3	49.8	51.3	52.5
3 : 6	42	47.2	48.4	49.9	51.4	52.6
3 : 7	43	47.2	48.4	49.9	51.4	52.7
3 : 8	44	47.3	48.5	50.0	51.5	52.7
3 : 9	45	47.3	48.5	50.1	51.6	52.8
3 : 10	46	47.4	48.6	50.1	51.6	52.8
3 : 11	47	47.4	48.6	50.2	51.7	52.9
4 : 0	48	47.5	48.7	50.2	51.7	53.0
4 : 1	49	47.5	48.7	50.3	51.8	53.0
4 : 2	50	47.5	48.8	50.3	51.8	53.1
4 : 3	51	47.6	48.8	50.4	51.9	53.1
4 : 4	52	47.6	48.9	50.4	51.9	53.2
4 : 5	53	47.7	48.9	50.4	52.0	53.2
4 : 6	54	47.7	49.0	50.5	52.0	53.3
4 : 7	55	47.7	49.0	50.5	52.1	53.3
4 : 8	56	47.8	49.0	50.6	52.1	53.4
4 : 9	57	47.8	49.1	50.6	52.2	53.4
4 : 10	58	47.9	49.1	50.7	52.2	53.5
4 : 11	59	47.9	49.2	50.7	52.2	53.5
5 : 0	60	47.9	49.2	50.7	52.3	53.5

Appendix XII Head circumference-for-age for girls birth to 5 years (percentiles)

Year : Month	Months	3rd	15th	Median	85th	97th
0 : 0	0	31.7	32.7	33.9	35.1	36.1
0 : 1	1	34.3	35.3	36.5	37.8	38.8
0 : 2	2	36.0	37.0	38.3	39.5	40.5
0 : 3	3	37.2	38.2	39.5	40.8	41.9
0 : 4	4	38.2	39.3	40.6	41.9	43.0
0 : 5	5	39.0	40.1	41.5	42.8	43.9
0 : 6	6	39.7	40.8	42.2	43.5	44.6
0 : 7	7	40.4	41.5	42.8	44.2	45.3
0 : 8	8	40.9	42.0	43.4	44.7	45.9
0 : 9	9	41.3	42.4	43.8	45.2	46.3
0 : 10	10	41.7	42.8	44.2	45.6	46.8
0 : 11	11	42.0	43.2	44.6	46.0	47.1
1 : 0	12	42.3	43.5	44.9	46.3	47.5
1 : 1	13	42.6	43.8	45.2	46.6	47.7
1 : 2	14	42.9	44.0	45.4	46.8	48.0

(Contd.)

Year : Month	Months	3rd	15th	Median	85th	97th
1 : 3	15	43.1	44.2	45.7	47.1	48.2
1 : 4	16	43.3	44.4	45.9	47.3	48.5
1 : 5	17	43.5	44.6	46.1	47.5	48.7
1 : 6	18	43.6	44.8	46.2	47.7	48.8
1 : 7	19	43.8	45.0	46.4	47.8	49.0
1 : 8	20	44.0	45.1	46.6	48.0	49.2
1 : 9	21	44.1	45.3	46.7	48.2	49.4
1 : 10	22	44.3	45.4	46.9	48.3	49.5
1 : 11	23	44.4	45.6	47.0	48.5	49.7
2 : 0	24	44.6	45.7	47.2	48.6	49.8
2 : 1	25	44.7	45.9	47.3	48.8	49.9
2 : 2	26	44.8	46.0	47.5	48.9	50.1
2 : 3	27	44.9	46.1	47.6	49.0	50.2
2 : 4	28	45.1	46.3	47.7	49.2	50.3
2 : 5	29	45.2	46.4	47.8	49.3	50.5
2 : 6	30	45.3	46.5	47.9	49.4	50.6
2 : 7	31	45.4	46.6	48.0	49.5	50.7
2 : 8	32	45.5	46.7	48.1	49.6	50.8
2 : 9	33	45.6	46.8	48.2	49.7	50.9
2 : 10	34	45.7	46.9	48.3	49.8	51.0
2 : 11	35	45.8	47.0	48.4	49.9	51.1
3 : 0	36	45.9	47.0	48.5	50.0	51.2
3 : 1	37	45.9	47.1	48.6	50.1	51.3
3 : 2	38	46.0	47.2	48.7	50.1	51.3
3 : 3	39	46.1	47.3	48.7	50.2	51.4
3 : 4	40	46.2	47.4	48.8	50.3	51.5
3 : 5	41	46.2	47.4	48.9	50.4	51.6
3 : 6	42	46.3	47.5	49.0	50.4	51.6
3 : 7	43	46.4	47.6	49.0	50.5	51.7
3 : 8	44	46.4	47.6	49.1	50.6	51.8
3 : 9	45	46.5	47.7	49.2	50.6	51.8
3 : 10	46	46.5	47.7	49.2	50.7	51.9
3 : 11	47	46.6	47.8	49.3	50.7	51.9
4 : 0	48	46.7	47.9	49.3	50.8	52.0
4 : 1	49	46.7	47.9	49.4	50.9	52.1
4 : 2	50	46.8	48.0	49.4	50.9	52.1
4 : 3	51	46.8	48.0	49.5	51.0	52.2
4 : 4	52	46.9	48.1	49.5	51.0	52.2
4 : 5	53	46.9	48.1	49.6	51.1	52.3
4 : 6	54	47.0	48.2	49.6	51.1	52.3
4 : 7	55	47.0	48.2	49.7	51.2	52.4
4 : 8	56	47.1	48.3	49.7	51.2	52.4
4 : 9	57	47.1	48.3	49.8	51.3	52.5
4 : 10	58	47.2	48.4	49.8	51.3	52.5
4 : 11	59	47.2	48.4	49.9	51.4	52.6
5 : 0	60	47.2	48.4	49.9	51.4	52.6

Appendix XII Head circumference-for-age for girls birth to 5 years (percentiles) *(Contd.)*

Appendix XIII Weight-for-length for boys birth to 2 years (percentiles)

cm	3rd	15th	Median	85th	97th
45.0	2.1	2.2	2.4	2.7	2.9
45.5	2.1	2.3	2.5	2.8	3.0
46.0	2.2	2.4	2.6	2.9	3.1
46.5	2.3	2.5	2.7	3.0	3.2
47.0	2.4	2.5	2.8	3.1	3.3
47.5	2.4	2.6	2.9	3.1	3.4
48.0	2.5	2.7	2.9	3.2	3.5
48.5	2.6	2.8	3.0	3.3	3.6
49.0	2.7	2.9	3.1	3.4	3.7
49.5	2.7	2.9	3.2	3.5	3.8
50.0	2.8	3.0	3.3	3.7	4.0
50.5	2.9	3.1	3.4	3.8	4.1
51.0	3.0	3.2	3.5	3.9	4.2
51.5	3.1	3.3	3.6	4.0	4.3
52.0	3.2	3.4	3.8	4.1	4.5
52.5	3.3	3.6	3.9	4.3	4.6
53.0	3.4	3.7	4.0	4.4	4.7
53.5	3.5	3.8	4.1	4.5	4.9
54.0	3.6	3.9	4.3	4.7	5.0
54.5	3.8	4.0	4.4	4.8	5.2
55.0	3.9	4.2	4.5	5.0	5.4
55.5	4.0	4.3	4.7	5.1	5.5
56.0	4.1	4.4	4.8	5.3	5.7
56.5	4.3	4.6	5.0	5.4	5.9
57.0	4.4	4.7	5.1	5.6	6.0
57.5	4.5	4.8	5.3	5.8	6.2
58.0	4.6	5.0	5.4	5.9	6.4
58.5	4.8	5.1	5.6	6.1	6.5
59.0	4.9	5.2	5.7	6.2	6.7
59.5	5.0	5.4	5.9	6.4	6.9
60.0	5.1	5.5	6.0	6.5	7.0
60.5	5.3	5.6	6.1	6.7	7.2
61.0	5.4	5.8	6.3	6.8	7.4
61.5	5.5	5.9	6.4	7.0	7.5
62.0	5.6	6.0	6.5	7.1	7.7
62.5	5.7	6.1	6.7	7.3	7.8
63.0	5.8	6.2	6.8	7.4	8.0
63.5	5.9	6.3	6.9	7.5	8.1
64.0	6.0	6.5	7.0	7.7	8.2
64.5	6.1	6.6	7.1	7.8	8.4
65.0	6.3	6.7	7.3	7.9	8.5
65.5	6.4	6.8	7.4	8.1	8.7
66.0	6.5	6.9	7.5	8.2	8.8
66.5	6.6	7.0	7.6	8.3	8.9
67.0	6.7	7.1	7.7	8.4	9.1
67.5	6.8	7.2	7.9	8.6	9.2

(Contd.)

		Appendix XIII Weight-for-length for boys birth to 2 years (percentiles) *(Contd.)*			
cm	*3rd*	*15th*	*Median*	*85th*	*97th*
68.0	6.9	7.3	8.0	8.7	9.3
68.5	7.0	7.4	8.1	8.8	9.5
69.0	7.1	7.5	8.2	8.9	9.6
69.5	7.1	7.6	8.3	9.1	9.7
70.0	7.2	7.7	8.4	9.2	9.9
70.5	7.3	7.8	8.5	9.3	10.0
71.0	7.4	8.0	8.6	9.4	10.1
71.5	7.5	8.1	8.8	9.6	10.3
72.0	7.6	8.2	8.9	9.7	10.4
72.5	7.7	8.3	9.0	9.8	10.5
73.0	7.8	8.4	9.1	9.9	10.7
73.5	7.9	8.4	9.2	10.0	10.8
74.0	8.0	8.5	9.3	10.1	10.9
74.5	8.1	8.6	9.4	10.3	11.0
75.0	8.2	8.7	9.5	10.4	11.2
75.5	8.2	8.8	9.6	10.5	11.3
76.0	8.3	8.9	9.7	10.6	11.4
76.5	8.4	9.0	9.8	10.7	11.5
77.0	8.5	9.1	9.9	10.8	11.6
77.5	8.6	9.2	10.0	10.9	11.7
78.0	8.7	9.3	10.1	11.0	11.8
78.5	8.7	9.3	10.2	11.1	12.0
79.0	8.8	9.4	10.3	11.2	12.1
79.5	8.9	9.5	10.4	11.3	12.2
80.0	9.0	9.6	10.4	11.4	12.3
80.5	9.1	9.7	10.5	11.5	12.4
81.0	9.1	9.8	10.6	11.6	12.5
81.5	9.2	9.9	10.7	11.7	12.6
82.0	9.3	10.0	10.8	11.8	12.7
82.5	9.4	10.1	10.9	11.9	12.8
83.0	9.5	10.1	11.0	12.0	13.0
83.5	9.6	10.3	11.2	12.2	13.1
84.0	9.7	10.4	11.3	12.3	13.2
84.5	9.8	10.5	11.4	12.4	13.3
85.0	9.9	10.6	11.5	12.5	13.5
85.5	10.0	10.7	11.6	12.7	13.6
86.0	10.1	10.8	11.7	12.8	13.7
86.5	10.2	10.9	11.9	12.9	13.9
87.0	10.3	11.0	12.0	13.1	14.0
87.5	10.4	11.2	12.1	13.2	14.2
88.0	10.6	11.3	12.2	13.3	14.3
88.5	10.7	11.4	12.4	13.5	14.4
89.0	10.8	11.5	12.5	13.6	14.6
89.5	10.9	11.6	12.6	13.7	14.7
90.0	11.0	11.7	12.7	13.8	14.9

		Appendix XIII Weight-for-height for boys 2 to 5 years (percentiles)			
cm	3rd	15th	Median	85th	97th
90.5	11.2	12.0	13.0	14.1	15.2
91.0	11.3	12.1	13.1	14.3	15.3
91.5	11.4	12.2	13.2	14.4	15.5
92.0	11.5	12.3	13.4	14.5	15.6
92.5	11.6	12.4	13.5	14.7	15.7
93.0	11.7	12.5	13.6	14.8	15.9
93.5	11.8	12.6	13.7	14.9	16.0
94.0	11.9	12.7	13.8	15.0	16.1
94.5	12.0	12.8	13.9	15.2	16.3
95.0	12.1	12.9	14.1	15.3	16.4
95.5	12.2	13.1	14.2	15.4	16.6
96.0	12.3	13.2	14.3	15.6	16.7
96.5	12.4	13.3	14.4	15.7	16.9
97.0	12.5	13.4	14.6	15.9	17.0
97.5	12.7	13.5	14.7	16.0	17.2
98.0	12.8	13.6	14.8	16.1	17.3
98.5	12.9	13.8	14.9	16.3	17.5
99.0	13.0	13.9	15.1	16.4	17.7
99.5	13.1	14.0	15.2	16.6	17.8
100.0	13.2	14.1	15.4	16.7	18.0
100.5	13.3	14.2	15.5	16.9	18.2
101.0	13.4	14.4	15.6	17.1	18.4
101.5	13.6	14.5	15.8	17.2	18.5
102.0	13.7	14.6	15.9	17.4	18.7
102.5	13.8	14.8	16.1	17.6	18.9
103.0	13.9	14.9	16.2	17.7	19.1
103.5	14.0	15.0	16.4	17.9	19.3
104.0	14.2	15.2	16.5	18.1	19.5
104.5	14.3	15.3	16.7	18.2	19.7
105.0	14.4	15.4	16.8	18.4	19.9
105.5	14.5	15.6	17.0	18.6	20.1
106.0	14.7	15.7	17.2	18.8	20.3
106.5	14.8	15.9	17.3	19.0	20.5
107.0	14.9	16.0	17.5	19.1	20.7
107.5	15.1	16.2	17.7	19.3	20.9
108.0	15.2	16.3	17.8	19.5	21.1
108.5	15.3	16.5	18.0	19.7	21.3
109.0	15.5	16.6	18.2	19.9	21.5
109.5	15.6	16.8	18.3	20.1	21.7
110.0	15.8	16.9	18.5	20.3	22.0
110.5	15.9	17.1	18.7	20.5	22.2
111.0	16.1	17.2	18.9	20.7	22.4
111.5	16.2	17.4	19.1	20.9	22.6
112.0	16.3	17.6	19.2	21.1	22.9
112.5	16.5	17.7	19.4	21.4	23.1
113.0	16.6	17.9	19.6	21.6	23.4

(Contd.)

Appendix XIII Weight-for-height for boys 2 to 5 years (percentiles) *(Contd.)*

cm	3rd	15th	Median	85th	97th
113.5	16.8	18.1	19.8	21.8	23.6
114.0	17.0	18.2	20.0	22.0	23.8
114.5	17.1	18.4	20.2	22.2	24.1
115.0	17.3	18.6	20.4	22.4	24.3
115.5	17.4	18.7	20.6	22.7	24.6
116.0	17.6	18.9	20.8	22.9	24.8
116.5	17.7	19.1	21.0	23.1	25.1
117.0	17.9	19.3	21.2	23.3	25.3
117.5	18.0	19.4	21.4	23.6	25.6
118.0	18.2	19.6	21.6	23.8	25.8
118.5	18.4	19.8	21.8	24.0	26.1
119.0	18.5	20.0	22.0	24.2	26.3
119.5	18.7	20.1	22.2	24.5	26.6
120.0	18.8	20.3	22.4	24.7	26.8

Appendix XIII Weight-for-length for girls birth to 2 years (percentiles)

cm	3rd	15th	Median	85th	97th
45.0	2.1	2.2	2.5	2.7	2.9
45.5	2.2	2.3	2.5	2.8	3.0
46.0	2.2	2.4	2.6	2.9	3.1
46.5	2.3	2.5	2.7	3.0	3.2
47.0	2.4	2.6	2.8	3.1	3.3
47.5	2.4	2.6	2.9	3.2	3.4
48.0	2.5	2.7	3.0	3.3	3.5
48.5	2.6	2.8	3.1	3.4	3.7
49.0	2.7	2.9	3.2	3.5	3.8
49.5	2.8	3.0	3.3	3.6	3.9
50.0	2.8	3.1	3.4	3.7	4.0
50.5	2.9	3.2	3.5	3.8	4.1
51.0	3.0	3.2	3.6	3.9	4.3
51.5	3.1	3.4	3.7	4.0	4.4
52.0	3.2	3.5	3.8	4.2	4.5
52.5	3.3	3.6	3.9	4.3	4.7
53.0	3.4	3.7	4.0	4.4	4.8
53.5	3.5	3.8	4.2	4.6	5.0
54.0	3.6	3.9	4.3	4.7	5.1
54.5	3.7	4.0	4.4	4.9	5.3
55.0	3.9	4.1	4.5	5.0	5.4
55.5	4.0	4.3	4.7	5.2	5.6
56.0	4.1	4.4	4.8	5.3	5.8
56.5	4.2	4.5	5.0	5.5	5.9
57.0	4.3	4.6	5.1	5.6	6.1
57.5	4.4	4.8	5.2	5.7	6.2
58.0	4.5	4.9	5.4	5.9	6.4
58.5	4.6	5.0	5.5	6.0	6.5
59.0	4.8	5.1	5.6	6.2	6.7

(Contd.)

Appendix XIII Weight-for-length for girls birth to 2 years (percentiles)

cm	3rd	15th	Median	85th	97th
59.5	4.9	5.2	5.7	6.3	6.9
60.0	5.0	5.4	5.9	6.5	7.0
60.5	5.1	5.5	6.0	6.6	7.2
61.0	5.2	5.6	6.1	6.7	7.3
61.5	5.3	5.7	6.3	6.9	7.5
62.0	5.4	5.8	6.4	7.0	7.6
62.5	5.5	5.9	6.5	7.2	7.8
63.0	5.6	6.0	6.6	7.3	7.9
63.5	5.7	6.1	6.7	7.4	8.0
64.0	5.8	6.2	6.9	7.5	8.2
64.5	5.9	6.3	7.0	7.7	8.3
65.0	6.0	6.5	7.1	7.8	8.5
65.5	6.1	6.6	7.2	7.9	8.6
66.0	6.2	6.7	7.3	8.0	8.7
66.5	6.3	6.8	7.4	8.2	8.9
67.0	6.4	6.9	7.5	8.3	9.0
67.5	6.5	7.0	7.6	8.4	9.1
68.0	6.6	7.1	7.7	8.5	9.2
68.5	6.7	7.2	7.9	8.6	9.4
69.0	6.7	7.3	8.0	8.8	9.5
69.5	6.8	7.3	8.1	8.9	9.6
70.0	6.9	7.4	8.2	9.0	9.7
70.5	7.0	7.5	8.3	9.1	9.9
71.0	7.1	7.6	8.4	9.2	10.0
71.5	7.2	7.7	8.5	9.3	10.1
72.0	7.3	7.8	8.6	9.4	10.2
72.5	7.4	7.9	8.7	9.5	10.3
73.0	7.4	8.0	8.8	9.6	10.4
73.5	7.5	8.1	8.9	9.7	10.6
74.0	7.6	8.2	9.0	9.9	10.7
74.5	7.7	8.3	9.1	10.0	10.8
75.0	7.8	8.3	9.1	10.1	10.9
75.5	7.8	8.4	9.2	10.2	11.0
76.0	7.9	8.5	9.3	10.3	11.1
76.5	8.0	8.6	9.4	10.4	11.2
77.0	8.1	8.7	9.5	10.5	11.3
77.5	8.2	8.8	9.6	10.6	11.4
78.0	8.2	8.9	9.7	10.7	11.5
78.5	8.3	8.9	9.8	10.8	11.7
79.0	8.4	9.0	9.9	10.9	11.8
79.5	8.5	9.1	10.0	11.0	11.9
80.0	8.6	9.2	10.1	11.1	12.0
80.5	8.7	9.3	10.2	11.2	12.1
81.0	8.8	9.4	10.3	11.3	12.2
81.5	8.8	9.5	10.4	11.4	12.4
82.0	8.9	9.6	10.5	11.6	12.5

(Contd.)

Appendix XIII Weight-for-length for girls birth to 2 years (percentiles) *(Contd.)*					
cm	*3rd*	*15th*	*Median*	*85th*	*97th*
82.5	9.0	9.7	10.6	11.7	12.6
83.0	9.1	9.8	10.7	11.8	12.8
83.5	9.2	9.9	10.9	11.9	12.9
84.0	9.3	10.0	11.0	12.1	13.1
84.5	9.4	10.1	11.1	12.2	13.2
85.0	9.5	10.2	11.2	12.3	13.3
85.5	9.6	10.4	11.3	12.5	13.5
86.0	9.8	10.5	11.5	12.6	13.6
86.5	9.9	10.6	11.6	12.7	13.8
87.0	10.0	10.7	11.7	12.9	13.9
87.5	10.1	10.8	11.8	13.0	14.1
88.0	10.2	10.9	12.0	13.2	14.2
88.5	10.3	11.0	12.1	13.3	14.4
89.0	10.4	11.2	12.2	13.4	14.5
89.5	10.5	11.3	12.3	13.6	14.7
90.0	10.6	11.4	12.5	13.7	14.8
90.5	10.9	11.7	12.8	14.0	15.2
91.0	11.0	11.8	12.9	14.2	15.3
91.5	11.1	11.9	13.0	14.3	15.5
92.0	11.2	12.0	13.1	14.4	15.6
92.5	11.3	12.1	13.3	14.6	15.8
93.0	11.4	12.2	13.4	14.7	15.9
93.5	11.5	12.3	13.5	14.9	16.1
94.0	11.6	12.4	13.6	15.0	16.2
94.5	11.7	12.6	13.8	15.1	16.4
95.0	11.8	12.7	13.9	15.3	16.5
95.5	11.9	12.8	14.0	15.4	16.7
96.0	12.0	12.9	14.1	15.6	16.9
96.5	12.1	13.0	14.3	15.7	17.0
97.0	12.2	13.1	14.4	15.8	17.2
97.5	12.3	13.3	14.5	16.0	17.3
98.0	12.4	13.4	14.7	16.1	17.5
98.5	12.6	13.5	14.8	16.3	17.7
99.0	12.7	13.6	14.9	16.4	17.8
99.5	12.8	13.8	15.1	16.6	18.0
100.0	12.9	13.9	15.2	16.8	18.2
100.5	13.0	14.0	15.4	16.9	18.3
101.0	13.1	14.1	15.5	17.1	18.5
101.5	13.3	14.3	15.7	17.2	18.7
102.0	13.4	14.4	15.8	17.4	18.9
102.5	13.5	14.5	16.0	17.6	19.1
103.0	13.6	14.7	16.1	17.8	19.3
103.5	13.8	14.8	16.3	17.9	19.5
104.0	13.9	15.0	16.4	18.1	19.7
104.5	14.0	15.1	16.6	18.3	19.9
105.0	14.2	15.3	16.8	18.5	20.1

(Contd.)

Appendix XIII Weight-for-length for girls birth to 2 years (percentiles) *(Contd.)*				
cm	*3rd*	*15th*	*Median*	*85th*	*97th*
105.5	14.3	15.4	16.9	18.7	20.3
106.0	14.5	15.6	17.1	18.9	20.5
106.5	14.6	15.7	17.3	19.1	20.7
107.0	14.7	15.9	17.5	19.3	21.0
107.5	14.9	16.1	17.7	19.5	21.2
108.0	15.0	16.2	17.8	19.7	21.4
108.5	15.2	16.4	18.0	19.9	21.6
109.0	15.4	16.6	18.2	20.1	21.9
109.5	15.5	16.7	18.4	20.3	22.1
110.0	15.7	16.9	18.6	20.6	22.4
110.5	15.8	17.1	18.8	20.8	22.6
111.0	16.0	17.3	19.0	21.0	22.8
111.5	16.2	17.4	19.2	21.2	23.1
112.0	16.3	17.6	19.4	21.5	23.4
112.5	16.5	17.8	19.6	21.7	23.6
113.0	16.7	18.0	19.8	21.9	23.9
113.5	16.8	18.2	20.0	22.2	24.1
114.0	17.0	18.4	20.2	22.4	24.4
114.5	17.2	18.5	20.5	22.6	24.7
115.0	17.3	18.7	20.7	22.9	24.9
115.5	17.5	18.9	20.9	23.1	25.2
116.0	17.7	19.1	21.1	23.4	25.5
116.5	17.9	19.3	21.3	23.6	25.7
117.0	18.0	19.5	21.5	23.8	26.0
117.5	18.2	19.7	21.7	24.1	26.3
118.0	18.4	19.9	22.0	24.3	26.5
118.5	18.6	20.1	22.2	24.6	26.8
119.0	18.7	20.3	22.4	24.8	27.1
119.5	18.9	20.5	22.6	25.1	27.4
120.0	19.1	20.6	22.8	25.3	27.6

Appendix XIV IAP body mass index percentiles for boys and girls (5–18 years)

IAP body mass index percentiles for boys

Age	3	5	10	25	50	23* Eq(71)	27* Eq(90)	SD	Age	3	5	10	25	50	23* Eq(71)	27* Eq(90)	SD
5.0	12.1	12.4	12.8	13.6	14.7	15.7	17.5	1.6	5.0	11.9	12.1	12.5	13.3	14.3	15.5	18.0	1.4
5.5	12.2	12.4	12.9	13.7	14.8	15.8	17.6	1.5	5.5	11.9	12.2	12.6	13.4	14.4	15.7	18.3	1.7
6.0	12.2	12.5	12.9	13.7	14.9	16.0	17.8	1.8	6.0	12.0	12.2	12.7	13.5	14.5	15.9	18.6	1.7
6.5	12.3	12.5	13.0	13.8	15.0	16.1	18.0	1.8	6.5	12.1	12.3	12.8	13.6	14.7	16.1	18.9	2.0
7.0	12.3	12.6	13.1	13.9	15.1	16.3	18.2	1.9	7.0	12.1	12.4	12.8	13.7	14.9	16.4	19.3	2.1
7.5	12.4	12.7	13.2	14.1	15.3	16.5	18.5	2.2	7.5	12.2	12.5	12.9	13.9	15.1	16.6	19.7	2.2
8.0	12.5	12.8	13.3	14.2	15.5	16.7	18.8	2.5	8.0	12.3	12.6	13.1	14.0	15.3	16.9	20.1	2.3
8.5	12.6	12.9	13.4	14.4	15.7	17.0	19.2	2.8	8.5	12.3	12.7	13.2	14.2	15.6	17.2	20.5	2.7
9.0	12.7	13.0	13.5	14.5	15.9	17.3	19.6	2.6	9.0	12.4	12.8	13.3	14.4	15.8	17.6	21.0	2.7
9.5	12.8	13.1	13.7	14.7	16.2	17.6	20.1	2.8	9.5	12.5	12.9	13.5	14.6	16.1	18.0	21.4	2.8
10.0	12.9	13.2	13.8	14.9	16.4	18.0	20.5	3.1	10.0	12.7	13.1	13.7	14.9	16.5	18.4	21.9	2.9
10.5	13.0	13.3	14.0	15.1	16.7	18.3	21.0	3.2	10.5	12.8	13.2	13.9	15.2	16.8	18.8	22.5	3.1
11.0	13.1	13.5	14.1	15.4	17.0	18.7	21.5	3.2	11.0	13.0	13.4	14.1	15.5	17.2	19.3	23.0	3.1
11.5	13.2	13.6	14.3	15.6	17.3	19.1	22.1	3.3	11.5	13.2	13.7	14.4	15.8	17.6	19.8	23.6	3.3
12.0	13.3	13.8	14.5	15.8	17.7	19.5	22.6	3.4	12.0	13.4	13.9	14.7	16.1	18.0	20.2	24.1	3.2
12.5	13.5	13.9	14.6	16.0	17.9	19.8	23.0	3.6	12.5	13.7	14.2	15.0	16.5	18.4	20.7	24.7	3.2
13.0	13.6	14.0	14.8	16.3	18.2	20.2	23.4	3.5	13.0	13.9	14.4	15.2	16.8	18.8	21.1	25.2	3.3
13.5	13.7	14.2	14.9	16.5	18.5	20.5	23.8	3.7	13.5	14.1	14.6	15.5	17.1	19.1	21.5	25.6	3.5
14.0	13.8	14.3	15.1	16.7	18.7	20.8	24.2	3.7	14.0	14.3	14.9	15.7	17.3	19.4	21.8	25.9	3.4
14.5	14.0	14.5	15.3	16.9	19.0	21.1	24.5	3.5	14.5	14.5	15.1	16.0	17.6	19.7	22.0	26.2	3.3
15.0	14.2	14.7	15.5	17.2	19.3	21.4	24.9	3.7	15.0	14.7	15.2	16.1	17.8	19.9	22.3	26.3	3.4
15.5	14.4	14.9	15.8	17.4	19.6	21.7	25.2	3.4	15.5	14.9	15.4	16.3	18.0	20.1	22.4	26.4	3.1
16.0	14.6	15.1	16.0	17.7	19.9	22.0	25.5	3.7	16.0	15.0	15.6	16.5	18.2	20.3	22.6	26.5	3.1
16.5	14.9	15.4	16.3	18.0	20.2	22.4	25.8	3.8	16.5	15.2	15.8	16.7	18.4	20.4	22.8	26.6	3.2
17.0	15.1	15.6	16.6	18.3	20.5	22.6	26.0	3.8	17.0	15.4	16.0	16.9	18.6	20.6	22.9	26.7	3.0
17.5	15.4	15.9	16.8	18.6	20.8	22.9	26.3	3.6	17.5	15.5	16.1	17.1	18.7	20.8	23.1	26.7	3.1
18.0	15.6	16.2	17.1	18.9	21.1	23.2	26.6	3.2	18.0	15.7	16.3	17.3	18.9	21.0	23.2	26.8	3.6

SD; standard deviation *23 and 27 adult equivalent BMI chart by IAP have 3rd, 5th, 10th, 25th, 50th percentiles and 23 adult equivalent (71st and 75th percentiles for boys and girls, respectively) and 27th adult equivalent (90th and 95th percentiles for boys and girls, respectively). Based on IAP BMI charts, underweight is defined as BMI below 3rd percentile, overweight as above 23 adult equivalent and obese as above 27 adult equivalent.

Index

Respiratory diseases 340

Respiratory distress syndrome 102

Resuscitation kit 63

Resuscitation of an asphyxiated newborn 61

Resuscitation protocol 64

Retinopathy of prematurity 307, 498

Retracted or inverted nipples 125

Rhesus hemolytic disease of the newborn 109

Rhesus isoimmunization 498

Rheumatic fever 321, 353, 498

Rheumatoid arthritis 499

Rice-congee, preparation of 330

Rickets 141, 316, 499

   clinical features of 317

   differential diagnosis of 319

   laboratory investigations of 319

   risk factors for development of 318

   treatment of 319

Rights of children 417

Ring worm 294

Road-to-health card 209

Rocking and head-banging 245

Role and responsibilities of nurses 29

Role of a nurse in keeping the babies warm 82

Role of a nurse in the OPD 32

Rotavirus vaccines 198

Rubella 170, 499

S

Salmon patch 75, 258

Scabies 293, 499

Scalds 402

School health program 28, 228

School phobia 238

Scorpion sting 412

Scurvy 141

Seborrhea capitis 290

Seizures 376

Septic arthritis 321

Septicemia in a neonate 105

   clinical features of 106

   diagnosis of 106

   nursing management of 106

Setting-sun sign 75

Severe acute malnutrition 151

Sexual abuse and exploitation 421

Sexual assault victims, handling of 422

Sexual development, stages of 225

Sexual maturation, disorders of 396

Sexually transmitted diseases 29, 398, 499

Shakir tape 468

Sickle cell anemia 370

Sinusitis 304, 499

Skin lesions, types of 290

Skin rash 292

Sleep problems 243

Sleep walking 245

Small-for-dates babies 96

Smarter child, correlates of 221

Snake bite 412

Sneezing 74

Solid tumors 374

Somnambulism 245

Southpaws 223

Spasmodic laryngitis, acute 341

Spastic child 269

Specific antidotes 411

Speech problems 243

Speech

   delayed 219

   regression of 220

Spina bifida 263, 499

Spinal abnormalities 326

Spinal tap 486

Spinal transection 80

Squint 309, 499

Stammering 243

Status epilepticus 378

Steam inhalation 457, 483

Sternomastoid 'tumor' 77

Stillbirth 16, 499

Stool sample 472

Stork bite 75, 258

Strabismus 309

Strategies for child survival 19

Strategies to improve newborn health and survival 434

Strawberry mark 258

Street children 423

Streptococcal pharyngitis 302

Stridor 340, 499

Stunting 499

Stuttering 243

Stye 308, 499

Subconjunctival hemorrhage 75

Substance abuse 29, 227

Successful nursing 9

Suctioning 482

Sunlight, exposure to 112

Superficial infections 71

Swabs 472

Swaddling 499

Swine flu 169, 340

Symptoms in children 275

Syncope 378, 499

Systemic lupus erythematosus 325

T

Talipes equinovarus 260

Tall child, correlates of 211

Tapeworms 188

Teeth and gums, care of 298

Teeth grinding 245

Teething 296

Television and behavior 234

Television viewing

   guidelines for 235

   hazards of 235

Temper tantrums 241

Terminally sick children 35

Tetanus 168

Tetanus neonatorum

   clinical features of 107

   nursing care of 107

   prevention of 108

Tetanus toxoid 197

Tetany 499

Thalassemias 369, 500

The child survival and safe motherhood program 428

The cold chain 201

Thermoneutral temperature 81

Thoracotomy 344

Thrush 305, 500

Tics 238, 378, 500

Tissue perfusion 92

Toe-walking 261, 500

Toilet training 242

Tongue tie 75, 305

Tonsillitis 500

Tonsils 500

Toothache 283

Torticollis 500

Toxic erythema 75

Traditional healthcare practices in children 255

Transient fever of the newborn 84

Transient synovitis 321